Quality of Life

From Nursing and Patient Perspectives

THEORY ▪ RESEARCH ▪ PRACTICE

THIRD EDITION

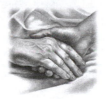

Edited by

Cynthia R. King, PhD, NP, MSN, CNL, FAAN

Professor and Nurse Scientist
Queens University at Charlotte
Charlotte, North Carolina

Pamela S. Hinds, PhD, RN, FAAN

Director, Department of Nursing Research
Children's National Medical Center
Professor of Pediatrics
The George Washington University
Washington, DC

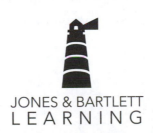

JONES & BARTLETT
LEARNING

World Headquarters
Jones & Bartlett Learning
40 Tall Pine Drive
Sudbury, MA 01776
978-443-5000
info@jblearning.com
www.jblearning.com

Jones & Bartlett Learning
Canada
6339 Ormindale Way
Mississauga, Ontario L5V 1J2
Canada

Jones & Bartlett Learning
International
Barb House, Barb Mews
London W6 7PA
United Kingdom

Jones & Bartlett Learning books and products are available through most bookstores and online booksellers. To contact Jones & Bartlett Learning directly, call 800-832-0034, fax 978-443-8000, or visit our website, www.jblearning.com.

Substantial discounts on bulk quantities of Jones & Bartlett Learning publications are available to corporations, professional associations, and other qualified organizations. For details and specific discount information, contact the special sales department at Jones & Bartlett Learning via the above contact information or send an email to specialsales@jblearning.com.

The authors, editors, and publisher have made every effort to provide accurate information. However, they are not responsible for errors, omissions, or for any outcomes related to the use of the contents of this book and take no responsibility for the use of the products and procedures described. Treatments and side effects described in this book may not be applicable to all people; likewise, some people may require a dose or experience a side effect that is not described herein. Drugs and medical devices are discussed that may have limited availability controlled by the Food and Drug Administration (FDA) for use only in a research study or clinical trial. Research, clinical practice, and government regulations often change the accepted standard in this field. When consideration is being given to use of any drug in the clinical setting, the health care provider or reader is responsible for determining FDA status of the drug, reading the package insert, and reviewing prescribing information for the most up-to-date recommendations on dose, precautions, and contraindications, and determining the appropriate usage for the product. This is especially important in the case of drugs that are new or seldom used.

Production Credits
Publisher: Kevin Sullivan
Acquisitions Editor: Amanda Harvey
Editorial Assistant: Sara Bempkins
Production Editor: Amanda Clerkin
Associate Marketing Manager: Katie Hennessy
V.P., Manufacturing and Inventory Control: Therese Connell
Composition: Paw Print Media
Cover Design: Scott Moden
Cover Image and Interior Illustrations: Marcia Smith
Printing and Binding: Malloy, Inc.
Cover Printing: Malloy, Inc.

Library of Congress Cataloging-in-Publication Data
Quality of life: from nursing and patient perspectives / [edited by] Cynthia R. King, PhD, NP, MSN, CNL, FAAN, Professor and Nurse Scientist, Queens University at Charlotte, Charlotte, North Carolina, Pamela S. Hinds, PhD, RN, FAAN, Professor of Pediatrics, The George Washington University, Washington, D.C. — Third edition.
    p. ; cm.
Includes bibliographical references and index.
ISBN-13: 978-0-7637-4943-9 (alk. paper)
ISBN-10: 0-7637-4943-5 (alk. paper)
1. Cancer—Nursing. 2. Quality of life. 3. Cancer—Psychological aspects. 4. Cancer—Social aspects. I. King, Cynthia R., editor. II. Hinds, Pamela S., editor.
[DNLM: 1. Neoplasms—nursing. 2. Quality of Life. 3. Neoplasms—psychology. WY 156]
RC266.Q35 2012
616.99'40231—dc22
                                    2010048643

6048

Printed in the United States of America
15 14 13 12 11   10 9 8 7 6 5 4 3 2 1

Dedication

We dedicate the third edition of this special book to our families (Michael, Martha, John, Ron, Ben, and Adam) and to our nursing colleagues, staff, seriously ill patients, and families at many hospitals and cancer centers who have taught us to look beyond the outcome of survival to quality of living and to remember the importance of hopefulness, courage, and love.

Contents

SECTION 3 RESEARCH

CHAPTER EIGHT

Quality of Life: Methodological and Measurement Issues....

Mel R. Haberman • Nigel E. Bush

CHAPTER NINE

Quality of Life and Symptoms ....

Tami Borneman • Denice Economou

CHAPTER TEN

Quality of Life of Family Caregivers of Cancer Patients.....

Bonnie Teschendorf • Carol Estwing Ferrans

CHAPTER FIFTEEN

Quality-of-Life Issues Related to Marrow Transplantation . . . 319

June G. Eilers • Cynthia R. King

CHAPTER SIXTEEN

A European Perspective on Quality of Life of Stem Cell Transplantation Patients 367

Monica C. Fliedner

CHAPTER SEVENTEEN

Fatigue and Sleep Disturbances: Symptoms that Cluster and Adversely Affect Quality of Life 393

Margaret Barton-Burke • Maria B. Carroll • Judith A. Headley • Judith Frain

Foreword

I have had the pleasure of writing the forewords for this book from the beginning. This third edition is a testimony to the remarkable strides made in the science related to quality of life, as illustrated by the positive reception and success of the previous editions. The diverse backgrounds of the two editors are reflected in the content, including the state of the science in quality of life for both adults and children. Much of the table of contents has remained the same in that it includes those dimensions of quality of life that are most applicable to ensuring improved outcomes for patients; however the editors have expanded our understanding of context by clarifying current chapters and adding chapters related to family caregivers and approaches for designing and analyzing complex and longitudinal health-related quality-of-life data. They have enlisted the help of authors who are experts on studying quality of life and its consequences—not only how to measure it, but also what strategies can be used to improve it. The contributors are seasoned researchers and experienced clinicians who are sensitive to the hard realities of trying to make a difference in clinical practice. Several authors have focused on the methodological and conceptual issues. Several chapters include issues related to quality of life in cancer treatment in general and some in relation to specific diagnoses, presented as prototypes for other less common diagnoses.

Some of what I have referred to previously in this foreword bears repeating here, for I believe that it is important to grasp that a concept so central to living with a disease like cancer evolved from a policy mandate. The term quality of life reached its outcome status when the Food and Drug Administration helped to promote its inclusion in cancer clinical trials in 1985. The federal guidelines were changed to include a favorable effect on either an individual's quality of life or survival when new anti-cancer drugs were approved for testing. Subsequently, quality-of-life research has proliferated as a result of this policy change. We now have journals devoted solely to quality-of-life research and special interest groups in many of our professional national and international organizations that help to establish research priorities, educational standards, and translation of evidence into practice.

Although the incidence of many cancers has remained relatively stable over the past century, long-term survival for many types of cancer has improved dramatically, resulting in an unprecedented number of survivors. This improvement in overall survival has gradually changed the image of cancer from a disease shrouded in overtones of death to a chronic illness with inherent, episodic, and often long-term needs. Dramatic changes in medical technology and healthcare delivery continue to impact patient care at every level. New, often toxic, multi-modal treatments have rendered previously fatal diseases treatable, although often with long-term consequences to patients, including varying degrees of symptomatic episodes and functional impairment. When cancer treatments are prescribed, the goal is to eliminate or control the cancer, but treatments often are accompanied by undesirable and lasting side effects. There is a need to weigh the negative and positive effects of a therapy when assessing its value, especially in the context of progressive disease. When put into the context of the patient's life situation, this overall balance is reflected by the concept of quality of life. As scientific progress in the fight against cancer continues, quality-of-life issues are an essential part of the equation when making treatment decisions, including when to halt treatment.

During my career as an oncology nurse I have been privileged to witness the extraordinary clinical and policy changes that have shaped the current treatment and management of cancer care over the past four decades. In the past 10 years, I have become cautiously optimistic that quality of life has finally achieved a position in clinical practice where it can no longer be easily dismissed. This change in position has lasting power because consumer groups have played a critical role in demanding that they have a voice in treatment decision making and the management of their care. The presence of this book underscores the importance of their voice, for it includes their perspectives.

This optimism was cemented even further when the committee of the Institute of Medicine (IOM) report, *Cancer Care for the Whole Patient: Meeting Psychosocial Needs* declared that the scientific evidence supports the standard that screening for psychological distress is integral to quality cancer care. The IOM developed a model for the delivery of psychosocial services that includes effective communication among patients, families, and care providers. Key aspects of the model include (1) identifying physical and psychosocial health needs, (2) linking patients and families to services they need, (3) supporting patients and families as they manage the illness, (4) coordinating psychosocial and biomedical care, and (5) following up on the delivery of care to determine its effectiveness, and making modifications as needed. Meeting these patient needs assumes that the patients' quality of life will be affected positively, whether from the patient or nurse's perspectives.

Our differences are reflected by our values. The experience of cancer holds different meanings and values for each of us and the experience can impact us on a range of quality-of-life dimensions. As a group we might have common responses across dimensions, but examination of an individual profile might show that any particular patient could be dramatically different from the overall group. Both perspectives—the individual and the group—are critical to include, and this book offers useful strategies for approaching these challenges. Cancer remains a devastating disease for patients and families and is likely to remain that way in our lifetime. The editors have taken an important step in giving educators, researchers, and clinicians a comprehensive guide of what is known and what can be done about ensuring quality of life for our patients and their families. King and Hinds are to be commended for expanding the context and increasing our understanding that quality of life permeates the total cancer experience for patients and families, making it explicit that it is not just limited to the effects of cancer treatment.

Ruth McCorkle, PhD, FAAN
The Florence S. Wald Professor of Nursing
Yale University School of Nursing
Director, Psychosocial Oncology Research
Yale Cancer Center
New Haven, Connecticut

Preface

For many lifetimes, patients and families have been telling nurses what is of special relevance or meaning to them, particularly during times of threatened health. Nurses have listened earnestly to these personal perspectives and reflections, realizing that significant information about the quality of these individuals' lives was being shared. Initially this information was used solely to individualize patient and family care in different healthcare settings. In the past few decades nurses have recognized that patients and families have similarities in their viewpoints on quality of life during health threats, and that they, as nurses, can use these to assist patients in order to have as positive a quality of life as possible. The combined patient/family and nurse points of view contribute to the ongoing effort to document the effectiveness of strategies that nurses use to try to contribute to patients' and families' quality of life. This provides rich opportunities to examine quality of life from nursing and patient/family perspectives that currently exist in oncology care and care of other chronic diseases.

From the time of inception of this book until this third edition, the purpose has always been to provide a reference on quality of life that reflects the voice of the patients and families who are receiving or have received care for cancer and the attention (in the form of research, theories, and practice) of their nurses. This book should be useful for oncology nurses in many healthcare settings, including inpatient units, outpatient clinics, ambulatory care centers, cancer centers, research centers, home care agencies, hospices, and many others. Furthermore, since the first edition we have discovered that many nurses have used this book and applied the quality-of-life information to patients dealing with many other chronic or life-threatening illnesses.

The book is divided into six sections for ease of use. The sections help the reader to find the pertinent information without reading the book from cover to cover. Section 1 provides an overview of the evolution of quality of life in oncology and oncology nursing as well as an overview of the controversial issues related to quality of life. Section 2 highlights theory development related to quality of life. Chapter 3 discusses theories and concepts and three additional chapters describe theory related to quality of life including "Spiritual Quality of Life" (Chapter 5), "Quality of Life, Health, and Culture" (Chapter 6), and "Health-Related Quality of Life in Children and Adolescents with Cancer" (Chapter 7).

The third section focuses on research and begins with an overview of methodological and measurement issues (Chapter 8). This is followed by Chapter 9, which illustrates the effects of symptoms on quality of life. Chapters 10 through 12 are new chapters in this edition. Chapter 10 is "Quality of Life of Family Caregivers of Cancer Patients," while Chapter 11 is "The Design, Conduct, and Analysis of HRQOL Studies: A Statistician's Perspective." This chapter is designed to help nurses understand the statistics related to quality-of-life research. Lastly, "Health-Related Quality-of-Life Studies Conducted Through the NCI Clinical Trials Networks" (Chapter 12) provides insight to conducting quality-of-life studies through the National Cancer Institute. Section 4 demonstrates the importance of quality of life in clinical practice. The section opens with a chapter focusing on quality-of-life issues related to individuals with breast or prostate cancer (Chapter 13). Afterward, there is a brief overview of the clinical implications of quality of life (Chapter 14), which is followed by two chapters on quality-of-life issues related to bone marrow transplantation (Chapter 15 and 16). One of these presents an international perspective. The last chapter in Section 4 examines fatigue and quality of life for individuals with cancer (Chapter 17).

Section 5 is a unique section with a chapter on cancer survivorship (Chapter 18) and a chapter with personal perspectives from patients and families (Chapter 19). Many nurses have copied and provided these chapters to their patients and families to read. Section 6 concludes the text with Chapter 20, which provides nursing and patient perspectives on quality of life.

In order to make this book particularly user-friendly for the majority of nurses, there are additional resources located in the appendices. The Appendix provides selected examples of quality-of-life measurement tools. The creators of these tools have provided permission for nurses to use these tools. However, it is always courteous to contact the author of the tool to describe how you plan to use the tool and share your results.

Many hours of thought and preparation have gone into making the third edition of this book as unique as the first two editions. Unique aspects of the book include the following: (1) its presentation of both nursing and patient/family perspectives; (2) quality-of-life issues related to specific diseases (e.g., breast or prostate cancer); (3) quality-of-life issues related to specific treatments (e.g., marrow transplantation); (4) quality-of-life issues related to specific populations (e.g., children and adolescents); (5) new research issues related to quality of life (e.g., statistics, studies at the National Cancer Institute); (6) quality-of-life issues related to family members; (7) an international perspective; and (8) discussion of theory, research, and practice throughout the book. We hope that one or more of these unique aspects will be helpful to the nurse reader whether currently a nursing student, a researcher, educator, administrator, or clinician.

Sincerely,

Cynthia R. King, PhD, NP, MSN, CNL, FAAN

Other recent books by Dr. King:

King, J. R., & King, C. R. (2009). *100 Questions and Answers About Communicating with Your Healthcare Provider*. Sudbury, MA: Jones & Bartlett.

Phillips, J., & King, C. R. (Eds.). (2009). *Advances in Oncology Nursing Research*. Pittsburgh, PA: ONS Press.

Acknowledgments

Many individuals contribute to the completion of a successful project, including the creation and revision of a book. Different members of our team (patients, families, nursing colleagues, editorial, and production staff) brought a variety of gifts, strengths, experiences, and expertise to the completion of this book. We wish to thank all who participated in its development, revision, and production. The list of individuals who have provided support, advice, and time is extensive and impressive. Although we are not able to adequately recognize everyone on the list, we would like to acknowledge a few of the individuals: (1) all of the contributing authors who provided their expertise, time, and special insight into quality-of-life issues for cancer patients; (2) Marcia Smith for her sensitive illustrations that portray the important aspects of quality of life and cancer care; (3) Ruth Wickersham Baldrige from Organizational Communication in Charlotte, North Carolina for her hours and dedication in editing; (4) all the staff at Jones & Bartlett Learning (from the first edition to this third edition) who guided us in our efforts, including Chris Davis, Kevin Sullivan, and Amanda Clerkin; (5) John, Martha, Michael, and Carla Gene for their amazing support and encouragement throughout the development of this edition; and lastly (6) in memory to Spirit Hope Knaus who provided unconditional love, attention, and taught us about quality of life during all three editions of this book.

Contributors

Editors

Cynthia R. King, PhD, NP, MSN, CNL, FAAN
Professor and Nurse Scientist
Presbyterian School of Nursing
Blair College of Health
Queens University of Charlotte
Charlotte, North Carolina

Pamela S. Hinds, PhD, RN, FAAN
Director, Department of Nursing Research and Quality Outcomes
Children's National Medical Center
Professor of Pediatrics
The George Washington University
Washington, D.C.

Contributors

Kimlin Tam Ashing-Giwa, PhD
Professor & Founding Director CCARE
Center of Community Alliance for Research and Education
Division of Population Sciences
City of Hope National Medical Center
Duarte, California

Margaret Barton-Burke, PhD, RN
Mary Ann Lee Endowed Professor of Oncology Nursing
Associate Professor
College of Nursing
University of Missouri, St. Louis
Research Scientist Siteman Cancer Center
St. Louis, Missouri

Tami Borneman, MSN, CNS, FPCN
Senior Research Specialist
Division of Nursing Research and Education
City of Hope
Duarte, California

Carrie Jo Braden, PhD, RN, FAAN
Professor and Associate Dean for Research
School of Nursing
University of Texas Health Science Center, San Antonio
San Antonio, Texas

Nigel E. Bush, PhD
Research Psychologist and Program Manager
National Center for Telehealth and Technology (T2)
Joint Base Lewis-McChord
Tacoma, Washington

Maria B. Carroll, MSN, RN, BC, GCNS
Gerontological Clinical Nurse Specialist
Barnes Jewish Hospital
St. Louis, Missouri

Faye Davenport, MN, MEd, BTheol, BA, RN
Nursing Lecturer, School of Nursing
Universal College of Learning
Palmerston North, New Zealand

Grace E. Dean, PhD, RN
Assistant Professor of Nursing
University at Buffalo
Adjunct Assistant Professor of Oncology
Roswell Park Cancer Institute
School of Nursing
Buffalo, New York

Denice Economou, RN, MN, CNS,
  AOCN
Senior Research Specialist
Director Survivorship Education for
  Quality Cancer Care
City of Hope National Medical Center
Duarte, California

June G. Eilers, PhD, APRN-CNS, BC
Clinical Nurse Researcher
The Nebraska Medical Center
Omaha, Nebraska

Diane L. Fairclough, PhD
Denver, Colorado

Carol Estwing Ferrans, PhD, RN, FAAN
Professor and Associate Dean for Research
  Co-Director
UIC Center for Excellence in Eliminating
  Health Disparities
University of Illinois, Chicago
College of Nursing
Chicago, Illinois

Monica C. Fliedner, RN, MSN
Clinical Nurse Specialist Oncology
Bern University Hospital (Inselspital)
Bern, Switzerland

Judith Frain, RN, MSN
Research Assistant and Doctoral Student
College of Nursing
University of Missouri, St. Louis
St. Louis, Missouri

Marcia M. Grant, RN, DNSc, FAAN
Director and Professor
Nursing Research
City of Hope
Duarte, California

Joan E. Haase, PhD, RN, FAAN
Holmquist Professor in Pediatric Oncology
  Nursing
Indiana University School of Nursing
Indianapolis, Indiana

Mel R. Haberman, PhD, RN, FAAN
Professor
Washington State University College of
  Nursing
Spokane, Washington

Judith A. Headley, PhD, RN
Adjunct Professor
College of Nursing
University of Missouri, St. Louis
St. Louis, Missouri

Annette Baker Hines, RN, MSN, PhD
  Student
Assistant Professor/Assistant Dean
Presbyterian School of Nursing
Queens University of Charlotte
Charlotte, North Carolina

Marjorie Kagawa-Singer, PhD, MN, RN,
  FAAN
Professor, UCLA School of Public Health
  and Professor, Department of Asian
  American Studies
Senior Editor, AAPI Nexus Journal
Los Angeles, California

Susan A. Leigh, BSN, RN
Breast Cancer Survivorship Navigator
Arizona Oncology, CASA Division
Tucson, Arizona

Ruth McCorkle, PhD, FAAN
The Florence S. Wald Professor of Nursing
Yale University School of Nursing
Director, Psychosocial Oncology Research
Yale Cancer Center
New Haven, Connecticut

Karen M. Meneses, PhD, RN, FAAN
Professor and Associate Dean for Research
School of Nursing
Senior Scientist, UAB Comprehensive
  Cancer Center
University of Alabama, Birmingham
Birmingham, Alabama

Ann M. O'Mara, PhD, RN, FAAN
Head, Palliative Care Research
Division of Cancer Prevention
National Cancer Institute
Bethesda, Maryland

Geraldine V. Padilla, PhD
Professor Emerita
School of Nursing
University of California, San Francisco
San Francisco, California

Judith K. Payne PhD, RN, AOCN
Associate Director, Nursing Research
  Planning and Development
MD Anderson Cancer Center
Houston, Texas

Lorrie L. Powel, PhD, RN
William and Berneice Castella
  Distinguished Professor in Aging Studies
Associate Professor

Department of Family Nursing, School of
  Nursing
Department of Urology, School of
  Medicine
University of Texas Health Science Center,
  San Antonio
San Antonio, Texas

Janna C. Roop, PhD, RN, CHPN
Assistant Professor (Clinical)
Wayne State University College of Nursing
Detroit, Michigan

Ellen L. Stovall
Senior Health Policy Advisor
National Coalition for Cancer
  Survivorship
Silver Spring, Maryland

Elizabeth Johnston Taylor, PhD, RN
Associate Professor, School of Nursing
Loma Linda University
Loma Linda, California
Research Director
Mary Potter Hospice
Wellington South, New Zealand

Bonnie Teschendorf, PhD
Director, Patient Reported Outcomes, US
Mapi Values
Boston, Massachusetts

April Hazard Vallerand, PhD, RN, FAAN
Associate Professor
Wayne State University College of Nursing
Detroit, Michigan

Overview

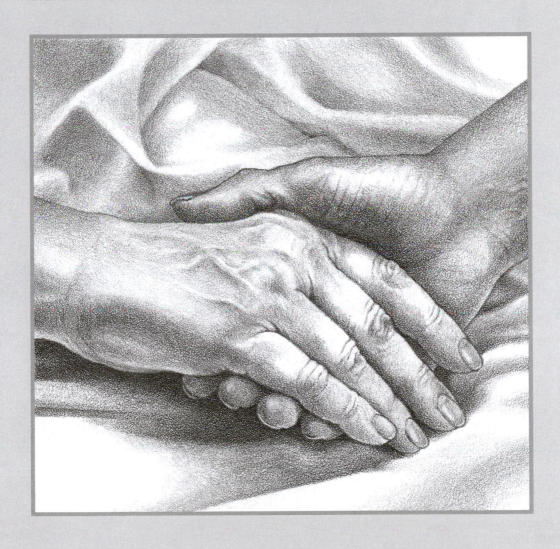

Chapter One

Evolution of Quality of Life in Oncology and Oncology Nursing

Marcia M. Grant • Grace E. Dean

There is no profit in curing the body if in the process we destroy the soul.
—SAM GOLTER, *CITY OF HOPE MEDICAL CENTER, DUARTE, CA*

Introduction

Health-related quality of life (HRQOL) assessment is an important aspect of the current care provided to cancer patients. This chapter discusses the theory, research, and practice related to quality-of-life (QOL) measurement, while addressing the role of oncology nurses in describing and promoting QOL for patients with cancer.

Evolution of Quality of Life as Oncology and Oncology Nursing Outcomes

Traditional medical evaluations of the outcomes of cancer treatments have included disease-free survival, tumor response, and overall survival (US Department of Health and Human Services, 1990). However, clinicians and researchers have come to realize these outcomes are inadequate for assessing the impact of cancer and its treatment on the patient and the patient's daily life, as well as for identifying interventions to improve or maintain the patient's QOL. Quality-of-life measurements provide valuable information to all members of the healthcare team. Quality-of-life assessment has been identified as an important nursing outcome variable for well over 20 years (Grant, 2000) and recently has been recognized as one of the primary patient-reported outcomes (PROs) used to provide the patient's perspective on the effects of treatment and disease (Revicki, 2006).

Interest in QOL assessment has continued to increase in recent years. Both national and international activities illustrate the increasing importance of QOL assessment and research. The US Food and Drug Administration now uses QOL measurements in the process of approving new anticancer drugs (Beitz, Gnecco, & Justice, 1996). National and international groups advocating QOL assessment in clinical trials research also have recognized its importance (Hoffman & Stovall, 2006; Johnson & Temple, 1985; Nayfield, Ganz, Moinpour, Cella, & Hailey, 1991; Osoba, 1992; US Department of Health and Human Services, 1990; World

Health Organization, 1993). Interest in QOL research has resulted in a major shift in randomized controlled clinical trials. The Oncologic Drugs Advisory Committee of the US Food and Drug Administration (FDA) has recommended that a positive effect on QOL and survival be the basis for approval of new anticancer drugs (Beitz et al., 1996). A favorable effect on QOL, in the absence of impact on survival, will carry more weight in the approval process than more traditional measures used to assess efficacy, such as objective tumor response. In addition to clinical trials, QOL assessment has evolved into a primary outcome measure in health services research, acute care, and chronic illness (Coleman, Krammer, Johnson, Eilersten, & Hothaus, 1999; Eiser & Morse, 2001; Mandelblatt & Eisenberg, 1995). This evolution has coincided with recent economic changes and pressures forcing healthcare providers to reconcile quality care and cost effectiveness (Zebrack, 2000).

More recently, the FDA developed a draft document outlining the PRO components evaluated by the FDA in providing efficacy endpoint information in labeling claims by the pharmaceutical industry (http://www.fda.gov/downloads/Drugs/GuidanceCompliance RegulatoryInformation/Guidances/UCM193282.pdf. Accessed May, 2011.) HRQOL could qualify as a PRO if the psychometric properties were well developed (Dueck, Halyard, Frost, & Sloan, 2006). This activity could result in PRO instruments and questionnaires providing evidence of effective endpoints for clinical trials and inclusion in product labeling. This FDA document will include qualities for acceptable PRO questionnaires and instruments.

In 2001, the National Cancer Institute created the Cancer Outcomes Measurement Working Group (COMWG). The purpose of this group was to evaluate and advance the science in patient-reported outcome measurement, especially as related to HRQOL. The group used medical outcomes trust (MOT) attributes and review criteria for evaluating HRQOL instruments (Lohr, 2002). The eight criteria included a conceptual and measurable model, reliability, validity, responsiveness, interpretability, burden, alternate modes of administration, and cultural and language adaptations. Analysis of current cancer instruments shows the need to evaluate PRO measures within the MOT framework, with a focus on prospectively designed studies (Lipscomb, Snyder, & Gotay, 2007).

The World Health Organization (WHO) has a global cancer control program based on knowledge currently available that, if appropriately implemented, can reduce cancer morbidity and mortality worldwide (Stjernswärd & Teoh, 1991). This program includes a focus on palliative care and its impact on the HRQOL of cancer patients. Because many of the world's cancer patients have no access to effective cancer therapy, only palliative care can be offered. Palliative care programs frequently focus on symptom management and can greatly improve HRQOL.

Interest in HRQOL is reflected also in international professional societies. The International Society for Quality of Life Research (ISQOL) was founded in 1994 to promote research in HRQOL and the scientific study of QOL relevant to health and health care throughout the world. This society promotes the rigorous investigation of HRQOL measurement from conceptualization to application and practice. The society's Web site is located at www.isoqol.org. Annual meetings are held throughout the world (see Table 1-1).

A second organization, the International Society for Quality of Life Studies (ISQOLS), has written into its bylaws its mission to promote and encourage research, discussion, and

Table 1-1.   **Annual Conferences of International Society for Quality of Life Research**

1994   Inaugural Meeting: Brussels, Belgium

1995   Montreal, Canada

1996   Manila, Philippines

1997   Vienna, Austria

1998   Baltimore, Maryland, USA

1999   Barcelona, Spain

2000   Vancouver, Canada

2001   Amsterdam, The Netherlands

2002   Toronto, Canada

2003   Prague, Czech Republic

2004   Hong Kong, People's Republic of China

2005   San Francisco, California, USA

2006   Lisbon, Portugal

2007   Toronto, Canada

2008   Montevideo, Uruguay

2009   New Orleans, Louisiana, USA

contributions to the research literature and teaching in HRQOL studies, and to provide a liaison among academic, public sector, and private sector researchers, scholars, and teachers in the managerial (policy), behavioral, social, medical, and environment sciences. Their Web site is located at www.isqols.org. Annual ISQOLS conferences have also been held internationally (Table 1-2).

Other international HRQOL activities include the following:

- The development of an integrated, modular approach to HRQOL assessment in oncology patients by the European Organization for Research and Treatment of Cancer (EORTC) (Aaronson et al., 1993)
- The translation of a HRQOL questionnaire into the eight languages spoken by members of the International Society for Chemo- and Immunotherapy (Tuchler et al., 1992)
- The cultural adaptation of HRQOL instruments with translations of various cancer and non-cancer HRQOL scales into more than 25 languages (Cultural Adaptation, 1996)
- The adoption of HRQOL outcomes in Canadian clinical trials in patients with cancer, including the development of a policy promoting HRQOL assessment in Phase III trials and the development of written guidelines to assist clinical trial investigators when developing protocols for proposed studies (Osoba, 1992)
- Multiple publications on HRQOL from developing countries

Table 1-2.   **Annual Conferences of International Society for Quality of Life Studies**

1997   Charlotte, North Carolina, USA

1998   Williamsburg, Virginia, USA

2000   Girona, Spain

2001   Washington, DC, USA

2002   Orlando, Florida, USA

2003   Frankfurt, Germany

2004   Philadelphia, Pennsylvania, USA

2006   Grahamstown, South Africa

2007   San Diego, California, USA

2009   Florence, Italy

Quality-of-life publications and organizations provide further proof of recent interest in HRQOL. The first listing of the term quality of life appeared in *Index Medicus* in 1972 with 15 citations. In 2006, there were over 27,000 citations on quality of life.

Defining Quality of Life

Quality-of-life assessment is complicated by the fact that there is no universally accepted definition for HRQOL. In the past, many researchers measured only one dimension, such as physical function, economic concern, or sexual function. Spilker (1990) described HRQOL assessment through three interrelated levels: overall assessment of well-being; broad domains such as physical, psychological, economic, spiritual, and social; and the components of each domain. This model, shown in Figure 1-1, demonstrates the multidimensional nature of HRQOL and the importance of assessing all three levels: overall HRQOL, each domain, and individual items. Further development of the concept has occurred by focusing on illness. Thus the definition of HRQOL has been limited to the subjective assessment of the impact of disease and its treatment across the physical, psychological, social, and somatic dimensions of functioning and well-being (Revicki et al., 2000).

The World Health Organization defines quality of life as "individuals' perceptions of their position in life in the context of the culture and value system in which they live and in relation to their goals, standards, and concerns" (WHO, 1993, p.1). This definition includes six broad domains: physical health, psychological state, levels of independence, social relationships, environmental features, and spiritual concerns.

In the report of the Workshop on Quality of Life Research in Cancer Clinical Trials cosponsored by the National Cancer Institute (NCI) and the Office of Medical Applications of Research at the National Institutes of Health (Nayfield et al., 1991), HRQOL also was identified as a multidimensional concept: "Health-related quality of life is the value assigned to duration of life as modified by impairments, functional states, perceptions, and

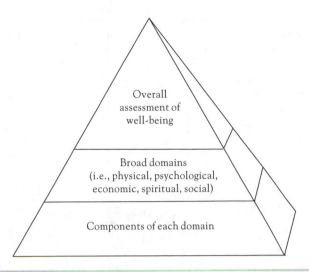

Figure 1-1.   **Three levels of quality of life. In their totality, these three levels constitute the scope (and definition) of quality of life.**

Source: Spilker, 1996, pp. 1–10. Used with permission of Lippincott-Raven Publishers.

social opportunities as influenced by disease, injury, treatment, or policy" (US Department of Health and Human Services, 1990, p. 3). The workshop recommended that HRQOL assessment at least include dimensions generally acknowledged to contribute to HRQOL (e.g., physical/role functioning, emotional/psychological functioning, social functioning, somatic/physiological complaints) and a global self-report of HRQOL.

Within the nursing literature, investigators' definitions of HRQOL parallel those of other disciplines with a focus on the multidimensionality of the concept. Ferrans's (1990) review of HRQOL literature in relation to conceptual issues identified five broad categories into which HRQOL definitions could be grouped. These categories focus on the patient's ability to live a normal life, the patient's happiness or satisfaction, the patient's achievement of personal goals, the patient's ability to lead a socially "useful" life, and the patient's physical and mental capabilities (actual or potential).

Research by Grant, Padilla, and Ferrell also emphasizes the need for a multidimensional definition for HRQOL, including an existential dimension (Grant, Ferrell, & Sakurai, 1994). These investigators have identified HRQOL as consisting of four dimensions or domains: physical well-being, psychological well-being, social well-being, and spiritual well-being. Each dimension consists of generic items of concern to all cancer patient populations, as well as items specific to a type of cancer or treatment. The model has been validated across studies in a number of cancer patient populations (Ferrell et al., 1992b; Ferrell, Grant, Funk, Otis-Green, & Garcia, 1997; Ferrell, Grant, Funk, Otis-Green, & Garcia, 1998a; Ferrell, Grant, Funk, Otis-Green, & Garcia, 1998b; Ferrell, Hassey Dow, Leigh, Ly, & Gulasekaram, 1995; Grant, 1999; Grant, Ferrell, Dean, Uman, Chu, & Krouse, 2004; Greimel, Padilla, & Grant, 1997; Padilla, Ferrell, & Grant, 1990; Padilla & Grant, 1985; Padilla et al., 1992; Padilla et

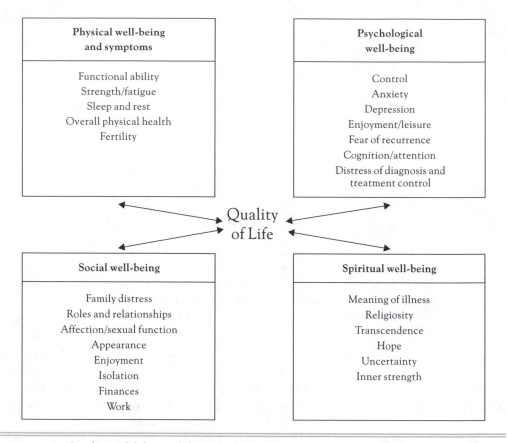

Physical well-being and symptoms
Functional ability
Strength/fatigue
Sleep and rest
Overall physical health
Fertility

Psychological well-being
Control
Anxiety
Depression
Enjoyment/leisure
Fear of recurrence
Cognition/attention
Distress of diagnosis and treatment control

Quality of Life

Social well-being
Family distress
Roles and relationships
Affection/sexual function
Appearance
Enjoyment
Isolation
Finances
Work

Spiritual well-being
Meaning of illness
Religiosity
Transcendence
Hope
Uncertainty
Inner strength

Figure 1-2. **Quality-of-life model applied to cancer survivors.**
Source: Ferrell, Hassey Dow et al., 1995. Used with permission of Oncology Nursing Press.

al., 1983; Padilla, Grant, Ferrell, & Presant, 1996). Figure 1-2 identifies the HRQOL model as it applies to cancer survivors. This model was identified in investigations involving cancer survivors who were members of the National Coalition of Cancer Survivors and who responded to a mailed HRQOL questionnaire. This model also is used to organize content in the Institute of Medicine report *From Cancer Patient to Cancer Survivor: Lost in Transition* (Hoffman & Stovall, 2006). The City of Hope Quality of Life model (Grant et al., 2004) acknowledges that HRQOL is subjective, based on the patient's self-report, always changing and dynamic, and a multidimensional concept.

Measuring Quality of Life

Many questionnaires and surveys have been developed for measuring HRQOL. Both general and disease-specific approaches have been used, resulting in the development of a multitude of instruments. The Mapi Research Institute in France has responded to the challenge of organizing information on the questionnaires by developing a HRQOL instrument database containing a list of 1000 instruments, descriptions of over 552 of them, copies of 375 original questionnaires, and copies of 500 translations. Information on this database is available at www.QOLID.org. Within the context of today's healthcare environment, the use of HRQOL as an outcome measure to allocate healthcare resources has been explored. Distribution of these resources based on expected HRQOL is tempting. However, because a gold standard for HRQOL assessment does not exist and the use of scientific methods to assess HRQOL is in its infancy, caution in applying HRQOL measures to allocate healthcare resources is imperative. Research has demonstrated differences between HRQOL assessments made by healthcare providers and made by patients (Fowlie, Berkeley, & Dingwall-Fordyce, 1989; King, Ferrell, Grant, & Sakurai, 1995; Slevin, Plant, Lynch, Drinkwater, & Gregory, 1988). Thus, healthcare providers are faced with the dilemma of whose HRQOL it is—society's, the healthcare provider's, the family's, or the patient's. When assessing HRQOL, researchers must respond to the following questions: Who should perform HRQOL assessment? When should HRQOL be assessed? Are the assessment instruments reliable, valid, and sensitive? For what purpose is the information being collected?

Relationship of Quality of Life to the Scope of Nursing

Quality-of-life perspectives are particularly relevant to the scope of nursing practice (King, 2006). Nurses are educated to provide the physical, psychosocial, spiritual, and cultural components of care. As such, nurses are keenly aware of the importance of the quality of their patients' lives and not simply the quantity. Padilla and Grant (1985) state that *quality of life* refers to "that which makes life worth living and connotes the caring aspects of nursing, because nursing is concerned not only with survival and decreased morbidity, but with the whole patient" (p. 45). Nursing is a caring practice in which nurses foster health promotion and maintenance, or restoration of function. Through these nursing activities, nurses promote patient well-being. Because cancer and its treatment impact the entire patient, including physical, psychological, social, and spiritual well-being, HRQOL information gathered by nurses can provide valuable nursing assessment data. In providing care to patients with cancer, nurses help patients manage the side effects of therapy and adjust to changes in body image, function, and appearance, and to living with a chronic disease. This holistic view of nursing care delivery can help the patient maintain or improve life and the quality of that life. The nurse can help the patient to make the changes necessary to adjust to a life with cancer.

Quality of life is affected by numerous factors including cultural variables, age, and diagnosis. However, many factors may not be amenable to nursing intervention (e.g., diagnosis, family illness history, predisposing characteristics, medical treatment) (Padilla & Grant, 1985). On the other hand, HRQOL is also influenced by factors over which nurses have influence, such as the environment of care, information provided to patients and family members, personal or social issues, symptom management, and nursing interventions.

Advances in cancer care have provided new opportunities for oncology nurses to improve the quality of their patients' lives. Cancer survivors face short- and long-term complications of cancer treatments, treatments designed to prevent secondary cancers, development of recurrent and secondary cancers, treatment of recurrent cancer, the use of rehabilitative services, and palliative and end-of-life care (Ayanian & Jacobsen, 2006; Korstjens, Mesters, van der Peet, Gijsen, & van den Borne, 2006; Morris, Grant, & Lynch, 2007).

In a study of bone marrow transplant survivors, respondents identified ways nurses and physicians can improve HRQOL, such as being accessible, discovering a cure, providing support groups, reinforcing current education, providing additional coping strategies, and increasing patient participation in decision making (Ferrell et al., 1992a). Other researchers have identified similar interventions in other cancer patient populations (Davis & Grant, 1994; Harrington, Lackey, & Gates, 1996; Stetz, McDonald, & Compton, 1996; Mock et al., 2001; Stanton et al., 2005; Yates et al., 2005).

Evidence of Nursing Interest in Quality of Life

Nursing has led the way for other scientific disciplines in identifying, measuring, promoting, and evaluating HRQOL in cancer patients. In the 1980s the relevance of HRQOL was identified as an appropriate outcome to measure the impact of nursing care (Padilla & Grant, 1985). The number of publications related to HRQOL has steadily increased since the term was first included in the *Cumulative Index of Nursing and Allied Health Literature* (CINAHL) as an indexed topic (Figure 1-3). These references span the specialties in nursing and include a large portion of nursing contributions to the cancer literature. Health-related quality of life has also been included as an evaluative component in acute care (Peters & Sellick, 2006), chronic care (Parikh et al., 2006), adult care (Tinker & White, 2006), pediatric care (Grilli et al., 2006), hospital care (Simpson & Pilote, 2005), home care (Friedman et al., 2005), and hospice care (Park et al., 2006).

Quality of life as a concept aligns well with the overall goals of nursing. Nurses believe that the most valid measure of HRQOL is whatever the individual believes it to be (King, Hinds, Dow, Schum, & Lee, 2002). Nurses learn about their patients' HRQOL through established therapeutic relationships with their patients. Nurse researchers are challenged to continue this scientific work and take an active part in the assessment, application, and evaluation of HRQOL for patients and families. Improving HRQOL is an area of research emphasis at the National Institute of Nursing Research (www.ninr.nih.gov). As the focus of health care continues to change, HRQOL, as an outcome of professional nursing care, may become one of the most important indicators of quality care. As a result, comparing HRQOL perceptions among patients, nurses, and family caregivers is essential for identifying differences and planning approaches to minimize those differences (King et al., 1995).

Relationship of Nursing HRQOL Studies to Other Disciplines

In the 2004 Oncology Nursing Society (ONS) Research Priorities Survey (Berger et al., 2005), the conduct of research on HRQOL was identified as the highest priority for research. This prioritization illustrates the continuing importance of nursing care for oncology patients. Additionally, over the years oncology nurses have been involved in HRQOL projects in collaboration with other disciplines.

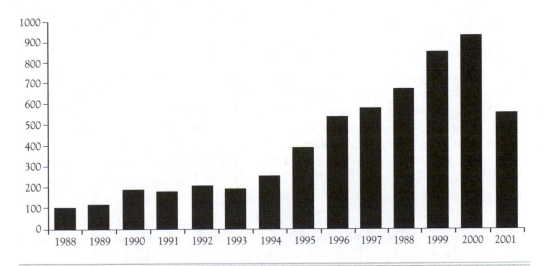

Figure 1-3.   **Citations in CINAHL using quality of life as an index term.**

The National Cancer Institute's clinical trials groups have included a HRQOL measurement in many of the Phase III trials. The Southwest Oncology Group (SWOG), the Gynecologic Oncology Group (GOG), and the National Surgical Adjuvant Project for Breast and Bowel Cancers (NSABP) have all incorporated HRQOL measures into multiple time periods to determine whether the difference in treatment arms can be described in terms of the impact on HRQOL. When implementing HRQOL studies, the medical protocol nurse typically is responsible for administering HRQOL questionnaires. Current approaches to including HRQOL measurements in these oncology groups may involve the development of an interdisciplinary HRQOL committee, which would be responsible for identifying HRQOL hypotheses, study methods, and analysis approaches. Interpretation of the analysis and writing manuscripts would be part of the committee members' responsibilities.

Grant and Ferrell at City of Hope National Medical Center in Duarte, California, have found the interdisciplinary approach valuable. In their research, they collaborated with physicians, psychologists, social workers, clergy, and others to explore HRQOL issues for bone marrow transplant patients (Grant, Cooke, Bhatia & Forman, 2005; Sherman, Cooke, & Grant, 2005,); for colorectal cancer patients (Grant et al., 2004; Krouse et al., 2006); for nursing home patients (Ferrell, Ferrell, & Rivera, 1995); for women with ovarian cancer (Ferrell, Melancon, Ervin, Smith, & Marek, 2002; Ferrell, Smith, Cullinane, & Melancon, 2003); in the home care setting (Ferrell & Borneman, 2002); and in pediatrics (Ferrell, Rhiner, Shapiro, & Dierkes, 1994).

Interdisciplinary approaches to HRQOL research have provided data important in expanding the perception of cancer and cancer treatment impact on HRQOL. As a broad outcome of patient care, HRQOL provides information valuable to physicians, nurses, social workers, psychologists, physical therapists, and pharmacists. As an outcome measure of the impact of health care, HRQOL will continue to provide valuable information in measuring the impact of healthcare changes on the lives of cancer patients.

Oncology Nursing Society Research Activities

The Oncology Nursing Society (ONS) and the Oncology Nursing Foundation (ONF) have demonstrated support for HRQOL research and clinical practice. From 1989 to the present, the ONF, in conjunction with corporate sponsors, funded many HRQOL research studies conducted by oncology nurse researchers (Table 1-3). Since 1988, the Upjohn Corporation, in conjunction with ONS, has supported an annual award to recognize nursing excellence in HRQOL issues (Table 1-4). Established in 1991, a QOL lectureship is delivered at ONS's Annual Fall Institute (now titled Institutes of Learning) and is published in *Oncology Nursing Forum* (Table 1-5). The purpose of this lectureship is as follows:

- Focus ONS membership attention on HRQOL issues in cancer care.
- Describe the contribution of oncology nurse clinicians, educators, administrators, and researchers to HRQOL in cancer care.
- Apply HRQOL-related information to nursing practice.
- Incorporate HRQOL philosophy into all aspects of cancer care.

In February 1995, AMGEN, USA, and AMGEN, Canada, sponsored the ONS QOL State-of-the-Knowledge Conference in San Diego, California, to address the current knowledge regarding HRQOL and the cancer experience (King et al., 1997). Oncology nurses and psychologists from the United States and Canada attended the conference.

Oncology Nursing Society Research Priorities

The ONS Research Committee or Research Special Interest Group has periodically surveyed membership to identify research priorities and provide a focus for nursing education programs and conferences. The organization uses the findings to advise the Oncology Nursing Foundation and federal agencies about priorities for research funding. Findings from the 2004 ONS Research Priorities Survey have been published in the *Oncology Nursing Forum* (Berger et al., 2005). Respondents ranked QOL studies as the highest priority for research by oncology nurses.

Quality-of-Life Research Issues

While progress has been made in defining HRQOL and developing qualitative, quantitative, and mixed methodologies to study HRQOL and identify HRQOL outcomes, many research challenges persist, including addressing conceptual and methodological issues.

Authors must include their definitions of assumptions about, and conceptual approaches to, HRQOL assessment. To combine findings across studies and synthesize what knowledge has been identified, it is essential to find clarity in defining and measuring HRQOL. Many quantitative instruments have been developed for measuring HRQOL,

Table 1-3.   **Quality-of-Life Research Projects Funded by the Oncology Nursing Foundation**

Small Grants Program

1989

Quality of Life Perceptions of Bone Marrow Transplant Recipients, Ruth Belec, RN, BSN, CCRN, Marquette University School of Nursing, Milwaukee, WI. Oncology Nursing Foundation/Lederle Research Award.

1990

Testing of a Trait-State Model for Quality of Life, Ann T. Foltz, RN, DNS, Duke University School of Nursing, Raleigh, NC. Oncology Nursing Foundation/Lederle Laboratories Research Grant.

1991

Effect of Pain and Quality of Life in Breast Cancer, Jeri Lynn Ashley, RN, MSN, Baptist Memorial Hospital, Memphis, TN. Oncology Nursing Foundation/Wyeth-Ayerst New Investigator's Research Grant.

1992

Side Effects of Quality of Life in Patients Receiving HDR Brachytherapy, Vickie K. Fieler, RN, MS, University of Rochester Cancer Center, Rochester, NY. Oncology Nursing Foundation/Wyeth-Ayerst New Investigator's Research Grant.

Quality of Life After Autologous Bone Marrow Transplantation, Marie Whedon, RN, MS, OCN, Dartmouth-Hitchcock Medical Center, Hanover, NH. Oncology Nursing Foundation/Wyeth-Ayerst New Investigator's Research Grant.

Quality of Life of Long Term Female Cancer Survivors, Gwen Wyatt, RN, PhD, Michigan State University, East Lansing, MI. Oncology Nursing Foundation/Bristol-Myers Research Grant.

1993

The Experience of Breast Cancer Survivorship, Diane G. Cope, RN, MSN, PhDc, Florida Atlantic University, Boca Raton, FL. Oncology Nursing Foundation/Wyeth Ayerst New Investigator's Research Grant.

Adaptation in Young Breast Cancer Survivors: A Pilot, Karen Hassey Dow, RN, PhD, Beth Israel Hospital, Boston, MA. Oncology Nursing Foundation/Lederle Laboratories Research Grant.

The Impact of Treatment of Endometrial Cancer on Quality of Life, Margaret Anne Lamb, RN, PhD, University of New Hampshire, Durham, NH. Oncology Nursing Foundation/Bristol-Myers Research Grant.

Development of a Nursing Intervention for Women with Breast Cancer-CMF, Roxanne W. McDaniel, RN, PhD, University of Missouri-Columbia, School of Nursing, Columbia, OH. Oncology Nursing Foundation/Smith Kline Beecham Research Grant.

continues

Table 1-3.   **Quality-of-Life Research Projects Funded by the Oncology Nursing Foundation (continued)**

Pain Relief and Pharmacokinetics of Rectal MS Contin, Cheryl Ann Mummy, RN, BSN, OCN, University of Iowa Hospital and Clinics, Iowa City, IA. Oncology Nursing Foundation/Purdue Frederick Research Grant.

Group Intervention to Home Bound Caregivers of Persons with Cancer and AIDS, Kathleen M. Stetz, RN, PhD, University of Washington, Bothell, WA. Oncology Nursing Foundation/Chiron Therapeutics Research Grant.

1994

The Experience of Being a Family Member of a Breast Cancer Survivor, Diane G. Cope, RN, PhD, OCN, Florida Atlantic University, College of Nursing, Boca Raton, FL. Oncology Nursing Foundation/Bristol-Myers Oncology Division Community Health Research Grant.

Predicting Adjustments in Hispanic Breast Cancer Survivors, Shannon R. Dirksen, RN, PhD, University of New Mexico, Albuquerque, NM. Oncology Nursing Foundation/Immunex Corporation Research Grant.

Black Women's Lived/Caring Experiences with Breast Cancer, Marie F. Gates, RN, PhD, University of Tennessee, College of Nursing, Memphis, TN. Oncology Nursing Foundation Research Grant.

Therapeutic Touch in Breast Cancer: Immune and Quality of Life Effects, Robin A. Meize Grochowski, RN, PhD, University of New Mexico, Albuquerque, NM. Oncology Nursing Foundation/Chiron Therapeutics Research Grant.

Quality of Life: Impact of Head and Neck Cancer, Mary E. Means, RN, BSN, CORLN, University of Iowa Hospital and Clinics, Department of Nursing, Iowa City, IA. Oncology Nursing Foundation Research Grant.

Quality of Life Considerations in Patients with Colon Polyps, Kimberly C. Phillips, RN, MSN, Bowman Gray School of Medicine, Department of Public Health Sciences, Winston-Salem, NC. Oncology Nursing Foundation/Wyeth New Investigator's Research Grant.

Quality of Life in Patients Receiving Monoclonal Antibody Therapy, Lindsey A. Trammell, RN, MSN, OCN, University of Alabama in Birmington, Comprehensive Cancer Center, Birmingham, AL. Oncology Nursing Foundation/Smith Kline Beecham Research Grant.

1995

Risks, Benefits, and Costs of Home and Hospital Care, Linda K. Birenbaum, RN, PhD, Walther Cancer Institute, Indianapolis, IN. Oncology Nursing Foundation/Cerenex Pharmaceuticals Research Grant.

Impact of Silicone Implants on the Lives of Women with Breast Cancer, Ann Coleman, RNP, PhD, OCN, University of Arkansas for Medical Sciences, College of Nursing, Little Rock, AR. Oncology Nursing Foundation/Oncology Nursing Certification Corporation Oncology Nursing Research.

Fear of Cancer Recurrence: A Phenomenological Study, Diane G. Cope, RN, PhD, OCN, University of North Carolina at Charlotte, College of Nursing, Charlotte, NC. Oncology Nursing Foundation Research Grant.

Table 1-3.   continued

Physiological Fatigue Indicators in Patients with Breast Cancer, Grace E. Dean, RN, MSN, City of Hope National Medical Center, Duarte, CA. Oncology Nursing Foundation/Ortho Biotech Research Grant.

Evaluation of a Hispanic Version of a Pain Education Intervention, Gloria Juarez, RN, MSN, City of Hope National Medical Center, Duarte, CA. Oncology Nursing Foundation Ethnic Minority Researcher and Mentorship Grant.

The Family Experience of Bone Marrow Transplant, Lynne M. Rivera, RN, BSN, City of Hope National Medical Center, Duarte, CA. Oncology Nursing Foundation/New Investigator's Research Grant.

Quality of Life in Persons with Multiple Myeloma, Mary Thomas, RN, MS, OCN, Department of Veteran's Affairs Medical Center, Palo Alto, CA. Oncology Nursing Foundation/Smith Kline Beecham Research Grant.

1996

Quality of Life in Brain Tumor Patients Undergoing Aggressive Therapy, Terri Armstrong, RN, MS, University of Pittsburgh Cancer Institute, Pittsburgh, PA. Oncology Nursing Foundation/American Brain Tumor Association Grant.

Forgiveness in Terminally Ill Cancer Patients, Jacqueline R. Mickley, RN, PhD, Kent State University, Hudson, OH. Oncology Nursing Foundation/Amgen, Inc. Research Grant.

Conservative Management of Urinary Incontinence Post Radical Prostatectomy: Impact on Urine Loss and Quality of Life, Katherine N. Moore, RN, MN, PhDc, University of Alberta, Edmonton, Alberta, Canada. Oncology Nursing Foundation/Hoechst Marion Roussel Research Grant.

The Relationship of Exercise and Fatigue to Quality of Life in Women with Breast Cancer, Anna L. Schwartz, RN, MS, FNP, University of Utah, College of Nursing, Salt Lake City, UT. Oncology Nursing Foundation/Glaxo Welcome Research Grant.

Taste Changes of Cancer Patients, Rita Wickman, RN, MS, AOCN, PhDc, Rush Presbyterian St. Luke's Medical Center, Chicago, IL. Oncology Nursing Foundation/Bristol-Myers Oncology Chapter's Grant.

1997

Uncertainty and Watchful Waiting with Prostate Cancer, Donald Bailey, Jr., RN, MN, University of North Carolina, Durham, NC. Oncology Nursing Foundation/Oncology Nursing Certification Corporation Research Grant.

Symptom Management and Successful Outpatient Transplant, Elizabeth Ann Coleman, PhD, RN, AOCN, University of Arkansas for Medical Sciences, College of Nursing, Little Rock, AR. Oncology Nursing Foundation/Smith Kline Beecham Research Grant.

Health Outcomes in Survivors of Breast Cancer, Denise M. Oleske, RN, PhD, Rush University, Chicago, IL. Oncology Nursing Foundation/Amgen, Inc. Research Grant.

continues

Table 1-3.   **Quality-of-Life Research Projects Funded by the Oncology Nursing Foundation (continued)**

Mutual Support Dyads and Quality of Life of Women with Breast Cancer, Laura B. Sutton, RN, MS, CS, University of Pittsburgh, Pittsburgh, PA. Oncology Nursing Foundation/Rhone-Poulence Rorer New Investigator's Research Grant.

1998

Determination of Preferences and Utilities for the Treatment of Prostate Cancer, Deborah W. Bruner, MSN, RN, Fox Chase Cancer Center, Philadelphia, PA. ONS Foundation/Amgen, Inc. Research Grant.

Evaluation of the Healing Odyssey Program, Nancy J. Raymon, MN, RN, Healing Odyssey, Inc., Irvine, CA. ONS Foundation Nursing Outcomes Research Grant.

1999

Exercise for Patients with Multiple Myeloma, Elizabeth Ann Coleman, PhD, RN, AOCN(r), University of Arkansas for Medical Sciences, College of Nursing, Little Rock, AR. ONS Foundation/Oncology Nursing Society Nursing Outcomes Research Grant.

Effects of Seated Exercise on Fatigue in Breast Cancer, Judith A. Headley, PhD, RN, AOCN(r), University of Texas Health Science Center-Houston School of Nursing, Houston, TX. ONS Foundation/Hoechst Marion Roussel Research Grant.

Quality of Life and Adjustment for Couples Experiencing Advanced Breast Cancer, Frances Marcus Lewis, PhD, RN, FAAN, University of Washington, School of Nursing, Seattle, WA. ONS Foundation/Amgen, Inc. Research Grant.

The Meaning of Incontinence and Impotence Postprostatectomy, Sally L. Maliski, PhD, RN, University of Pennsylvania, School of Nursing, Philadelphia, PA. ONS Foundation/Ortho Biotech Research Grant.

Prevention of Osteoporosis in Breast Cancer Survivors, Nancy L. Waltman, PhD, RN, University of Nebraska Medical Center, College of Nursing, Omaha, NE. ONS Foundation/Janssen Pharmaceutica Research Grant.

Quality of Life with Photodynamic Therapy vs. Conservative Treatment, Kathy B. Wright, MS, RN, CGRN, CS, Parkland Health and Hospital System, Dallas, TX. ONS Foundation Smith Kline Beecham Research Grant.

2000

Smoking, Alcohol Intake, and Depression in Head/Neck Cancer Patients, Sonia Duffy, PhD, RN, HSR&D Field Program, Ann Arbor, MI. ONS Foundation and Sigma Theta Tau International Research Grant.

Symptom Management of Chemotherapy via Telephone Outreach, Janet S. Fulton, PhD, RN, Wright State University, Cincinnati, OH. ONS Foundation/Smith Kline Beecham Research Grant.

African American Women: The Experience of Breast Cancer and Menopause, M. Tish Knobf, PhD, RN, FFAN, Yale University, New Haven, CT. ONS Foundation/Genetech Research Research Grant.

Table 1-3. **continued**

Effects of Symptom Combination on Quality End of Life, Barbara M. Raudonis, PhD, RN, CS, University of Texas at Arlington, Arlington, TX. ONS Foundation/Roxanne Laboratories Research Grant.

In-Home Pain Education for Cancer Patients-A Pilot Study, Mary Anne Reynolds, PhD, RN, CS, Washington State University Tri-Cities, Richland, WA. ONS Foundation/Knoll Pharmaceutical Research Grant.

2001

Surviving Prostate Cancer and Treatment: Impact on Couples, Michael E. Galbraith, PhD, RN, Loma Linda University School of Nursing, Loma Linda, CA. ONS Foundation/Aventis Research Grant.

Building a Story: Word Patterns in Writing and Quality of Life, Margaret Saul Laccetti, MSN, RN, AOCN(r), Salem State College, Salem, MA. ONS Foundation/Aventis New Investigator Research Grant.

Factors Influencing Quality of Life Following Autologous Bone Marrow Transplantation, Usama S. Saleh, MSN, RN, PhD candidate, University of Kentucky College of Nursing, Lexington, KY. ONS Foundation Ethnic Minority Researcher and Mentorship Grant.

Late Effects and Quality of Life in Long-Term Survivors of Testis Cancer, Linda A. Jacobs, PhD, CRNP, AOCN(r), CS, University of Pennsylvania, Philadelphia, PA. ONS Foundation/Bristol-Myers Oncology Research Grant.

2002

Quality of Life in Older Cancer Survivors: Impact of Age and Culture, Kimberly A. Christopher, PhD, RN, OCN(r), University of Massachusetts, South Dartmouth, MA. ONS Foundation, Ortho Biotech Research Grant.

Quality of Life in Women Who Carry a BRCA Mutation, Sarah M. McCaffrey, MS, RN, City of Hope National Medical Center, Duarte, CA. ONS Foundation/Genetech Research Grant.

Treatment Decision-Making for the Primary Treatment of Early-Stage Breast Cancer in Chinese American Women, Shiu-yu C. Lee, MSN, RN, Yale University, New Haven, CT. ONS Foundation Ethnic Minority Research Grant.

Prophylactic Skin Care for Patients Undergoing Radiation Therapy, Tracy K. Gosselin, MSN, RN, AOCN(r), Duke University Medical Center, Durham, NC. ONS Foundation/Aventis Oncology Research Grant.

Fatigue and Physical Activity in Stem Cell Transplant Patients, Eileen Hacker, PhD, RN, AOCN(r), University of Illinois at Chicago College of Nursing, Chicago, IL. ONS Foundation/Ortho Biotech Inc. Research Grant.

The Cancer Pain Experience of Israeli Elders, Catherine F. Musgrave, DNS(c), RN, University of Pennsylvania, Philadelphia, PA. ONS Foundation/Purdue Frederick Trish Greene Research Grant.

Breast Biopsy and Distress: Testing a Reiki Intervention, Pamela J. Potter, APRN, CS, MSN, MA, Yale University School of Nursing, New Haven, CT. ONS Foundation/Ortho Biotech Inc. Research Grant.

continues

Table 1-3.   Quality-of-Life Research Projects Funded by the Oncology
              Nursing Foundation (continued)

Symptoms of Dying Children in the Last Week of Life, Michele Pritchard, MSN, RN, CPNP, St. Jude Children's Research Hospital, Memphis, TN. ONS Foundation/Aventis Oncology New Investigator Research Grant.

2003

Biopsychosocial Impact of Parental Cancer on Schoolagers, Ying-Hwa Su, RN, BSN, MS. Funded by the ONS Foundation/Aventis Pharmaceuticals New Investigator Research Grant.

The Experience of Hope in Women with Advanced Ovarian Cancer, Anne M. Reb, MS, NP. ONS Foundation/Oncology Nursing Certification Corporation (ONCC).

Growth Patterns and Gastrointestinal Symptoms in Children Post Bone Marrow Transplant, Cheryl Rodgers, MSN, CPNP, CPON(r), Baylor College of Medicine, Houston, TX. ONS Foundation/Ortho Biotech Products, L.P. Research Grant.

Experiences of Colorectal Cancer Patients and Their Caregivers, Arlene D. Houldin, PhD, RN, CS, University of Pennsylvania, Philadelphia, PA. ONS Foundation/Genentech, Inc. Research Grant.

2004

Partners' Survivorship from the Effects of Prostate Cancer, Jean Boucher, PhD, RN, NP, AOCN(r), University of Massachusetts. ONS Foundation/Bristol-Myers Squibb Oncology Research Grant.

Functional Status and Quality of Life in Children with Medulloblastoma, Patricia L. Cullen, MEd, CPNP, Regis University. ONS Foundation/Aventis Pharmaceuticals Research Grant.

End of Life Decisions in Intensive Care Units, Michael H. Limerick, MSN, RN, APRN, BC, University of Texas, Austin, TX. ONS Foundation/Aventis Pharmaceuticals Research Grant.

2005

Quality of Life of Jordanians Post Stem Cell Transplantation, Fawwaz Alaloul, MSN, RN, University of Kentucky.

Sleep Disturbance in Patients with Head and Neck Cancer, Maria Cho, PhD, RN

University of California–San Francisco. ONS Foundation/Oncology Nursing Society/Sigma Theta Tau International Research Grant.

Family Management and Survivors of Childhood Brain Tumors, Janet A. Deatrick, PhD, RN, FAAN, University of Pennsylvania, Philadelphia, PA. ONS Foundation/American Brain Tumor Association Research Grant.

Psychosocial Outcomes in Online Cancer Support Groups, Paula R. Klemm, DNSc, RN, OCN(r), University of Delaware, Newark, DE. ONS Foundation/Oncology Nursing Society Research Grant.

Symptom Concerns and QOL in Hepatobiliary Cancers, Virginia Sun, MSN, RN, City of Hope National Medical Center, Duarte, CA. ONS Foundation/Purdue Pharma, L.P. Research Grant.

Table 1-3. **continued**

2006

Fatigue and Related Factors during Colorectal Cancer Chemotherapy, Ann M. Berger, PhD, RN, AOCN(r), University of Nebraska Medical Center, Omaha, NE. ONS Foundation/Bristol-Myers Squibb Oncology Research Grant.

Impact of Fatigue Education in Patients with NSCLC During RT, Michele E. Gaguski, MSN, RN, AOCN(r), APN-C, Ocean Medical Center, Brick, NJ. ONS Foundation/Oncology Nursing Society and Sigma Theta Tau International Foundation for Nursing Research Grant.

The Meaning of Dignity to the Urban Poor with Advanced Disease, Anne M. Hughes, RN, MN, AOCN(r), FAAN, University of California, San Francisco, CA. ONS Foundation/Oncology Nursing Certification Corporation Research Grant.

Frequency, Intensity and Distress Associated with Chemotherapy Symptom, Jacquelyn A. Keehne-Miron, RN, MSN, AOCN(r), Michigan State University, East Lansing, MI. ONS Foundation/Purdue Pharma L.P, Trish Greene Research Grant.

Melanoma High-Risk Patients' Perceived Risk, Worry, Risk Communications, Lois J. Loescher, PhD, RN, University of Arizona, Tucson, AZ. ONS Foundation/Oncology Nursing Society Research Grant.

2007

Palliative Care and End-of-Life Communication Experiences of Pediatric Oncology Nurses, Verna Hendricks-Ferguson, DNSc, RN, Indiana University, Indianapolis, IN. ONS Foundation/Oncology Nursing Society Nursing Research Grant.

Counter-Stimulation for Post Mastectomy Pain Syndrome, Jean M. Rosiak, RN, MSN, APRN, BC, AOCNP, Aurora Health Care, Milwaukee, WI. ONS Foundation/Oncology Nursing Society and Sigma Theta Tau International Foundation for Nursing Research Grant.

The Family Experience Following Bone Marrow/Blood Cell Transplant, Linda K. Young, MSN, CNS, RN, University of Wisconsin-Madison, Madison, WI. ONS Foundation Nursing Research Grant.

2008

Spirituality in Mexican American Cancer Caregivers, Carolyn S. Cagle, PhD, RNC, Texas Christian University, Fort Worth, TX. ONS Foundation/Oncology Nursing Society/Sigma Theta Tau International Foundation for Nursing Research Grant.

Characteristics and Prevalence of Sudden Fatigue in Cancer, Horng-Shiuann Wu, PhD, RN, Wayne State University, Detroit, MI. ONS Foundation/Novartis Nursing Research Grant.

Major Grants Program

ONS Foundation Center for Leadership, Information, and Research

1999

Living with Lung Cancer: The Women's Perspective, Linda Sarna, DNSc, RN, University of California, Los Angeles, CA. ONS Foundation/Bristol-Myers Squibb Foundation Inc.

continues

Table 1-3.   **Quality-of-Life Research Projects Funded by the Oncology Nursing Foundation (continued)**

2000

A Behavioral Randomized Trial for Patients on Interferon, Anna L. Schwartz, PhD, ARNP, Oregon Health Sciences University, Portland, OR. ONS Foundation/Schering Oncology Biotherapy Research Grant.

2001

Telephone Intervention Project: Rural Women with Cancer & Their Partners, Terry A. Badger, PhD, RN, University of Arizona College of Nursing, Tucson, AZ. ONS Foundation/Ortho Biotech, Inc. Symptom Management Phase I Research Grant.

Computerized Cancer Symptom and Quality of Life Assessment, Donna L. Berry, PhD, RN, AOCN(r), University of Washington, Seattle, WA. ONS Foundation/Ortho Biotech Inc. Symptom Management Phase I Research Grant.

2004

Outcomes of a Ovarian Cancer Quality of Life Intervention, Betty R. Ferrell, PhD, FAAN, City of Hope National Medical Center, Duarte, CA.

Effect of Endurance Exercise on Biobehavioral Outcomes of Fatigue, Sadeeka Al-Majid, PhD, Virginia Commonwealth University, Richmond, VA.

2005

Management of Skin Toxicities Following Biotherapy, Kyra Whitmer, PhD, RN, University of Cincinnati, Cinncinnati, OH.

Development of a Chronic Graft Versus Host Disease Symptom Inventory, Lori A. Williams, DSN, RN, CNS, AOCN, The University of Texas, MD Anderson Cancer Center, Houston, TX.

2006

Paclitaxel-Induced Peripheral Neuropathy in Breast Cancer, Judith A. Paice, PhD, RN, Director, Cancer Pain Program, Northwestern University, Feinberg School of Nursing, Chicago IL.

Neuropenia Symptoms: Communication and Self-Monitoring. Margaret H. Crighton, PhD, RN, Assistant Professor, University of Pittsburgh, School of Nursing, Pittsburgh, PA.

2007

Intervention to Improve Adherence and Symptoms from Oral Agents, Barbara Given, PhD, RN, FAAN, Michigan State University, East Lansing, MI.

2008

Sleep-Wake Disturbances in Lung Cancer: A Mixed Method Study, Grace E. Dean, PhD, RN, SUNY University at Buffalo, Buffalo, NY.

A "Finding Balance" Nursing Intervention for Bereaved Caregivers, Lorraine F. Holtslander, PhD, RN, CHPCN, University of Saskatchewan, Saskatoon, Canada.

Table 1-4.   **Recipients of the Annual Quality-of-Life Award Sponsored by the Oncology Nursing Society and Corporations**

1988   *Pregnancy and Parenthood after Treatment for Breast Cancer.* Karen M. Hassey, RN, MS, presented this paper at the 14th Annual Oncology Nursing Society Congress in Pittsburgh, PA. She was the first recipient of the ONS/Upjohn Company QOL Award.

1989   *Effects of Controlled-Release Morphine on Quality of Life for Cancer Pain,* Betty R. Ferrell, RN, PhD; Cheryl Wisdom, RN, MS; Carol Wenzel, RN, MEd; and Judy Brown, RN, MS. Dr. Ferrell presented this paper at the 15th Annual Oncology Nursing Society Congress in San Francisco, CA. The paper was selected for the 1989 ONS/Upjohn Company QOL Award.

1990   *Delirium in Patients with Cancer: Nursing Assessment and Intervention,* Marianne Zimberg, RN, MA, and Susan Berenson, RN, MS. Ms. Zimberg presented this paper at the 16th Annual Oncology Nursing Society Congress in Washington, DC. The paper was selected for the 1990 ONS/Upjohn Company QOL Award.

1991   *Self-Transcendence and Emotional Well-Being in Women with Advanced Cancer.* Doris D. Coward, PhD, RN, presented this paper at the 17th Annual Oncology Nursing Society Congress in San Antonio, TX. The paper was selected for the 1991 ONS/Upjohn Company QOL Award.

1992   *The Oncology Nurse's Role in Patient Advance Directives.* Eileen Parinisi Dimond, MS, RN, OCN, presented this paper at the 17th Annual Oncology Nursing Society Congress in San Diego, CA. The paper was selected for the 1992 ONS/Upjohn Company QOL Award.

1993   *Return-to-Work Experiences of People with Cancer.* Donna L. Berry, RN, PhD, presented this paper at the 18th Annual Oncology Nursing Society Congress in Orlando, FL. The paper was selected for the 1993 ONS/Upjohn Company QOL Award and for the 1993 ONS/ Schering Corporation Excellence in Cancer Nursing Research Award.

1994   *Living with Cancer: Children with Extraordinary Courage,* Marilyn Hockenberry-Eaton, RN, PhD, and Ptlene Minick, RN, PhD. Dr. Hockenberry-Eaton presented this paper at the 19th Annual Oncology Nursing Society Congress in Cincinnati, OH. The paper was selected for the 1994 ONS/Upjohn Company QOL Award.

1995   *Quality of Life in Long-Term Cancer Survivors,* Betty R. Ferrell, RN, PhD, RN; Karen Hassey Dow, RN, PhD; Susan Leigh, RN, BSN. Dr. Ferrell presented this paper at the 20th Annual Oncology Nursing Society Congress in Anaheim, CA. The paper was selected for the 1995 ONS/Upjohn Company QOL Award and for the 1995 ONS/ Schering Corporation Excellence in Cancer Nursing Research Award.

1996   *Addressing Sexual Dysfunction Following Radiation Therapy for a Gynecologic Malignancy.* Frances Cartwright-Alcarese presented this paper at the 21st Annual Oncology Nursing Society Congress in Philadelphia, PA. The paper was selected for the 1996 ONS/Upjohn Company QOL Award.

1997   *Getting Back to Normal: The Family Experience During Early Stage Breast Cancer.* B. Ann Hilton presented this paper at the 22nd Annual Oncology Nursing Society Congress in Washington, DC. The paper was selected for the 1997 ONS/Upjohn Company QOL Award.

continues

Table 1-4.　**Recipients of the Annual Quality-of-Life Award Sponsored by the Oncology Nursing Society and Corporations (continued)**

1998　*Quality of Life and the Cancer Experience: The State-of-the-Knowledge.* Cynthia R. King presented this paper at the 23rd Annual Oncology Nursing Society Congress in Dallas, TX. The paper was selected for the 1998 ONS/Upjohn Company QOL Award.

1999　*End of Life Confusion in Patients.* Deborah A. Boyle presented this paper at the 24th Annual Oncology Nursing Society Congress in Atlanta, GA. The paper was selected for the 1999 ONS/Upjohn Company QOL Award.

2000　*The Meaning of Quality of Life in Cancer Survivorship.* Karen Hassey Dow, Betty R. Ferrell, Mel R. Haberman, and Linda Eaton presented this paper at the 25th Annual Oncology Nursing Society Congress in San Antonio, TX. The paper was selected for the 2000 ONS/Upjohn Company QOL Award.

2001　*Quality of Life, Survivorship, and Psychosocial Adjustment of Young Women with Breast Cancer after Breast-Conserving Surgery and Radiation Therapy.* Karen Hassey Dow and Patricia Lafferty presented this paper at the 26th Annual Oncology Nursing Society Congress in San Diego, CA. The paper was selected for the 2001 ONS/Upjohn Company QOL Award.

2002　*Posttraumatic Stress, Quality of Life, and Psychological Distress in Young Adult Survivors at Childhood Cancer.* Kathleen Meeske presented this paper at the 27th Annual Oncology Nursing Society Congress in Washington, DC. The paper was selected for the 2002 ONS/Upjohn Company QOL Award.

2003　*Restoring the Spirit at the End of Life: Music as an Intervention for Oncology Nurses.* Marilyn Tuls Halstead and Sherry Tuls Roscoe presented this paper at the 28th Annual Oncology Nursing Society Congress in Denver, CO. The paper was selected for the 2003 ONS/UP John Company QOL Award

2004　*Self-Surveillance for Genetic Predisposition to Cancer: Behaviors and Emotions.* Ellen Giarelli presented this paper at the 29th Annual Oncology Nursing Society Congress in Anaheim, CA. The paper was selected for the 2004 ONS/UP John Company QOL Award.

2005　*Supporting the Gift of Oncology.* Jane Clark presented this paper at the 30th Annual Oncology Nursing Society Congress in Orlando, FL. The paper was selected for the 2005 ONS/UP John Company QOL Award.

2006　*Quality of Life and Meaning of Illness of Women with Lung Cancer and Family Members.* Linda Sarna, Mary Cooley, Jean Brown, Roma Williams, Cynthia Chernecky, Geraldine Padilla, Leda Layo Danao, presented this paper at the 31st Annual Oncology Nursing Society Congress in Boston, MA. The paper was selected for the 2006 ONS/UP John Company QOL Award.

2007　*Advances in How Clinical Nurses Can Evaluate and Improve Quality of Life for Individuals with Cancer.* Cynthia R. King. presented this paper at the 32 Annual Oncology Nursing Society Congress in Las Vegas, NV. The paper was selected for the 2007 ONS/Up John Company QOL Award.

2008　*Pain Management: Nurses in Jeopardy.* Jeri L. Ashley presented this paper at the 33rd Annual Oncology Nursing Society Congress in Philadelphia, PA. The paper was selected for the 2008 ONS/Up John Company QOL Award.

Table 1-5.   **ONS Quality-of-Life Lectureships**

1991   *The Healthcare Implications of Cancer Rehabilitation in the 21st Century.* Presented by Deborah Mayer, RN, MSN, OCN, at the Second Annual Fall Institute in Atlanta, GA. Sponsored by CIBA-GIEGY Pharmaceuticals.

1992   *Myths, Monsters, and Magic: Personal Perspectives and Professional Challenges of Survival.* Presented by Susan Leigh, RN, BSN, at the Third Annual Fall Institute in Minneapolis, MN. Sponsored by CIBA-GIEGY Pharmaceuticals.

1993   *To Know Suffering.* Presented by Betty R. Ferrell, PhD, RN, at the Fourth Annual Fall Institute in Seattle, WA. Sponsored by CIBA-GIEGY Pharmaceuticals.

1994   *Quality of Life Through the Eyes of Survivors of Breast Cancer.* Presented by Carol Estwing Ferrans, PhD, RN, FAAN, at the Fifth Annual Fall Institute in Pittsburgh, PA. Sponsored by the Purdue Frederick Company.

1995   *Patient-Induced Dehydration: Can It Ever Be Therapeutic?* Presented by Shirley Anne Smith, MSN, RN, OCN, at the Sixth Annual Fall Institute in Nashville, TN. Sponsored by the Purdue Frederick Company.

1996   *Sexuality Issues: Keeping Your Cool.* Presented by Mary K. Hughes, MSN, RN, at the Seventh Annual Fall Institute in Phoenix, AZ. Sponsored by the Purdue Frederick Company.

1997   *Light Your World.* Presented by Rosanne M. Radziewica, RN, MSN, CA, at the Sixth Annual Fall Institute in Washington, DC. Sponsored by Purdue Frederick Company.

1998   *Changing Seasons of Care: Harvesting Hope in the Autumn of Life.* Presented by Terri Armstrong, RN, MS, ANP, CS at the Seventh Annual Fall Institute in Dallas, TX. Sponsored by Purdue Frederick Company.

1999   *Silence Is Not Golden: Conversations with the Dying.* Presented by Karen J. Stanley, RN, MSN, AOCN, at the Eighth Annual Fall Institute in Salt Lake City, UT. Sponsored by Purdue Frederick Company.

2000   *The Dance of Life.* Presented by Cynthia R. King, PhD, NP, MSN, RN, FAAN, at the First Annual Institute of Learning in Charlotte, NC. Sponsored by Purdue Pharma L.P.

2001   *Revisiting the Road: Integrating Palliative Care into Oncology Nursing.* Presented by Marie Bakitas Whedon, ARNP, AOCN(r), CHPN, FAAN, at the Second Annual Institute of Learning in St. Louis, MO. Sponsored by Purdue Pharma L.P.

2002   *In My House Are Many Rooms: A Proposed Model to Examine Self Concept.* Presented by June Eilers, PhD, RN, CS, at the Third Annual Institute of Learning in Seattle, WA. Sponsored by Purdue Pharma L.P.

2003   *Managing from the Middle: Integrating Midlife Challenges of Children, Elder Parents, and Cancer.* Presented by Brenda M. Nevidjon, RN, MSN, at the Fourth Annual Fall Institute of Learning in Philadelphia, PA. Sponsored by Purdue Pharma L.P.

2004   *Healing Odyssey: Stepping Beyond "The Edge" of Traditional Cancer Support.* Presented by Nancy J. Raymon, RN, MN, AOCN, at the Fifth Annual Institute of Learning in Nashville, TN. Sponsored by Purdue Pharma L.P.

continues

Table 1-5.   **ONS Quality-of-Life Lectureships (continued)**

2005   *Dance as a Metaphor for Quality of Life in Patients with Cancer.* Presented by Lois A. Almadrones, RN, MS, C, FNP, MPA, at the Sixth Annual Institute of Learning in Phoenix, AZ. Sponsored by Purdue Pharma L.P

2006   *Therapeutic Decisions and Quality of Life in Patients with Prostate Cancer.* Presented by Maureen O'Rourke, PhD, RN, at the Seventh Annual Institute of Learning in Pittsburgh, PA. Sponsored by Purdue Pharma L.P.

2007   *Quality of Life for Our Patients: How Media Images and Messages Influence Their Perceptions* Presented by Ellen R. Carr, RN, MSN, AOCN, at the Eighth Annual Institute of Learning in Chicago, IL. Sponsored by Purdue Pharma L.P.

2008   *Exercise and Quality of Life: Strengthening the Connections.* Presented by Eileen Danaher Hacker, PhD, APN, AOCN, at the Nineth Annual Institute of Learning in Seattle, WA. Sponsored by Purdue Pharma L.P.

some of which show early evidence of reliability, validity, and sensitivity. Future research should focus on the application of these instruments to a variety of patient populations by a variety of researchers. It is unlikely new instruments are needed.

Selection of an appropriate instrument should be related specifically to the questions posed in the research study. One HRQOL instrument may be valuable in measuring HRQOL over medical treatment periods, while another may be appropriately suited for evaluating survivors' concerns. Because no gold standard of HRQOL has been developed, researchers should select instrumentation based on the nature of the study, the population, the purpose, and the setting (Cooley et al., 2005).

Although assumptions are unstated in many research publications, specifying them in HRQOL research will assist in interpreting findings and building appropriate science. Is it assumed that all items in the selected HRQOL questionnaire have equal weight? Is it assumed that a baseline value can be gathered any time before treatment starts? Is it assumed that follow-up evaluation can be obtained any time after treatment ends? These and other assumptions must be carefully identified so studies can be grouped and synthesized.

Missing data in HRQOL studies is an important issue. In some instances, clinicians have been reluctant to collect HRQOL data when patients are ill, feeling that questions on HRQOL may prove upsetting. However, without acute-phase data, follow-up data cannot be compared; the true impact of the disease and treatment on HRQOL may never be known. To measure HRQOL during acute treatment periods, it may be necessary to use experienced nurses who are sensitive to the patient's needs but still able to obtain needed information. Qualitative approaches may be valuable in these situations as a measure of providing individualized approaches. A number of statistical approaches to handling missing data during analysis have been successfully applied (Sloan, 2005). Because this is a specialized area in statistical analysis, providing resources for qualified statistical consultation is essential in the analysis of HRQOL research, particularly in longitudinal studies.

Several challenges have surfaced in the interpretation of HRQOL study results. One of these is the tension between statistical differences in pre- and post-HRQOL scores, as well as what relationship these differences have to clinical differences. Formal discussions on ways to identify clinically significant differences in HRQOL measures have begun to explore methods to determine this important clinical application (Wyrwich et al., 2005). This challenge illustrates the necessity of combining research and clinical expertise when conducting and interpreting HRQOL studies. Another challenge is the adaptation humans make to changes in health statuses and how this adaptation affects their perceptions of HRQOL. The response-shift concept has been explored and developed to assist in discussing these changes, as well as in designing research to demonstrate and assess such shifts. The theoretical underpinnings of the response-shift construct, methodology for assessment in primary and secondary analyses, and application to treatment outcomes research have been described by Schwartz & Sprangers (2000).

Now that assessment of HRQOL is possible, intervention studies and hypothesis-driven studies are needed. Studies are needed that test interventions directed toward improving the patient's HRQOL, maintaining HRQOL during acute treatment periods, and maintaining HRQOL in cancer survivors and terminally ill patients. Such studies will provide meaningful information for those planning cancer programs, as well as provide sound evidence for appropriating resources for cancer patients in general.

CONCLUSION

Quality of life continues to be a concept relevant to the discipline of nursing. Nurses, and specifically oncology nurses, have contributed actively to the development of the HRQOL concept through instrument development, population description, and intervention testing. Challenges to conducting research on this concept are many and include the development of an agreement on what constitutes the domains of HRQOL, as well as timing and number of measurements to improve precision while reducing excessive patient dropout from undue data assessment burden. Although these and other challenges will persist, research opportunities are abundant and provide fertile ground for continued work.

Nurses also have promoted HRQOL through clinical nursing activities by promoting patient well-being, beginning with diagnosis and continuing throughout the disease/treatment trajectory. In both research and clinical practice, nurses have collaborated with those in other disciplines to expand the knowledge regarding the impact of cancer and cancer treatment on HRQOL. Lastly, through the Oncology Nursing Society and Oncology Nursing Foundation, oncology nurses have demonstrated support for QOL research and clinical practice.

As interest in quality-of-life issues continues to increase, nurses will continue to be involved actively, locally, regionally, nationally, and internationally. Oncology nurses will continue to assess the impact of cancer and cancer treatment on HRQOL and implement strategies to decrease adverse physical, psychological, social, and spiritual effects on the lives of patients with cancer.

References

Aaronson, N. K., Ahmedzai, S., Bergman, B., Bullinger, M., Cull, A., Duez, N. J., Filiberti, A., et al. (1993). The European Organization for Research and Treatment of Cancer QLQ-C30: A quality-of-life instrument for use in international clinical trials in oncology. *Journal of the National Cancer Institute, 85,* 365–376.

Ayanian, J. Z., & Jacobsen, P. B. (2006). Enhancing research on cancer survivors. *Journal of Clinical Oncology, 24*(32), 5149–5153.

Beitz, J., Gnecco, C., & Justice, R. (1996). Quality-of-life end points in cancer clinical trials: The US Food and Drug Administration perspective. *Journal of National Cancer Institute Monograph, 20,* 7–9.

Berger, A. M., Berry, D. L., Christopher, K. A., Greene, A. L., Maliski, S., Swenson, K. K., et al. (2005). Oncology Nursing Society year 2004 research priorities survey. *Oncology Nursing Forum, 32*(2), 281–290.

Coleman, E. A., Krammer, A. M., Johnson, M., Eilertsen, T. B., & Holthaus, D. (1999). Quality measure in post-acute care: The need for a unique set of measures. *Abstract Book of Association of Health Service Research, 16,* 78.

Cooley, M., McCorkle, R., Knaft, G. J., Rimar, J., Barbieri, M. J., Davies, M., et al. (2005). Comparison of health-related quality of life questionnaires in ambulatory oncology. *Quality of Life Research, 14,* 1239–1249.

Cultural adaptation of quality of life (QOL) instruments. (1996). *MAPI Research Institute, 13–14,* 5.

Davis, L. L., & Grant, J. S. (1994). Constructing the reality of recovery: Family home care management strategies. *Advances in Nursing Science, 17*(2), 66–76.

Dueck, A., Halyard, M. Y., Frost, M. H., & Sloan, J. A. (2006). Meeting on the FDA draft guidance on patient-reported outcomes. *Patient Reported Outcomes, 36,* 1–4.

Eiser, C., & Morse, R. (2001). A review of measures of quality of life for children with chronic illness. *Archives of Disease in Childhood, 84*(3), 205–211. www.fda.gov/cder/guidance/7478fnl.pdf. Retrieved July 26, 2007.

Ferrans, C. E. (1990). Development of a quality of life index for patients with cancer. *Oncology Nursing Forum, 17*(3 Suppl), 15–19; discussion 20.

Ferrell, B., & Borneman, T. (2002). Community implementation of a home care palliative care education program. *Cancer Practice, 10*(1), 20–27.

Ferrell, B., Grant, M., Schmidt, G. M., Rhiner, M., Whitehead, C., Fonbuena, P., & Forman, S. J. (1992a). The meaning of quality of life for bone marrow transplant survivors. Part 2: Improving quality of life for bone marrow transplant survivors. *Cancer Nursing, 15*(4), 247–253.

Ferrell, B., Grant, M., Schmidt, G. M., Rhiner, M., Whitehead, C., Fonbuena, P., & Forman, S. J. (1992b). The meaning of quality of life for bone marrow transplant survivors. Part 1: The impact of bone marrow transplant on quality of life. *Cancer Nursing, 15*(3), 153–160.

Ferrell, B., Melancon, C., Ervin, K., Smith, S., & Marek, T. (2002). Family perspectives of ovarian cancer. *Cancer Practice, 10*(6), 269–276.

Ferrell B., Smith, S., Cullinane, C., & Melancon, C. (2003). Symptom concerns in ovarian cancer. *Journal of Pain and Symptom Management, 25*(6), 528–538.

Ferrell, B. A., Ferrell, B. R., & Rivera, L. (1995). Pain in cognitively impaired nursing home patients. *Journal of Pain and Symptom Management, 10*(8), 591–598.

Ferrell, B. R., Grant, M., Funk, R., Otis-Green, S., & Garcia, N. (1997). Quality of life in breast cancer, Part I: Physical and social well being. *Cancer Nursing, 20*(6), 398–408.

Ferrell, B. R., Grant, M., Funk, R., Otis-Green, S., & Garcia, N. (1998a). Quality of life in breast cancer, Part II: Psychological and spiritual well being. *Cancer Nursing, 21*(1), 1–9.

Ferrell, B. R., Grant, M. M., Funk, B., Otis-Green, S. A., & Garcia, N. (1998b). Quality of life in breast cancer survivors: Implications for developing support services. *Oncology Nursing Forum, 25*(5), 887–895.

Ferrell, B. R., Hassey Dow, K., Leigh, S., Ly, J., & Gulasekaram, P. (1995). Quality of life in long-term cancer survivors. *Oncology Nursing Forum, 22*(6), 915–922.

Ferrell, B. R., Rhiner, M., Shapiro, B., & Dierkes, M. (1994). The experience of pediatric cancer pain, Part I: Impact of pain on the family. *Journal of Pediatric Nursing, 9*(6), 368–379.

Fowlie, M., Berkeley, J., & Dingwall-Fordyce, I. (1989). Quality of life in advanced cancer: The benefits of asking the patient. *Palliative Medicine, 3,* 55–59.

Friedman, L. C., Brown, A. E., Romero, C., Dulay, M. F., Peterson, L. E., Wehrman, P., et al. (2005). Depressed mood and social support as predictors of quality of life in women receiving home health care. *Quality of Life Research, 14*(8), 1925–1929.

Grant, M. (1999). Quality of life issues in colorectal cancer. *Developments in Supportive Cancer Care, 3*(1), 4–9.

Grant, M. (2000). Fatigue and quality of life with cancer. In M. L. Winningham & M. Barton-Burke (Eds.), *Fatigue in Cancer: A Multidimensional Approach* (pp. 353–364). Sudbury, MA: Jones and Bartlett Publishers.

Grant, M., Cooke, L., Bhatia, S., & Forman, S. (2005). Discharge and unscheduled readmissions of adult hematopoietic cell transplant. Patients: Implications for developing nursing interventions. *Oncology Nursing Forum, 32*(1), E1–E8.

Grant, M., Ferrell, B., Dean, G., Uman, G., Chu, D., & Krouse, R. (2004). Revision and psychometric testing of the city of hope quality of life – Ostomy questionnaire. *Quality of Life Research, 13*(8), 1445–1458.

Grant, M., Ferrell, B. R., & Sakurai, C. (1994). Defining the spiritual dimension of quality of life assessment in bone marrow transplant survivors [Abstract]. *Oncology Nursing Forum, 21*(2), 376.

Greimel, E. R., Padilla, G. V., & Grant, M. M. (1997). Physical and psychosocial outcomes in cancer patients: A comparison of different age groups. *British Journal of Cancer, 76*(2), 251–255.

Grilli, L. Feldman, D. E., Majnemer, A., Couture, M., Azoulay, L., & Swaine, B. (2006). Associations between a functional independence measure (WeeFIM) and the pediatric quality of life inventory (PedsQL4.0) in young children with physical disabilities. *Quality of Life Research, 15*(6), 1023–1031.

Harrington, V., Lackey, N. R., & Gates, M. F. (1996). Needs of caregivers of clinic and hospice cancer patients. *Cancer Nursing, 19*(2), 118–125.

Hoffman, B., & Stovall, E. (2006). Survivorship perspectives and advocacy. *Journal of Clinical Oncology, 24*(32), 5154–5159.

Johnson, J. R., & Temple, R. (1985). Food and Drug Administration requirements for approval of new anti-cancer drugs. *Cancer Treatment Reports, 69,* 1155–1157.

King, C. R. (2006). Advances in how clinical nurses can evaluate and improve quality of life for individuals with cancer. *Oncology Nursing Forum, 33*(1), Supp., 5–12.

King, C. R., Ferrell, B. R., Grant, M., & Sakurai, C. (1995). Nurses' perceptions of the meaning of quality of life for bone marrow transplant survivors. *Cancer Nursing, 18*(2), 118–129.

King, C. R., Haberman, M., Berry, D. L., Bush, N., Butler, L., Dow, K. H., et al. (1997). Quality of life and the cancer experience: The state-of-the-knowledge. *Oncology Nursing Forum, 24*(1), 27–41.

King, C. R., Hinds, P., Dow, K. H., Schum, L., & Lee C. (2002). The nurse's relationship-based perceptions of patient quality of life. *Oncology Nursing Forum Online, 29*(10), E118–E126.

Korstjens, I., Mesters, I., van der Peet, E., Gijsen, B., & van den Borne, B. (2006). Quality of life of cancer survivors after physical and psychosocial rehabilitation. *European Journal of Cancer Prevention. 15*(6), 541–547.

Krouse, R. S., Mohler, M. J., Wendel, C. S., Grant, M., Baldwin, C. M., Rawl, S. M., et al. (2006). The VA ostomy health-related quality of life study: Objectives, methods, and patient sample. *Current Medical Research and Opinion, 22*(4), 781–791.

Lipscomb, J., Snyder, C. F., & Gotay, C. C. (2007). Cancer outcomes measurement: Through the lens of the medical outcomes trust framework. *Quality of Life Research, 16*(1), 143–164.

Lohr, K. N. (2002). Assessing health status and quality-of-life instruments: Attributes and review criteria. *Quality of Life Research. 11*(3), 193–205.

Mandelblatt, J. S., & Eisenberg, J. M. (1995). Historical and methodological perspectives on cancer outcomes research. *Oncology, 9*(11 Suppl), 23–32.

Mock, V., Pickett, M., Ropka, M. E., Lin, E. M., Stewart, K. J., Rhodes, V. A., et al. (2001) Fatigue and quality of life outcomes of exercise during cancer treatment. *Cancer Practice: A Multidisciplinary Journal of Cancer Care, 9*(3), 119–127.

Morris, M. E., Grant, M., & Lynch, J. C. (2007). Patient-reported family distress among long-term cancer survivors. *Cancer Nursing, 30*(1), 1–8.

National Institute of Nursing Reseach. *Areas of research emphasis.* Retrieved February 26, 2007 from http://www.ninr.nih.gov/NR/rdonlyres/F85C02CA-1EE3-40F7-BDA4-3901F2284E96/0/StrategicAreas ofResearchEmphasis.pdf.

Nayfield, S. G. Karp, J. E., Ford, L. G., Dorr, F. A., & Kramer, B. S. (1991). Potential role of tamoxifen in prevention of breast cancer. *Journal of the National Cancer Institute, 83*(20), 1450–1459.

Nayfield, S. G., Hailey, B. J., McCabe, M. (1991). Quality of life assessment in cancer clinical trials. *Report of the Workshop on Quality of Life Research in Cancer Clinical Trials; July 16–17, 1990; Bethesda (MD):US DHHS.*

Nayfield, S. G., Ganz, P. A., Moinpour, C. M., Cella, D. F., & Hailey, B. J. (1992). Report from a National Cancer Institute (USA) workshop on quality of life assessment in cancer clinical trials. *Quality of Life Research, 1*(3), 203–210.

Osoba, D. (1992). The Quality of Life Committee of the Clinical Trials Group of the National Cancer Institute of Canada: Organization and functions. *Quality of Life Research, 1,* 211–218.

Padilla, G. V., Ferrell, B., & Grant, M. M. (1990). Defining the content domain of quality of life for cancer patients with pain. *Cancer Nursing 13*(2), 108–115.

Padilla, G. V., & Grant, M. M. (1985). Quality of life as a cancer nursing outcome variable. *ANS Advances in Nursing Science, 8*(1), 45–60.

Padilla, G. V., Grant, M., Ferrell, B. F., & Presant, G. A. (1996). Quality of life—cancer. In B. Spilker (Ed.), Quality of life and pharmacoeconomics in clinical trials (2nd ed.) (pp. 301–308). Philadelphia, PA: Lippincott-Raven.

Padilla, G. V., Grant, M. M., Lipsett, J., Anderson, P. R., Rhiner, M. & Bogen, C. (1992). Health quality of life and colorectal cancer. *Cancer Suppl 70*(5), 1450–1456.

Padilla, G. V., Presant, C., Grant, M., Metter, G., Lipsett, J., & Heide, F. (1983). Quality of life index for patients with cancer. *Research in Nursing and Health, 6,* 117–126.

Parikh, C. R., Coca, S. G., Smith, G. L., Vaccarino, V., & Krumholz, H. M. (2006). Impact of chronic kidney disease on health-related quality-of-life improvement after coronary artery bypass surgery. *Archives of Internal Medicine, 166*(18), 2014–2019.

Park, S. M., Park, M. H., Won, J. H., Lee, K. O., Choe, W. S., Heo, D. S., et al. (2006). EuroQol and survival prediction in terminal cancer patients: A multicenter prospective study in hospice-palliative care units. *Supportive Care in Cancer, 14*(4), 329–333.

Peters, L., & Sellick, K. (2006). Quality of life of cancer patients receiving inpatient and home-based palliative care. *Journal of Advanced Nursing, 53*(5), 524–533.

Revicki, D. A. (2006) The importance of PRO's and the FDA Draft Guidelines. *Research News: A Publication of United Biosource Corporation, X11*(2), 5.

Revicki, D., Osoba, D., Fairclough, D. L., Barofsky, I., Berzon, R., Leidy, N. M., & Rothman, M. (2000). Recommendations in health-related quality of life research to support labeling and promotional claims in the United States. *Quality of Life Research 9,* 887–900.

Schwartz, C. E., & Sprangers, M. A. G. (2000). Adaptation to changing health: Response shift in quality-of-life research. Washington, DC: American Psychological Association.

Sherman, R. S., Cooke, L., & Grant, M. (2005). Dialogue among survivors of hematopoietic cell transplantation: Support-group themes. *The Journal of Psychosocial Oncology, 23*(1), 1–24.

Simpson, E., & Pilote, L. (2005). Quality of life after acute myocardial infarction: A comparison of diabetic versus non-diabetic acute myocardial infarction patients in Quebec acute care hospitals. *Health & Quality of Life Outcomes, 3*, 80.

Slevin, M. L., Plant, H., Lynch, D., Drinkwater, J., & Gregory, W. M. (1988). Who should measure quality of life, the doctor or the patient? *British Journal of Cancer, 57*, 109–112.

Sloan, J. (2005). Statistical issues in the application of cancer outcome measures. In J. Lipscomb, C. Gotany, & C. Snyder (Eds.), *Outcomes assessment in cancer* (pp. 362–385). Cambridge, England: Cambridge University Press.

Spilker, B. (1990). Introduction. In B. Spilker (Ed.), *Quality of life assessments in clinical trials* (pp. 3–9). New York, NY: Raven Press.

Stanton, A. L., Ganz, P. A., Kwan, L., Meyerowitz, B. E., Bower, J. E., Krupnick, et al. (2005). Outcomes from Moving Beyond Cancer psychoeducational, randomized, controlled trial with breast cancer patients. *Journal of Clinical Oncology, 23*(25), 6009–6018.

Stetz, K. M., McDonald, J. C., & Compton, K. (1996). Needs and experiences of family caregivers during marrow transplantation. *Oncology Nursing Forum, 23*(9), 1422–1427.

Stjernswärd, J., & Teoh, N. (1991). Perspectives on quality of life and the global cancer problem. In D. Osoba (Ed.), *Effect of cancer on quality of life* (pp. 1–5). Boca Raton, FL: CRC Press.

Tinker, R., & White, A. (2006). Promoting quality of life for patients with moderate to severe COPD. *British Journal of Community Nursing, 11*(7), 278–284.

Tuchler, H., Hofmann, S., Bernhart, M., Brugiatelli, M., Chrobak, L., Franke, A., et al. (1992). A short multilingual quality of life questionnaire—practicability, reliability, and interlingual homogeneity. *Quality of Life Research, 1*(2), 107–117.

US Department of Health and Human Services, Public Health Service, National Institutes of Health. (1990). Quality of life assessment in cancer clinical trials. *Report of the workshop on quality of life research in cancer clinical trials*. Bethesda, MD.

World Health Organization, Division of Mental Health. (1993). *WHO-QOL Study protocol: The development of the World Health Organization quality of life assessment instrument* (MNG/PSF/93.9). Geneva, Switzerland.

Wyrwich, K. W., Bullinger, M., Aaronson, N., Hays, R. D., Patrick, D., & Symonds, T. (2005). Estimating clinically significant differences in quality of life outcomes: The clinical significance consensus meeting group. *Quality of Life Research 14*, 285–295.

Yates, P., Aranda, S., Hargraves, M., Mirolo, B., Claravino, A., McLachlan, S., & Skerman, H. (2005). Randomized controlled trial of an educational intervention for managing fatigue in women receiving adjuvant chemotherapy for early-stage breast cancer. *Journal of Clinical Oncology, 23*(25), 6027–6036.

Zebrack, B. (2000). Cancer survivors and quality of life: A critical review of the literature. *Oncology Nursing Forum, 27*(9), 1395–1401.

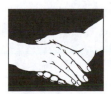

Overview of Quality of Life and Controversial Issues

Cynthia R. King

Introduction

For centuries individuals have been concerned with seeking the good life. In that search, the prevailing question has been what is the quality of any individual life? As treatments for cancer become more aggressive and are associated with greater toxicities, and survival time is lengthened significantly by new therapies, there is an increasing need to move beyond the focus of morbidity and mortality and evaluate the nursing and patient perspectives on quality of life (QOL). Both nursing and patient perspectives are important when assessing QOL for individuals with cancer. Oncology nurses, and nurses in general, are committed to obtaining patients' views on QOL in order to improve nursing care and ultimately the outcomes of care. This chapter highlights the numerous controversies related to QOL and the importance of nursing and patient perspectives.

Many controversies currently exist regarding quality of life and its measurement. How we define and measure the QOL of individuals with cancer reflects much of the ongoing debates related to QOL in general. A more basic question is, "Why should we study or use the concept of QOL in cancer care?" The answer may be examined at the levels of the individual, the healthcare provider, or national healthcare policy. When addressing the question at the level of the patient, the response is to improve the quality of the individual's life and treatment. When evaluating a particular therapy, healthcare providers may evaluate QOL in clinical trials to differentiate between two therapies with similar survival rates. Healthcare providers are concerned with QOL because it may alter prescribing habits, treatment regimens, and decisions to continue or cease treatment. At the national healthcare policy level, QOL is an important concept used to improve the allocation of appropriate healthcare resources, to solve all the healthcare problems (Grusenmeyer & Wong, 2007; Weinfurt, 2007).

Despite the excessive costs of obtaining health care and the number of Americans with health insurance, the US Census Bureau reported that, in 2000, there were 39 million uninsured Americans. This number exceeded the aggregate population of 22 states, plus the District of Columbia. In 2009, there were reports that this number increased to 47 million uninsured Americans (20% of the population) (National Coalition on Healthcare, 2009). This number is estimated to increase by 1 million each year. Kaplan (1995) describes three major problems with the healthcare system in the United States: healthcare costs are excessive, thus employers and the government can no longer provide the same level of payment;

the system is inequitable, as many individuals are without insurance or adequate resources to cover medical care; and individuals are failing to be good consumers (e.g., individuals may buy unnecessary or ineffective services in an attempt to achieve good health). These problems are labeled as affordability, accessibility, and accountability. Overall, QOL becomes an important concept when examining health care and cancer care at the levels of the individual, the healthcare practitioner, and the national healthcare policy.

The concept of QOL is increasing in importance as a valid indicator of whether a given medical treatment is beneficial. Quality of life now represents a descriptor of the overall results of diagnostic and treatment efforts that makes sense to individuals with cancer and to healthcare professionals (particularly nurses). Quality of life is one of only two validated quality measurements applied to cancer care in women (Schachter et al., 2006). Quality of life appears to be a relevant goal, even in palliative care (Hølen et al., 2006; McCahill et al., 2002).

Definitions

In order to conduct valid QOL studies or adequately describe, assess, or discuss QOL, a clear definition of quality of life is required. Unfortunately, many individuals, including healthcare professionals and researchers, have used this term without establishing a common definition. Heathcare professionals or researchers may fail to define QOL because they believe an accepted meaning exists already or the term is too amorphous to be described adequately. For many years, there has been a lack of agreement on how to define and describe QOL for patients with cancer (Aaronson, 1990; Clinch & Schipper, 1993; King et al., 1997; Reid & Renwick, 1994; Schipper, Clinch, & Powell, 1990; Semple et al., 2004; Zebrack, 2000). A number of authors and researchers have attempted to define QOL. These definitions reflect how QOL has been defined for adults, adolescents, and children, and how the definitions vary. Nurses have been involved actively in attempting to define QOL and have found multiple conceptualizations to be helpful.

When discussing QOL, it is important to distinguish QOL from related, but different, concepts including well-being, health status, life satisfaction, and hope. In Chapter 4, Haase and Braden discuss the need to clarify the concept of QOL and provide guidelines for obtaining clarity in QOL conceptualization, assessment, and measurement. One method for clarifying this concept is through the use of concept analysis. Whatever method is used, it is crucial to distinguish QOL from other related concepts.

Cella and Tulsky (1991) recommend avoiding the term "quality of life" when discussing or measuring a single dimension of the concept, because experts in QOL may determine one definition cannot adequately describe all the changes in QOL throughout the course of the disease. Additionally, concept analyses may be needed by various healthcare disciplines. In fact, the meaning and importance of QOL may be discipline-specific or population-specific (King et al., 1997). Also, QOL is an attribute nurses and other healthcare professionals may evaluate in themselves as part of their ability to care for others (Nevidjon, 2004). Unfortunately, patients have been involved in defining the concept of QOL only rarely; thus, it is not appropriate to assume that patients, survivors, and healthcare professionals share a common understanding of the term. Despite the challenges related to defining QOL, there are areas of conceptual agreement among experts. Most would agree that QOL is a multidimensional concept comprised of both positive and negative facets of life. Additionally, many experts agree on the subjectivity and dynamism of the concept (Grant, Padilla, Ferrell, & Rhiner, 1990; Hinds, 1990; Holmes & Dickerson, 1987; Hyland, Kenyon, & Jacobs, 1994; King et al., 1997; Mellon, 2002; Moinpour et al., 1989; Zebrack, 2000; Zhao, Kanda, Liu, & Mao, 2003). The multidimensional aspect of QOL is demonstrated in the numerous dimensions identified as part of the concept, including physical, psychological, social, somatic, and spiritual. Although some studies include objective measures of QOL, many rely on subjective, self-report instruments. The trend toward using patients' self-reports, rather than reports of proxies, has developed after various studies demonstrated a lack of strong agreement among the ratings of QOL given by patients, family members, and healthcare providers (Epstein, Hall, Tognetti, Son, & Conant, 1989; King, Ferrell, Grant, & Sakurai, 1995; Mellon, 2002; Osoba, 1994). This is because the QOL assessment by a proxy is biased by the proxy's subjective standards of what comprises a desirable QOL (Mellon, 2002; Osoba, 1994). Dynamism reflects the need to measure perceptions of QOL along a continuum, as an individual's perception or definition of QOL may change over time.

Considerable work remains to be done in order to develop consensus definitions of QOL for specific populations or specific disciplines. Until consensus is reached, it is advisable to identify the definition of QOL in research and publications, as well as in educational or clinical settings.

Dimensions

Despite intensive work by many experts, controversies remain regarding the dimensions that comprise quality of life. These controversies are discussed also by Haase and Braden in Chapter 4, and by Haberman and Bush in Chapter 8. Generally, there has been little theoretical basis for the dimensions reflected in the health-related QOL (HRQOL) literature (Aaronson, 1991; Padilla et al., 1983). In some instances, researchers developing scales combined factors that were *assumed* to indicate QOL, and then chose dimensions to represent those factors.

Most experts agree there are four to five generally accepted QOL dimensions: physical, psychological, social, somatic/disease- and treatment-related symptoms, and spiritual (Aaronson, 1991; Ferrans, 1990; Ferrell, Smith, Juarez, & Melancon, 2003; King et al., 1997; Schipper, 1991). The physical dimension most closely approximates the outcome measures traditionally used. Questions asked in QOL studies regarding physical aspects include questions about strength, energy, ability to perform activities of daily living (ADL), and self-care. These facts generally correlate with the physicians' estimates of the patient's well-being and functional status (Aaronson, 1991; Padilla, Ferrell, Grant, & Rhiner, 1990; Schipper et al., 1990; Zebrack, 2000). Psychological well-being often is problematic for healthcare professionals, who are usually poor estimators of patients' psychological state. Often, nurses, social workers, and psychologists are better at estimating the psychological state of patients than other healthcare providers. The most frequently studied psychological symptoms are anxiety, depression, and fear. Unfortunately, many of the tests used to study these factors were developed for use with healthy populations or persons with diagnosed mental or psychological disabilities (Aaronson, 1991; Schipper et al., 1990), rather than for those populations or persons diagnosed with cancer. Social well-being refers to how individuals carry on relationships with family, friends, colleagues at work, and the general community (Aaronson, 1991; Ferrell et al., 1992a; Ferrell et al., 1992b; Padilla et al., 1990; Schipper et al., 1990). Somatic refers to disease symptoms and treatment side effects, such as pain, nausea, vomiting, while spiritual well-being refers to the perception that one's life has purpose and meaning (Aaronson, 1991; Ferrell et al., 1992a, Ferrell et al., 1992b; Ferrell et al., 2003; Schipper et al., 1990; Williams & Schreier, 2004).

As with the definition of quality of life, it is important to specify and fully describe the domains of QOL when evaluating QOL in education, research, or clinical practice contexts. Additionally, a rationale for the use of these specifically described dimensions should be included within the evaluation results. Some nurses in education, research, or clinical practice include a model that depicts QOL, its dimensions, and associated variables (e.g., Eilers and King, Chapter 15). In the future, nurses should elicit more information from patients and survivors regarding the dimensions of QOL and the associated variables, as work has been limited in this area. Ferrell and colleagues (1992a; 1992b) did evaluate bone marrow transplant recipients' perceptions of QOL and its dimensions and discovered that spiritual well-being was an important, separate domain of QOL and was not considered a part of the psychological dimension.

Measurement

Quality of life studies can provide comprehensive and sensitive methods for communicating information on the burden of the disease and effectiveness of treatment if they are designed and implemented well. The impact of cancer and progress in treatment cannot be adequately measured by mortality rates, incidence and prevalence, or average length of stay in the hospital. Cancer affects many dimensions of health and well-being. Ideally, treatment should not only prolong survival and disease-free intervals, but also decrease symptoms associated with disease, not cause noxious side effects, and improve an individual's ability to return to a normal lifestyle. The use of QOL assessments in clinical trials can improve clinical practice by leading to suggestions for changes in treatment, and survivor and rehabilitation needs (Moinpour, Savage, Hayden, Sayers, & Upchurch, 1995; Schachter et al., 2006; Schuttiga, 1995; Zhao et al., 2003). Overall, the purpose of assessing QOL is to consider the patient perspective of the disease, identify benefits and risks of treatment choices, and determine the contribution of therapeutic and nursing interventions to QOL (Berry et al., 2004; Bowling, 1991; de Haes & van Knippenberg, 1985; Faden & Leplege, 1992).

The potential applications of QOL measures fall into three categories: prediction, discrimination, and evaluation. Prediction is used when the gold standard is available; this method is used to classify individuals into a set of predefined measurement categories. Then a gold standard is used to determine if individuals have been classified correctly (Guyatt &

Jaeschke, 1990). Discrimination is used to distinguish between individuals or groups with respect to an underlying dimension when none is available. An evaluation index is used to measure the magnitude of longitudinal change in an individual or group. These tools have provided the main focus for existing QOL clinical trials.

Instruments used to measure QOL in patients with cancer should have reproducibility (reliability), validity, and responsiveness. Reliability is important to ensure that the same results are obtained with repeated measures when the status has not changed. Validity or accuracy is essential for the tool to measure what it is intended to measure. This is easy if there is a gold standard, but currently no gold standard for quality-of-life measurement exists. Responsiveness or sensitivity refers to the ability to detect clinically important changes. The instrument must register changes in the score when the subject's QOL increases or decreases (Guyatt & Jaeschke, 1990).

Measurement issues are discussed more thoroughly by Haberman and Bush in Chapter 8, yet some QOL controversies deserve mentioning, as follows:

1. The use of generic versus specific measurement tools
2. The use of a single QOL instrument versus a battery of questionnaires
3. The use of dimension scores versus a total score
4. The use of self-administered tools versus those of proxies
5. Quantitative versus qualitative tools
6. Measurement at one time point versus measurements on multiple occasions
7. Whether assessments are culturally sensitive

Specific vs. Generic Measurement Tools

There is an ongoing controversy regarding the use of a generic versus a specific measurement tool. The generic instrument is designed to measure the complete spectrum of dimensions relevant to QOL and can be used to measure QOL for numerous chronic illnesses (e.g., heart disease, pulmonary disease, arthritis, AIDS, cancer). The two types of generic instruments are health profiles and utility measures. Health profiles are single instruments that measure different aspects of QOL, such as the effect of the disease and/or treatment on everyday functioning. Health profiles are designed for use in a wide variety of conditions and do not reflect a specific disease or treatment. Examples of these instruments are the Sickness Impact Profile (SIP), the Nottingham Health Profile, and the Medical Outcomes Study Short Form-36 (MOS SF-36). Many generic health profile tools can be both lengthy and difficult to use if individuals are seriously ill (Aaronson, 1991; Moinpour et al., 1995; Semple et al., 2004; Stewart et al., 1989). Although health profile tools are often reliable and valid, many do not focus adequately on specific aspects of QOL. Utility instruments, on the other hand, are derived from economic decision theory. With utility instruments, QOL is measured as a single number along a continuum of full health (10) to death (0). Some researchers have questioned whether a single measurement has the ability be responsive to small, but clinically important, changes (Guyatt & Jaeschke, 1990). There is also a problem in using a single overall score for QOL. With this method, different dimensions of QOL may yield different results or lead to less informative results. For example, treatment I may be more effective than treatment II in two out of four domains, while treatment II may be more effective than treatment I in the other two domains (Spilker, 1990). Haberman and Bush provide a list of generic questionnaires in Table 8-3.

Specific instruments focus on problems that are applicable only to certain individuals. These instruments may be specific to a disease, a population (e.g., individuals with cancer), a specified dimension of QOL (e.g., psychological), or a given condition (e.g., pain). These instruments are usually more responsive to small but clinically important changes. Unfortunately, specific instruments are seldom comprehensive and cannot be used to compare results across diseases or conditions (Aaronson, 1991; Guyatt & Jaeschke, 1990; Semple et al., 2004).

Single Instrument vs. Battery of Tests

Some researchers administer a battery of tests to achieve comprehensive results. The advantage of this approach is that rich data on multiple dimensions of QOL may be recollected. This method is problematic, however, if the researcher uses only one section of a tool in the battery of tests (Guyatt & Jaeschke, 1990). When using a battery of tests, it is impossible to combine all test score results. Also, patients may assign different weights to different dimensions based on their beliefs, which are influenced by the severity of their disease, their cultural background, religion, and past experiences (Spilker, 1990). Other problems that may be encountered when using a battery of tests include small sample sizes (a large sample size is needed if, for example, researchers are using multiple QOL tests) and the use of univariate statistical techniques to analyze multiple measures of QOL. Additionally, analyzing change across time is difficult when multiple tools are used (Shumaker, Anderson, & Czajkowski, 1990).

Dimension Scores vs. Total Score

Another controversy exists regarding the use of a total score versus use of individual dimension scores. Some instruments provide single scores with a total score. Examples of these types of measurement tools include the Cancer Rehabilitation Evaluation System (CARES), the Functional Living Index-Cancer (FLIC), and the Functional Assessment of Cancer Therapy (FACT) (Cella et al., 1993; Ganz, Rofessart, Polinsky, Schag, & Heinrich, 1986; Morrow, Lindke, & Black, 1992). Another method for gathering data combines several separate tools into a QOL test. In this example, each dimension may be measured using a different scale. This approach is used with the Southwest Oncology Group (SWOG) QOL questionnaire, which combined generic (MOS SF) scales, symptom scales (Symptom Distress Scale), and side effects of treatment (treatment-specific items). The treatment-specific scales are revised for each clinical trial depending on the disease site and treatment evaluation in the trial (Moinpour et al., 1995).

Recommendations on Tools

There are a vast number of scales used to evaluate QOL issues and no consensus has been reached yet as to which are the best. It is possible consensus will be reached on a few widely accepted scales for each domain, or we may be able to better identify specific conditions under which to use certain scales (Spilker, 1990).

Several experts have developed a "core plus module" that is administered to measure QOL. This means a global QOL index is administered as the core tool that assesses multiple dimensions, then a smaller additional module is administered specific to a particular disease, population, or condition. The European Organization for Research and Treatment of Cancer (EORTC) QOL Core Questionnaire (QLQ-C30) is an example of a core plus module approach (Aaronson et al., 1993; Aaronson et al., 1991; Aaronson et al., 1987; Aaronson, Bullinger, & Ahmedzai, 1988; Schipper et al., 1990). The SWOG Quality of Life Questionnaire is another example of a core plus module (Moinpour et al., 1989; Moinpour, Hayden, Thompson, Feigl, & Metch, 1990). Haberman and Bush discuss more specific modules that have been developed in Chapter 8.

Regardless of other factors, a successful QOL instrument should be brief and easy to read, understand, score, and analyze. The success of any instrument or series of tests will be related, in part, to the burden imposed on respondents and their willingness to participate (King et al., 1997).

Self-Report vs. Proxies

Most instruments are designed to be self-administered. Frequently, when physicians are used as proxies, the physician emphasizes physiological data. Nurses, social workers, and families, used as proxies, place more emphasis on psychosocial measures (Schipper et al., 1990; Sneeuw et al., 1999; Zhao et al., 2003). Other researchers have found that proxy respondents tend to underestimate patients' QOL (King et al., 1995; King, 2001; Sprangers & Aaronson, 1992). Although it is generally accepted that QOL information is most accurate when it is directly obtained from the patient or survivor, in some situations (e.g., very young children, very ill patients, comatose patients), it is appropriate to include the evaluation of QOL from healthcare professionals or significant others. It is also important for researchers to consider the inherent limitations of self-reported data, which include missing data, language problems, cultural differences, and patient burden.

Quantitative vs. Qualitative

A phenomenological approach to QOL may be useful because it stresses the importance of individuals' subjective perceptions of their current ability to function as it compares to their internalized standards of what is possible or ideal. Patients may change expectations and standards throughout treatment and their disease process (Lutgendorf, Antoni, Schneiderman, Ironson, & Fletcher, 1995). A qualitative approach makes use of more open-ended questions and typically collects very rich data. However, a qualitative approach may be more burdensome and time-consuming for the patient. A quantitative approach, by contrast, typically employs a closed-question format and categorical scaling and is less time consuming for the respondent. More recently, nurses in research and clinical settings have begun to combine the two approaches in what is now called a mixed methods design.

Measurements at One vs. Multiple Time Points

Previously, much of the QOL research involved measurements at a single time point. Unfortunately, measurement of QOL at one time point has not provided a thorough understanding of the nature of QOL or how to improve outcomes through clinical care. More recently, experts have recognized the dynamism of QOL and the need for multiple measurement points with the same respondents, or a cross-sectional approach. As advances in the treatment of cancer continue, multiple measurements are needed to demonstrate improvements over time as a result of new therapies. It should be recognized, however, that the burden for patients and survivors might increase as the number of measurements of their QOL increases. Researchers will have to strike a balance between providing an opportunity for patients to express their perceptions regarding QOL and not overburdening the patient.

Culture

The question of whether assessments and measurements of QOL are culturally sensitive must be raised. It is important to evaluate the relationship between QOL and culture because QOL perceptions of an individual are heavily influenced by culture, varying from society to society. In Chapter 6, Padilla, Ashing-Giwa, and Kagawa-Singer discuss how culture is an important determinant of QOL. Despite recent research (Hastie, Riley, & Fillingim, 2005; Phillips & Weekes, 2002), multiculturalism has been incorporated more into oncology nursing research between 1999 and 2000. Little effort has been made to address cultural issues in QOL research and to assess the impact of culture on QOL perceptions. Healthcare practitioners must be sure they are analyzing QOL beliefs within the context of the patient's culture. Additionally, researchers must avoid ethnocentrism—that is, interpreting the behaviors of patients with cancer within a framework of the researchers' personal feelings, beliefs, and cultural values. Future research should include translating QOL measures into multiple languages, conducting studies to examine the cross-cultural applicability of theoretical frameworks used to explain QOL, and determining the impact of cultural variables on perceived QOL (Campos & Johnson, 1990; King et al., 1997).

CONCLUSION

Advances in cancer care and increases in patient survival have led to nurses taking an interest in quality of life and its relationship to practice, education, and research. Despite the many ongoing controversies related to QOL, QOL appears to be an important concept from both a nursing and patient perspective. As the controversies are resolved and our QOL knowledge base increases, both education and clinical practices will improve. If QOL is a major outcome variable in nursing research, many methodological issues must be addressed and resolved. Schipper and colleagues (1990) provide ten recommendations for conducting QOL research (see Table 2-1). Additionally, Hinds and King (Chapter 20) provide recommendations for future research or projects to ensure nursing and patient perspectives are

Table 2-1. **Recommendations for Conducting QOL Research**

Research an aspect of QOL in which you expect a substantial difference in outcome.

Measure QOL and overall survival in addition to other clinical parameters.

You may not need a large sample size as each patient contributes repeated measures over time.

Use tools that are reliable and valid.

Define when the initial measurement of QOL will be performed.

Repeat the measurements at intervals that will allow tracking of the treatment.

Time periods should be 2–4 weeks as this allows for accurate recall.

Follow patients until all influence of treatment is likely to have passed or the endpoint of their disease.

Do not simply average your data; use multivariate ANOVA.

Be modest with extrapolations from the data.

Source: Adapted from Schipper et al., 1990.

reflected sufficiently. These recommendations are helpful for all nurse researchers. As an outcome of a State-of-the-Knowledge Conference on Quality of Life and the Cancer Experience, King and colleagues (1997) listed recommended topics and questions for future research on QOL. It will become even more crucial to include nursing and patient perspectives when conducting future research and attempting to influence clinical care and outcomes.

REFERENCES

Aaronson, N. K. (1990). Quality of life research in clinical trials: A need for common rules and language. *Oncology, 4*(5), 59–66.

Aaronson, N. K. (1991). Quality of life research in cancer clinical trials: A need for common rules and language. In N. S. Tchekmedyian & D. F. Cella (Eds.), *Quality of life in oncology practice and research* (pp. 33–42). Williston Park, NY: Dominus Publishing Company.

Aaronson, N. K., Ahmedzai, S., Bergman, B., Bullinger, M., Cull, A., Duez, N. J., et al. (1993). The European Organization for Research and Treatment of Cancer QLQ-C30: A quality of life instrument for use in international clinical trials in oncology. *Journal of the National Cancer Institute, 85,* 365–376.

Aaronson, N. K., Ahmedzai, S., Bullinger, M., Crabeels, D., Estape, J., Filiberti, A., et al. (1991). The EORTC Core quality-of-life questionnaire: Interim results on an international field study. In D. Osoba (Ed.), *Effect of cancer on quality of life* (pp. 293–305). Boca Raton, FL: CRC Press.

Aaronson, N. K., Bakker, W., Stewart, A. L., van Dam, F. S. A. M., van Zandwijk, N., Yarnold, J. R., & Kirkpatrick, A. (1987). Multidimensional approach to the measurement of quality of life in lung cancer clinical trials. In N. K. Aaronson & J. H. Beckman (Eds.), *Monograph series of the European Organization for Research and Treatment of Cancer* (Vol. 17, pp. 63–82). New York, NY: Raven Press.

Aaronson, N. K., Bullinger, M., & Ahmedzai, S. (1988). A modular approach to quality-of-life assessment in cancer clinical trials. *Recent Results in Cancer Research, 111,* 231–249.

Berry, D. L., Trigg, L. J., Lober, W. B., Karras, B. T., Galligan, M. L., Austin-Seymour, M., Martin, S. (2004). Computerized symptom and quality-of-life assessment for patients with cancer part I: Development and pilot testing. *Oncology Nursing Forum, 31*(5), E75–E83.

Bowling, A. (1991). Health care research: Measuring health status. *Nursing Practice, 4*(4), 2–8.

Campos, S. S., & Johnson, T. M. (1990). Cultural considerations. In B. Spilker (Ed.), *Quality of life assessments in clinical trials* (pp. 163–170). New York, NY: Raven Press.

Cella, D. F., & Tulsky, D. S. (1991). Measuring quality of life today: Methodological aspects. In N. S. Tchekmedyian & D. F. Cella (Eds.), *Quality of life in oncology practice and research* (pp. 9–18). Williston Park, NY: Dominus Publishing Company.

Cella, D. F., Tulsky, D. S., Gray, G., Sarafian, B., Linn, E., Bonomi, A., et al. (1993). The functional assessment of cancer therapy scale: Development and validation of the general measure. *Journal of Clinical Oncology, 11,* 570–579.

Clinch, J. J., & Schipper, H. (1993). Quality of life assessment in palliative care. In D. Doyle, G. W. C. Hanks, & N. MacDonald (Eds.), *Oxford Textbook of Palliative Medicine* (pp. 61–70). Oxford: Oxford University Press.

de Haes, J. C., & van Knippenberg, F. C. E. (1985). The quality of life instruments for cancer patients: A review of the literature. *Social Science and Medicine, 20*(8), 809–817.

Epstein, A. M., Hall, J. A., Tognetti, J., Son, L. H., & Conant, L. (1989). Using proxies to evaluate quality of life. *Medical Care, 27,* 591–598.

Faden, R., & Leplege, A. (1992). Assessing quality of life: Moral implications for clinical practice. *Medical Care, 30*(Suppl. 5), MS166–MS175.

Ferrans, C. C. (1990). Quality of life: Conceptual issues. *Seminars in Oncology Nursing, 6,* 248–254.

Ferrell, B., Grant, M., Schmidt, G. M., Rhiner, M., Whitehead, C., Fonbuena, P., & Forman, S. J. (1992a). The meaning of quality of life for bone marrow transplant survivors: Part 1: The impact of bone marrow transplant on quality of life. *Cancer Nursing, 15*(3), 153–160.

Ferrell, B., Grant, M., Schmidt, G. M., Rhiner, M., Whitehead, C., Fonbuena, P., & Forman, S. J. (1992b). The meaning of quality of life for bone marrow transplant survivors: Part 2: Improving quality of life for bone marrow transplant survivors. *Cancer Nursing, 15*(4), 247–253.

Ferrell, B. R., Smith, S. L., Juarez, G., & Melancon, C. (2003). Meaning of illness and spirituality in ovarian cancer survivors. *Oncology Nursing Forum, 30*(2), 249–257.

Ganz, P. A., Rofessart, J., Polinsky, M. L., Schag, C. C., & Heinrich, R. L. (1986). A comprehensive approach to the assessment of cancer patient's rehabilitation needs: The cancer inventory of problem situation and a companion interview. *Journal of Psychosocial Oncology, 4,* 27–42.

Grant, M. M., Padilla, G. V., Ferrell, B. R., & Rhiner, M. (1990). Assessment of quality of life with a single instrument. *Seminars in Oncology Nursing, 6,* 260–270.

Grusenmeyer, P. & Wong, Y. N. (2007). Interpreting the economic literature in oncology. *Journal of Clinical Oncology, 25*(2), 196–202.

Guyatt, G. H., & Jaeschke, R. (1990). Measurements in clinical trials: Choosing the appropriate approach. In B. Spilker (Ed.), *Quality of life assessments in clinical trials* (pp. 37–46). New York, NY: Raven Press.

Hastie, B. A., Riley, J. L.,& Fillingim, R. B. (2005). Ethnic differences and responses in pain in healthy young adults. *Pain Medicine, 6*(1), 61–71.

Hinds, P. S. (1990). Quality of life in children and adolescents with cancer. *Seminars in Oncology Nursing, 6,* 285–291.

Hølen, J. C, Hjermstad, M. J., Loge, J. H., Fayers, P. M., Caraceni, A., De Conno, F., Forbes, K., Fürst, C. J., Radbruch, L., & Kaasa, S. (2006). Pain assessment tools: Is the content appropriate for use in palliative care? *Journal of Pain and Symptom Management, 32*(6), 567–580.

Holmes, S., & Dickerson, J. (1987). The quality of life: Design and evaluation of a self-assessment instrument for use with cancer patients. *International Journal of Nursing Studies, 24*(1), 15–24.

Hyland, M. E., Kenyon, C. A. P., & Jacobs, P. A. (1994). Sensitivity of quality of life domains and constructs to longitudinal change in a clinical trial comparing almeterol with placebo in asthmatics. *Quality of Life Research, 3,* 121–126.

Kaplan, R. M. (1995). Quality of life resource allocation and health-care crisis. In J. E. Dimsdale & A. Baum (Eds.), *Quality of life in behavioral medical research* (pp. 3–30). Hillsdale, NJ: Lawrence Erlbaum Associates.

King, C. R. (2001). The dance of life. *Clinical Journal of Oncology Nursing, 5*(1), 29–33.

King, C. R., Ferrell, B. R., Grant, M., & Sakurai, C. (1995). Nurses' perceptions of the meaning of quality of life for bone marrow transplant survivors. *Cancer Nursing, 18,* 118–129.

King, C. R., Haberman, M., Berry, D., Bush, N., Butler, L., Dow, K. H., et al. (1997). Quality of life and the cancer experience: The state-of-the knowledge. *Oncology Nursing Forum, 24*(1), 27–41.

Lutgendorf, S., Antoni, M. H., Schneiderman, N., Ironson, G., & Fletcher, M. A. (1995). Psychosocial interventions and quality of life changes across the HIV spectrum. In J. E. Dimsdale & A. Baum (Eds.), *Quality of life in behavioral medical research* (pp. 205–240). Hillsdale, NJ: Lawrence Erlbaum Associates.

McCahill, L. E., Krouse, R., Chu, D., Juarez, G., Uman, G. C., Ferrell, B., & Wagman, L. D. (2002). Indications and use of palliative surgery—results of society of surgical oncology survey. *Annals of Surgical Oncology, 9*(1), 104–112.

Mellon, S. (2002). Comparisons between cancer survivors and family members on meaning of the illness and family quality of life. *Oncology Nursing Forum, 29*(70), 1117–1125.

Moinpour, C. M., Feigl, P., Metch, B., Hayden, K. A., Meyskens, F. L., Jr., & Crowley, J. (1989). Quality of life endpoints in cancer clinical trials: Review and recommendations. *Journal of the National Cancer Institute, 81,* 485–495.

Moinpour, C. M., Hayden, K. A., Thompson, J. M., Feigl, P., & Metch, B. (1990). Quality of life assessment in southwest oncology group trials. *Oncology, 4,* 79–89.

Moinpour, C. M., Savage, M., Hayden, K. A., Sayers, J., & Upchurch, C. (1995). Quality of life assessment in cancer clinical trials. In J. E. Dimsdale & A. Baum (Eds.), *Quality of life in behavioral medical research* (pp. 79–96). Hillsdale, NJ: Lawrence Erlbaum Associates.

Morrow, G. R., Lindke, J., & Black, P. (1992). Measurement of quality of life in patients: Psychometric analyses of the functional living index-cancer (FLIC). *Quality of Life Research, 1,* 287–296.

National Coalition on Healthcare. (2009). Facts on healthcare insurance. Retrieved from http://www.nchc.org/facts/coverage.shtml.

Nevidjon, B. (2004). Managing from the middle: Integrating midlife challenges of children, elder parents and career. *Clinical Journal of Oncology Nursing, 8*(1), 72–75.

Osoba, D. (1994). Lessons learned from measuring health-related quality of life in oncology. *Journal of Clinical Oncology, 12,* 608–616.

Padilla, G. V., Ferrell, B., Grant, M., & Rhiner, M. (1990). Defining the content domain of quality of life for cancer patients with pain. *Cancer Nursing, 13*(2), 108–115.

Padilla, G. V., Presant, C., Grant, M. M., Metter, G., Lipsett, J., & Heide, F. (1983). Quality of life index for patients with cancer. *Research in Nursing and Health, 6*(3), 117–126.

Phillips, J., & Weekes, D. (2002). Incorporating multiculturalism into oncology nursing research: The last decade. *Oncology Nursing Forum, 29*(5), 807–816.

Reid, D., & Renwick, R. (1994). Preliminary validation of a new instrument to measure life satisfaction in adolescents with neuromuscular disorders. *International Journal of Rehabilitation Research, 17,* 184–188.

Schachter, H. M., Mamaladze, V., Lewin, G., Graham, I. D., Brouwers, M., Sampson, M., Morrison, A., Zhang, L., O'Blenis, P., Garritty, C.(2006). Many quality measurements, but few quality measures assessing the quality of breast cancer in women: A systematic review. *BMC Cancer, 18*(6), 291.

Schipper, H. (1991). Guidelines and caveats for quality of life measurement in clinical practice and research. In N. S. Tchekmedyian & D. F. Cella (Eds.), *Quality of life in oncology practice and research* (pp. 25–31). Williston Park, NY: Dominus Publishing Company.

Schipper, H., Clinch, J., & Powell, V. (1990). Definitions and conceptual issues. In B. Spilker (Ed.), *Quality of life assessments in clinical trials* (pp. 11–24). New York, NY: Raven Press.

Schuttiga, J. A. (1995). Quality of life from a federal regulation perspective. In J. E. Dimsdale & A. Baum (Eds.), *Quality of life in behavioral medical research* (pp. 31–42). Hillsdale, NJ: Lawrence Erlbaum Associates.

Semple, C. J., Sullivan, K., Dunwoody, L., & Kernohan, W. G. (2004). Psychosocial interventions for patients with head and neck cancer: Past, present and future. *Cancer Nursing, 27*(6), 434–441.

Shumaker, S. A., Anderson, R. T., & Czajkowski, S. M. (1990). Psychological tests and scales. In B. Spilker (Ed.), *Quality of life assessments in clinical trials* (pp. 95–114). New York, NY: Raven Press.

Sneeuw, K. C., Aaronson, N. K., Sprangers, M. A., Detmar, S. B., Wever, L. D., Schornagel, J. H. (1999). Evaluating the quality of life of cancer patients: Assessments by patients, significant others, physicians, and nurses. *British Journal of Cancer, 81*(1), 87–94.

Spilker, B. (1990). Introduction. In B. Spilker (Ed.), *Quality of life assessments in clinical trials* (pp. 3–9). New York, NY: Raven Press.

Sprangers, M. A. G., & Aaronson, N. K. (1992). The role of health care providers and significant others in evaluating the quality of life of patients with chronic disease: A review. *Journal of Clinical Epidemiology, 45*, 743–760.

Stewart, A. L., Greenfield, S., Hays, R. D., Wells, K., Rogers, W. H., Berry, D. S., McGlynn, E. A., & Ware, J. E., Jr. (1989). Functional status and well-being of patients with chronic conditions: Results from the medical outcomes study. *Journal of the American Medical Association, 262*, 907–913.

Weinfurt, K. P. (2007). Value of high cost cancer care: A behavioral science perspective, *Journal of Clinical Oncology, 25*(2), 223–227.

Williams, S. A. & Schreier, A. M. (2004). The effects of education in managing side effects in women receiving chemotherapy for treatment of breast cancer. *Oncology Nursing Forum, 31*(1), E16–E23.

Zebrack, B. (2000). Cancer survivors and quality of life: A critical review of the literature. *Oncology Nursing Forum, 27*(9), 1395–1401.

Zhao, H., Kanda, K., Liu, S. J., & Mao, X. Y. (2003). Evaluation of quality of life in chinese patients with gynecological cancer: Assessments by patients and nurses. *International Journal of Nursing Practice, 9*(1),40–48.

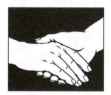

Theory

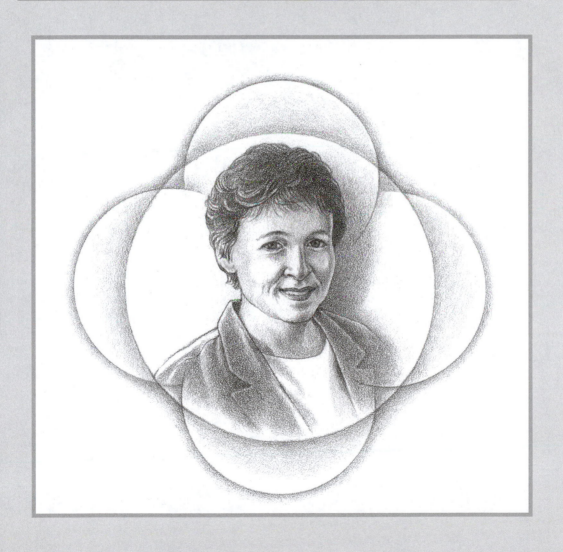

Theories and Conceptual Models to Guide Quality-of-Life Research

Janna C. Roop • Judith K. Payne •
April Hazard Vallerand

Introduction

In the last century, the life expectancy in the United States increased by almost 30 years, from 49.2 to 77.7 years (Xu, Kochanek, & Tejada-Vera, 2009). This remarkable change is due largely to improved sanitation, eradication and control of communicable diseases, development of antibiotics, and increasingly effective treatment of chronic diseases. Comparatively, in 1900, most people were relatively healthy for most of their lives and succumbed to death rather quickly after experiencing a severe illness or injury. Today many people can expect to live with sequelae of serious injury or chronic illness for several years before they die (Morrison & Morrison, 2006). In the second half of the 20th century, the concept of *quality of life* gained increasing interest, as some began to realize increased *quantity* of life is not always desirable if the quality of that life is poor.

Quality of life (QOL) is a concept that has been used from the time of Aristotle to the current day (Mandzuk & McMillan, 2005). Today, QOL is a term used in contexts as varied as political arenas, educational settings, environmental and sociological studies, advertising, and, of course, health care. In the 1960s, objective measures such as income, housing, employment, and education were the foci of most QOL studies (Morrison & Morrison, 2006). Currently, greater emphasis is placed on self-reported measures. Even within the scholarly community, however, there is no consensus on exactly what QOL means or how it is to be conceptualized. Authors define QOL in different ways, conceptualize QOL as having differing dimensions or domains, and use study-specific measures, which often are not subjected to psychometric testing (Vallerand & Payne, 2003). This lack of consensus hinders efforts to compare findings and develop a sound theory of QOL that can predict patient outcomes and inform practice. For example, if one study defines and measures QOL in one way and another uses different definitions and measures, how are the studies to be compared and synthesized?

As nursing science has increased in sophistication, it has appreciated anew the need for theoretical foundations in its knowledge base, practice, and research (Vallerand & Payne, 2003). Theories and conceptual frameworks move knowledge beyond mere observation, important as that is. Theoretical ontologies begin to organize the knowledge of a discipline into a framework and propose relationships among concepts. Those relationships can be tested and, eventually, knowledge can be generated to guide future practice and research. As we shall see in the ensuing discussion about QOL, it is the differing conceptualizations of what QOL *is* that lead to different methods of studying and measuring the phenomenon.

Dimensions of QOL

QOL is conceived almost always as having several dimensions. Even when a single item instrument is used to measure quality of life, the underlying assumption is that the participant's response will include an evaluation of several related dimensions. The most frequently cited dimensions are physiological, psychological, and sociological (Donovan, Sanson-Fisher, & Redman, 1989; Fawcett, 2005; Ferrell, Wisdom, & Wenzl, 1989a); Padilla, Ferrell, Grant, & Rhiner, 1990). Many scholars include a spiritual or existential domain as well (Fawcett, 2005; Padilla, Grant, & Martin, 1988).

In the early 1960s, objective measures such as income and employment were used to determine QOL. Over the last 40 years, however, the trend has shifted strongly toward subjective self-report to rate one's own QOL. This trend has been motivated by many studies that have found poor correlations between ratings of family members or healthcare providers and ratings of the patients themselves (Bishop, 2005; Drotar, 2004; Finlayson, Moyer, & Sonnad, 2004; Fitzsimmons, George, Payne, & Johnson, 1999; Ware, 1991). A particularly vivid example is offered by Albrecht and Devlieger (1999) in their study of 153 people with serious disabilities. They found that 54.3% of the 153 respondents in their study rated their QOL as "good" or "excellent" despite the fact that 93% of the sample acknowledged their disability had a moderate to serious effect on their daily lives. Analysis of the interviews revealed what Albrecht and Devlieger termed "a balance framework among body, mind, and spirit" (p. 985). Respondents who reported a high QOL had reevaluated this balance, placing greater importance on the faculties still intact (mind and spirit) and less emphasis on their physical disabilities. This re-ordering of the balance enabled respondents to feel satisfied with their lives, even though an outsider might believe their QOL to be low. The notion that personal evaluations of balance can affect self-ratings of QOL is illustrated by Haas's example (1999b) suggesting that two patients, both rating a symptom of nausea as 8 on a scale of 1–10, might report very different levels of QOL if one patient's nausea was caused by a long awaited pregnancy and the other's by chemotherapy treatments.

The idea that QOL is determined not only by an evaluation of several domains but also by the person's evaluation of the importance of those domains contributes to the complexity of the construct (Cella, 1992; 1994). People in similar circumstances and health states can nevertheless rate their QOL at different levels. Thus, Bishop (2005) defines QOL as "the subjective and personally derived assessment of overall well-being that results from evaluation of satisfaction across an aggregate of personally or clinically important domains" (p. 7). Similarly, as we shall see, Ferrans and Power's Quality of Life Index (1985) measures not only the domains of a person's QOL, but also how important each domain is to that individual.

Haas (1999b), while acknowledging that QOL is primarily a subjective rating, is not content to exclude objective measures entirely. She notes that proxies commonly assess the QOL of people unable to self-report, such as elderly people with dementia, people in persistent vegetative states, and critically ill neonates and children. Haas asserts that concepts of the construct of QOL must include objective measures such as adequate safety and living conditions.

In the early 1980s, the term *health-related quality of life* (HRQOL) came into use (Ware, 1984). The term is meant to exclude influences on QOL such as cultural, political, and environmental factors less directly influenced by health care. As Ferrans, Zerwic, Wilbur, and Larson (2005) point out, however, it can be very difficult to differentiate health-related factors from other factors. Political factors can influence one's access to health care; cultural factors can have a strong influence on use of contraception or adherence to guidelines for routine cancer screening (especially cervical and breast cancers); and the environment (e.g., air and water quality) also influences health. Nevertheless, the term remains in use (Ferrans et al., 2005; Gregory, Gibson, & Robinson, 2005; Resnick et al., 2005).

Early Work in QOL

When a construct as complex as QOL is defined and its domains delineated, the next step is to describe the relationships within the construct by creating a conceptual model. In 1985, Padilla and Grant (1985) created a theoretical model that illustrated the relationship between the nursing process and the dimensions of QOL (Figure 3-1). Padilla and Grant viewed QOL as a multidimensional concept that encompassed the dimensions of psychological well-being, social concerns, body image concerns, physical well-being, and response to diagnosis or treatment. The model depicted the dimensions of QOL as dependent outcome variables and nursing process activities manipulated by the investigator as independent variables. Thus, the model attempted to explain which nursing interventions had a positive effect on QOL. Padilla and Grant recognized that QOL is affected by nursing interventions and by variables within the individual. They called these mediating variables *cognitive variables*. They grouped them into *perceived caring attitude* (whether or not the individual perceived the caring attitude of the nurse) and *perceived self-care ability* (to what extent did the client believe that he or she was capable of self-care). Nursing care can influence the mediating variables, but it is the mediating variables that determine the QOL. Therefore, nursing care has an indirect effect on QOL. The model also recognizes extraneous variables, or those variables that are not manipulated by the investigator but that may affect the outcomes, such as treatment characteristics, diagnostic characteristics, and personal characteristics. (In tests of the model, extraneous variables usually are controlled directly or through statistical control).

Another model that emerged in the 1980s was derived from the Medical Outcomes Study (MOS). The MOS was designed for two broad purposes. First is to "determine whether variations in patient outcomes are explained by differences in system of care, clinical specialty, and clinicians' technical and interpersonal styles and (2) develop more practical tools for the routine monitoring of patient outcomes in medical practice." (Tarlov et al., 1989, p. 925) The MOS also was designed to develop a standardized practical measurement tool that

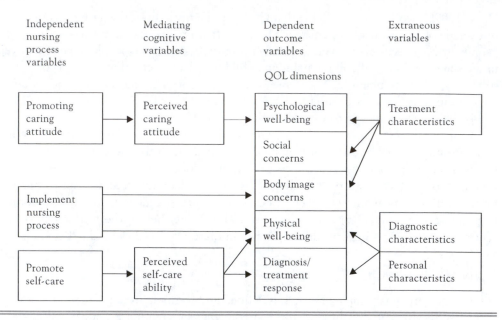

Figure 3-1. **A model of the relationship between the nursing process and the dimensions of quality of life.**

Source: Reprinted with permission from *Advances in Nursing Science*, "Quality of life as a cancer nursing outcome variable," Padilla & Grant, vol. 8, no. 1, p. 53. © 1985 Aspen Publishers, Inc.

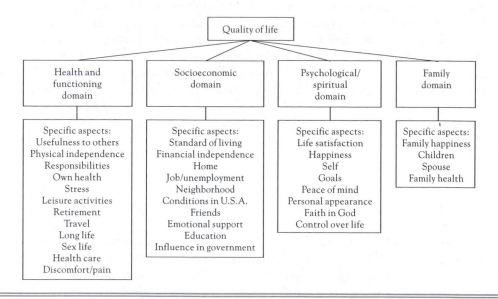

Figure 3-2. **Hierarchical relationship between the global construct of quality of life, four major domains, and specific aspects of the domains.**

Source: Ferrans, 1990b. Used with permission from Dr. Carol Estwing Ferrans.

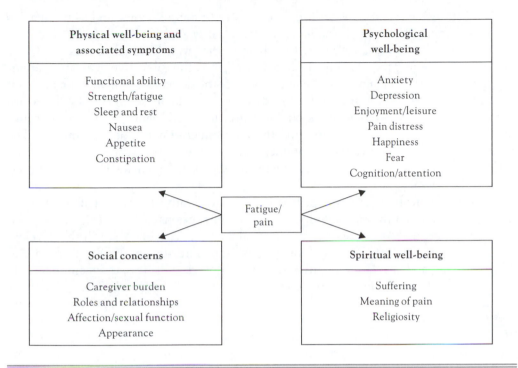

Figure 3-3.   The impact of fatigue and pain on the dimensions of quality of life.

Source: Modified from Ferrell, Grant, Padilla, Vemuri, & Rhiner, 1991; Ferrell, Grant, Dean, Funk, & Ly, 1996. Used with permission from Oncology Nursing Press.

could be easily and routinely used in clinical settings to develop a large database. Such a database would permit comparisons of outcomes across widely different diseases and treatments. Work has continued on the measurement tool, advancing it from a tool that was taking approximately 20 minutes to complete to short forms that can be completed in minutes (Ware, 1991).

Two other conceptual models frequently used to guide research and practice regarding QOL in clients with cancer are Ferrans and Powers' QOL Model (1985) (Figure 3-2) and the City of Hope Model (Figure 3-3). (Ferrell, Grant, Padilla, Vermuri, & Rhiner, 1991). Both models were developed initially to generate theory that defines the domains of QOL in clients with cancer; both models have since been modified to use with clients with disorders other than cancer. Both models view QOL from a multidimensional, subjective perspective. The implicit assumptions underlying these models are based on individualistic ideologies and view individuals as complex beings, health as a multidimensional construct, and QOL as dependent on the unique perspective of the individual. The models also reflect the definition of QOL used by the researchers.

Ferrans and Powers (1992) defined QOL as "a person's sense of well-being that stems from satisfaction or dissatisfaction with the areas of life that are important to him/her"

(p. 29). Ferrans's framework was based on extensive literature review and factor analysis using data from clients on hemodialysis. The Quality of Life Index (QLI) (Ferrans, 1990a; Ferrans & Powers, 1992) used in these studies was designed to measure QOL, while acknowledging the life domains noted by experts, the subjective evaluation of satisfaction within the domains, and the importance of the domains to the individual. Their conceptual model of QOL has evolved to describe four major domains of QOL: health and functioning, socioeconomic, psychological/spiritual, and family. The four domains encompass 35 aspects of life, conveying the multidimensionality of the concept. The conceptual model illustrates the hierarchical relationships between the global construct of QOL, the four major domains, and specific aspects of the domains (Figure 3-2) (Ferrans, 1990b, 1996).

The theoretical model developed by Padilla and Grant (1985) that illustrated the relationship between the nursing process and the dimensions of QOL (Figure 3-1) was used as a conceptual framework by Ferrell, Wisdom, and Wenzl (1989a) in the development and testing of the QOL survey instrument. In this instrument, QOL was defined as the prevention and alleviation of physical and psychological distress, the maintenance of physical/mental functioning, and the presence of a supportive network. The QOL survey was designed to measure QOL as an outcome variable in the management of cancer pain. After the reliability and validity of the QOL survey were determined (Ferrell, Wisdom, Wenzl, & Brown, 1989b), the instrument was revised, and testing was extended to gather data about the relationship between pain and QOL (Padilla et al., 1990). From these studies, a conceptual model, commonly referred to as the City of Hope Model, emerged to illustrate the influence of pain on the dimensions of QOL (Figure 3-3 [Ferrell et al., 1991; Ferrel, et al., 1992]). The four dimensions included in this model are physical well-being and symptoms, psychological well-being, social well-being, and spiritual well-being. The City of Hope Model demonstrates that pain influences all dimensions of QOL. Subsequently, fatigue has also been identified as a variable influencing all four dimensions of QOL (Ferrell, Grant, Dean, Funk, & Ly, 1996). Although developed independently and simultaneously in diverse samples, both Ferrans' QLI and the City of Hope Model identify four common domains or dimensions.

Cella (1994) contended that although there are many diverse conceptualizations of the concept of QOL, "most can be grouped into one of four correlated but distinct areas: physical, functional, emotional, and social" (p. 188). The two fundamental characteristics of the definition of QOL are multidimensionality and subjectivity. Multidimensionality of QOL refers to a broad range of content that includes physical, functional, emotional, and social well-being. The assumption is that, by combining measures of these aspects, one can approximate a single index of QOL. Subjectivity refers to the fact that QOL can be understood only from the patient's perspective. The underlying processes that comprise the patient's perspective include perception of illness, perception of treatment, expectation of self, and appraisal of risk or harm. A complex relationship exists between treatment and effects. The two distinct aspects of the relationship between symptoms and overall QOL are symptom intensity and symptom duration.

Current Conceptualization Work in Quality of Life

Quality of life has been studied extensively in the context of oncology, but studies about chronic illness and pain are also well represented in the literature (Baas, Fontana, & Bhat, 1997; Bailey, 2001; Bishop, 2005; Coutu et al., 2005; Houlihan et al., 2004; Jakobsson & Hallberg, 2006; Khan, Otter, & Springett, 2006; Rains & Hunt, 2006; Ribu et al., 2006; Vas et al., 2004). The evolving nature of the concept of QOL is illustrated in two other articles (Mandzuk & McMillan, 2005; Ferrans et al., 2005). Mandzuk and McMillan (2005) undertook an analysis of the concept of quality of life for the *Journal of Orthopaedic Nursing*. Using Walker and Avant's framework, they examined definitions, uses, critical attributes, and cases to explicate current renditions of quality of life. Mandzuk and McMillan (2005) identified three critical attributes of quality of life:

> (1) individuals make a subjective appraisal of their own lives, (2) individuals identify their satisfaction with their lives as it pertains to the physical [health and functioning], psychological [emotional well-being, spirituality, fulfillment, and personal satisfaction], and social [social support, social roles, friendship, family, feelings of belonging] domains of their life, and (3) objective measures [housing, finances, education] may supplement people's subjective evaluations of the QOL. (p. 15)

Although concept analysis is essential for theoretical and conceptual foundations of knowledge, it is instructive to note how unsatisfying Mandzuk and McMillan's (2005) description of empirical referents is; they state: "If individuals are satisfied, happy, and healthy within physical, psychological, and social contexts, they probably have a high level of QOL" (p. 16).

Also in 2005, Ferrans and colleagues undertook the revision of a model of health-related quality of life (HRQOL) published in 1995 by Wilson and Cleary. Wilson and Cleary's model moved beyond identifying domains of the construct to suggest causal relationships among the domains. They labeled arrows specifying which domains of quality of life were affected by individual characteristics and which were affected by environmental characteristics. Ferrans and colleagues (2005) expanded the conceptualization of the domains in the original model and integrated it with work of other theorists, including McLeroy, Bibeau, Steckler, Glanz, Eyler, Wilcox, Matson-Koffman, Evenson, Sanderson, Thompson, and others (Ferrans et al., 2005). Ferrans and colleagues (2005) refined the original model by more clearly differentiating the individual factors from environmental factors described by McLeroy (interpersonal factors, institutional factors, community factors, and public policy). They added arrows illustrating that patient outcomes are influenced by both individual and environmental factors, but eliminated the labels on the arrows in the Wilson and Cleary model, believing the labels on the arrows to be too restrictive. They subsumed "nonmedical factors" into individual and environmental factors, but retained the five categories of patient outcomes: biological function, symptoms, functional status, general health perceptions, and quality of life. Ferrans and colleagues (2005) provided theoretical grounding for the patient outcome categories and suggested instruments for measuring each. The revised model advances the conceptualization of QOL by suggesting causal relationships among domains and guides future research.

Hinds, Burghen, Haase, and Phillips (2006) have addressed the topic of QOL in adolescents and adults. They published a review of the work that has been done in defining, conceptualizing, and measuring QOL in pediatric and adolescent patients with cancer. As might be expected, children and adolescents envision QOL differently from adults. The definition that emerged from studies with 36 pediatric patients was "an overall sense of well-being based on being able to participate in usual activities; to interact with others and feel cared about; to cope with uncomfortable physical, emotional, and cognitive reactions; and to find meaning in the illness experience" (Hinds et al., 2006, p. 24). The definition includes six dimensions: symptoms, usual activities, social and family interactions, health status, mood, and the meaning of being ill. The authors also described several emerging models, including the Adolescent Resilience Model (ARM), the Self-Sustaining Model for Adolescents, and the Pediatric QOL at End-of-Life Model, all of which are being used to guide research. The Pediatric QOL at End-of-Life Model is intriguing in particular because it addresses the critical transition from curative to palliative goals and captures the interplay between children and parents, both of whose QOL is affected strongly by concern for the other. Children need to be assured that their surviving family members' needs will be met before and after the child's death; parents' QOL is influenced partly by their desire to make appropriate decisions for the child that are congruent with their values. Hinds and colleagues (2006) further note the number of instruments for measuring QOL in pediatric patients has increased so much that researchers actually are being asked to stop producing new tools in order to develop the testing of existing instruments.

Application of Quality of Life in the Research Literature

Since 1993, the National Institute of Nursing Research (NINR) has designated improving quality of life as a priority for research. In the most recently published strategic plan, NINR (2006) states: "Improving quality of life is the *ultimate goal of research* in the fields of self-management, symptom management, and caregiving (p. 15, emphasis added)." Clearly, researchers have responded to these priorities. A recent search of the Cumulative Index of Nursing and Allied Health Literature (CINAHL) using "quality of life" as a keyword resulted in 26,522 citations. Limiting that set to research articles published between 2004 and 2009 still yielded 10,173 articles.

Investigators from various disciplines, such as medicine (Cella, 1992, 1994; Cella & Tulsky, 1990; Ware, 2003), nursing (Ferrell, Wisdom, & Wenzl, 1989a; Ferrell et al., 1989b, 1992, 1996; Ferrans & Powers, 1985; Ferrans, 1990a, 1990b, 1996; Ferrell et al., 1991; Ferrans et al., 2005; Ferrans & Powers, 1992), and sociology (Albrecht & Devlieger, 1999; Gregory, Gibson, & Robinson, 2005), are studying QOL in multiple populations, including patients diagnosed with COPD (Kaplan & Ries, 2005); HIV/AIDS (Holzemer, Spicer, Wilson, Kemppainen, & Coleman, 1998; Tann, Sousa, & Kwok, 2005); heart disease (Clark et al., 2003; Rector, 2005); in caregivers of patients (Mellon, Northous, & Weiss, 2006; White, Lauzon, Yaffe, & Wood-Dauphinee, 2004); and in settings as diverse as the

Table 3-1.   **A Sample of Recent Studies in QOL**

Reference	Definition	Model/Instruments	Research Purpose/ Question
Borsbo, Peolsson, & Gerdle (2009)	No definition explicitly stated, but see instrument.	Quality of Life Scale (QLS-S) (Swedish version) "composed of 16 items that together describe the quality of life concept (p. 1607)." Concepts include several unique to this instrument including helping or encouraging others, participation in political organizations or public affairs, or public affairs, learning, understanding yourself, expressing yourself creatively, participating in active recreation, and independence. Missing is a direct explication of the spiritual domain.	"To identify subgroups of patients with chronic pain based on the occurrence of depression, anxiety, and catastrophising, and the duration of pain and pain intensity. In addition to this, the relationship between the subgroups with respect to background variables, diagnosis, pain-related disability, and perceived quality of life are investigated (p. 1605)."

Netherlands (Ormel, Lindenberg, Steverink, & Vonkorff, 1997), Sweden (Borsbo, Peolsson, & Gerdle, 2009), Korea (Han et al., 2005), and sub-Saharan Africa (Phaladze et al., 2005). Given the breadth of the settings and the increasing attention to cultural influence on health care and patient outcomes, Ashing-Giwa and Kagawa-Singer (2006) have presented a model to increase cultural competence in oncology research. As noted in the previous section, Hinds and colleagues (2006) have expanded the work in pediatric and adolescent populations. Byrne-Davis, Bennett, and Wilcock (2006) have demonstrated that even people with advanced dementia can provide meaningful subjective evaluations of their quality of life. Table 3-1 highlights a small sample of the plethora of recent studies.

CONCLUSION

The emerging consensus described in the previous edition of this book has been sustained (Vallerand & Payne, 2003). Quality of life continues to be seen as a multidimensional, dynamic construct that involves the evaluation of both positive and negative factors and is best determined subjectively. Although conceptual work has been accomplished that can guide future research, many studies continue to develop study-specific definitions and measures. Future knowledge development will be enhanced as scholars continue to offer conceptual definitions for the major concepts in their studies and delineate the theoretical foundations of their work. Given the dynamic and evolving nature of QOL, we should heed Mount and Cohen's (Haas, 1999b) suggestion that "we let the people whose QOL we are attempting to measure teach us what QOL means to them." (p. 218)

References

Albrecht, G. L., & Devlieger, P. J. (1999). The disability paradox: High quality of life against all odds. *Social Science and Medicine, 48*, 977–988.

Ashing-Giwa, K., & Kagawa-Singer, M. (2006). Infusing culture into oncology research on quality of life. *Oncology Nursing Forum, 33*(1), Current Approaches to Quality of Life in Patients with Cancer: 31–36.

Baas, L. S., Fontana, J. A., & Bhat, G. (1997). Relationships between self-care resources and the quality of life of persons with heart failure: A comparison of treatment groups. *Progress in Cardiovascular Nursing, 12*(1), 25–38.

Bailey, C. B. (2001). Testing an asthma quality of life model. *Journal of Theory Construction & Testing, 5*(2), 38–44.

Bishop, M. (2005). Quality of life and psychosocial adaptation to chronic illness and acquired disability: A conceptual and theoretical synthesiss [sic]. *Journal of Rehabilitation, 71*(2), 5–13.

Borsbo, B., Peolsson, M., & Gerdle, B. (2009). The complex interplay between pain intensity, depression, anxiety and catastrophising with respect to quality of life and disability. *Disability & Rehabilitation, 31*(19), 1605–1613.

Byrne-Davis, L. M. T., Bennett, P. D., & Wilcock, G. K. (2006). How are quality of life ratings made? Toward a model of quality of life in people with dementia. *Quality of Life Research, 15*, 855–865.

Cella, D. F. (1992). Quality of life: The concept. *Journal of Palliative Care, 8*(3), 8–13.

Cella, D. F. (1994). Quality of life: Concepts and definitions. *Journal of Pain and Symptom Management, 9*(186–192).

Cella, D. F., & Tulsky, D. S. (1990). Measuring quality of life today: Methodological Aspects. *Oncology, 4*(5), 29–38.

Clark, D. O., Tu, W., Weiner, M., & Murray, M. D. (2003). Correlates of health-related quality of life among lower-income, urban adults with congestive heart failure. *Heart & Lung, 32*(6), 391–401.

Clark, E. H. (2004). Quality of life: a basis for clinical decision-making in community psychiatric care. *Journal of Psychiatric and Mental Health Nursing, 11*(6), 725–730.

Coutu, M., Durand, M., Loisel, P., Dupuis, G., & Gervais, S. (2005). Measurement properties of a new quality of life measure for patients with work disability associated with musculoskeletal pain. *Journal of Occupational Rehabilitation, 15*(3), 295–312.

Donovan, K., Sanson-Fisher, R. W., & Redman, S. (1989). Measuring quality of life in cancer patients. *Journal of Clinical Oncology, 7*(7), 959–968.

Drotar, D. (2004). Validating measures of pediatric health status, functional status, and health-related quality of life: Key methodological challenges and strategies. *Ambulatory Pediatrics, 4*(4), Supplement: 358–364.

Fawcett, J. (2005). *Contemporary nursing knowledge. Analysis and evaluation of nursing models and theories* (2nd ed.). Philadelphia, PA: F. A. Davis Company.

Ferrans, C. E. (1990a). Development of a quality of life index for patients with cancer. *Oncology Nursing Forum, 17*(3, Supp), 15–21.

Ferrans, C. E. (1990b). Quality of life: Conceptual issues. *Seminars in Oncology Nursing, 6*(4), 248–254.

Ferrans, C. E. (1996). Development of a conceptual model of quality of life. *Scholarly Inquiry for Nursing Practice, 10*(3), 293–304.

Ferrans, C. E., & Powers, M. J. (1985). Quality of life index: Development and psychometric properties. *Advances in Nursing Science, 8*(7), 15–24.

Ferrans, C. E., & Powers, M. J. (1992). Psychometric assessment of the quality of life index. *Research in Nursing and Health, 15,* 29–38.

Ferrans, C. E., Zerwic, J. J., Wilbur, J. E., & Larson, J. L. (2005). Conceptual model of health-related quality of life. *Journal of Nursing Scholarship, 37*(4), 336–342.

Ferrell, B., Grant, M., Dean, G., Funk, B., & Ly, J. (1996). "Bone tired": The experience of fatigue and its impact on quality of life. *Oncology Nursing Forum, 23*(10), 1539–1547.

Ferrell, B. R., Grant, M. M., Padilla, G., Vermuri, S., & Rhiner, M. (1991). The experiences of pain and perceptions of quality of life: Validation of a conceptual model. *The Hospice Journal, 7*(3), 9–24.

Ferrell, B. R., Grant, M. M., Rhiner, M., & Padilla, G. V. (1992). Home care: Maintaining quality of life for patient and family. *Oncology, 6*(2), 136–140.

Ferrell, B. R., Wisdom, C., & Wenzl, C. (1989a). Quality of life as an outcome variable in the management of cancer pain. *Cancer, 63*(2321–2327).

Ferrell, B. R., Wisdom, C., Wenzl, C., & Brown, J. (1989b). Effects of controlled-release morphine on quality of life for cancer pain. *Oncology Nursing Forum, 26,* 521–526.

Finlayson, T. L., Moyer, C. A., & Sonnad, S. S. (2004). Assessing symptoms, disease severity, and quality of life in the clinical context: A theoretical framework. *American Journal of Managed Care, 10*(5), 336–344.

Fitzsimmons, D., George, S., Payne, S., & Johnson, C. D. (1999). Differences in perception of quality of life issues between health professionals and patients with pancreatic cancer. *Psycho-Oncology, 8*(2), 135–143.

Fox, S. W., & Lyon, D. E. (2006). Symptom clusters and quality of life in survivors of lung cancer. *Oncology Nursing Forum, 33*(5), 931–936.

Green, H. J., Pakenham, K. I., Headley, B. C., & Gardiner, R. A. (2002). Coping and health-related quality of life in men with prostate cancer randomly assigned to hormonal medication or close monitoring. *Psycho-Oncology, 11*(5), 401–414.

Gregory, J., Gibson, B., & Robinson, P. G. (2005). Variation and change in the meaning of oral health related quality of life: A 'grounded' systems approach. *Social Science & Medicine, 60*(8), 1859–1868.

Haas, B. K. (1999b). A multidisciplinary concept analysis of quality of life. *Western Journal of Nursing Research, 21*(6), 728–742.

Hahn, E. A., Cella, D., Dobrez, D. G., Weiss, B. D., Du, H., Lai, J., et al. (2006). The impact of literacy on health-related quality of life measurement and outcomes in cancer outpatients. *Quality of Life Research, 16*(3), 495–507.

Han, K. S., Lee, S. J., Park, E. S., Park, Y., & Cheol, K. H. (2005). Structural model for quality of life of patients with chronic cardiovascular disease in Korea. *Nursing Research, 54*(2), 85–96.

Hinds, P. S., Burghen, E. A., Haase, J. E., & Phillips, C. R. (2006). Advances in defining, conceptualizing, and measuring quality of life in pediatric patients with cancer. *Oncology Nursing Forum, 33*(1), Current Approaches to Quality of Life in Patients with Cancer: 23–29.

Holzemer, W. L., Spicer, J. G., Wilson, H. S., Kemppainen, J. K., & Coleman, C. (1998). Validation of the quality of life scale: Living with HIV. *Journal of Advanced Nursing, 28*(3), 622–630.

Houlihan, C. M., O'Donnell, M., Conaway, M., & Stevenson, R. D. (2004). Bodily pain and health-related quality of life in children with cerebral palsy. *Developmental Medicine & Child Neurology, 46*(5), 305–310.

Jakobsson, U. L. F., & Hallberg, I. R. (2006). Quality of life among older adults with osteoarthritis: An explorative study. *Journal of Gerontological Nursing, 32*(8), 51–60.

Kaplan, R. M., & Ries, A. L. (2005). Quality of life as an outcome measure in pulmonary diseases. *Journal of Cardiopulmonary Rehabilitation, 25*(6), 321–331.

Khan, S., Otter, S., & Springett, K. (2006). The effects of reflexology on foot pain and quality of life in a patient with rheumatoid arthritis: A case report. *The Foot: International Journal of Clinical Foot Science, 16*(2), 112–116.

Mandzuk, L. L., & McMillan, D. E. (2005). A concept analysis of quality of life. *Journal of Orthopaedic Nursing, 9*(1), 12–18.

Mellon, S., Northous, L. L., & Weiss, L. K. (2006). A population-based study of the quality of life of cancer survivors and their family caregivers. *Cancer Nursing, 29*(2), 120–133.

Morrison, L. J., & Morrison, S. (2006). Palliative care and pain management. *The Medical Clinics of North America, 90,* 983–1004.

National Institute of Nursing Research. (2006). *NINR strategic plan 2006–2010* (DHHS Publication No. 06-4832, p. 15).

Ormel, J., Lindenberg, S., Steverink, N., & Vonkorff, M. (1997). Quality of life and social production functions: A framework for understanding health effects. *Social Science & Medicine, 45*(7), 1051–1063.

Padilla, G. V., Ferrell, B. R., Grant, M. M., & Rhiner, M. (1990). Defining the content domain of quality of life for cancer patients with pain. *Cancer Nursing, 13*(2), 108–115.

Padilla, G. V., & Grant, M. M. (1985). Quality of life as a cancer nursing outcome variable. *Advances in Nursing Science, 8*(1), 45–60.

Padilla, G. V., Grant, M. M., & Martin, L. (1988). Rehabilitation and quality of life measurement issues. *Head & Neck Surgery, 10*(Suppl. 11), S156–S160.

Phaladze, N. A., Human, S., Dlamini, S. B., Hulela, E. B., Mahlubi Hadebe, I., Sukati, N. A., et al. (2005). Quality of life and the concept of "living well" with HIV/AIDS in sub-Saharan Africa. *Journal of Nursing Scholarship, 37*(2), 120–126.

Rains, G. A., & Hunt, F. E. (2006). Quality of life, pain, and spirituality in end-stage congestive patients. *Progress in Cardiovascular Nursing, 21*(2), 112–113.

Rector, R. S. (2005). A conceptual model of quality of life in relation to heart failure. *Journal of Cardiac Failure, 11*(3), 173–176.

Resnick, B., Orwig, D., Wehren, L., Hawkes, W., Hebel, R., Zimmerman, S., et al. (2005). Health-related quality of life: Is it a good indicator of function post THR?...total hip replacement. *Rehabilitation Nursing, 30*(2), 46–54.

Ribu, L., Rustoen, T., Birkeland, K., Hanestad, B. R., Paul, S. M., & Miaskowski, C. (2006). The prevalence and occurrence of diabetic foot ulcer pain and its impact on health-related quality of life. *Journal of Pain, 7*(4), 290–299.

Tann, S. S., Sousa, K. H., & Kwok, O. (2005). 16th International Nursing Research Congress. Testing a quality of life model in Latinos living with HIV/AIDS. *Sigma Theta Tau International,* 1p.

Tarlov, A. R., Ware, J. E., Jr., Greenfield, S., Nelson, E. C., Perrin, E., & Zubkoff, M. (1989). The Medical Outcomes Study. An application of methods for monitoring the results of medical care. *JAMA, 262*(7), 925–930.

Tsay, S.-L., Lee, Y.-C., & Lee, Y.-C. (2005). Effects of an adaptation training programme for patients with end-stage renal disease. *Journal of Advanced Nursing, 50*(1), 39–46.

Vallerand, A. H., & Payne, J. K. (2003). Theories and conceptual models to guide *quality of life* related research. In E. C. R. King & P. S. Hinds (Eds.), *Quality of life. From nursing and patient perspectives. Theory. Research. Practice* (2nd ed.). Sudbury, MA: Jones and Bartlett Pubishers.

Vas, J., Mendez, C., Perea-Milla, E., Vega, E., Panadero, M. D., Leon, J. M., et al. (2004). Acupuncture as a complementary therapy to the pharmacological treatment of osteoarthritis of the knee: Randomised controlled trial. *BMJ, 329*(7476), 1216–1219.

Ware, J. E., Jr. (1984). Conceptualizing disease impact and treatment outcomes. *Cancer, 53,* 2316–2323.

Ware, J. E., Jr. (1991). Conceptualizing and measuring generic health outcomes. *Cancer, 67*(3 Suppl.), 774–779.

Ware, J. E., Jr. (2003). Conceptualization and measurement of health-related quality of life: Comments on an evolving field. *Archives of Physical Medicine and Rehabilitation, 84*(4), Suppl 2: S43–51.

White, C. L., Lauzon, S., Yaffe, M. J., & Wood-Dauphinee, S. (2004). Toward a model of quality of life for family caregivers of stroke survivors. *Quality of Life Research, 13,* 625–638.

Wilson, I. B., & Cleary, P. D. (1995). Linking clinical variables with health-related quality of life. A conceptual model of patient outcomes. *The Journal of the American Medical Association, 273*(1), 59–65.

Xu, J., Kochanek, K. D., & Tejada-Vera, B. (2009). Deaths: Preliminary Data for 2007. *National Vital Statistics Reports, 58*(1), 1. Retrieved from http://www.cdc.gov/nchs/data/nvsr/nvsr58/nvsr58_01.pdf

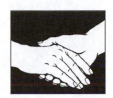

Conceptualization and Measurement of Quality of Life and Related Concepts: Progress to Date and Guidelines for Clarity

Joan E. Haase • Carrie Jo Braden

Introduction

The purposes of this chapter are to examine progress made in efforts to clarify health-related quality of life (HRQOL) conceptualization and measurement issues that make it difficult to distinguish concepts *related* to HRQOL from concepts that are *indicators* of HRQOL, and to provide guidelines for achieving conceptual clarity. (Aaronson et al., 1991; Ballatori, 2001; Cella & Tulsky, 1990; Costain, Hewison, & Howes, 1993; de Haes & van Knippenberg, 1989; Dow, Ferrell, Haberman, & Eaton, 1999; Goodinson & Singleton, 1989; Grumann & Schlag, 2001; Hinds & Haase, 2003; Holzner et al., 2001a; Leplege & Hunt, 1997; Moons, Budts, & De Geest, 2006; Mosconi, Colozza, De Laurentiis, De Placido, & Maltoni, 2001; Murphy, 2003; Padilla, Ferrell, Grant, & Rhiner, 1990; Sousa & Chen, 2002; Thorne & Paterson, 2000). Based on recent HRQOL discussions, the logic or validity link between definition and measurement of HRQOL remains weak. That is, no definition to date has been established that identifies the essential characteristics or attributes that form the conceptual parameters of HRQOL (Dijkers, 2007; Moons et al., 2006).

Quality-of-Life Conceptualization and Measurement Issues

There are three major HRQOL conceptualization and measurement issues: reaching consensus on a definition of quality of life (QOL), deciding on core components of HRQOL, and deciding on measurement approaches and types of measurements used. The conceptualization issues for HRQOL are long standing. One set of exchanges among researchers in the late 1980s regarding HRQOL was likened to the Tower of Babel (de Haes & van Knippenberg, 1989; Mor & Guadagnoli, 1988). Another described HRQOL as a primitive term with a few directly observable and clearly identifying characteristics (Mast, 1995). Discussion continued throughout the 1990s about whether defining and measuring HRQOL even is possible, given the complexity of situational and demographic variables between patients and within patients over time (Albert, 1998; Frank et al., 1998; Leplege & Hunt, 1997).

More recently, and despite some advancement, scholars continue to express discouragement over the lack of debate related to the underlying assumptions for various conceptualizations of HRQOL (Dijkers, 2007). The concern is that, despite its elusive and complex nature, HRQOL is now so "fashionable" that researchers often do not thoughtfully define HRQOL or specify their purpose for measuring it. They also often simply use "off-the-shelf" instruments to measure HRQOL (Dijkers, 2007).

Without consensus regarding what HRQOL means, it is likely HRQOL will continue to be communicated primarily by variables or instances that *illustrate rather than define or specify the essential attributes of the concept*. For example, a healthcare provider concerned with the impact of illness treatment on physical functioning may focus on side effect characteristics as illustrative of the patients' HRQOL. Another healthcare provider with a desire to understand more about the impact of the illness on patients' overall happiness or satisfaction with life may focus on role performance or spirituality as illustrative of HRQOL. The number of potential illustrative indicators is large. Given the lack of clearly identified essential characteristics of HRQOL, the problem remains how to provide a meaningful way to differentiate related concepts from the possible indicators that clearly identify the essential components of HRQOL. Health-related quality of life will cease to be a primitive term only when there is consensus about a set of clearly identifiable characteristics or attributes that will be consistently used as the basis for definition and measurement.

The number of articles on the quality of life for cancer patients has increased steadily. The proportion of HRQOL articles listed in *PubMed* increased from 0.002% in 1996 to 1.36% in 2005 (Moons et al., 2006). There is general acceptance of a core set of broad domains that constitute HRQOL and are useful in evaluating clinical trails (Gunnars, Nygren, & Glimelius, 2001); however, specific domains vary widely and measures are not always comparable (Holzner et al., 2001b). The HRQOL domains more or less agreed upon as broad domains in adult clinical trial HRQOL studies include physical functioning, disease-related and treatment-related symptoms, and psychological and social functioning (Aaronson et al., 1991; Baker et al., 1994; Ferrell, 1990; King et al., 1997; Moinpour, 1994). Examples of other domains include satisfaction with care, a sense of well-being, and general life satisfaction. Aaronson and da Silva (1987) and Schipper (1990b) describe a HRQOL paradigm consisting of four components: physical and occupational function, psychological function, social interaction, and somatic sensation. Patrick and Erickson (1993) organized four core domains within which nine associated concepts were subsumed. The four core domains and nine component concepts form an HRQOL framework. Opportunity, functional status, impairment, and death or duration of life are the relevant domains for identifying variables that are indicators of HRQOL. More recently, there is an increasing call for including spirituality in the basic list of domains for health-related quality of life (Brady, Peterman, Fitchett, Mo, & Cella, 1999; Mytko & Knight, 1999; Peterman, Fitchett, Brady, Hernandez, & Cella, 2002).

In addition to variations in the domains that constitute HRQOL, there is still much debate about methods appropriate for defining the domains and variables that illustrate HRQOL (Gunnars et al., 2001; King et al., 1997; Koopmans, 2002). The level of consensus remains very general with the only solid source of agreement being the assumption that health-related quality of life is a multidimensional construct.

Moons and colleagues describe a unique approach intended to help scientists arrive at consensus about HRQOL conceptualization (Moons et al., 2006). First, these researchers used Ferrans (1990) taxonomy of six HRQOL conceptual groupings, and expanded them to eight groupings, based on the literature. These eight broad HRQOL conceptualizations included normal life, social utility, cost-based utility, happiness/affect, satisfaction with life, satisfaction with specific domains of life, achievement of personal goals, and natural capacity. Definitions were provided for each grouping. Next, the researchers identified six HRQOL issues and presented their conclusions related to each HRQOL conceptualization, with rationale based on the literature and specific patient examples. The issues were quality of life vs. health status and functioning; objective vs. subjective dimensions; distinctions between indicators and determinants; changes over time; negative vs. positive components; and health-related quality of life definitions. Next, the eight broad conceptualizations were evaluated dichotomously (with a *yes* or *no*) in relation to whether or not each HRQOL conceptualization adequately addressed each issue. From that comparative evaluation, they concluded HRQOL is defined most appropriately in terms of satisfaction with life. While this unique approach is an admirable first attempt to arrive systematically at consensus regarding HRQOL terms and definitions, the approach is somewhat simplistic in that conclusions were reached on the basis of a *yes* or *no* scoring dichotomy of whether the conceptual issue was "solved" in the direction they had concluded was accurate. Still, the boldness of their conclusions about the "best" conceptualization for addressing the issues has already served an important function by renewing the much needed debate of HRQOL conceptualization issues (Dijkers, 2007).

For the most part, the domains identified in HRQOL frameworks (Aaronson et al., 1991; Cummins, 2005; Padilla, Presant, Grant, Baker, & Metter, 1981; Padilla et al., 1990; Patrick & Guttmacher, 1983) continue to have little theoretical basis. Even when a theoretical framework is identified to evaluate HRQOL, as was done with social cognitive therapy (Graves, 2003), the usual, function-based outcomes still are most often used to define the HRQOL domains (Cummins, 2005). Most commonly, sets of factors thought to indicate HRQOL are grouped together and items believed to represent the factors are developed or taken from existing instruments designed to measure some other variable. Validity is assessed sometimes by exploratory factor analyses to deduce factors or to interpret agreement of the factors that emerge without a theoretical structure (Aaronson & da Silva, 1987; Bliss, Selby, Robertson, & Powles, 1992; Jenkins, Jono, Stanton, & Stroup-Benham, 1990). For instance, several studies comparing commonly used quality-of-life measures, scales, or subscales found the measures were not comparable across one or more domains (Cella, Hahn, & Dineen, 2002; Holzner et al., 2001b; Kemmler et al., 1999; Kuenstner et al., 2002). Frequently, there is no assessment made of the sensitivity of the factors to detect meaningful changes in a patient's HRQOL (Donovan, Sanson-Fisher, & Redman, 1989; Gunnars et al., 2001; Testa & Simonson, 1996) and few studies address logistics such as the timing of measurement (Hakamies-Blomqvist et al., 2001). And, illustrative of "HRQOL as function," Smith and Huntington (2006) attempted to assist clinicians to select HRQOL measures to include in clinical trials through an acceptance-by-default approach. The authors described an algorithm that included no definition or conceptual framework of HRQOL. What patients view as meaningful and important to their HRQOL, such as goals, dreams, and hopes, are mostly left out of the multidimensional formulations developed by healthcare professionals (Costain et al., 1993; Dijkers, 2003; Zebrack, 2000).

Acknowledgment that HRQOL is multidimensional is an insufficient basis with which to justify treatment choices and make judgments about the effects of therapeutic interventions when a biomedical-focused framework of HRQOL is primarily used (Corner, 1997; Costain et al., 1993; Molassiotis & Morris, 1998; Schipper, 1990). Such a focus results in reliance on a functional living perspective with HRQOL domains selected on the basis of professional concerns about physical and psychological morbidity and the patient's capacity for active and independent function. By contrast, a patient-focused approach to HRQOL is based on the notion of the *meaning* of the cancer experience to the patient and its subsequent treatment. The patient perspective includes concerns about information, ideas about the nature of supportive and nonsupportive contacts, the nature of choice in treatment decision making, and the changing perceptions of experience as the treatment continues or comes to an end. These perspectives go beyond merely the presence or absence of function. A meaning-based model can be used also as a basis for selecting treatment choices and for determining the effectiveness of therapeutic intervention (Levine & Ganz, 2002; Moinpour, 1994). A meaning-based model also may be a better perspective for guiding the development of multidimensional frameworks for HRQOL (Costain et al., 1993; Somerfield, 2001). Additionally, meanings of experiences may provide a useful framework for survivorship (Zebrack, 2000).

For effective decision making, it is necessary to identify the most powerful predictors of HRQOL, beyond those measuring function (Bliss et al., 1992; Levine & Ganz, 2002). Bliss and colleagues (1992) concluded further use of factor analysis would not help define HRQOL factors more precisely in cancer patients, because the findings are so similar to other measures that include psychological as well as physical distress domains. Thus, the problem with the existing general consensus about categories of variables represented in most HRQOL frameworks is one of an increasing gap between sophisticated statistical analysis of data obtained from multidimensional instruments and the lack of conceptual sophistication reflected in the operational definition of variables thought to be illustrative of HRQOL (Costain et al., 1993). The narrower conceptualization of HRQOL in terms of domains that illustrate HRQOL does not resolve theoretical dilemmas about the nature or meaning of HRQOL (Faden & Leplege, 1992). The various measures and methods currently used to assess HRQOL do not have congruent theoretical constructs or philosophic views yet.

Inductive, patient-generated approaches to define the illustrative domains of HRQOL have also been described (Ferrell et al., 1992a, 1992b; Padilla et al., 1990). The lists of categories and subcategories emerging from the application of the essentially descriptive surveys converge on four very broad categories: physical, psychological, interpersonal well-being and, most recently added, spiritual well-being (Padilla et al., 1990). Attention to subcategories under each of the broad domains emerging from their survey data provides some insight about which domains are most critical from the patient's point of view during the kind of life-changing events that cancer patients experience. These findings also support the idea that there is a middle road where a meaning-based model and a function-based model complement one another. For example, the data indicated that social role functioning composed of the themes of making others happy (e.g., satisfying others, giving of self, helping others) and fulfilling one's role (e.g., good parent, community member, church-goer) are central to most patients' perception of what constitutes HRQOL in bad times, as well as in good times. This finding aligns well with several later conceptualizations, such as the social well-being dimension that includes roles and relationships, affection and sexual function, leisure activities, and return-to-work aspects (Ferrell et al., 1992b). It is also similar to the HRQOL concept of social function that fits within a broader domain of functional status (Patrick & Erickson, 1993). Patrick and Erickson defined roles in terms of social function (i.e., major activities), integration through participation in the community, contact (i.e., interaction with others) and intimacy, and sexual function.

The studies that used specific inductive approaches to collect data to obtain the depth, meaning, and experience of cancer treatment needed to understand HRQOL, especially as a way to discern contextual patterns of quality of life, are promising:

- McBride's (1993) description of adult role outcomes as pivotal to the management of chronic illness conditions
- Braden's (1993) definition of self-help outcomes in terms of involvement in the things one finds important in life, specifically social role activities
- Leidy and Haase's (1999) conceptualization of being able and being with as a means of preserving integrity or wholeness in chronic illness
- Cohen and Leis' (2002) five broad domains of HRQOL in the context of palliative care (the patient's own state, including physical and cognitive functioning, psychological state, and physical condition; quality of palliative care; physical environment; relationships; and outlook).

There is broad agreement on the importance of considering human experiences when studying HRQOL (Faden & Leplege, 1992). Yet few first-person descriptions of such experiences are available. From their first-person experiences as patients, patient advocates and cancer patient group facilitators (Chauhan & Eppard, 2005) give an important and missing voice to discussions of quality of life. They clearly illustrate the differences in perspectives of providers and patients regarding what HRQOL means; they also suggest face-to-face communication about HRQOL is likely the most promising way to clinically assess HRQOL (Chauhan & Eppard, 2005). Research supports the importance of such provider–patient communication as well (Detmar, Muller, Schornagel, Wever, & Aaronson, 2002).

Family relationships and social role performance as meaningful concepts for HRQOL frameworks are supported by Costain and associates' comparison study of function-based and meaning-based perspectives on HRQOL (Costain et al., 1993). The focus of the meaning-based perspective of an illness experience includes personal relationships with others. The measure contains nine items for family relationships and four for social life. By contrast, the measure used to index a function-based model (representing professional definitions of optimum functional status) contains one global item for family relationships. Results demonstrate a lack of fit between the two measures on family relationships and social life with the meaning-based measure providing more information about the context of family relationships, including feelings of usefulness, expressing love and affection, sharing one's experience with others, and contact with children and parents. Additionally, the meaning-focused measure was more sensitive to detecting dissatisfaction in the domain, providing a better tool for problem identification and focusing of oncology support services. Another example of differences in function-based and meaning-based findings was demonstrated by Mackworth and colleagues (Mackworth, Fobair, & Prados, 1992). They used a multidimensional HRQOL instrument that provides a more definitive assessment of HRQOL than the assessment provided by the Karnofsky Performance Scale (KPS) (Karnofsky & Burchenal, 1949). Specifically, the KPS was not sufficiently discriminatory to be sensitive enough to find distinctions for two thirds of the subjects (Mackworth et al., 1992).

The issue of measure sensitivity or responsiveness to change is very important, given that a primary purpose for including HRQOL endpoints in clinical assessments of cancer treatment is to include the patient, as well as the disease, when assessing effectiveness of treatment (Costain et al., 1993; Moinpour et al., 1989; Ward et al., 1999). Measures that are insensitive because they do not represent patients' views about their HRQOL during their cancer experience fail in two regards: they do not inform clinicians about where and for whom intervention efforts need to be focused, and they cannot assess treatment effectiveness from the patient's perspective. Some researchers now involve patients in the development of instruments through interviews and focus groups as a way to address this concern (Zebrack, Ganz, Bernaards, Petersen, & Abraham, 2006).

Being sensitive to patients' cultures obliges instrument developers to assess whether items are biased against one demographic group compared to another (Teresi et al., 1995; Teresi, Kleinman, & Ocepek-Welikson, 2000). Tests of differential item functioning (DIF) represent a promising set of statistical methods that provide bias (Holland & Wainer, 1993) useful in measuring HRQOL in different groups. Differential item functioning methods compare two or more groups on an item score, after adjusting for a measure of overall trait (such as total score or a latent trait estimate).

Guidelines for Obtaining Clarity in Quality-of-Life Conceptualization and Measurement

A number of investigators offer criteria or guidelines that, if followed, improve efforts to assess HRQOL for the purposes of justifying treatment choice and determining therapeutic intervention effectiveness. Several are discussed here and synthesized in Table 4-1.

Goodinson and Singleton (1989) list six criteria for assessing HRQOL:

- Data need to be based on patients' self-reports in order to reflect a patient perspective.

Table 4-1. **Guidelines for Achieving Clarity in QOL Assessment**

1. Specify the purpose(s) for use of the QOL assessment
   a. Designate the population(s) of interest considering the following:
      - Diagnostic groups
      - Treatment option groups
      - Groups experiencing specific phenomena such as specific symptoms
      - Demographic characteristics such as gender, ethnicity, and age
      - Consumer-focused populations such as HMO-targeted populations
   b. Determine if the assessment is process or endpoint focused:
      - Make decisions regarding issues of identifying and defining endpoints such as when the endpoint occurs and whose perspective of the endpoint will be measured.
      - Make decisions regarding issues of identifying and defining processes such as when data will be obtained and whose perspective(s) will be measured at each point.
   c. Identify design alternatives based on the state of knowledge development and the philosophical context of science:
      - Options include: exploration, description, prediction, and evaluation
      - Contexts include: discovery or justification

2. Select a conceptual orientation or theoretical framework
   a. Variable (concept) specifications should be consistent with decision criteria about whether concept is "part of" or has a validity (logic) link to defining attributes of quality of life:
      - Decide on methods for clarification of variables (concept analysis, derivation, and synthesis; retrodiction process in middle range theory development; structural analysis of underlying measurement model to test alternative item sets)
   b. Relationship (statement) specification should be consistent with decision criteria about whether concepts are "illustrative of" QOL in terms of antecedents of ("cause of") or consequences of ("result of") QOL:
      - Decide on methods for clarification of relationships (statement analysis, derivation, and synthesis; alternative theory testing of multiple hypotheses using structural equation analysis or other methods)

3. Specify measurement criteria to include
   a. The current status of measurement of selected concepts
   b. The measurement burden
   c. Multiple stakeholders' perspective:
      - Critical multiplism
      - Resources/access to multiple stakeholders

- The conceptual orientation needs to give recognition to the fact that a patient's perspective cannot be abstracted from the individual in isolation from coping strategies, past experiences of illness, and other variables.
- The weighing of dimension importance must reflect what is important to the patient.
- The dimensions included should have both a history of contribution to HRQOL and a definition base from which it is developed.
- The design should ensure the selected way of assessing HRQOL will be applicable across a range of times (e.g., in states of wellness, during illness diagnosis and treatment phases, following treatment completion).
- Studies of HRQOL should fit within an ongoing investigative framework that seeks to establish the influence of adaptation phenomenon and coping strategies on HRQOL.

Three of the four key policies adapted by the Cancer Control Research Committee of the Southwest Oncology group for guiding HRQOL definition demonstrate incorporation of many of the criteria offered by Goodinson and Singleton (1989):

- Measure physical functioning, symptoms and global HRQOL separately.
- Include measures of social functioning and additional protocol-specific measures if resources permit.
- Use patient-based instruments with psychometric properties that have been documented in published studies.

Gunnars and associates (2001) provide an overview of the most commonly used quality-of-life instruments, including a discussion of the major characteristics of each instrument, with number of items, scaling model, reliability and validity, differences in versions, and limited information on the specific subscales contained within each instrument. These authors conclude there is little need for development of additional instruments. In addition to describing the instruments, this group also provides several conclusions:

- Assessments are increasingly utilized and should primarily be done by self-reports.
- A predicted hypothesis should determine the most appropriate instruments.
- Despite difficulties in interpreting the relationship of objective endpoints in light of subjective data, both perspectives are valuable.
- HRQOL assessment continues to require methodological improvement. Timing, response shift, missing data, and difficulty comparing across protocols are all examples of the method problems that make the current state of knowledge tentative.
- HRQOL assessments demand resources and should be used primarily in studies motivated by comparisons of treatments without major differences in objective endpoints.

A nursing state-of-the-knowledge conference on quality of life and the cancer experience resulted in guidelines related to both theory and measurement (King et al., 1997). Recommendations included the following:

- The underlying mechanisms that explain how quality of life "works" should be considered.
- Sources of items should be derived from patient-generated data.
- Respondents should have the opportunity to weigh the importance, as well as the occurrence, of items in HRQOL instruments.
- In addition to meeting established criteria for reliability and validity, instruments should be selected to fit the specific aims of the study.
- Consideration should be given to the impact of culture and life experiences on basic perceptions of HRQOL.

As previously mentioned, general guidelines for achieving conceptual clarity in HRQOL assessment are outlined in Table 4-1. Three general steps are suggested: specify the purpose, identify the theoretical or conceptual framework, and specify additional measurement criteria.

Specify the Purpose

Three general purposes for assessing HRQOL appear in the literature. Many authors (Compas, Connor-Smith, Saltzman, Thomsen, & Wadsworth, 2001; Leplege & Hunt, 1997; Moinpour, 1994; Moinpour et al., 1989; Sloan et al., 2006) indicate the primary purpose for including HRQOL in clinical assessments of cancer treatment is to consider the patient as well as the disease when assessing treatment effectiveness or identifying treatment choices. Thus, the broad purposes are to provide a patient perspective of the cancer experience, identify treatment choices, and determine the effectiveness of therapeutic interventions. Examination of the goals for undertaking HRQOL assessment is essential as different goals can lead to different choices of measures, as well as implications for respondent and administrative burdens (Koller, Klinkhammer-Schalke, & Lorenz, 2005; Schag, Ganz, & Heinrich, 1991; Somerfield, 2001).

Reasons for undertaking HRQOL assessment include "(1) justifying or refuting different forms of medical treatment; (2) resolving disputes concerning different therapeutic approaches; (3) identifying the sequelae of disease or treatment, which may be resolved by other therapeutic interventions (e.g., nursing) and with regard to quality adjusted life year (QALY); and (4) providing a basis for allocating resources to those treatments judged to be most cost effective" (Goodinson & Singleton, 1989, p. 327).

Goodinson and Singleton (1989) and others (Cascinu, Labianca, Daniele, Beretta, & Salvagni, 2001; Langenhoff, Krabbe, Wobbes, & Ruers, 2001) also suggest HRQOL assessments should serve as a basis for treatment selection between individuals, with preference given to those who have the potential for maximum benefit. The economic perspective inherent in HRQOL assessment as a basis for treatment selection clearly raises ethical issues that are a part of purpose identification (Goodwin, 2001; Sherbourne et al., 2001). However, there are moral issues surrounding any HRQOL assessment, regardless of purpose, which are not being addressed (Faden & Leplege, 1992; Leplege & Hunt, 1997). Thus, specifying the purpose for the HRQOL assessment is an important first step in working toward clarity, not only because of conceptual and measurement concerns but also because of significant ethical concerns. Specifying the purpose of HRQOL assessment is enhanced further when there is clarification of the population of interest, the focus as either process or endpoint, and the research design. Also, assessment of quality of life actually may foster enhanced quality of life in the social domain, especially with healthcare providers.

Population of Interest

One criterion used to evaluate the adequacy of measures of HRQOL is items based on patient perspectives (Donovan et al., 1989). Population-specific patient perspectives are beginning to be reflected in measures, and there is evidence HRQOL definitions and measures may change dramatically when the population characteristics are considered (Quill et al., 2006; Zebrack et al., 2006). Quality-of-life populations are most often defined based on specific diagnoses and treatment groups (El-Serag, Olden, & Bjorkman, 2002; Trippoli et al., 2001). And, despite the lack of consensus in conceptualization or measurement, for some disease-specific groups, HRQOL assessment has influenced the nature of treatment. For example, Priestman concluded that studies of psychiatric morbidity associated with breast cancer patients clearly have influenced treatment decisions for surgeons toward lumpectomy and irradiation rather than disfiguring procedures (Priestman, 1987).

Less frequently, HRQOL studies define populations based on experiences with specific phenomena, often physical symptoms such as fatigue (Mast, 1998; Nail & Jones, 1995; Piper, 1991) and pain (Ferrell, Ferrell, Ahn, & Tran, 1994). Although nurses have studied and developed instruments for elusive but important concepts for patients with cancer, such as hope (Herth, 1989; Owen, 1989), courage (Haase, 1987), suffering (Gregory, 1994; Steeves & Kahn, 1987), spirituality (Kaczorowski, 1989), and self-transcendence (Coward, 1991), few studies have been conducted to study cancer patients by defining the population as those experiencing such phenomena. Yet, when such studies have been done, they yield important information on HRQOL, often identifying interventions specifically within nursing's domain. The importance of defining populations of interest in the study of HRQOL based on culture or ethnic group is well documented (Leininger, 1994; Marshall, 1990). When a cultural group is defined as the population of interest, it is important that studies are culturally sensitive and appropriate, because interpretation of results is clearly dependent on meanings within the culture. Quality of life itself is likely to be defined differently in different cultures (Iwamoto, 1994). Measures developed for one population may be inappropriate in another. Erroneous conclusions can result from cultural bias about HRQOL, such as there are no differences attributable to culture or that there are extreme differences, which make cross-cultural studies futile (Bonomi et al., 1996; Cella, 1992).

Other demographic characteristics, such as age and gender, require special consideration. Developmental issues are important, especially for children and adolescents, when longitudinal studies are planned. For example, changes in functional status are difficult to track when the indicators of what a child can do change over the course of lengthy treatment periods (Bradlyn, Harris, & Spieth, 1995). Consumer-focused populations, such as those in Health Maintenance Organizations (HMO), are rapidly increasing. Although dissatisfaction with the quality of care may be expressed in studies of HRQOL, important information also may be obtained from which healthcare delivery systems can be revised.

For example, HRQOL studies of cancer survivors imply long-term survivors may have a continued need for psycho-oncologic support (Decker, Haase, & Bell, 2007; Holzner et al., 2001b; Kiss et al., 2002; Kopp et al., 1998; Tomich & Helgeson, 2002).

People at later stages of cancer or in palliative care raise very different HRQOL questions than long-term survivors or those in early stages (Coates et al., 2000; Frost, Bonomi, Ferrans, Wong, & Hays, 2002; Tassinari, Panzini, Ravaioli, Maltoni, & Sartori, 2002). Although some understanding of quality of life in palliative care has been gained, there are no well established and validated HRQOL tools available to date (Tassinari et al., 2002).

Process or Outcome Focus

A second means of clarifying the purpose of HRQOL assessment is to delineate whether HRQOL issues are process- or outcome-focused. While HRQOL factors are often labeled as endpoints or outcomes, many would be labeled more appropriately as treatment-related processes. Symptom distress and alterations in functional status—core domains in most cooperative group studies and most general HRQOL measures—occur most frequently during active treatment. While knowledge about the amount of symptom distress or the inability to carry out usual activities is important, patients may consider these conditions endurable with a perspective that the condition is temporary and accompanied by a hope of cure. Endpoint concerns might focus on concepts such as transcendence, role changes, and altered body image. Quality-of-life-assessments that are meaning-based, rather than function-based, may yield very different information depending on whether variables are assessed as process or outcome. For example, patients' perspectives of their cancer experience, and the meanings they derive from the experience, often change following the initial diagnosis and treatment phase. Even after completion of treatments the meaning of the experience may be evolving (Haase & Rostad, 1994).

One approach to addressing lack of sensitivity to the subtleties and complexities of human perception relative to quality of life is to incorporate the construct of response shift in HRQOL studies. Response shift is defined as the change in individuals' internal standards, values, and conceptualizations of HRQOL that accompany a change in an individual's health state (Schwartz & Sprangers, 2000). A test of two models of response shift effects on HRQOL in men treated for prostate cancer concluded response shifts may be an identifiable process of accommodation to disease-induced deterioration that preserves social and emotional well-being (Lepore & Eton, 2000). Similar conclusions were found in a study of patients with colon cancer who had radical resection with or without adjuvant chemotherapy (Bernhard, Hurny, Maibach, Herrmann, & Laffer, 1999). Further exploratory investigation of response shift in perception of health among newly diagnosed colon cancer patients indicated patients substantively reframed their internal standards of health, as well as their perceived HRQOL (Bernhard, Lowy, Maibach, & Hurny, 2001). Such studies offer a promising approach to researchers who seek to strengthen understanding of HRQOL as a standard outcome for oncology care.

In decisions about process and outcomes, timing and perspective are key factors (Huisman, van Dam, Aaronson, & Hanewald, 1987). In order to assess process, HRQOL factors must be assessed more than once and at times when the process is likely to vary. Relevant times depend on whose perspective is sought and for what purpose. As an example, from a physician's perspective, if the purpose for evaluation is to determine which treatment produces the least symptom distress, the timing of measures should be based on anticipated times of exacerbation following alternative treatments. A patient, on the other hand, may view HRQOL in terms of an ability to resume desired activities. Relevant timing to assess symptom distress from a patient's perspective may be dictated, for example, on whether an adolescent is able to go to a desired party on the weekend.

Clearly delineating processes by identifying phases of disease and treatment may increase the sensitivity of instruments as well as dictate variables of importance. A good example of differences in patient perspectives of HRQOL is based on the phases of acute leukemia disease and treatment (Zittoun, 1987). In the first phase, (i.e., hospitalization and induction treatment) social context, hospital milieu, personality, and other individual psychological factors are considered. In the remission phase, when consolidation and maintenance treatments are administered, the struggle for cure and quality of survival are key issues. During the remission phase, side effects and returning to normal life are important. Failures of induction treatment or relapse present very different HRQOL issues, often marked by prolonged exacerbations of uncertainty. The end-of-life phase is also unique. Quality of life in the dying process requires a clear change of focus for the patient, his or her family, and healthcare providers. In one study, HRQOL was often affected in this phase by feelings of abandonment when physicians identified there was "nothing more to do" (Gregory, 1994). In fact, as physical condition deteriorates, spiritual issues commonly gain importance as determinants of HRQOL, yet they are rarely studied (Gotay, 1985).

Identify a Conceptual or Theoretical Framework

The second step in achieving clarity in HRQOL assessment is to lay explicit claim to and describe the conceptual or theoretical basis for the assessment. One way of dealing with very basic differences in concept about the nature of HRQOL is to identify for self and others the assumptions that guide dimensions and the importance each is given.

By itself, a multidimensional approach to HRQOL assessment does not provide a conceptual basis for the HRQOL assessment. In a comparative study of two HRQOL models, even though measures selected to index each model were multidimensional and both models assessed psychological, social, and physical function aspects of oncologic HRQOL, the resulting assessments produced markedly divergent information on some of the dimensions (Costain et al., 1993). There are also merits and drawbacks of multidimensional scaling as a tool for analyzing HRQOL data (Kemmler et al., 2002). If the conceptual or theoretical basis across all HRQOL studies were explicit, it would be possible to compare findings in a way that would expand the understanding of HRQOL as a construct (Costain et al., 1993). The result could be a change in the designation of HRQOL as a primitive construct to one with definable and predictable attributes in its own right and the potential to provide a basis for development of a measure that could become the "gold standard" for indexing HRQOL in the future. King and colleagues (1997) provide a useful overview of initial attempts to link concepts in explanatory models. Examples of emerging explanatory models include Mishel's uncertainty in illness theory (Mishel, 1990), discrepancy between expected and actual outcomes (Michalos, 1986), internalized standards (Breetvelt & Van Dam, 1991), distinctions between affective and cognitive components of HRQOL (de Haes & van Knippenberg, 1989), and meaning-making processes (Northouse & Northouse, 1987).

Variable Specification

As noted in the background section of this chapter, the only way to index HRQOL at this point is through identified dimensions that are illustrative of, rather than definers of, the construct. Although it may be safe to assume that persons who have fewer symptoms, more happiness, and better functioning in daily activities have a better HRQOL, it cannot be said that these concepts are components of HRQOL (Stewart, 1992). For example, social well-being concepts appear to be predictors of HRQOL rather than a direct part of HRQOL. To date, the conceptual muddiness across HRQOL studies has precluded identifying critical attributes of HRQOL. There are processes or methods available for clarifying the defining characteristics, in this case concepts, of an amorphous construct such as HRQOL.

A variety of methods for clarifying concepts are found in nursing literature. Although it is beyond the scope of this chapter to describe each, we identify several in Table 4-1 (e.g., concept analysis, derivation, synthesis). Inductive research approaches, such as *grounded theory* and *phenomenology*, have been used to study processes and experiences of cancer patients and concepts related to HRQOL. Examples include studies of quality-of-life concerns of African American breast cancer survivors (Kooken, Haase, & Russell, 2007), cancer symptom experiences of children and families (Woodgate & Degner, 2004) and among different cultural groups (Barkwell, 2005), and quality of life at end of life (Coyle, 2006). *Concept analysis*, in which critical attributes of the concept are identified and distinguished from antecedents and outcomes of the concept, has been used to clarify concepts relevant to HRQOL (Haase, Britt, Coward, Leidy, & Penn, 1992). *Simultaneous concept analysis* provides a way of teasing out subtle differences in concepts such as hope, self-transcendence, acceptance, and spiritual perspective (Haase et al., 1992). Deductive strategies also hold promise for clarifying concepts. *Structural analyses* of an underlying measurement model provides evidence about items that constitute specific domains in instrument development (Loehlin, 1992). Whatever method or methods are used, the goal is to distinguish the concept from all other concepts—related, contrary, antecedent, and outcome concepts—and specify the relationships among the related concepts.

Relationship Specification

Because most of the dimensions now specified to illustrate HRQOL represent variables that are related to, rather than definers of, HRQOL, description of patterns of relationships among the dimensions is particularly important for clarity. Again, the explicit identification of the underlying conceptual or theoretical perspective enables meaningful interpretation of the HRQOL assessment. An atheoretical approach to conceptualizing HRQOL as a multidimensional construct results in a laundry list of variables, as can be

Table 4-2.   **Atheoretical Dimensions of QOL**

Dimensions Related to Physical Problems	Dimensions Related to Psychological, Social, and Spiritual Factors	Wider Dimensions
Physical	Psychological	Individual
Toxicity	Interpersonal	Cultural
Body image	Happiness	Political
Mobility	Spiritual	Philosophic
	Financial	Time

seen in Table 4-2. Even though such a specification of variables is said to be atheoretical, there is an implied theoretical assumption underlying the specification that can be used as a framework for specifying relationships. An ontological perspective of humans made up of biological, psychological, sociological, spiritual, and cultural elements forms the belief system for this particular type of multidimensional depiction of HRQOL. In this synergistic view, the whole of HRQOL is a compilation of the parts, a particulate–deterministic view that says every variable listed contributes to one's HRQOL. The relationship patterns implied in a laundry list of domains consist of multiple single-order associations with no means of indicating relationship patterns among the parts. Because each variable is considered necessary to predict the whole, there is no designation of which variables are *illustrative of* HRQOL versus which variables are *related to* the illustrative variables.

There are many middle range theories consistent with the ontological belief that human experience is represented best by patterns that reflect reciprocal interaction of person and environment, an unfolding of life and context. Such theories seek to specify experience in terms of processes that move through and interact with a particular time and space frame. In this perspective, the selected dimensions of HRQOL are related in ways that represent a simultaneous stochastic process (Jones, Fayers, & Simons, 1987), whereby the choice of endpoint depends on what the particular theory identifies as the ultimate focus of concern. Thus, many psychosocial theories, such as Anderson and colleagues' model of cancer stress and psychosocial course specify psychosocial adjustment as the endpoint (Andersen, Kiecolt-Glaser, & Glaser, 1994). In this model, HRQOL is a construct that is specified as affecting coping behaviors. However, one confounding problem that emerges from the relationship specifications posed is that the choice of measures for HRQOL as a construct include coping instruments. Such confounding issues are a common problem in HRQOL studies because of the conceptual difficulties, but an explicit description of the models that underpin thinking about HRQOL assessment provides a way to identify sources of confounding and to rethink relationship specifications or measure choices.

Braden's Self-Help Model (Figure 4-1) provides an example of a model that specifies relationships among variables that influence HRQOL with the outcome, global HRQOL,

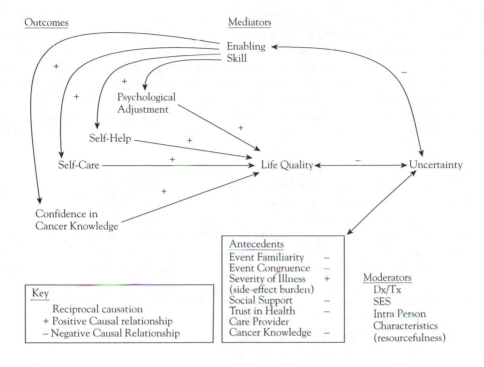

Figure 4-1.   **Combined self-help/uncertainty in illness model: Essential variables and relationships of learned response to chronic illness experience and of uncertainty in illness.**

Dx = diagnosis; Tx = treatment; SES = socioeconomic status

defined as overall satisfaction with one's current circumstance. Thus, HRQOL conceptualized as a global variable is the ultimate endpoint of a learned response to chronic illness within a specific time and space frame. Self-help and self-care are other, interrelated outcome variables that contribute to overall life satisfaction. Self-help is defined in terms of social role function and self-care is defined in terms of adult role behaviors devoted to enhancing or maintaining health. The model variables often listed *within* a symptom or side effect dimension of a multidimensional HRQOL perspective measure the concept of severity of illness, which is the primary antecedent for the initiation of learning in the cancer experience. Variables often listed in a physical functional status dimension of a multidimensional HRQOL perspective measure the concept of dependency, one of the adversities that can come with illness experience. Uncertainty is the other adversity that accompanies illness experience. Braden's theory identifies a positive relationship between symptom and side effects and uncertainty. Dependency levels increase in situations where perceived severity of illness leads individuals to feel that they have to rely on others to carry out the functional activities of daily life. Thus, dependency (Eiser, Havermans, Craft, &

Kernahan, 1995) operates as an adversity only in some, not all, illness experiences. For example, for most women, younger women in particular, the diagnosis and early treatment phase of breast cancer presents greater adversity for uncertainty than for dependency. Dependency becomes a stronger aversive aspect of cancer experience with increased illness severity and/or more aggressive treatment protocols (e.g., late stage at time of diagnosis, recurrence, bone marrow transplant, aggressive chemotherapy protocols). As previously noted, patient demographic characteristics, such as age, can also moderate the relationship between severity of illness and dependency and the relationship between severity of illness and uncertainty.

In Braden's (1993) model symptoms and side effects are not related directly to overall life satisfaction. Rather, the relationship of symptoms and side effects with global life quality is mediated by uncertainty and dependency. That is, dependency and uncertainty have specified relationships with life quality that directly undermine one's satisfaction with life. The undermining effect of symptoms and side effects relative to life quality is increased by the adversities operating in the particular situation. If the model contained only the four concepts—severity of illness, dependency, uncertainty, and life quality—and relational statements linking severity of illness to dependency and to uncertainty and linking dependency and uncertainty to life quality, the model would address only negative aspects of illness experience. Thus, the model incorporates personality and coping abilities as additional mediators. These potentially reduce the negative effect of uncertainty and dependency on life quality.

Enabling skills, the primary positive mediator in the Braden model, represent the opportunity dimension of a multidimensional HRQOL framework as described by Patrick and Erickson (1993). Thus, across the process of learning to live with illness as depicted by the Self-Help Model (Figure 4-1), many of the dimensions commonly used in HRQOL frameworks are addressed. The relationships among the dimensions are also specified. The problem of confounding is dealt with through clear definition and measure choice. For example, the measure for life quality is a global inventory of well-being instruments. Additionally, the model incorporates feedback loops to depict the learning process over time and allow assessment of variables illustrative of HRQOL over the cancer experience, from diagnosis to long-term survival phases.

Specify Measurement Criteria

Desirable characteristics of HRQOL measures include having been developed from an appropriate conceptual or theoretical framework; adequate evidence of validity and reliability; responsive to changes; based on client-generated data; and acceptable to clients, health providers, and researchers (Donovan et al., 1989). In applying these criteria to specific HRQOL instruments, Donovan and colleagues (1989) concluded many HRQOL instruments clearly were inadequate, some met many of the criteria, but none met all criteria. The situation is not different for concepts related to HRQOL. For example, in a review of the state of knowledge about fatigue, the authors concluded there is lack of theoretical models of fatigue (Winningham et al., 1994). It then follows that most fatigue measures lack a conceptual basis. The instruments do not clearly distinguish fatigue from depression or other mood situations. In order for instruments to be responsive to change, they must have reasonable total numbers of items and at least five items per domain (Donovan et al., 1989). These criteria often require a greater response burden, especially if several concepts related to HRQOL are of interest. To be acceptable to respondents and healthcare providers, HRQOL instruments need to be able to be completed in a reasonable amount of time, easily administered and scored, readily understandable, and perceived as relevant and meaningful to the respondents (Donovan et al., 1989).

CONCLUSION

The conceptualization issues that continue to interfere with the ability to adequately and appropriately assess the HRQOL of oncology clients are, firstly, *conceptual inadequacy* relative to domains selected as illustrative of HRQOL and, secondly, *psychometric inadequacy* of measures with failure to use client-generated data to develop or to confirm instrument items and to test reliability, validity, and sensitivity or responsiveness to change. Conceptual inadequacy can be attributed to the failure to use a client perspective, rather than that of a healthcare provider, about what is important for domain specification and the continued, unquestioned selection of existing instruments that are not sensitive to context. There is also failure to use theory to guide domain selection, which decreases the ability to identify whether variables illustrating HRQOL are of equal weight relative to overall life satisfaction, cost, and quality-of-care outcomes. Theoretical approaches fail in several ways. First, one cannot assess if or how domains are related to one another. Second, there is no way to interpret the meaning of relationship patterns. Third, there is no basis for specifying whether the dimensions are moderated or mediated by person-, disease-, and/or treatment-related factors relative to overall life satisfaction, cost, and quality-of-care outcomes. Psychometric inadequacy contributes to problems with credibility of findings, which then further undermine inclusion of HRQOL assessment in clinical trials.

Guidelines for achieving conceptual clarity include specification of the purpose of HRQOL assessment, specifically designating the population of interest, and identifying whether the focus is on process or endpoint. Additionally, a conceptual or theoretical framework should be utilized. This requires identification of clearly defined concepts and the relationships between them.

Finally, criteria for measurement should be specified. Instruments selected to measure concepts should have not only well established psychometric properties, but should also include criteria regarding response burden.

REFERENCES

Aaronson, N. K., & da Silva, F. C. (1987). Prospects for the future: Quality of life evaluation in prostatic cancer protocols. *Prog Clin Biol Res, 243B*, 501–512.

Aaronson, N. K., Meyerowitz, B. E., Bard, M., Bloom, J. R., Fawzy, F. I., Feldstein, M., et al. (1991). Quality of life research in oncology. Past achievements and future priorities. *Cancer, 67*(3 Suppl), 839–843.

Albert, S. M. (1998). Defining and measuring quality of life in medicine. *Jama, 279*(6), 429; author reply 431.

Andersen, B., Kiecolt-Glaser, J., & Glaser, R. A. (1994). A biobehavioral model of cancer stress and disease course. *American Psychologist, 49*, 319–404.

Baker, F., Wingard, J. R., Curbow, B., Zabora, J., Jodrey, D., Fogarty, L., et al. (1994). Quality of life of bone marrow transplant long-term survivors. *Bone Marrow Transplant, 13*(5), 589–596.

Ballatori, E. (2001). Unsolved problems in evaluating the quality of life of cancer patients. *Ann Oncol, 12 Suppl 3*, S11–S13.

Barkwell, D. (2005). Cancer pain: Voices of the Ojibway people. *J Pain Symptom Manage, 30*(5), 454–464.

Bernhard, J., Hurny, C., Maibach, R., Herrmann, R., & Laffer, U. (1999). Quality of life as subjective experience: Reframing of perception in patients with colon cancer undergoing radical resection with or without adjuvant chemotherapy. Swiss Group for Clinical Cancer Research (SAKK). *Ann Oncol, 10*(7), 775–782.

Bernhard, J., Lowy, A., Maibach, R., & Hurny, C. (2001). Response shift in the perception of health for utility evaluation. An explorative investigation. *Eur J Cancer, 37*(14), 1729–1735.

Bliss, J. M., Selby, P. J., Robertson, B., & Powles, T. J. (1992). A method for assessing the quality of life of cancer patients: Replication of the factor structure. *Br J Cancer, 65*(6), 961–966.

Bonomi, A. E., Cella, D. F., Hahn, E. A., Bjordal, K., Sperner-Unterweger, B., Gangeri, L., et al. (1996). Multilingual translation of the Functional Assessment of Cancer Therapy (FACT) quality of life measurement system. *Qual Life Res, 5*(3), 309–320.

Braden, C. J. (1993). Research program on learned response to chronic illness experience: Self-help model. *Holist Nurs Pract, 8*(1), 38–44.

Bradlyn, A. S., Harris, C. V., & Spieth, L. E. (1995). Quality of life assessment in pediatric oncology: A retrospective review of phase III reports. *Soc Sci Med, 41*(10), 1463–1465.

Brady, M. J., Peterman, A. H., Fitchett, G., Mo, M., & Cella, D. (1999). A case for including spirituality in quality of life measurement in oncology. *Psychooncology, 8*(5), 417–428.

Breetvelt, I. S., & Van Dam, F. S. (1991). Underreporting by cancer patients: The case of response-shift. *Soc Sci Med, 32*(9), 981–987.

Cascinu, S., Labianca, R., Daniele, B., Beretta, G., & Salvagni, S. (2001). Survival and quality of life in gastrointestinal tumors: Two different end points? *Ann Oncol, 12 Suppl 3*, S31–S36.

Cella, D., Hahn, E. A., & Dineen, K. (2002). Meaningful change in cancer-specific quality of life scores: Differences between improvement and worsening. *Qual Life Res, 11*(3), 207–221.

Cella, D. F. (1992). Quality of life: The concept. *J Palliat Care, 8*(3), 8–13.

Cella, D. F., & Tulsky, D. S. (1990). Measuring quality of life today: Methodological aspects. *Oncology (Williston Park), 4*(5), 29–38; discussion 69.

Chauhan, C., & Eppard, W. (2005). The impact of quality of life measurements on the patient. *Curr Probl Cancer, 29*(6), 332–342.

Coates, A. S., Hurny, C., Peterson, H. F., Bernhard, J., Castiglione-Gertsch, M., Gelber, R. D., et al. (2000). Quality-of-life scores predict outcome in metastatic but not early breast cancer. International Breast Cancer Study Group. *J Clin Oncol, 18*(22), 3768–3774.

Cohen, S. R., & Leis, A. (2002). What determines the quality of life of terminally ill cancer patients from their own perspective? *J Palliat Care, 18*(1), 48–58.

Compas, B. E., Connor-Smith, J. K., Saltzman, H., Thomsen, A. H., & Wadsworth, M. E. (2001). Coping with stress during childhood and adolescence: Problems, progress, and potential in theory and research. *Psychol Bull, 127*(1), 87–127.

Corner, J. (1997). Beyond survival rates and side effects: Cancer nursing as therapy. The Robert Tiffany Lecture. 9th International Conference on Cancer Nursing, Brighton, UK, August 1996. *Cancer Nurs, 20*(1), 3–11.

Costain, K., Hewison, J., & Howes, M. (1993). Comparison of function-based model and a meaning-based model of quality of life in oncology: Multidimensionality examined. *Journal Psychosocial Oncology, 11*(4), 17–37.

Coward, D. D. (1991). Self-transcendence and emotional well-being in women with advanced breast cancer. *Oncol Nurs Forum, 18*(5), 857–863.

Coyle, N. (2006). The hard work of living in the face of death. *J Pain Symptom Manage, 32*(3), 266–274.

Cummins, R. A. (2005). Moving from the quality of life concept to a theory. *J Intellect Disabil Res, 49*(Pt 10), 699–706.

de Haes, J. C., & van Knippenberg, F. C. (1989). Quality of life instruments for cancer patients: "Babel's Tower revisited." *J Clin Epidemiol, 42*(12), 1239–1241.

Decker, C. L., Haase, J. E., & Bell, C. J. (2007). Uncertainty in adolescents and young adults with cancer. *Oncology Nursing Forum, 34*(3), 681–688.

Detmar, S. B., Muller, M. J., Schornagel, J. H., Wever, L. D., & Aaronson, N. K. (2002). Health-related quality-of-life assessments and patient-physician communication: A randomized controlled trial. *Jama, 288*(23), 3027–3034.

Dijkers, M. (2007). "What's in a name?" The indiscriminate use of the "Quality of life" label, and the need to bring about clarity in conceptualizations. *Int J Nurs Stud, 44*(1), 153–155.

Dijkers, M. P. (2003). Individualization in quality of life measurement: Instruments and approaches. *Arch Phys Med Rehabil, 84*(4 Suppl 2), S3–S14.

Donovan, K., Sanson-Fisher, R. W., & Redman, S. (1989). Measuring quality of life in cancer patients. *J Clin Oncol, 7*(7), 959–968.

Dow, K. H., Ferrell, B. R., Haberman, M. R., & Eaton, L. (1999). The meaning of quality of life in cancer survivorship. *Oncol Nurs Forum, 26*(3), 519–528.

Eiser, C., Havermans, T., Craft, A., & Kernahan, J. (1995). Development of a measure to assess the perceived illness experience after treatment for cancer. *Arch Dis Child, 72*(4), 302–307.

El-Serag, H. B., Olden, K., & Bjorkman, D. (2002). Health-related quality of life among persons with irritable bowel syndrome: A systematic review. *Aliment Pharmacol Ther, 16*(6), 1171–1185.

Faden, R., & Leplege, A. (1992). Assessing quality of life. Moral implications for clinical practice. *Med Care, 30*(5 Suppl), MS166–MS175.

Ferrans, C. E. (1990). Quality of life: Conceptual issues. *Semin Oncol Nurs, 6*(4), 248–254.

Ferrell, B., Grant, M., Schmidt, G. M., Rhiner, M., Whitehead, C., Fonbuena, P., et al. (1992a). The meaning of quality of life for bone marrow transplant survivors. Part 1. The impact of bone marrow transplant on quality of life. *Cancer Nurs, 15*(3), 153–160.

Ferrell, B., Grant, M., Schmidt, G. M., Rhiner, M., Whitehead, C., Fonbuena, P., et al. (1992b). The meaning of quality of life for bone marrow transplant survivors. Part 2. Improving quality of life for bone marrow transplant survivors. *Cancer Nurs, 15*(4), 247–253.

Ferrell, B. R. (1990). Development of a quality of life index for patients with cancer. *Oncology Nursing Forum, 17*(3(Suppl)), 15–19.

Ferrell, B. R., Ferrell, B. A., Ahn, C., & Tran, K. (1994). Pain management for elderly patients with cancer at home. *Cancer, 74*(7 Suppl), 2139–2146.

Frank, L., Kleinman, L., Leidy, N. K., Legro, M., Shikiar, R., & Revicki, D. (1998). Defining and measuring quality of life in medicine. *Jama, 279*(6), 429–430; author reply 431.

Frost, M. H., Bonomi, A. E., Ferrans, C. E., Wong, G. Y., & Hays, R. D. (2002). Patient, clinician, and population perspectives on determining the clinical significance of quality-of-life scores. *Mayo Clin Proc, 77*(5), 488–494.

Goodinson, S. M., & Singleton, J. (1989). Quality of life: A critical review of current concepts, measures and their clinical implications. *Int J Nurs Stud, 26*(4), 327–341.

Goodwin, P. J. (2001). Economics, quality of life and breast cancer outcomes—is balance possible? *Breast, 10*, 190–198.

Gotay, C. C. (1985). Why me? Attributions and adjustment by cancer patients and their mates at two stages in the disease process. *Soc Sci Med, 20*(8), 825–831.

Graves, K. D. (2003). Social cognitive theory and cancer patients' quality of life: A meta-analysis of psychosocial intervention components. *Health Psychol, 22*(2), 210–219.

Gregory, D. (1994). *Narratives of suffering in the cancer experience.* Unpublished Dissertation, University of Arizona College of Nursing, Tucson.

Grumann, M., & Schlag, P. M. (2001). Assessment of quality of life in cancer patients: Complexity, criticism, challenges. *Onkologie, 24*(1), 10–15.

Gunnars, B., Nygren, P., & Glimelius, B. (2001). Assessment of quality of life during chemotherapy. *Acta Oncol, 40*(2-3), 175–184.

Haase, J. E. (1987). Components of courage in chronically ill adolescents: A phenomenological study. *ANS Adv Nurs Sci, 9*(2), 64–80.

Haase, J. E., Britt, T., Coward, D. D., Leidy, N. K., & Penn, P. E. (1992). Simultaneous concept analysis of spiritual perspective, hope, acceptance and self-transcendence. *Image J Nurs Sch, 24*(2), 141–147.

Haase, J. E., & Rostad, M. (1994). Experiences of completing cancer therapy: Children's perspectives. *Oncol Nurs Forum, 21*(9), 1483–1492; discussion 1493–1494.

Hakamies-Blomqvist, L., Luoma, M. L., Sjostrom, J., Pluzanska, A., Sjodin, M., Mouridsen, H., et al. (2001). Timing of quality of life (QoL) assessments as a source of error in oncological trials. *J Adv Nurs, 35*(5), 709–716.

Herth, K. A. (1989). The relationship between level of hope and level of coping response and other variables in patients with cancer. *Oncol Nurs Forum, 16*(1), 67–72.

Hinds, P., & Haase, J. (2003). Theory development in quality of life for children and adolescents with cancer. In C. King & P. Hinds (Eds.), *Quality of life from nursing and patient perspectives: Theory, research, and practice* (2nd ed., pp. 143–168). Sudbury, MA: Jones and Bartlett.

Holland, P. W., & Wainer, H. (1993). *Differential item functioning.* Hillsdale, NJ: Lawrence Erlbaum.

Holzner, B., Kemmler, G., Kopp, M., Moschen, R., Schweigkofler, H., Dunser, M., et al. (2001b). Quality of life in breast cancer patients—not enough attention for long-term survivors? *Psychosomatics, 42*(2), 117–123.

Holzner, B., Kemmler, G., Sperner-Unterweger, B., Kopp, M., Dunser, M., Margreiter, R., et al. (2001a). Quality of life measurement in oncology—a matter of the assessment instrument? *European Journal of Cancer, 37*(18), 2349–2356.

Huisman, S., van Dam, F., Aaronson, N. K., & Hanewald, G. (1987). On measuring complaints of cancer patients: Some remarks on the time span of the question. In N. K. Aaronson & J. Beckman (Eds.), *Quality of life of cancer patients* (pp. 101–109). New York, NY: Raven Press.

Iwamoto, R. (1994). Cultural influences on quality of life. *Quality of Life: A Nursing Challenge, 3*(4), 68–73.

Jenkins, C. D., Jono, R. T., Stanton, B. A., & Stroup-Benham, C. A. (1990). The measurement of health-related quality of life: Major dimensions identified by factor analysis. *Soc Sci Med, 31*(8), 925–931.

Jones, D. R., Fayers, P. M., & Simons, J. (1987). Measuring and analyzing quality of life in cancer clinical trials. In N. K. Aaronson & J. Beckman (Eds.), *Quality of life of cancer patients* (pp. 41–61). New York, NY: Raven Press.

Kaczorowski, J. M. (1989). Spiritual well-being and anxiety in adults diagnosed with cancer. *Hosp J, 5*(3–4), 105–116.

Karnofsky, D. A., & Burchenal, J. H. (1949). The clinical evaluation of chemotherapeutic agents in cancer. In C. M. McCleod (Ed.), *Evaluation of chemotherapeutic agents.* New York, NY: Columbia University Press.

Kemmler, G., Holzner, B., Kopp, M., Dunser, M., Greil, R., Hahn, E., et al. (2002). Multidimensional scaling as a tool for analysing quality of life data. *Qual Life Res, 11*(3), 223–233.

Kemmler, G., Holzner, B., Kopp, M., Dunser, M., Margreiter, R., Greil, R., et al. (1999). Comparison of two quality-of-life instruments for cancer patients: The functional assessment of cancer therapy-general and the European Organization for Research and Treatment of Cancer Quality of Life Questionnaire-C30. *J Clin Oncol, 17*(9), 2932–2940.

King, C. R., Haberman, M., Berry, D. L., Bush, N., Butler, L., Dow, K. H., et al. (1997). Quality of life and the cancer experience: The state-of-the-knowledge. *Oncol Nurs Forum, 24*(1), 27–41.

Kiss, T. L., Abdolell, M., Jamal, N., Minden, M. D., Lipton, J. H., & Messner, H. A. (2002). Long-term medical outcomes and quality-of-life assessment of patients with chronic myeloid leukemia followed at least 10 years after allogeneic bone marrow transplantation. *J Clin Oncol, 20*(9), 2334–2343.

Koller, M., Klinkhammer-Schalke, M., & Lorenz, W. (2005). Outcome and quality of life in medicine: A conceptual framework to put quality of life research into practice. *Urol Oncol, 23*(3), 186–192.

Kooken, W. C., Haase, J. E., & Russell, K. M. (2007). "I've been through something": Poetic explorations of African American women's cancer survivorship. *West J Nurs Res, 29*(7), 896–919; discussion 920–899.

Koopmans, P. P. (2002). Clinical endpoints in trials of drugs for cancer: Time for a rethink? *Bmj, 324*(7350), 1389–1391.

Kopp, M., Schweigkofler, H., Holzner, B., Nachbaur, D., Niederwieser, D., Fleischhacker, W. W., et al. (1998). Time after bone marrow transplantation as an important variable for quality of life: Results of a cross-sectional investigation using two different instruments for quality-of-life assessment. *Ann Hematol, 77*(1–2), 27–32.

Kuenstner, S., Langelotz, C., Budach, V., Possinger, K., Krause, B., & Sezer, O. (2002). The comparability of quality of life scores. A multitrait multimethod analysis of the EORTC QLQ-C30, SF-36 and FLIC questionnaires. *Eur J Cancer, 38*(3), 339–348.

Langenhoff, B. S., Krabbe, P. F., Wobbes, T., & Ruers, T. J. (2001). Quality of life as an outcome measure in surgical oncology. *Br J Surg, 88*(5), 643–652.

Leidy, N. K., & Haase, J. E. (1999). Functional status from the patient's perspective: The challenge of preserving personal integrity. *Res Nurs Health, 22*(1), 67–77.

Leininger, M. (1994). Quality of life from a transcultural nursing perspective. *Nurs Sci Q, 7*(1), 22–28.

Leplege, A., & Hunt, S. (1997). The problem of quality of life in medicine. *JAMA, 278*(1), 47–50.

Lepore, S. J., & Eton, D. T. (2000). Response shifts in prostate cancer patients: An evaluation of suppressor and buffer models. In C. E. Schwartz & M. A. Sprangers (Eds.), *Adaptation to Changing Health Response Shift in Quality-of-Life Research* (pp. 37–51). Washington, DC: American Psychological Association.

Levine, M. N., & Ganz, P. A. (2002). Beyond the development of quality-of-life instruments: Where do we go from here? *J Clin Oncol, 20*(9), 2215–2216.

Loehlin, J. C. (1992). *Latent variable models: An introduction to factor, path, and structural analysis* (2nd ed.). Hillsdale, NJ: Lawrence Erlbaum Associates, Inc.

Mackworth, N., Fobair, P., & Prados, M. D. (1992). Quality of life self-reports from 200 brain tumor patients: Comparisons with Karnofsky performance scores. *J Neurooncol, 14*(3), 243–253.

Marshall, P. A. (1990). Cultural influences on perceived quality of life. *Semin Oncol Nurs, 6*(4), 278–284.

Mast, M. E. (1995). Definition and measurement of quality of life in oncology nursing research: Review and theoretical implications. *Oncol Nurs Forum, 22*(6), 957–964.

Mast, M. E. (1998). Correlates of fatigue in survivors of breast cancer. *Cancer Nurs, 21*(2), 136–142.

McBride, A. B. (1993). Managing chronicity: The heart of nursing care. In S. Funk, E. Tornquist, M. Champagne & R. Wiese (Eds.), *Key Aspects of Caring for the Chronically Ill.* New York, NY: Springer.

Michalos, A.C. (1986). Job satisfaction, marital satisfaction and quality of life: A review and a preview. In F. M. Andrews (Ed.), *Research on the quality of life* (pp. 57–83). Ann Arbor, MI: University of Michigan Press.

Mishel, M. H. (1990). Reconceptualization of the uncertainty in illness theory. *Image J Nurs Sch, 22*(4), 256–262.

Moinpour, C. M. (1994). Measuring quality of life: An emerging science. *Semin Oncol, 21*(5 Suppl 10), 48–60; discussion 60-43.

Moinpour, C. M., Feigl, P., Metch, B., Hayden, K. A., Meyskens, F. L., Jr., & Crowley, J. (1989). Quality of life end points in cancer clinical trials: Review and recommendations. *J Natl Cancer Inst, 81*(7), 485–495.

Molassiotis, A., & Morris, P. J. (1998). The meaning of quality of life and the effects of unrelated donor bone marrow transplants for chronic myeloid leukemia in adult long-term survivors. *Cancer Nurs, 21*(3), 205–211.

Moons, P., Budts, W., & De Geest, S. (2006). Critique on the conceptualisation of quality of life: A review and evaluation of different conceptual approaches. *Int J Nurs Stud, 43*(7), 891–901.

Mor, V., & Guadagnoli, E. (1988). Quality of life measurement: A psychometric tower of Babel. *J Clin Epidemiol, 41*(11), 1055–1058.

Mosconi, P., Colozza, M., De Laurentiis, M., De Placido, S., & Maltoni, M. (2001). Survival, quality of life and breast cancer. *Ann Oncol, 12 Suppl 3*, S15–S19.

Murphy, S. B. (2003). Research involving long-term survivors of childhood and adolescent cancer: Issues impacting design and conduct of clinical trials. *Curr Probl Cancer, 27*(4), 225–235.

Mytko, J. J., & Knight, S. J. (1999). Body, mind and spirit: Towards the integration of religiosity and spirituality in cancer quality of life research. *Psychooncology, 8*(5), 439–450.

Nail, L., & Jones, L. (1995). Fatigue as a side effect of cancer treatment: Impact on quality of life. *Quality of Life: A Nursing Challenge, 4*, 8–13.

Northouse, P. G., & Northouse, L. (1987). Communication and cancer: Issues confronting patients, health professionals and family members. *Journal of Psychosocial Oncology, 5*(3), 17–46.

Owen, D. C. (1989). Nurses' perspectives on the meaning of hope in patients with cancer: A qualitative study. *Oncol Nurs Forum, 16*(1), 75–79.

Padilla, G., Presant, C. A., Grant, M., Baker, C., & Metter, G. (1981). *Assessment of quality of life in cancer patients.* Paper presented at the Proceedings American Association of Cancer Research.

Padilla, G. V., Ferrell, B., Grant, M. M., & Rhiner, M. (1990). Defining the content domain of quality of life for cancer patients with pain. *Cancer Nurs, 13*(2), 108–115.

Patrick, D. L., & Erickson P. (1993). *Health Status and Health Policy.* New York, NY: Oxford University Press.

Patrick, D. L., & Guttmacher, S. (1983). Socio-political issues in the uses of health indicators *Health indicators* (pp. 165–173). Oxford, England: Martin Robertson and Company.

Peterman, A. H., Fitchett, G., Brady, M. J., Hernandez, L., & Cella, D. (2002). Measuring spiritual well-being in people with cancer: The functional assessment of chronic illness therapy—Spiritual Well-being Scale (FACIT-Sp). *Ann Behav Med, 24*(1), 49–58.

Piper, B. F. (1991). Alterations in energy: The sensation of fatigue. In S. Baird & R. McCorkle (Eds.), *Cancer nursing: A comprehensiver textbook* (pp. 1461). Philadelphia, PA: W.B. Sauders.

Priestman, T. (1987). Evaluation of quality of life in women with breast cancer. In N. K. Aaronson & J. Beckman (Eds.), *Quality of life of cancer patients* (pp. 193–199). New York, NY: Raven Press.

Quill, T., Norton, S., Shah, M., Lam, Y., Fridd, C., & Buckley, M. (2006). What is most important for you to achieve?: An analysis of patient responses when receiving palliative care consultation. *J Palliat Med, 9*(2), 382–388.

Schag, C. A., Ganz, P. A., & Heinrich, R. L. (1991). Cancer Rehabilitation Evaluation System—short form (CARES-SF). A cancer specific rehabilitation and quality of life instrument. *Cancer, 68*(6), 1406–1413.

Schipper, H. (1990). Definition and conceptual issues. In B. Spilker (Ed.), *Quality of life assessments in clinical trials* (pp. 11–24). New York, NY: Raven Press.

Schipper, H. (1990b). Quality of life. *Journal of Psychosocial Oncology, 8*(2–3), 171–185.

Schwartz, C. E., & Sprangers, M. A. (2000). Introduction. In C. E. Schwartz & M. A. Sprangers (Eds.), *Adaptation to Changing Health Response Shift in Quality-of-Life Research* (pp. xiii–xvi). Washington, DC: American Psychological Association.

Sherbourne, C. D., Unutzer, J., Schoenbaum, M., Duan, N., Lenert, L. A., Sturm, R., et al. (2001). Can utility-weighted health-related quality-of-life estimates capture health effects of quality improvement for depression? *Medical Care, 39*(11), 1246–1259.

Sloan, J. A., Frost, M. H., Berzon, R., Dueck, A., Guyatt, G., Moinpour, C., et al. (2006). The clinical significance of quality of life assessments in oncology: A summary for clinicians. *Support Care Cancer, 14*(10), 988–998.

Smith, D. J. & Huntington, J. (2006). Choosing the "correct" assessment tool. *Curr Probl Cancer, 30*(6), 272–282.

Somerfield, M. (2001). Hazards of quality-of-life data for clinical decision making. *J Clin Oncol, 19*(2), 594–595.

Sousa, K. H., & Chen, F. F. (2002). A theoretical approach to measuring quality of life. *J Nurs Meas, 10*(1), 47–58.

Steeves, R. H., & Kahn, D. L. (1987). Experience of meaning in suffering. *Image J Nurs Sch, 19*(3), 114–116.

Stewart, A. (1992). Conceptual and methodological issues in defining quality of life: State of the art. *Progress in Cardiovascular Nursing, 7*, 3–10.

Tassinari, D., Panzini, I., Ravaioli, A., Maltoni, M., & Sartori, S. (2002). Quality of life at the end of life: How is the solution far away? *J Clin Oncol, 20*(6), 1704–1705.

Teresi, J. A., Golden, R. R., Cross, P., Gurland, B., Kleinman, M., & Wilder, D. (1995). Item bias in cognitive screening measures: Comparisons of elderly white, Afro-American, Hispanic and high and low education subgroups. *J Clin Epidemiol, 48*(4), 473–483.

Teresi, J. A., Kleinman, M., & Ocepek-Welikson, K. (2000). Modern psychometric methods for detection of differential item functioning: Application to cognitive assessment measures. *Stat Med, 19*(11–12), 1651–1683.

Testa, M. A., & Simonson, D. C. (1996). Assesment of quality-of-life outcomes. *N Engl J Med, 334*(13), 835–840.

Thorne, S. E., & Paterson, B. L. (2000). Two decades of insider research: What we know and don't know about chronic illness experience. *Annu Rev Nurs Res, 18*, 3–25.

Tomich, P. L., & Helgeson, V. S. (2002). Five years later: A cross-sectional comparison of breast cancer survivors with healthy women. *Psychooncology, 11*(2), 154–169.

Trippoli, S., Vaiani, M., Linari, S., Longo, G., Morfini, M., & Messori, A. (2001). Multivariate analysis of factors influencing quality of life and utility in patients with haemophilia. *Haematologica, 86*(7), 722–728.

Ward, W. L., Hahn, E. A., Mo, F., Hernandez, L., Tulsky, D. S., & Cella, D. (1999). Reliability and validity of the Functional Assessment of Cancer Therapy-Colorectal (FACT-C) quality of life instrument. *Qual Life Res, 8*(3), 181–195.

Winningham, M. L., Nail, L. M., Burke, M. B., Brophy, L., Cimprich, B., Jones, L. S., et al. (1994). Fatigue and the cancer experience: The state of the knowledge. *Oncol Nurs Forum, 21*(1), 23–36.

Woodgate, R. L., & Degner, L. F. (2004). Cancer symptom transition periods of children and families. *J Adv Nurs, 46*(4), 358–368.

Zebrack, B. J. (2000). Cancer survivor identity and quality of life. *Cancer Pract, 8*(5), 238–242.

Zebrack, B. J., Ganz, P. A., Bernaards, C. A., Petersen, L., & Abraham, L. (2006). Assessing the impact of cancer: Development of a new instrument for long-term survivors. *Psychooncology, 15*(5), 407–421.

Zittoun, R. (1987). Quality of life in adults with acute leukemia. In N. K. Aaronson & J. Beckman (Eds.), *Quality of Life in Cancer Patients* (pp. 183–192). New York, NY: Raven Press.

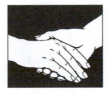

Spiritual Quality of Life

ELIZABETH JOHNSTON TAYLOR • FAYE DAVENPORT

Introduction

Mrs. Brown is a 57-year-old woman who is receiving chemotherapy for colorectal cancer. When asked about the quality of her life, she reports that she is adversely affected by nausea, sluggishness, worry, and sadness. She wistfully describes how her cancer and its treatments have limited her social interactions. She doesn't have the energy to romp with her grandkids or to have sex with her husband. Her once weekly lunch dates with friends are on hold; she is unable to cook or clean now, and she is very disappointed that a planned vacation cruise with her husband had to be cancelled. Mrs. Brown then confides, "what's really getting to me is the part that people can't see—the questions I have inside. Like, what's the purpose for this happening to me? Why would God allow this to happen to me? And some days, all I do is lie in bed, and as you stare at the ceiling, you wonder a lot of things. But I do keep praying, and I sometimes do get a feeling that God is out there watching out for me."

Mrs. Brown's descriptive statements and questions illustrate how spirituality is connected with the quality of the life of a person living with cancer. Her questions also demonstrate how a person's religious background can provide him or her with helpful coping strategies such as prayer, as well as distressing questions like "Why would God allow this to happen to me?" Mrs. Brown also demonstrates how overtly spiritual concerns often are difficult for individuals to voice because personal spirituality can be such an intimate topic.

The spiritual aspect of quality of life (QOL) increasingly is being recognized as an important domain of health-related quality of life (HRQOL). Until the 1990s, core dimensions of HRQOL included physical, emotional, social, and functional well-being (Brady, Peterman, Fitchett, Mo, & Cella, 1999). Now that researchers report qualitative data indicating spirituality is considered by clients to be essential to their overall quality of life, a spiritual domain is being included in concepts of HRQOL and HRQOL instruments.

Included in this chapter is a discussion about the spiritual domain of HRQOL and its importance to those who receive cancer care. Also included are a description of the elements of spiritual quality of life (SpQOL), a review of the available research about SpQOL in individuals receiving cancer care, and a description of the clinical implications that are derived from this research. Additionally, this chapter is concluded by a discussion of how SpQOL can be empirically investigated.

Conceptualizing Spiritual Quality of Life

Because the term *spiritual* is an abstraction that carries varied and personalized connotations, it is important that it be defined before any discussion of spiritual quality of life occurs. Spirituality refers to that part of being human that seeks meaningfulness through intra-, inter-, and transpersonal connection (Reed, 1992). Or, as Dossey and Guzzetta (2000) define it, spirituality is that "unifying force of a person . . . [that involves] interconnectedness with self, others, nature, and God/Life" (p. 7). As part of a process to develop a measure of SpQOL for palliative care patients, a QOL work group of the European Organization for Research and Treatment of Cancer (Vivat, 2008) reviewed literature and constructed this definition:

> Spirituality is the search for meaning in one's life and (includes) the living of one's life on the basis of one's understanding of that meaning. It may involve some or all of the following: having or finding (i) sustaining relationships with self and others; (ii) meaning beyond one's self; (iii) meaning beyond immediate events; (iv) explanations for events and/or experiences (p. 860).

Martsolf and Mickley (1998) reviewed nursing definitions of spirituality and observed five frequently reported elements of spirituality: meaning (i.e., having purpose, making sense of life), value (i.e., having cherished beliefs and standards), transcendence (i.e., appreciating a dimension that is beyond self), connecting (i.e., relating), and becoming (i.e., involving reflection, allowing life to unfold, and knowing who one is).

SpQOL of life research sometimes measures aspects of religiosity. In contemporary nursing literature, religiosity often is conceptualized as a narrower perception that is observed more easily and directly. Religions are systems of beliefs and practices that reflect spiritualities; they can also function as a bridge for developing spiritual awareness. Whether or not a person's religion is of an organized form, religion offers a participant a specific worldview and answers questions about ultimate meaning. Religion responds to, and provides mechanisms for, attending to spiritual yearnings (Taylor, 2002).

As with physical, social, and other domains of HRQOL, spiritual quality of life is comprised of several elements. Table 5-1 presents the elements of SpQOL identified by three research teams who interviewed cancer patients to develop or refine their models of HRQOL. The identification of existential well-being as an important determinant of HRQOL by Cohen, Mount, Tomas, and Mount (1996) elucidates how issues of existence and meaning can occur regardless of client religiosity. Ferrans' model (2000) does not distinguish clearly between what is spiritual and what is psychological, illustrating how great the overlap or interrelatedness of the spiritual and psychosocial domains can be. Ferrell and colleagues' (Ferrell, Dow, Leigh, Ly, & Gulasekaram,1995; Ferrell, Grant, Funk, Otis-Green, & Garcia, 1998; Ferrell, Cullinane, Ervine, Melancon, Uman, & Juarez, 2005) model confirms a reciprocal relationship between spiritual well-being and HRQOL, equating spiritual well-being with SpQOL.

Research investigating the spiritual dimensions of HRQOL utilizes a variety of terms or concepts that intend to measure SpQOL (Johnson et al., 2007; Vivat, 2008). These terms

Table 5-1.   **Elements of Spiritual Quality of Life**

Researcher/Terminology for Domain	Elements
Cohen, Mount, Tomas, & Mount (1996)/ Existential Well-being	• Concerns regarding death (existential obliteration) • Freedom (the absence of external structure) • Isolation (the unbridgeable gap separating self from all else) • Questions of meaning (the dilemma of recognizing the possibility of a cosmos without meaning)
Ferrans (2000)/ Psychological/Spiritual Domain	• Satisfaction with life • Happiness in general • Satisfaction with self • Achievement of personal goals • Peace of mind • Personal appearance • Faith in God
Ferrell & Grant (e.g., Ferrell, Grant, Funk, Otis-Green, & Garcia, 1998; in Ferrans, 2000)/ Spiritual Well-being	• Hopefulness • Suffering • Meaning of illness • Religiosity • Transcendence • Feelings of uncertainty

or concepts not only include aspects of religiosity, but also existential and spiritual well-being. Although there is no published conceptual analysis teasing out the differences between SpQOL, existential, and spiritual well-being, this author will equate the concepts, even though some conceptual differences are probable. Vivat's team (2008), for instance, differentiated between approaching spirituality as substantive (i.e., exploring the content of spiritual beliefs and experiences) and functional (i.e., how beliefs and behaviors relate to ultimate concerns). They viewed spiritual well-being and health as aspects of a functional approach to spirituality.

While research evidence documents religiousness as an important aspect of QOL for many patients and family living with cancer (Balboni et al., 2007; Hampton, Hollis, Lloyd, Taylor, & McMillan, 2007; Ka'opua, Gotay, & Boehm, 2007), Edmondson, Park, Blank, Fenster, and Mills (2008) observed while using an established 12-item tool comprised of two subscales measuring existential and religious well-being, that existential well-being fully mediated religious well-being's effect on QOL; religious well-being did not predict QOL. Indeed, research untangling the complex relationship between spirituality and religiousness in relation to QOL is needed.

Indicators of Spiritual Quality of Life

Because of the subjective nature of HRQOL (Brady et al., 1999) and because spirituality is a particularly ethereal phenomenon, it is helpful to understand what phenomenon may reveal SpQOL among persons with cancer. In addition to research investigating cancer patients' perceptions of what quality of life encompasses, research about what comprises spiritual needs for cancer patients will be reviewed.

Ferrell's research teams (Ersek, Ferrell, Dow, & Melancon, 1997; Ferrell et al., 1998b; Ferrell et al., 2005) have studied what cancer patients think quality of life means. Content analysis of 130 ovarian cancer patients' written responses to a questionnaire revealed the following themes that explicitly show the interrelatedness of spirituality and HRQOL:

- To have happiness and enjoyment, to live life to its fullest, to appreciate the small things (this is the most frequently cited theme, with 46 respondents)
- To engage in relationships, to love and be loved; to be close to God, to be spiritual, to have meaning in life, to have hope
- To be able to make a contribution, to feel worthwhile, to participate, to feel useful
- To prioritize what's important in life, to maintain balance
- To let go of control

During interviews with 161 breast cancer survivors, 83% identified that spirituality contributed to their mood and QOL (Levine, Yoo, Aviv, Ewing, & Au, 2007). Those identified included God as a comforting presence, questioning faith, anger at God, spiritual transformation of self and attitude toward others, recognition of one's own mortality, deepening faith, acceptance, and prayer. This study, as well as others (Fatone, Moadel, Floey, Fleming, & Jandorf, 2007), suggests spirituality is especially significant for Latinos and African Americans coping with cancer.

Research findings about what constitutes spiritual needs of cancer patients also offer information about what may contribute to SpQOL, assuming satisfied spiritual needs indicate SpQOL. For example, from interviews with 20 British patients with life-threatening disease (mostly cancer), Grant, Murray, Kendall, Boyd, Tilley, and Ryan (2004) identified the following spiritual needs: losing roles and self-identity, fearing death, and needing to make sense of life. These findings are mirrored by a quantitative study ($n=248$), which ranked how important such spiritual needs were to cancer patients (Moadel et al., 1999). Moadel et al. (1999) noted 51% of respondents wanted help with overcoming fears, 42% finding hope, and 40% finding meaning in life.

Data from in-depth interviews with 28 cancer patients and family caregivers suggest seven categories of spiritual needs that would determine SpQOL (Taylor, 2003b). These needs involved the following:

- Relating to God (the language of these informants): Examples of such needs include needing to know God's will, remembering how God has guided, getting right with God, believing God has or will heal, and resigning to God being in control of the illness.
- Having hope, gratitude, and being positive: Examples of such needs include needing to have hope for healing, keep a positive outlook, and count blessings.
- Giving and receiving love from other persons: Examples of such needs include needing to make the world a better place, help others, and get right with others.
- Reviewing beliefs: Examples of such needs include wondering if your beliefs about God are correct, and asking "why?" questions.
- Creating meaning and finding purpose: Examples of such needs include needing to get past asking "why me?," become aware of positive things that have come with illness, reevaluate life, and sense that there is a reason for being alive now.
- Having religious needs met: Examples of such needs include needing to pray or receive a religious ritual from a religious leader, or have quiet time or space to reflect or meditate.
- Preparing for death: Examples of such needs include needing to make sure personal business is in order, and balance thoughts about dying with hoping for health.

For both cancer patients and family caregivers ($n=224$), of the spiritual needs listed here, the most important needs included maintaining a positive perspective, loving others, being able to relate to God, and finding meaning (Taylor, 2006).

Indeed, how one satisfactorily finds meaning and positive perspective is a salient indicator of SpQOL. An increasing amount of research evidence describes spiritual transformation or stress-related personal growth that occurs for many with a history of cancer (Andrykowski et al., 2005; McGrath, 2004). Several qualitative studies, mostly of women with breast or ovarian cancer, describe how these specific illnesses can often changes one's attitude about life, self, and God. Living with cancer can prompt a survivor to live in the present more fully, reprioritize values and behave more congruently with these values, intensify spiritual awareness, appreciate life and nature more fully, and gain self-awareness and self-respect along with increased sensitivity for the suffering of others (Ferrell et al., 1998a, 1998b; McGrath, 2004).

While qualitative data suggest this spiritual transformation and personal growth are indicators of SpQOL, quantitative studies lend support as well and suggest it may be distinctive in cancer survivors. A study of 662 hematopoietic stem cell transplant survivors showed personal growth is significantly greater for cancer survivors than for healthy matched peers, and that this personal growth can last for many years after a transplant (Andrykowski et al., 2005).

These research findings provide a rich description of many of the spiritual needs that persons living with cancer experience. These needs reflect spiritual experiences that can be either distressful or euphoric. These negative and positive spiritual needs can occur simultaneously. Individuals can, for example, concurrently be engaged in a spiritually distressing wrestle with God about what is the purpose of their suffering, while experiencing forgiveness with and of others or while sensing God's providence. These spiritual needs, in concert, are what determine an individual's state of spiritual health or well-being, hence SpQOL.

Degree of Spiritual Quality of Life

The levels and patterns of SpQOL among persons with cancer are being documented now. Because several instruments for quantitatively measuring HRQOL among persons with cancer include items assessing SpQOL, it is becoming possible to identify a person's level or degree of SpQOL and to compare SpQOL with other domains of HRQOL. These data are helpful for clinicians who seek to understand who may need additional spiritual support or when an individual may be at risk for spiritual distress.

Several studies have found persons with cancer rank SpQOL first or second in importance within the domains of HRQOL. For persons facing death, two studies suggest that SpQOL ranks first or second as most important aspect of HRQOL (Kutner et al., 2003; McMillan & Weitzner, 1998; McMillan, & Weitzner, 2000; Thomson, 2000). For long-term survivors of cancer, SpQOL remains important—but not quite as important—ranking second after physical well-being (Ersek, Ferrell, Dow, & Melancon, 1997; Heiney et al., 2003; Saleh & Brockopp, 2001; Wyatt & Friedman, 1996). Other studies of persons with cancer ranking SpQOL with other HRQOL domains do not separate out those with active disease from long-term survivors, yet still report SpQOL as second (Cohen et al., 1996; Ferrell et al., 2005).

Observed together, these data may suggest that SpQOL is very important to cancer patients; even when it is not ranked as high, patients report high degrees of SpQOL. It is intriguing that even when physical symptoms become less of a concern, spiritual aspects of having lived with cancer can remain. When survivors are told their cancer is cured, they may savor the spiritual blessings that accompany a serious illness, such as increased inner strength, improved relationships, or a new or invigorated sense of mission and purpose for life. Or, they may wonder still why God allows cancer to happen.

Although there is growing evidence SpQOL may rank consistently first or second among the various domains of HRQOL, there is conflicting evidence about whether SpQOL remains constant during the cancer trajectory. That is, studies have found minimal or no differences between SpQOL measured at various times during the illness or survival trajectory (Ferrell et al., 2005), or between persons with cancer and healthy controls (Andrykowski et al., 2005; McMillan & Weitzner, 2000; Ersek et al., 1997). Other studies, however, provide evidence to question this stability of SpQOL. Patients with no impairment in their performance status were found to have significantly higher SpQOL than those with symptom distress (Heiney et al., 2003), and survivors who lived more than five years had higher SpQOL than their recently diagnosed counterparts (Ferrell et al., 1995). Two studies of women with early stage cancer may also support the contention that change in SpQOL does occur. An intervention study of 66 women being treated for stage I or stage II breast cancer reported SpQOL as most important (Heiney et al., 2003), while 49 disease-free, early stage, ovarian cancer survivors ranked SpQOL as the least important of four QOL domains, while also reporting high levels of SpQOL (Wenzel et al., 2002).

This small amount of evidence describing the patterns of SpQOL among cancer patients suggests that it either remains constant or it adapts quickly. Whether these findings reflect the response shift phenomenon observed in other HRQOL research, social desirability, optimism, or the indomitable nature of the human spirit, it may be more impressive given that small gains in HRQOL reflect significant change (Cella, Hahn, & Dineen, 2002). Regardless, it is impressive that SpQOL can remain high despite declines in physical functioning (see especially, Brady et al., 1999).

Factors Related to Spiritual Quality of Life

Certain demographic factors have been found to be associated with SpQOL among persons with cancer. When evaluating the psychometric properties of the Functional Assessment of Chronic Illness–Spiritual Well-Being scale using a sample of 1617 (83% of whom had cancer), Peterman, Fitchett, Brady, Hernandez, and Cella (2002) found that SpQOL was associated with age, gender, marital status, ethnicity, religious affiliation, and performance status. Other studies validate these findings. That is, younger cancer patients (especially those less than mid-40 years of age) have lower SpQOL (Gioiella, Berkman, & Robinson, 1998; Wyatt & Friedman, 1996) or spiritual health (Highfield, 1992). Women have higher SpQOL than do men (Ferrans, 2000; Kutner et al., 2003), as do those who are married (Ferrell et al., 1995; Gioiella et al., 1998). African Americans and Latinos have also been found to have higher SpQOL than those of Euro or Asian American ethnicities (Ashing-Giwa et al., 2004; Fatone et al., 2007; Tarakeshwar et al., 2006; Levine et al., 2007.)

The relationship between SpQOL and overall HRQOL for persons with cancer is positive and moderately strong. Researchers have observed correlations ranging from 0.25 to 0.70 for SpQOL and overall HRQOL (Brady et al., 1999; Cohen et al., 1996; Ersek et al., 1997; Ferrell et al., 1998a; Leak, Hu, & King, 2008; Manning-Walsh, 2005; Whitford, Olver, & Peterson, 2008). Brady and colleagues (1999) observed that even controlling for physical, social, and emotional HRQOL, regression analysis indicated SpQOL remained a significant contributor to HRQOL (n=1610; see also Cotton, Levine, Fitzpatrick, Dold, & Targ, 1999).

Spirituality and religiosity also predict or correlate directly and modestly with quality of life among cancer patients (Canada et al., 2006; Rabkin, McElhiney, Moran, Acree, & Folkman, 2009; Riley et al.,1998; Romero et al., 2006; Tarakeschwar et al., 2006; Tate & Forchheimer, 2002). For example, two European studies showed that cancer patients who believed in God had higher HRQOL (Becker et al., 2006; Slovacek, Slovackova, & Jebavy, 2005). Romero and colleagues (2006) documented that spirituality and a self-forgiving attitude predicted HRQOL (Beta=.44, $p<.001$) among 81 women undergoing treatment. However, Manning-Walsh (2005), did not find that having social relationships with religious congregation members affected HRQOL.

Various specific spiritual and religious factors have been explored in relation to SpQOL:

- Positive religious coping (e.g., using benevolent religious appraisals for challenging situations, sensing security with God) contributed to SpQOL (Beta=.26, $p=.005$) whereas negative religious coping, such as feeling punished or abandoned by God, lent to poorer SpQOL (Beta=−.21, p=.01) among 170 persons with advanced cancer (Tarakeschwar et al., 2006).

- Belief in an afterlife was associated with greater SpQOL among terminally ill cancer patients (n=276; p=.0001); when controlling for SpQOL, however, the afterlife beliefs did not predict end-of-life despair, further supporting the prevalent impact of SpQOL (McClain-Jacobson et al., 2004).

- Spiritual support, whether from a religious community or the medical system, was found to be associated with QOL for patients with advanced cancer (n=230) (Balboni et al., 2007).

- SpQOL was positively correlated with intrinsic religiosity (i.e., how one lives one's religion; r=.77), and negatively with extrinsic religiosity (i.e., how one uses one's religion; r=.30) in a study of 100 elderly cancer patients (Fehring, Miller, & Shaw, 1997).

- Personal growth (r=.61) and spiritual change (r=.65), as well as mental health, were related to SpQOL in a study of 49 ovarian cancer survivors (Wenzel et al., 2002).

- "Being at peace" was highly correlated with SpQOL (r=.60) among terminally ill patients (56% of these 248 had cancer), leading those observing to suggest that asking "Are you at peace?" may be a valid method for a brief assessment (Steinhauser et al., 2006).

These findings suggest a positive, internalized spirituality that provides comfort and purposefulness contributes to SpQOL. Likewise, the absence of such or emotionally disturbing religious beliefs can hinder SpQOL.

SpQOL has been linked also to other more specific physical and psychological indicators of HRQOL. The presence of distressing symptoms, such as pain, appears to negatively impact SpQOL (Fernsler, Klemm, & Miller, 1999; Wyatt & Friedman, 1996), and those with high physical well-being tend to have high spiritual well-being. Several studies show inverse relationships between SpQOL and depression, negative mood, hopelessness or helplessness, and anxiety (Cotton et al., 1999; Fehring et al., 1997; Nelson, Rosenfeld, Breitbart, & Galietta, 2002; Whitford et al., 2008; Kaczorowski, 1989). Likewise, SpQOL has been found to be directly related to psychological well-being, positive moods, hope, and a fighting spirit (Cohen et al., 1996; Fehring et al., 1997; Ferrell et al., 1998a; Cotton et al., 1999; Rabkin et al., 2009).

Spirituality or SpQOL has been linked with family caregiver QOL as well (Colgrove, Kim, & Thompson, 2007; Ka'opua et al., 2007; Tang, 2009). For example, in a study of 403 spouses of cancer survivors, spirituality was observed to play a stress-buffering role in caregiver stress (Colgrove et al., 2007). Even a cancer patient's SpQOL is indirectly correlated with the amount of strain their family caregiver experiences (r=−.65) (Redinbaugh, Baum, Tarbell, & Arnold, 2003). Interviews by Ka'opua and colleagues (2007) with elderly wives of prostate cancer patients (n=28) revealed that spiritual resources helped these women to remain connected with their community, grow personally and transformationally, have positive health attitudes and behaviors, and gain support for issues encountered in marriage. These studies provide ample support for the importance of considering SpQOL in HRQOL discussions in clinical practice.

Clinical Implications

In part because of the swelling chorus of research findings demonstrating that SpQOL is a significant contributor to HRQOL, nursing literature is replete with affirmations for nurses to support spiritual well-being in their patients and provide spiritual care. The Joint Commission (2008) now mandates spiritual assessments be completed for all patients, and that spiritual support be made available to those who request it. Furthermore, HRQOL intervention studies have begun to document that holistic interventions that include teaching patients about spiritual health are effective (Borman et al., 2005; Kristeller, Rhodes, Cripe, & Sheets, 2005; Rummans et al., 2006).

Because of the nature of nursing—the intimacy and availability required of a nurse to provide nursing care—the nurse can be an ideal professional for supporting SpQOL. This section will discuss not only some specific strategies nurses can employ to support SpQOL, but client perspectives on what promotes SpQOL. This section ends with a summary of institutional approaches to supporting SpQOL.

Client Perspectives

Before discussing what nurses can do to support SpQOL, nurses must understand the client perspective. The study of breast cancer survivors by Ferrell and colleagues (1998) directly documents the spiritual care some perceive will improve HRQOL. When asked what aspects of care were most helpful in improving their HRQOL, respondents first indicated supportive, cheerful, positive, caring hospital staff (154 of 243 patients), then identified support from family and friends (n=45) and spiritual support (n=30) as the next most important aspects of care. Yet when asked what resources they did not receive that were most necessary to improving HRQOL, only 5 of 72 respondents indicated spiritual support. Griesinger, Lorimor, Aday, Winn, and Baile (1997), however, learned from 74 terminally ill cancer patients that existential and spiritual aspects of illness are rarely the focus of care and that patients wish they were.

Nurse researchers have obtained evidence that while some cancer patients do want spiritual support from a nurse, others may *not* expect or want their nurses to address their spiritual needs (Reed, 1991). A survey of cancer patients and family caregivers (n=224) found no statistical differences between these two groups for how much they desired a nurse's spiritual caregiving; these respondents welcomed most spiritual care that was traditional, not overtly religious, and did not involve much intimacy. An exception to this observation, however, was the finding that two thirds of the respondents wanted their nurse to "pray privately" for them and 56% of caregivers wanted their loved one's nurse to pray *with* them (Taylor & Mamier, 2005). Oncology nurses need to remember patients do not view them as primary spiritual care providers. Indeed, nurses are ranked fourth (after family, friends, and clergy) as spiritual resources (Highfield, 1992). Although clients rarely identify nurses as primary spiritual resource persons, clients do recognize them as potential spiritual caregivers.

Numerous survey studies document the complementary and alternative medicine (CAM) approaches cancer patients use. Spiritual healing, faith, and prayer are often identified as some of the more frequently utilized CAM approaches (see Taylor, 2005 for a review). Studies of CAM use among persons with cancer indicate that such approaches may be especially prevalent. For example, VandeCreek, Rogers, and Lester, (1999) learned from 112 outpatients with breast cancer that 85% used prayer and 48% used spiritual healing of some type. Similarly, Sparber and colleagues (2000) found spirituality to be the most used CAM in a sample of 100 cancer patients.

Parallel findings are found in studies exploring coping strategies used by cancer patients (Pargament, 1997). When investigating spiritual coping strategies, in particular, there is evidence that spiritual beliefs and practices are fundamental, cherished, and influential mechanisms for coping with cancer (McIllmurray et al., 2003; Taylor & Outlaw, 2002; Walton & Sullivan, 2004; Zaza, Sellick, & Hillier, 2005).

Nursing Approaches to Promoting SpQOL

Although recipients of cancer care may not expect spiritual support from nurses, they do desire it and seek it out privately. Individuals who are not overtly aware of personal spirituality or receptive to spiritual care likely still want care that "boosts their spirits," gives them a "fighting spirit," or inner peace, meaningfulness, and hope. So how can nurses support their patients in developing or maintaining spiritual well-being?

The nursing literature that describes approaches to nurturing the spirit is filled with a variety of interventions that include spiritual care. Some examples of these approaches or mechanisms for nurturing the spirit are as follows:

- Presencing
- Being empathic and respectful
- Story listening or storytelling
- Encouraging self-expression through art (e.g., drawing, singing, dancing, flower arranging) or journal writing
- Facilitating recreation through play and sabbatarian rest periods
- Prayer, meditation, and guided spiritual imagery
- Providing spiritually edifying reading material or music or visual focal points
- Humor
- Facilitating religious practices
- Encouraging dream analysis
- Introducing nature
- Healing rituals
- Respecting spiritual beliefs

For in-depth descriptions of these approaches to spiritual care, readers are encouraged to consult nursing texts on spiritual care (for example, Taylor, 2002).

Because a comprehensive discussion of how to promote spiritual well-being or SpQOL is beyond the scope of this chapter, a brief review of a few specific approaches that are perhaps most pertinent to persons living with cancer are offered. Research findings suggest that assisting cancer patients to transcend their suffering and find meaning, supporting their spiritual beliefs and practices, and "simply" being caring may be especially helpful (Feher & Maly, 1999; Ferrell et al., 1998b; Taylor, 2003a).

Transcending Suffering: Finding Meaning

Persons experiencing cancer often ask spiritually painful questions in an attempt to find meaning. These questions can include questions of causality (e.g., "Why do bad things happen?"), selective incidence (e.g., "Why me—instead of someone else?"), responsibility (e.g., "Did I do something to allow this to happen to me?"), and significance (e.g., "How can I become a better person because of this?") (Taylor, 2002). Although some persons with cancer may get "stuck" in the process of searching for meaning, many are able to transcend this suffering and ascribe some positive meaning (Taylor, 2000).

Although nurses cannot make a patient find meaning, they can encourage or facilitate activities that promote a sense of meaningfulness. Activities that can help a person sense that his or her life is meaningful include altruistic deeds of service to others or the world, dedication to a cause, creative experiences of any type, and pleasurable activities. For example, bored, bedridden patients can find some meaning when they write a poem, taste gourmet food, pray for others, donate time or money for a campaign, or call to encourage another cancer survivor.

A nurse can also facilitate meaning-making by allowing patients to discuss their search for meaning. Nurses who ask thoughtful questions and listen attentively to responses may help clients to gain self-awareness. A nurse might ask, for example, "What are some of the good things that have come out of your cancer experience?" or "What sorts of lessons about life have you learned from this experience?" Sensitive responses to patients asking questions about meaning must not be superficial or avoidant; questions of meaning are ultimately unanswerable. According to Rilke in Wismer (1995), by compassionately being present to those who seek meaning, the nurse can support patients as they attempt to "be patient towards all that is unsolved . . . and . . . to love the questions themselves. . . . [to] live the questions. . . . [and] then gradually, without noticing it, live along some distant day into the answer" (p. 149).

A recent intervention, Dignity Therapy, which incorporates life review and open questions for participants, encourages reflection about what is purposeful in life and has been tested in several settings. This therapeutic approach has been found to contribute significantly to improving quality of life (Chochinov et al., 2005). Other interventions aimed at enhancing meaning (seen as an element of SpQOL) include a psychologist-led interview (Ando, Morita, Lee, & Okamoto, 2008) and short-term life review (Ando, Morita, Okamoto, & Ninosaka, 2008) (both developed in Japan), and brief, manualized intervention aimed at helping patients prepare emotionally and spiritually for end-of-life concerns (Steinhauser et al., 2008).

Supporting Spiritual Beliefs and Practices

Supporting spiritual beliefs does not require that a nurse alter or devalue personal spiritual beliefs. Neither does it mean that a nurse impose his or her beliefs unethically (Taylor, 2002). Rather, the nurse can allow the patient to explore spiritual beliefs, remember how these beliefs are helpful, and determine what beliefs may need revision. The nurse accomplishes this by remaining present, actively listening and, when appropriate, asking questions that allow the patient to probe further within. When a patient recognizes discordant beliefs, it is likely that the services of a trained chaplain will be beneficial. Indeed, nurses often support spiritual beliefs by involving chaplains, clergy, or other spiritual care experts in the care of their patients.

Supporting spiritual practices may involve assisting a patient with prayer or devotional practices, educating them about how to attend religious services when neutropenic, or safeguarding religious clothing, talismans, or other personal objects. Several recent studies have explored the efficacy of spiritual practices such as transcendental meditation (Nidich et al., 2009), prayer (Johnson et al., 2009; Levine, Aviv, Yoo, Ewing, & Au, 2009), and yoga (Duncan, Leis, & Taylor-Brown, 2008). Each of these studies has linked the spiritual practice with SpQOL and offered positive assessments for the practice. A nurse does not need to be an expert in comparative religions. Rather, the nurse only need allow the patient to give instructions for how to help and follow them respectfully. While some religious practices may be difficult for a nurse to support personally, many are rituals that a nurse who shares similar beliefs can participate in or support (Taylor, 2002).

To participate with a patient in a religious practice in a way that is healing, it is imperative the nurse do so ethically. Observing the following guidelines can help nurses to employ religious rituals with clients in an ethical manner:

- Try to understand the client's spiritual needs, resources, and preferences.
- Employ religious practices with permission.
- Respect the client's expressed wishes.
- Do not prescribe or push religious beliefs or practices.
- Strive to understand your own spiritual beliefs and needs before addressing others'.
- Employ religious practices with patients when it is appropriate, doing so in a manner that is authentic and in harmony with your spiritual beliefs (Winslow & Wehtje-Winslow, 2007).

Being Caring

Although being caring may appear to be an obvious suggestion for enhancing SpQOL, it is not easy given current healthcare system stressors and the psycho-spiritually challenging work of oncology nursing. Findings from a qualitative study of cancer patients' and family caregivers' (n=28) perspectives on how a nurse can provide spiritual care support this approach (Taylor, 2003b). When asked how a nurse could help them with their spiritual needs, these respondents almost invariably first replied with statements like "just be nice," "it's the little things," and "show care and concern."

Respondents in this study also described how they wanted to have a degree of connectedness with their nurse. Symmetry (e.g., "I want her to not be my nurse, but be my friend"), physical presence (e.g., "Just stay for a few minutes"), and authenticity (e.g., "Be genuine . . . if you're talking and connecting [with the nurse], it's a spiritual thing") were all important desired aspects of the nurse–patient relationship (Taylor, 2002). These statements underscore what chaplains and spiritual care nurse experts have often suggested: spiritual care is ultimately about *being*, not *doing*.

Institutional Approaches

A number of cancer clinicians recently have studied the efficacy of structured programs for improving HRQOL, including SpQOL (Bormann et al., 2005; Kristeller et al., 2005; Rummans et al., 2006). Kristeller and colleagues (2005) have studied the impact of a 5–7 minute discussion of spirituality in oncologist–patient conferences on HRQOL. This research team observed HRQOL improved for the cancer patients in the experimental group receiving this intervention ($p=.05$; $n=118$). Rummans and colleagues (2006) conducted a clinical trial as well, to determine whether an 8-session psycho-educational intervention would improve HRQOL. The intervention was tailored to patients present at each meeting. A chaplain discussed various issues over the course of the meetings, including grief, guilt, hope, death and afterlife, challenged beliefs, rituals, and meaning and purpose. The participants who received the intervention had a nearly significant increase in SpQOL compared to the control group ($p=.06$; $n=103$). These findings offer hope that healthcare institutions can provide care that improves SpQOL.

Empirically Investigating Spiritual Quality of Life

Studying any concept presents challenges and studying SpQOL is no exception. Whether investigating SpQOL qualitatively or quantitatively, the researcher must address certain challenges to enhance the credibility of study findings. A few of these challenges are described and several instruments for quantifying SpQOL are presented. Suggestions for future research on SpQOL are also offered.

Qualitative Research

Three of the issues pertaining specifically to qualitative research that explores SpQOL are confusion about terminology, cultural bias, and social desirability. Not only do professionals confuse religiosity with spirituality, but laypersons do so as well. While asking about spiritual well-being, for example, informants may limit responses to include only descriptions of personal religiosity. Even for informants who distinguish spirituality from religiosity, it is often difficult to identify what comprises the spiritual domain. Concepts such as meaning in life and transcendence are complex to think about, let alone put into language.

The interviewer is the instrument for collecting data during a qualitative study. The researcher(s) who designs the study and analyzes the data, likewise, personally influences the research process. Those who conduct qualitative research about SpQOL are especially prone to biasing their findings with their own cultural backgrounds. A white, educated, Christian researcher will inevitably design research, use language, and interpret data using this personal cultural framework. Trustworthiness of findings will depend on the researcher's openness, flexibility, and ability to recognize and control personal bias. Soliciting informants' feedback on preliminary analyses of data may be helpful, especially when the researcher and informant represent significantly different cultural or religious backgrounds.

Although social desirability plagues much social research, it may be a special threat to research about SpQOL. For many, recognizing spiritual distress or concerns is disconcerting personally and embarrassing socially. A sensitive, respectful interviewer's prolonged engagement may allow an informant to verbalize such private spiritual pain.

Quantitative Research

Quantitative research investigating SpQOL is tainted by conceptual muddiness. Typically, SpQOL is equated with spiritual well-being, as this author has done in this chapter. No one has clarified how spiritual well-being, health, needs, concerns, and so forth are related to SpQOL. Furthermore, what comprises a spiritual phenomenon could often be confused with a psychosocial phenomenon. HRQOL instruments that have been analyzed are often composed of items that could be argued as reflective of either the spiritual or psychosocial domain.

During the last two decades, several instruments were developed to measure quality of life with subscales that recognized the spiritual domain. These subscales are summarized in Table 5-2. McMillan and Weitzner's (2000) and Ferrans and Powers' (1992) subscales combine the spiritual domain with other psychosocial quality-of-life concerns. The Functional Assessment of Chronic Illness Therapy (Brady et al., 1999; Peterman et al., 2002), McGill (Cohen et al., 1996), World Health Organization (Brady et al., 1999), and Ferrell, and colleagues' (1998) quality-of-life instruments all include a subscale dedicated to spiritual well-being. Some SpQOL measures, like the FACIT-Sp (Peterman et al., 2002) and Spirituality Index of Well-Being (Daalman & Frey, 2004), are psychometrically strong as standalone scales.

During the past quarter century, dozens of quantitative measures for assessing spirituality or aspects of spirituality and religiosity have been developed by social scientists and healthcare professionals. These instruments measure concepts as diverse as purpose in life, hope, mysticism, daily spiritual experience, prayer experience, religious beliefs and practices, spiritual or religious coping, and forgiveness. Some of these tools may measure a concept similar to SpQOL, spiritual well-being (Brady et al., 1999).

Until the new millennium, the gold standard for measuring spiritual well-being was the 20-item Spiritual Well-Being (SWB) scale developed by Paloutzian and Ellison (Ellison, 1983). This scale has been used in over 300 studies. The scale consists of two subscales: the "vertical" dimension (i.e., how one relates to God) is measured by religious well-being (RWB); and the "horizontal" dimension of spirituality (i.e., how well one relates to self, community, and environment) is measured by the existential well-being (EWB) subscale. The RWB items use the term "God," which can be problematic for the less than 10% of Americans who avow they do not believe in a "God" (Taylor & Mamier, 2005). Each subscale contains 10 items with 6-point Likert response options. Satisfactory psychometric properties have been observed when the tool was used with cancer patients. (Permission to use the SWB can be addressed to Life Advance, Inc., 81 Front St., Nyack, NY 10960.)

Although the SWB scale is used still, the new standard for measuring SpQOL among persons with cancer is the 12-item Functional Assessment of Chronic Illness Therapy-Spiritual Well-Being Scale (FACIT-Sp) (Peterman et al., 2002). Often used and available in multiple languages, this psychometrically sound tool is presented as an appendix in Peterman and

Table 5-2. **Instruments for Measuring Spiritual Quality of Life**

Authors/Instrument/ Subscale Title	Basic Descriptors	Examples of Content for Items
Cohen, Mount, Tomas, & Mount (1996)/McGill Quality-of-Life Questionnaire (MQOL)/MQOL Existential Well-being	<ul><li>6 items with 10-point response options</li><li>Cronbach alpha = 0.87</li></ul>	<ul><li>Existence meaningful</li><li>Achieve goals</li><li>Life worthwhile</li><li>Control over life</li><li>Like self</li><li>Every day a gift</li></ul>
Daaleman & Frey (2004)/Spirituality Index of Well-being	<ul><li>12 items with 5-point response options</li><li>2 subscales: self-efficacy (6 items), life scheme (6 items)</li><li>Chronbach's alpha = .86</li><li>Test-retest reliability = .77</li></ul>	<ul><li>There is not much I can do to help myself</li><li>I can't begin to understand my problems</li><li>I haven't yet found my life's purpose</li><li>There is a great void in my life at this time</li><li>In this world, I don't know where I fit in</li></ul>
Ferrell & Grant (e.g., in Ferrell et al., 1998)/Quality-of-Life-Spiritual Well-being	<ul><li>7 items with 10-point response options</li><li>Cronbach alpha = 0.71</li></ul>	<ul><li>Feelings of hopefulness</li><li>Sense of purpose</li><li>Positive changes because of illness</li><li>Spiritual life changed</li><li>Importance of church or temple</li><li>Importance of meditation or praying</li><li>Uncertainty about the future</li></ul>
McMillan (in McMillan and Weitzner, 2000)/Hospice Quality-of-Life Index/HQLI social/spiritual domain	<ul><li>8 items, some of which may be tangential to spirituality</li><li>0–10-point response options</li><li>Cronbach alpha between 0.82 and 0.86</li></ul>	<ul><li>Meaning in life</li><li>Spiritual support from healthcare team</li><li>Support from family and friends</li><li>Emotional support</li><li>Relationship with God (however defined)</li></ul>

continues

Table 5-2. **Instruments for Measuring Spiritual Quality of Life (continued)**

Authors/Instrument/ Subscale Title	Basic Descriptors	Examples of Content for Items
Ferrans & Powers (1992)/Quality-of-Life Index (QLI)/Psychological/Spiritual domain	• Factor analysis confirmed four domains, including 7 items reflecting emotional and spiritual concerns • 6-point response scales • Original testing done with dialysis patients • Cronbach alpha for this subscale = 0.90	• Satisfaction with life • Happiness in general • Satisfaction with self • Achievement of personal goals • Peace of mind • Personal faith in God • Personal appearance
Canada, Murphy, Fitchett, Peterman, & Schover (2008)/Functional Assessment of Chronic Illness Therapy-Spiritual Well-being Scale(FACIT-Sp)	• 12 items with 5-point response scales • 3 factors, labeled: Peace (an affective component), Meaning (existential), and Faith (generic spiritual beliefs); these subscales have demonstrated internal reliability (coefficients between 0.84–0.85).	• I have a reason for living • My life has been productive • I have trouble feeling peace of mind • I feel a sense of purpose in my life • I am able to reach down deep into myself for comfort • I feel a sense of harmony within myself • My life lacks meaning and purpose • I find comfort in my faith or spiritual beliefs • I find strength in my faith or spiritual beliefs • My illness has strengthened my faith or spiritual beliefs • I know that whatever happens with my illness, things will be okay

colleagues' report (Peterman et al., 2002). The original factor analysis of the FACIT-Sp demonstrated two factors: meaning or peace, and faith. A weak, positive correlation was noted between the FACIT-Sp and Marlowe-Crowne Social Desirability Scale (r=.27). Convergent validity was supported by moderate relationships between the FACIT-Sp and related concepts of spirituality and religiosity (e.g., intrinsic religiosity, religious activity, beliefs, mood). The tool's brevity, reliability, and validity all undoubtedly contribute to its current popularity in HRQOL research. More recently, the FACIT-Sp authors have reevaluated the instrument and proposed a more psychometrically sound three-factor model (using meaning, peace, and faith)(Canada et al., 2006).

Two recent studies have examined the validity of using a single-item linear analogue scale assessment (LASA) to measure QOL, including SpQOL, among persons with cancer (Johnson et al., 2007; Yates, Chalmer, St. James, Follansbee, & McKegney, 1981). Both studies concluded the SpQOL LASA showed evidence of validity. While these are positive findings for clinicians wanting a simple assessment tool, the researchers recommend more detailed instrumentation for any study desiring better assessment of the complexity of SpQOL.

Future Research

While most study findings present strong, unified support for SpQOL contributing significantly to HRQOL, there remains opportunity for further investigation. Some discrepant findings across studies illuminate the need for improved research design and methodologies for understanding SpQOL in relation to other HRQOL phenomena. For example, there is minimal evidence regarding the relationship between SpQOL and physical well-being. Is SpQOL associated with physical pain or well-being? Ferrell and colleagues (1998) observed no relationship, while Yates and colleagues (1981) observed significant low–moderate correlations between aspects of religiosity and pain (r=–0.22 to –0.33). Also, longitudinal research can document how SpQOL may fluctuate over time or in relation to symptom distress and other salient aspects of illness.

There is evidence that intrinsic religiosity (religiosity that is motivated by internal yearnings, in contrast to socially-driven, extrinsic religiosity) is associated highly with spiritual well-being among cancer patients (Fehring et al., 1997). But what other characteristics supported by nurses may contribute to SpQOL?

Additionally, oncology nurse researchers should explore how to best support client SpQOL. What spiritual care therapeutics can nurses offer? How can they most effectively be delivered? Further support can be gained for spiritual care if research evidence documents economic and health outcomes of supporting SpQOL.

CONCLUSION

This literature review provides overdue recognition for a domain of HRQOL that is extremely important to persons with cancer. Spirituality, an interior and integrative aspect of human life, contributes fundamentally to overall HRQOL. Oncology nurses, therefore, must provide spiritual care in clinical arenas that cultivate SpQOL. Additionally, oncology nurse researchers must investigate further what promotes SpQOL and how nurses can effectively nurture spiritual well-being.

REFERENCES

Andrykowski, M. A., Bishop, M. M., Hahn, E. A., Cella, D. F., Beaumont, J. L., Brady, M. J., et al. (2005). Long-term health-related quality of life, growth, and spiritual well-being after hematopoietic stem-cell transplantation. *Journal of Clinical Oncology, 23*(3), 599–608.

Ando, M., Morita, T., Lee, V., & Okamoto, T. (2008). A pilot study of transformation, attributed meanings to the illness, and spiritual well-being for terminally ill cancer patients. *Palliative & Supportive Care, 6*(4), 335–340.

Ando, M., Morita, T., Okamoto, T., & Ninosaka, Y. (2008). One-week short-term life review interview can improve spiritual well-being of terminally ill cancer patients. *Psycho-Oncology, 17*(9), 885–890.

Ashing-Giwa, K. T., Padilla, G., Tejero, J., Kraemer, J., Wright, K., & Coscarelli, A. (2004). Understanding the breast cancer experience of women: A qualitative study of African American, Asian American, Latina and Caucasian cancer survivors. *Pscyho-Oncology, 13*(6), 408–428.

Balboni, T. A., Vanderwerker, L. C., Block, S. D., Paulk, M. E., Lathan, C. S., Peteet, J. R., et al. (2007). Religiousness and spiritual support among advanced cancer patients and associations with end-of-life treatment preferences and quality of life. *Journal of Clinical Oncology, 25*(5), 555–560.

Becker, G., Momm, F., Xander, C., Bartelt, S., Zander-Heinz, A., Budischewski, K., et al. (2006). Religious belief as a coping strategy: An explorative trial in patients irradiated for head-and-neck cancer. *Strahlenther Onkol, 182*(5), 270–276.

Bormann, J. E., Smith, T. L., Becker, S., Gershwin, M., Pada, L., Grudzinski, A. H., et al. (2005). Efficacy of frequent mantram repetition on stress, quality of life, and spiritual well-being in veterans: A pilot study. *Journal of Holistic Nursing, 23*(4), 395–414.

Brady, M. J., Peterman, A. H., Fitchett, G., Mo, M., & Cella, D. (1999). A case for including spirituality in quality of life measurement in oncology. *Psycho-Oncology, 8*, 417–428.

Canada, A. L., Parker, P. A., de Moor, J. S., Basen-Engquist, K., Ramondetta, L. M., & Cohen, L. (2006). Active coping mediates the association between religion/spirituality and quality of life in ovarian cancer. *Gynecological Oncology, 101*(1), 102–107.

Canada, A. L., Murphy, P. E., Fitchett, G., Peterman, A. H. & Schover, L. R. (2008). A 3-factor model for the FACIT-Sp. *Psychooncology, 17*(9), 908–916.

Cella, D., Hahn, E. A., & Dineen, K. (2002). Meaningful change in cancer-specific quality of life scores: Differences between improvement and worsening. *Quality of Life Research, 11*(3), 207–221.

Chochinov, H. M., Hack, T., Hassard, T., Kristjanson, L. J., McClement, S., & Harlos, M. (2005). Dignity therapy: A novel psychotherapeutic intervention for patients near the end of life. *Journal of Clinical Oncology, 23*(24), 5520–5525.

Cohen, S. R., Mount, B. M., Tomas, J. J. N., & Mount, L. F. (1996). Existential well-being is an important determinant of quality of life. *Cancer, 77*, 576–586.

Colgrove, L. A., Kim, Y., & Thompson, N. (2007). The effect of spirituality and gender on the quality of life of spousal caregivers of cancer survivors. *Annals of Behavioral Medicine, 33*(1), 90–98.

Cotton, S. P., Levine, E. G., Fitzpatrick, C. M., Dold, K. H., & Targ, E. (1999). Exploring the relationships among spiritual well-being, quality of life, and psychosocial adjustment in women with breast cancer. *Psycho-Oncology*, 8, 429–438.

Daaleman, T. P., & Frey, B. B. (2004). The spirituality index of well-being: A new instrument for health-related quality of life research. *Annals of Family Medicine*, 2(5), 499–503.

Dossey, B. M., & Guzzetta, C. E. (2000). Holistic nursing practice. In B. M. Dossey, L. Keegan, & C. E. Guzzetta (Eds.), *Holistic nursing: A handbook for practice* (3rd ed., pp. 5–26). Rockville, MD: Aspen.

Duncan, M. D., Leis, A., & Taylor-Brown, J. W. (2008). Impact and outcomes of an iyengar yoga program in a cancer centre. *Current Oncology*, 15(Suppl. 2), 72–78.

Edmondson, D., Park, C. L., Blank, T. O., Fenster, J. R., & Mills, M. A. (2008). Deconstructing spiritual well-being: Existential well-being and HRQOL in cancer survivors. *Psycho-Oncology*, 17, 161–169.

Ellison, C. W. (1983). Spiritual well-being: Conceptualization and measurement. *Journal of Psychology and Theology*, 11, 330–340.

Ersek, M., Ferrell, B. R., Dow, K. H., & Melancon, C. H. (1997). Quality of life in women with ovarian cancer. *Western Journal of Nursing Research*, 19(3), 334–350.

Fatone, A. M., Moadel, A. B., Foley, F. W., Fleming, M., & Jandorf, L. (2007). Urban voices: The quality-of-life experience among women of color with breast cancer. *Palliative & Supportive Care*, 5(2), 115–125.

Feher, S., & Maly, R. C. (1999). Coping with breast cancer in later life: The role of religious faith. *Psychooncology*, 8, 408–416.

Fehring, R. J., Miller, J. F., & Shaw, C. (1997). Spiritual well-being, religiosity, hope, depression, and other mood states in elderly people coping with cancer. *Oncology Nursing Forum*, 24, 663–671.

Fernsler, J. I., Klemm, P., & Miller, M. A. (1999). Spiritual well-being and demands of illness in people with colorectal cancer. *Cancer Nursing*, 22, 134–140.

Ferrans, C. E. (2000). Quality of life as an outcome of cancer care. In C. H. Yarbro, M. H. Frogge, M. Goodman, & S. L. Groenwald (Eds.), *Cancer nursing: Principles and practice* (5th ed.). Sudbury, MA: Jones and Bartlett.

Ferrans, C. E., & Powers, M. (1992). Psychometric assessment of the Quality of Life Index. *Research in Nursing and Health*, 15(1), 29–38.

Ferrell, B., Cullinane, C. A., Ervine, K., Melancon, C., Uman, G. C., & Juarez, G. (2005). Perspectives on the impact of ovarian cancer: Women's views of quality of life. *Oncology Nursing Forum*, 32, 1143–1149.

Ferrell, B. R., Dow, K. H., Leigh, S., Ly, J., & Gulasekaram, P. (1995). Quality of life in long-term cancer survivors. *Oncology Nursing Forum*, 22, 915–922.

Ferrell, B. R., Grant, M. M., Funk, B., Otis-Green, S., & Garcia, N. (1998a). Quality of life in breast cancer survivors: Implications for developing support services. *Oncology Nursing Forum*, 25, 887–895.

Ferrell, B. R., Grant, M., Funk, B., Otis-Green, S., & Garcia, N. (1998b). Quality of life in breast cancer: Part II: Psychological and spiritual well-being. *Cancer Nursing*, 21(1), 1–9.

Gioiella, M. E., Berkman, B., & Robinson, M. (1998). Spirituality and quality of life in gynecologic oncology patients. *Cancer Practice*, 6, 333–338.

Grant, E., Murray, S. A., Kendall, M., Boyd, K., Tilley, S., & Ryan, D. (2004). Spiritual issues and needs: Perspectives from patients with advanced cancer and non-malignant disease: A qualitative study. *Palliative Support Care*, 2(4), 371–378.

Griesinger, A. J., Lorimor, R. J., Aday, L. A., Winn, R. J., & Baile, W. F. (1997). Terminally ill cancer patients: Their most important concerns. *Cancer Practice*, 5, 147–154.

Hampton, D. M., Hollis, D. E., Lloyd, D. A., Taylor, J., & McMillan, S. C. (2007). Spiritual needs of persons with advanced cancer. *American Journal of Hospice & Palliative Medicine*, 24(1), 42–48.

Heiney, S. P., McWayne, J., Hurley, T. G., Lamb, L. S., Jr., Bryant, L. H., Butler, W., et al. (2003). Efficacy of therapeutic group by telephone for women with breast cancer. *Cancer Nursing*, 26(6), 439–447.

Highfield, M. F. (1992). Spiritual health of oncology patients: Nurse and patient perspectives. *Cancer Nursing, 15*(1), 1–8.

Johnson, M. E., Dose, A. M., Pipe, T. B., Petersen, W. O., Huschka, M., Gallenberg, M. M., et al. (2009). Centering prayer for women receiving chemotherapy for recurrent ovarian cancer: A pilot study. *Oncology Nursing Forum, 36*(4), 421–428.

Johnson, M. E., Piderman, K. M., Sloan, J. A., Huschka, M., Atherton, P. J., Hanson, J. M., et al. (2007). Measuring spiritual quality of life in patients with cancer. *The Journal of Supportive Oncology, 5*(9), 437–442.

Kaczorowski, J. M. (1989). Spiritual well-being and anxiety in adults diagnosed with cancer. *Hospice Journal, 5*(3–4), 105–116.

Ka'opua, L. S., Gotay, C. C., & Boehm, P. S. (2007). Spiritually based resources in adaptation to long-term prostate cancer survival: Perspectives of elderly wives. *Health & Social Work, 32*(1), 29–39.

Kristeller, J. L., Rhodes, M., Cripe, L. D., & Sheets, V. (2005). Oncology Assisted Spiritual Intervention Study (OASIS): Patient acceptability and initial evidence of effects. *International Journal of Psychiatry in Medicine, 35*(4), 329–347.

Kutner, J. S., Nowels, D. E., Kassner, C. T., Houser, J., Bryant, L. L., & Main, D. S. (2003). Confirmation of the "disability paradox" among hospice patients: Preservation of quality of life despite physical ailments and psychosocial concerns. *Palliative and Supportive Care, 1*(3), 231–237.

Leak, A., Hu, J., & King, C. R. (2008). Symptom distress, spirituality, and quality of life in African American breast cancer survivors. *Cancer Nursing, 31*(1), E15–E21.

Levine, E. G., Aviv, C., Yoo G., Ewing, C., & Au A. (2009). The benefits of prayer on mood and well-being of breast cancer survivors. *Supportive Care in Cancer, 17*(3), 295–306.

Levine, E. G., Yoo, G., Aviv, C., Ewing, C., & Au, A. (2007). Ethnicity and spirituality in breast cancer survivors. *Journal of Cancer Survivorship, 1*(3), 212–225.

Locke, D. E., Decker, P. A., Sloan, J. A., Brown, P. D., Malec, J. F., Clark, M. M., et al. (2007). Validation of single-item linear analog scale assessment of quality of life in neuro-oncology patients. *Journal of Pain & Symptom Management, 34*(6), 628–638.

Manning-Walsh, J. (2005). Social support as a mediator between symptom distress and quality of life in women with breast cancer. *Journal of Obstetric, Gynecological, and Neonatal Nursing, 34*(4), 482–493.

Martsolf, D. S., & Mickley, J. R. (1998). The concept of spirituality in nursing theories: Differing worldviews and extent of focus. *Journal of Advanced Nursing, 27*, 294–303.

McClain-Jacobson, C., Rosenfeld, B., Kosinski, A., Pessin, H., Cimino, J. E., & Breitbart, W. (2004). Belief in an afterlife, spiritual well-being and end-of-life despair in patients with advanced cancer. *General Hospital Psychiatry, 26*(6), 484–486.

McGrath, P. (2004). Positive outcomes for survivors of haematological malignancies from a spiritual perspective. *International Journal of Nursing Practice, 10*, 280–291.

McIllmurray, M. B., Francis, B., Harman, J. C., Morris, S. M., Soothill, K., & Thomas, C. (2003). Psychosocial needs in cancer patients related to religious belief. *Palliative Medicine, 17*(1), 49–54.

McMillan, S. C., & Weitzner, M. (1998). Quality of life in cancer patients: Use of a revised hospice index. *Cancer Practice, 6*, 282–288.

McMillan, S. C., & Weitzner, M. (2000). How problematic are various aspects of quality of life in patients with cancer at the end of life? *Oncology Nursing Forum, 27*, 817–823.

Mickley, J. R., Soeken, K., & Belcher, A. (1992). Spiritual well-being, religiousness, and hope among women with breast cancer. *Image, 24*, 267–272.

Moadel, A., Morgan, C., Fatone, A., Grennan, J., Carter, J., Laruffa, G., et al. (1999). Seeking meaning and hope: Self-reported spiritual and existential needs among an ethnically-diverse cancer patient population. *Psycho-Oncology, 8*, 378–385.

Nelson, C. J., Rosenfeld, B., Breitbart, W., & Galietta, M. (2002). Spirituality, religion, and depression in the terminally ill. *Psychosomatics, 43*(3), 213–220.

Nidich, S. I., Fields, J. Z., Rainforth, M. V., Pomerantz, R., Cella, D., Kristeller, J., et al. (2009). A randomized controlled trial of the effects of transcendental meditation on quality of life in older breast cancer patients. *Integrative Cancer Therapies, 8*(3), 228–234.

Pargament, K. I. (1997). *The psychology of religion and coping.* New York, NY: Guilford.

Peterman, A. H., Fitchett, G., Brady, M. J., Hernandez, L., & Cella, D. (2002). Measuring spiritual well-being in people with cancer: The Functional Assessment of Chronic Illness Therapy—Spiritual Well-Being Scale (FACIT-Sp). *Annals of Behavioral Medicine, 24*(1), 49–58.

Rabkin, J. G., McElhiney, M., Moran, P., Acree, M., & Folkman, S. (2009). Depression, distress and positive mood in late-stage cancer: A longitudinal study. *Psycho-Oncology, 18*(1), 79–86.

Redinbaugh, E. M., Baum, A., Tarbell, S., & Arnold, R. (2003). End-of-life caregiving: What helps family caregivers cope? *Journal of Palliative Medicine, 6,* 901–909.

Reed, P. G. (1991). Preferences for spiritually related nursing interventions among terminally ill and non-terminally ill hospitalized adults and well adults. *Applied Nursing Research, 4,* 122–128.

Reed, P. G. (1992). An emerging paradigm for the investigation of spirituality in nursing. *Research in Nursing and Health, 15,* 349–357.

Riley, B. B., Perna, R., Tate, D., Forchheimer, M., Anderson, C., & Luera, G. (1998). Types of spiritual well-being among persons with chronic illness: Their relation to various forms of quality of life. *Archives of Physical Medicine and Rehabilitation, 79,* 258–264.

Romero, C., Friedman, L. C., Kalidas, M., Elledge, R., Chang, J., & Liscum, K. R. (2006). Self-forgiveness, spirituality, and psychological adjustment in women with breast cancer. *Journal of Behavioral Medicine, 29*(1), 29–36.

Rummans, T. A., Clark, M. M., Sloan, J. A., Frost, M. H., Bostwick, J. M., Atherton, P. J., et al. (2006). Impacting quality of life for patients with advanced cancer with a structured multidisciplinary intervention: A randomized controlled trial. *Journal of Clinical Oncology, 24*(4), 635–642.

Saleh, U. S., & Brockopp, D. Y. (2001). Quality of life one year following bone marrow transplantation: Psychometric evaluation of the Quality of Life Bone Marrow Transplant Survivors Tool. *Oncology Nursing Forum, 28,* 1457–1464.

Slovacek, L., Slovackova, B., & Jebavy, L. (2005). Global quality of life in patients who have undergone the hematopoietic stem cell transplantation: Finding from transversal and retrospective study. *Exp Oncol, 27*(3), 238–242.

Sparber, A., Bauer, L., Curt, G., Eisenberg, D., Levin, T., Parks, S., et al. (2000). Use of complementary medicine by adult patients participating in cancer clinical trials. *Oncology Nursing Forum, 27,* 623–632.

Steinhauser, K. E., Alexander, S. C., Byock, I. R, George, L. K., Olsen, M. K., & Tulsky, J. A. (2008). Do preparation and life completion discussions improve functioning and quality of life in seriously ill patients? Pilot randomized control trial. *Journal of Palliative Medicine, 11*(9), 1234–1240.

Steinhauser, K. E., Voils, C. I., Clipp, E. C., Bosworth, H. B., Christakis, N. A., & Tulsky, J. A. (2006). "Are you at peace?" One item to probe spiritual concerns at the end of life. *Archives of Internal Medicine, 166*(1), 101–105.

Tang, W. (2009). Hospice family caregivers' quality of life. *Journal of Clinical Nursing. 18,* 2563–2572.

Tarakeshwar, N., Vanderwerker, L. C., Paulk, E., Pearce, M. J., Kasl, S. V., & Prigerson, H. G. (2006). Religious coping is associated with the quality of life of patients with advanced cancer. *Journal of Palliative Medicine, 9*(3), 646–657.

Tate, D. G., & Forchheimer, M. (2002). Quality of life, life satisfaction, and spirituality. *American Journal of Physical and Medical Rehabilitation, 81,* 400–410.

Taylor, E. J. (2000). Transformation of tragedy among women surviving breast cancer. *Oncology Nursing Forum, 27,* 781–788.

Taylor, E. J. (2002). *Spiritual care: Nursing theory, research, and practice.* Upper Saddle River, NJ: Prentice Hall.

Taylor, E. J. (2003a). Nurses caring for the Spirit: Patients with cancer and family caregiver expectations. *Oncology Nursing Forum, 30,* 585–590.

Taylor, E. J. (2003b). Spiritual needs of cancer patients and family caregivers. *Cancer Nursing, 26,* 260–266.

Taylor, E. J. (2005). Spiritual complementary therapies in cancer care. *Seminars in Oncology Nursing, 21*(3), 159–163.

Taylor, E. J. (2006). Prevalence of spiritual needs among cancer patients and family caregivers. *Oncology Nursing Forum, 33*(4), 729–735.

Taylor, E. J., & Mamier, I. (2005). Spiritual care nursing: What cancer patients and family caregivers want. *Journal of Advanced Nursing, 49*(3), 260–267.

Taylor, E. J., & Outlaw, F. H. (2002). Use of prayer among persons with cancer. *Holistic Nursing Practice, 16*(3), 46–60.

The Joint Commission. (2008, November 24). *Spiritual assessment.* Retrieved December 6, 2009, from http://www.jointcommission.org/AccreditationPrograms/LongTermCare/Standards/09_FAQs/PC/Spiritual_Assessment.

Thomson, J. E. (2000). The place of spiritual well-being in hospice patient's overall quality of life. *Hospice Journal, 15*(2), 13–27.

Vachon, M. L. (2008). Meaning, spirituality, and wellness in cancer survivors. *Seminars in Oncology Nursing, 24*(3), 218–225.

VandeCreek, L., Rogers, E., & Lester, J. (1999). Use of alternative therapies among breast cancer outpatients compared with the general population. *Alternative Therapies in Health and Medicine, 5*(1), 71–76.

Vivat, B. (2008). Measures of spiritual issues for palliative care patients: A literature review. *Palliative Medicine, 22,* 859–868.

Walton, J., & Sullivan, N. (2004). Men of prayer: Spirituality of men with prostate cancer: A grounded theory study. *Journal of Holistic Nursing, 22*(2), 133–151.

Wenzel, L. B., Donnelly, J. P., Fowler, J. M, Habbal, R., Taylor, T. H., Aziz, N., et al. (2002). Resilience, reflection, and residual stress in ovarian cancer survivorship: A gynecologic oncology group study. *Psycho-Oncology, 11,* 142–153.

Whitford, H. S., Olver, I. N., & Peterson, M. J. (2008). Spirituality as a core domain in the assessment of quality of life in oncology. *Psycho-Oncology, 17,* 1121–1128.

Winslow, G. R., & Wehtje-Winslow, B. W. (2007). Ethical boundaries of spiritual care. *Medical Journal of Australia, 186*(10, Suppl.), S63–S66.

Wismer, P. (1995). For women in pain: A feminist theology of suffering. In A. O. Graff (Ed.), *In the embrace of God: Feminist approaches to theological anthropology.* Maryknoll, NY: Orbis Books.

Wyatt, G., & Friedman, L. L. (1996). Long-term female cancer survivors: Quality of life issues and clinical implications. *Cancer Nursing, 19,* 1–7.

Yates, J. W., Chalmer, B. J., St. James, P., Follansbee, M., & McKegney, F. P. (1981). Religion in patients with advanced cancer. *Medical and Pediatric Oncology, 9,* 121–128.

Zaza, C., Sellick, S. M., & Hillier, L. M. (2005). Coping with cancer: What do patients do. *Journal of Psychosocial Oncology, 23*(1), 55–73.

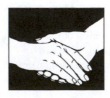

Chapter Six

Quality of Life, Health, and Culture

GERALDINE V. PADILLA • MARJORIE KAGAWA-SINGER •
KIMLIN TAM ASHING-GIWA

Introduction

Health-related quality of life (HRQOL) is an important benchmark of nursing care and medical treatment effectiveness. Culture influences perceptions of illness, of cognitive impairment, and of other physical and mental health problems. Negative perceptions and stigmatization of these conditions, in turn, influence HRQOL as demonstrated in a cohort study of HIV-positive persons from five African countries. The study showed that increases in HIV-related stigma over one year were significantly associated with decreases in life satisfaction with rates of change differing by country (Greeff et al., 2010). Life satisfaction was reflected in reduced living enjoyment, loss of control in life, decreased social interaction, and decreased perceived health status. Likewise, HIV-positive Hispanics who reported feeling stigmatized when receiving medical care had poorer psychological and physical functioning, and a decreased ability to complete daily activities (Larios, Davis, Gallo, Heinrich, & Talavera, 2009).

Considering the need for research, we think it worthwhile to briefly review what is known about quality of life (QOL) in the context of health and culture to better understand the relationship between these constructs. This chapter begins with explanations of culture, differentiating it from ethnicity and race. It continues with HRQOL conceptual and operational definitions used across cultures, models of determinants and dimensions of the construct, and issues relevant to cross-cultural research in HRQOL.

Culture, Ethnicity, and Race

Culture

The Center for Advanced Research on Language Acquisition defines culture as ". . . the shared patterns of behaviors and interactions, cognitive constructs, and affective understanding that are learned through a process of socialization. These shared patterns identify the members of a culture group while also distinguishing those of another group." (Center for Advanced Research on Language Acquisition, 2010, p. 1). Culture is purposeful. It prescribes the ways of life for a group to ensure its survival and well-being. It provides beliefs and values to give meaning and purpose to life (Kagawa-Singer, 2000, 2006; Spector, 2004). Culture addresses three basic and universal needs: safety and security, sense of integrity and meaning or purpose in life, and sense of belonging as an integral member of one's social network (Kagawa-Singer & Chung, 1994). Culture is fundamental to life and is an important determinant of quality of life in the context of health because it defines the purpose of and prescriptions for living a meaningful life in wellness and sickness.

A comprehensive operationalization of culture would measure health, ethnicity, and socio-demographic variables (Kagawa-Singer, 2006). Health characteristics include diet, physical activity, and alternative health practices (e.g., healers, parallel or complementary health practices). Ethnic factors are parental heritage, ethnic self-identity (i.e., generation, degree of integration into mainstream society, language proficiencies, beliefs and practices, degree of personal identification and public identity, number of identity groups, and degree of overlap), interethnic social interaction choices (e.g., by circumstances or choice, by regional or community geographic residence), and religiosity and spirituality (e.g., beliefs, practices, internal/external locus of control). Sociodemographic variables consist of family structure and support system (e.g., composition, age), socioeconomic status (e.g., wealth, education, percent of money sent to home country or to support other households), and generation in the United States and reason for immigration.

Race and Racism

Racial categories are based on phenotypes expressed as physical or biochemical characteristics. However, the scientific basis for making racial distinctions is weak (Hirschman, Alba, & Farley, 2000; Kagawa-Singer & Blackhall, 2001; Montagu, 1962, 1997). Many traits cross over "races," and "racial" identity can change over time. Data from the Human Genome Project and from human genome variation dispute the validity of the term "race" (Royal & Dunston, 2004). Foster and Sharp (2004, p. 790) said it well:

> Race and other preexisting population definitions (ethnicity, religion, language, nationality, culture and so on) tend to be contentious concepts that have polarized discussions about the ethics and science of research into population-specific human genetic variation. By contrast, a broader consideration of the multiple historical sources of genetic variation provides a whole-genome perspective on the ways in which existing population definitions do, and do not, account for how genetic variation is distributed among individuals.

Studies of health and quality-of-life disparities continue to use race and racial group categories to predict and understand why some people are better or worse off than others, what genetic variations exist between groups, and what behavioral, social, and environmental factors put some racial or ethnic groups at greater or lesser risk than others for poor health and HRQOL outcomes. Racism, the belief in the superiority of one group over another because of genetic traits, justifies the exertion of power and discriminatory action by the "superior" group over the "less superior" group. Disparities in care and reduced health and quality-of-life outcomes result from racially related beliefs and actions (Institute of Medicine, 2001).

Ethnicity

Ethnicity is that which holds a group together because of a common identity based on some or all of the following shared characteristics: culture, history, language, religion, genealogy, and ancestry. Ethnicity encompasses both culture and "race." Members of multicultural societies form ethnic bonds for solidarity. These bonds assure their way of life and meaning in life, particularly when the universal needs of safety and security, sense of integrity and meaning or purpose in life, and sense of belonging as an integral member of one's social network are threatened (Kagawa-Singer & Chung, 1994). Ethnic mores also specify behaviors to promote or maintain health, to prevent disease or illness, and to manage seemingly random events.

Theories of culture, race, or ethnicity can contribute to strategies to promote or maintain health and well-being (Kagawa-Singer, 1995, 2006). The cultural beliefs and values that bind an ethnic group in their approach to health, and the racial identity that places an ethnic group in a position of more or less power and status in their ability to access and use the healthcare system, ultimately influence HRQOL (Kagawa-Singer, 2001).

Concepualization of Quality of Life and Health-Related Quality of Life

Conceptual Definitions

An important philosophical question preceding the study of quality of life asks what it is to be human. Cultural in origin, beliefs about humanness include values about life and about the quality of life compared to other desirable outcomes. Fletcher (1990, p. 12) lists fifteen positive human criteria: minimal human intelligence, self-awareness, self-control, a sense of time, a sense of futurity, a sense of the past, the capability to relate to others, concern for others, communication, control of existence, curiosity, change and changeability, balance of rationality and feeling, idiosyncrasy, and neocortical function. This view of humanness means that HRQOL assessments are made by conscious-thinking, socio-emotional individuals who view their health condition or that of others in a time span encompassing past, current, and potential future health states, who view life events as not totally random but somewhat controllable, and who are unique from others.

Pertinent to this chapter is whether people from diverse cultures view humanness similarly. The indicators of humanhood listed previously stem from a Judeo-Christian orientation, which is neither more nor less valid than other views. Perhaps, Buddhism, Islam, or other religions or philosophies would change, add, or otherwise revise Fletcher's list (Fletcher, 1990). The uniqueness of a culture is less about the array of indicators of humanhood, but rather what a culture singles out and emphasizes as key components of humanness. A culture for which control of existence is the most important aspect of humanness would value health-related research differently than a culture for which balance of rationality and feeling is the key component of humanness. The first culture might emphasize cure, while the second might balance cure with care research. The cultural view of what it is to be human informs the relevant dimensions of quality of life for that culture, and the level of well-being for an individual, a group, a society, and a nation.

In a sense, HRQOL is not only an outcome of care, treatment, or medical decisions, but also a prescriber of behavior based on cultural beliefs, values, and norms. In the case of an infant born with severe health conditions or deformities that require extensive and prolonged medical treatment, parents and health professionals may believe that the infant has no chance for a meaningful life with even minimal quality. The parents and professionals may decide to do nothing and let the infant die. This is a painful, terrifying decision fraught with ethical challenges, but a decision ultimately based on cultural norms that define a minimally acceptable HRQOL. These types of culturally rooted HRQOL decisions are made every day.

Despite the relationship between culture and HRQOL, few of the many definitions of quality of life and HRQOL mention culture. This omission is understandable, because culture is a factor that shapes the meaning of, but is not an attribute or dimension of, quality of life. In the 1980s and 1990s, most definitions of HRQOL focused on personal perceptions of what made one's life worthwhile given certain health conditions. For example, Shumaker and Naughton (1995), after reviewing the theoretical, clinical, and research literature concerning quality of life in the context of health summarized the defining characteristic of the concept as the subjective evaluation of one's ability to pursue valued life goals. This ability is influenced by one's health status, health care, health-promoting activities, and level of function. The important functions include social, physical, and cognitive function, as well as mobility, self-care, and emotional well-being. Culture may be implied by the characteristics of subjectivity and valued life goals.

An international group of behavioral scientists and healthcare providers representing white Euro American cultures met in 1992 to discuss client-based measures of individual function, well-being, and satisfaction within the context of cross-cultural, clinical research. This group acknowledged the influence of culture on variations in perceptions of health and sickness, interpretations of symptoms, the meaning of quality of life, and expectations of care (Berzon & Shumaker, 1995). Considering cultural diversity in the definition, measurement, and use of HRQOL in cross-national clinical trials, the group identified four fundamental dimensions of HRQOL: physical, mental/psychological, social, and global perceptions of function and well-being. Additional possible attributes were described as pain, energy/vitality, sleep, appetite, and symptoms associated with the disease or treatment.

Later, others added the component of spiritual/existential well-being (Ashing-Giwa et al., 2004; Ashing-Giwa et al., 2006; Brady, Peterman, Fitchett, Mo, & Cella, 1999; Edmondson, Park, Blank, Fenster, & Mills, 2007) as a dimension of quality of life. The spiritual/existential dimension of the HRQOL construct addresses the meaning of illness for an individual and may include personal beliefs about the meaning and value of life, spiritual needs, uncertainty and hope concerning the future, life priorities, and transcendence from life to death (Ferrell, Grant, Funk, Otis-Green, & Garcia, 1998).

Parker and Fox-Rushby believed that it was inappropriate to assume that dimensions of health are identical or comparable across cultures (Parker & Fox-Rushby, 1995). They questioned "...whether it is appropriate to assume that there is a cultural universality in the definition of HRQOL, and whether the research methods used to date have been capable of unearthing universal dimensions of HRQOL" (Parker & Fox-Rushby, 1995, p. 154).

Given this concern, a broad definition is preferable because quality of life can mean different things to people of different cultural backgrounds. For example, Higuchi (1985, p. 89) emphasized the importance of ". . . the patient's harmony with the world, with others, with himself, and with death" when considering quality of life and health. We have not come across an English language measure of quality of life that includes items on harmony. Yet, in 1988, Kagawa-Singer found from ethnographic interviews that both Japanese American and Anglo American cancer patients reported that a life of quality was one that maintained their sense of self-integrity and allowed them to continue to fulfill their role responsibilities. Instead of harmony, concepts of acceptance, adjustment, and adaptation in relation to illness and quality of life are more commonly used in research and illustrate different cultural orientations. For example, Japanese Americans view side effects of treatment as expected outcomes to be endured, while Anglo Americans view side effects as problems to be eliminated or overcome (Kagawa-Singer, 1993).

The World Health Organization Quality of Life Group (WHOQOL), a set of cross-cultural investigators working under the auspices of the Division of Mental Health of the World Health Organization (World Health Organization, 1993), developed a landmark definition of quality of life that explicitly identified culture as a determinant of the construct. WHOQOL defined quality of life as, "An individual's perception of their position in life in the context of the culture and value systems in which they live, and in relation to their goals, expectations, standards, and concerns. It is a broad ranging concept, affected in a complex way by the person's physical health, psychological state, level of independence, social relationships, and their relationship to salient features of their environment" (WHOQOL Group, 1995, p. 1404).

Personal meaning of illness and HRQOL are related (Sherman, Simonton, Latif, & Bracy, 2010), but the conditions that give meaning to life in the context of illness may be perceived differently in diverse cultures (Kirkham, Pesut, Meyerhoff, & Sawatzky, 2004; Taylor, 2001). The transcultural framework of QOL (Kagawa-Singer, 1988) includes broad domains that consider important human needs for safety and security (i.e., food, shelter, clothing, physical comfort), sense of integrity, meaning or purpose in one's life (i.e., perceiving oneself to be a contributing member of one's group), and sense of belonging (i.e., connection to others). The WHOQOL definition (WHOQOL Group, 1995) together with the Kagawa-Singer transcultural framework (Kagawa-Singer, 1988) provide a broad, practical, descriptive, and prescriptive definition of quality of life as related to health that is likely to be valid in similar and diverse cultures.

Issues in the Conceptualization of QOL and HRQOL

In 1995, Shumaker and Naughton identified some issues surrounding the construct HRQOL that persist today (Shumaker & Naughton, 1995). These issues concern the distinction between quality of life and HRQOL, between determinants (predictors) and dimensions (attributes) of HRQOL, and between conceptual models of HRQOL.

In addressing the first issue, it is necessary to describe how the concepts of QOL and HRQOL differ (Gill & Feinstein, 1994; Moons, Van Deyk, Budts, & De Geest, 2004). An overall, holistic definition of QOL takes into account multiple and diverse domains of one's life and need not focus specifically on health. Focusing on the individual, QOL is defined as a subjective, multidimensional experience that involves a summary evaluation of the positive and negative attributes that characterize one's life (Padilla, Grant, Ferrell, & Presant,

1996). It is a dynamic construct affected by one's ability to adapt to discrepancies between expected and experienced well-being (Padilla et al., 1996), as well as one's ability to maintain an overall level of functioning that allows the individual to pursue valued life goals and enjoy general well-being (Shumaker & Naughton, 1995).

HRQOL means that a summary evaluation of attributes that characterize one's life is made at a point in time when health, illness, and treatment conditions are relevant (Padilla et al., 1996). The pertinent characteristics of a healthy person's quality of life may not include physically, emotionally, or biomedically defined health, but rather social relationships, financial success, and a satisfying job. On the other hand, a person whose health is threatened by acute or chronic illness will likely attribute certain dimensions of life quality to the influence of health problems, health status, health care, and health-promoting activities. A review of the literature on quality of life in congenital heart disease patients revealed that only 1 out of 70 articles distinguished between overall QOL and HRQOL (Moons et al., 2004). These results likely apply to QOL and HRQOL studies for other health problems.

The definition of health should not be limited to the biomedical model of physiologic integrity. Instead, health should be viewed in the context of self-integrity along the dimensions of physical status and social function (Kagawa-Singer, 1993). The WHO defines health as "a state of complete physical, mental, and social well-being and not merely the absence of disease or infirmity" (World Health Organization, 1946, p. 100). This definition is based on the WHO principles of health, happiness, harmonious relations, and security of all people. An attempt to include a fourth dimension of health—spiritual well-being—was not successful (Sein, 2002). The inclusion of spiritual well-being would have acknowledged the role of meaning in one's life in determining HRQOL. The ability to make meaning of one's life would account for why ill persons can maintain a sense of self-integrity by perceiving themselves as healthy in one HRQOL dimension, for instance psychological well-being, while acknowledging the effects of their illness on their physical well-being (Kagawa-Singer, 1993).

A second issue concerns the distinction between determinants (predictors) and dimensions (attributes) of HRQOL (Shumaker & Naughton, 1995; Stewart, 1992; Strickland, 1991). The lack of distinction between determinants and dimensions of HRQOL in definitions of the construct can lead to conceptual and operational confusion and circularity. For example, pain is identified as a symptom of cancer or side effect of treatment that has an impact on HRQOL. At the same time, evaluations of pain distress, intensity, and frequency are used as a basis for HRQOL scores. Pain should not be treated as both the cause and effect. The distinction between predictors and attributes is important to future understanding of interventions that can maintain or improve HRQOL in persons with acute or chronic illness. Published studies on QOL need to provide a clear, unequivocal definition of the construct and its domains, to distinguish between overall QOL and HRQOL, to select measures of HRQOL that fit the definition of the construct (Gill & Feinstein, 1994; Moons et al., 2004), and to ensure that there is no conceptual or operational overlap between HRQOL and its predictors.

What attributes of HRQOL are most salient to persons who are ill? How do these characteristics differ between persons of different cultural orientations? What aspects of culture are most likely to affect elements of HRQOL? These questions are associated with the third HRQOL definitional issue—conceptual models and measures of HRQOL (Shumaker & Naughton, 1995). At issue is the kind of relationship that exists between determinants and dimensions of HRQOL. How specific are these relationships? Are current HRQOL instruments able to measure these relationships? For example, do the instruments include the specific dimensions of HRQOL (e.g., perceived physical or psychological support from family and friends) that can be affected by the predictors (e.g., network of actual social resources)? Keeping in mind that investigators revise their models of HRQOL as they learn more about the construct, the models described here are not all inclusive, but rather illustrative of different ways of viewing the relationships between determinants and dimensions of HRQOL.

Models of QOL and HRQOL

In 1985, Padilla and Grant included a number of process, mediating cognitive, extraneous, and HRQOL outcome variables in their model of quality of life (Figure 6-1) (Padilla & Grant, 1985). The relationships between process, mediating, or extraneous variables to HRQOL outcomes are specific. For example, extraneous variables concerning diagnosis (e.g., stage of cancer) are predicted to have their most immediate impact on physical well-being and the diagnosis and treatment response. On the other hand, implementing the nursing process (e.g., colostomy care) has a direct impact on body image concerns surrounding the colostomy as well as on physical well-being. Padilla and Grant's model includes examples of the kinds of measures required and predicts the specific relationships between determinants and dimensions of HRQOL.

The 1996 Spilker model (Figure 6-2) illustrates how medical treatments can result in adverse reactions (safety measures), benefits (efficacy measures), and costs (other measures) (Spilker, 1996). These, in turn, are filtered through the client's belief, value, and judgment structure before affecting the quality-of-life domains of physical status and abilities, psychological well-being, social interactions, and economic status and factors. Beliefs, values, and judgments are influenced by the patient's culture.

The model proposed by Ferrell and colleagues in 1991 conceptualized pain from cancer and its treatment as having an independent impact on the QOL dimensions of physical well-being and symptoms, psychological, social, and spiritual well-being (Ferrell, Grant, Padilla, Vemuri, & Rhiner, 1991). Later, Ferrell, Grant, and colleagues amplified the QOL model for pain and specified additional QOL models for fatigue, family caregivers, cancer survivorship, and others (City of Hope Pain and Palliative Care Resource Center, 2010). The QOL model related to pain (Figure 6-3) is illustrated here for the following reasons. Quality-of-life dimensions are based on information from Hispanic (Juarez, Ferrell, & Borneman, 1998) and non-Hispanic white (Ferrell et al., 1991; Padilla, Ferrell, Grant, & Rhiner, 1990) cancer patients with pain. The model illustrates how the pain experience as predictor (e.g., frequency, intensity, type) is distinguished from pain distress (psychological well-being domain) and pain suffering and meaning attributes (spiritual well-being

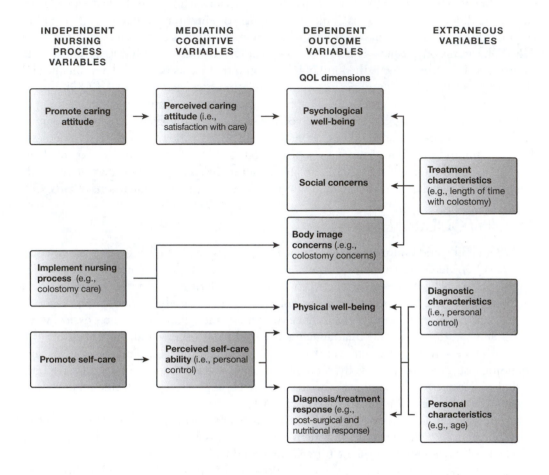

Figure 6-1. **Padilla and Grant model of nursing process and quality-of-life outcomes.**
Source: Padilla, G. V., & Grant, M. M. (1985) "Quality of life as a cancer nursing outcome variable."*Advances in Nursing Science, 8*(1), 45–60.

domain) of QOL. The model includes a spiritual well-being domain that provides measurable attributes such as suffering, meaning of pain, and transcendence, as well as religiosity. All the City of Hope models share the same four clearly delineated quality-of-life domains with specific outcomes that can be influenced by nursing care.

In 1999, Sprangers and Schwartz proposed a theoretical model of response shift and HRQOL (Figure 6-4). Response shift concerns an alteration in the meaning of one's assessment of a construct because of a change in one's (a) internal standards of measurement concerning the construct (i.e., scale recalibration); (b) values relative to the construct (i.e., the

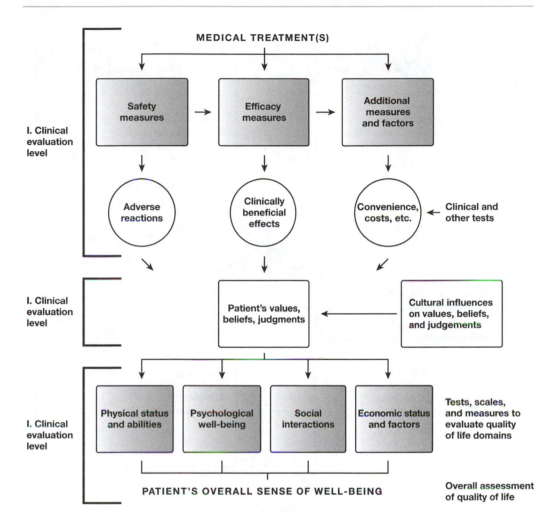

Figure 6-2.   **Spilker model of clinical evaluation, integration/assessment, and quality of life.**

Source: Spilker B. (1996). Introduction. In Spilker B. (Ed.), Quality of Life and Pharmacoeconomics in Clinical Trials.(p. 1–10). New York: Lippincott-Raven. Fig 2. p. 6

relative worth of aspects of one's life in relation to the construct); or (c) definition of the construct (i.e., reconceptualization of the construct)(Schwartz & Sprangers, 1999). The theoretical model of response shift and quality of life includes five components. A catalyst such as a diagnosis of cancer activates behavioral, cognitive, or affective mechanisms. These mechanisms may include goal reordering or reframing of expectations or other accommodation

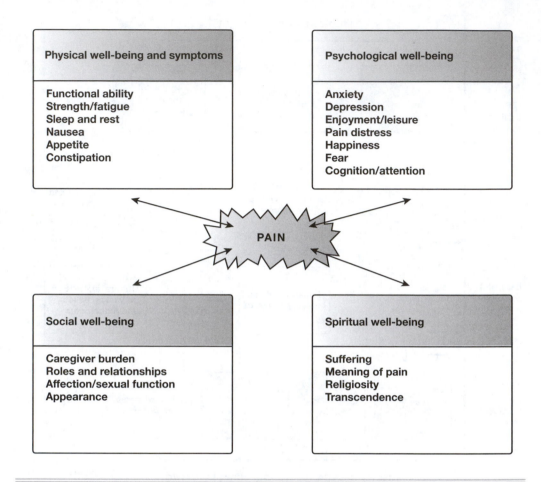

Figure 6-3.   **Ferrell and Grant quality-of-life model.**

> *Source:* Used with permission of Informa Medical and Pharmaceutical Science, from "The Experience of Pain and Perceptions of Quality of Life: Validation of a Conceptual Model", Ferrell BR, Grant M, Padilla G, Vemuri S, Rhiner M, The Hospice Journal, 7(3): 9–24 (1991), permission conveyed through Copyright Clearance Center, Inc.veyed through Copyright Clearance Center, Inc.

processes that are used to adjust to the catalyst. Successful accommodation mechanisms result in a response shift, meaning a change in one's internal standards, values, or conceptualizations. Response shift permits the individual to maintain or improve health-related quality of life despite the catalytic negative change in health status. The relationships between the catalyst and accommodation mechanisms and response shift can be affected by antecedent factors like sociodemographics (e.g., age), personality (e.g., optimism), expectations, and spiritual identity. The elements of response shift, meaning internal standards, values, and conceptualizations, are subjective as well as culturally based cognitive behaviors. The response

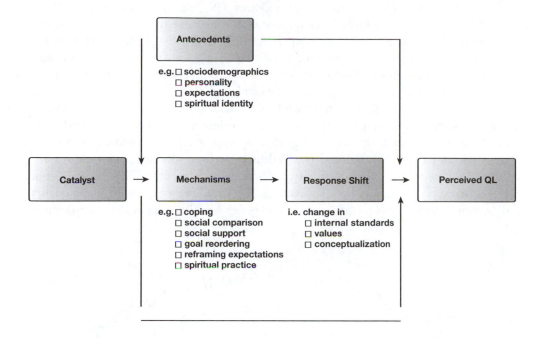

Figure 6-4.   **Sprangers and Schwartz theoretical model of response shift and quality of life (QOL).**

Source: Reprinted from Social Science and Medicine, Vol. 48, Sprangers MAG, Schwartz CE, Integrating response shift into health-related quality of life research: a theoretical model, 1507–1515, Copyright (1999), with permission from Elsevier.

shift model fits the Kagawa-Singer transcultural framework of QOL with its emphasis on self-integrity and meaning in life (Kagawa-Singer, 1988).

The original model of response shift (Sprangers & Schwartz, 1999) was thought to be useful in hypothesizing relationships between quality of life and relevant predictors. However, counterintuitive findings such as improvements in HRQOL in the face of deteriorating health underscored the need to expand the model to include an appraisal process. Appraisal of QOL is subjective, differs across individuals, and changes over time within individuals (Rapkin & Schwartz, 2004). In fact, Rapkin and Schwartz (2004, p. 14) emphasized the importance and feasibility of measuring the appraisal process itself by assessing: "1) induction of a frame of reference; 2) recall and sampling of salient experiences; 3) standards of comparison used to appraise experiences; and 4) subjective algorithms used to prioritize and combine appraisals to arrive at a QOL rating." These investigators concluded that by measuring the appraisal process itself, we could better understand quality-of-life change mechanisms.

In 2005, Ashing-Giwa published a model of HRQOL (Ashing-Giwa, 2005) that included macro- and individual-level factors that constitute the contextual framework within which HRQOL is assessed and experienced. In her model (Figure 6-5), HRQOL is defined as a multidimensional construct consisting of physical (bodily concerns from disease and treatments), functional (ability to carry out responsibilities like work and activities of daily living), psychological and emotional (positive and negative affect), social (ability to participate in family and network activities), spiritual (spiritual and existential experiences), and sexual well-being (sexuality and intimacy related to one's health status). Macro-level contextual components include socio-ecological (i.e., socio-economic status, life burden, social support), cultural (i.e., ethnicity, ethnic identify, acculturation, interconnectedness, worldview, and spirituality), demographic (i.e., chronological age, gender), and healthcare system factors (i.e., access to health care, quality of health care, quality of relationship). Individual level factors consist of general health (i.e., health status), medical

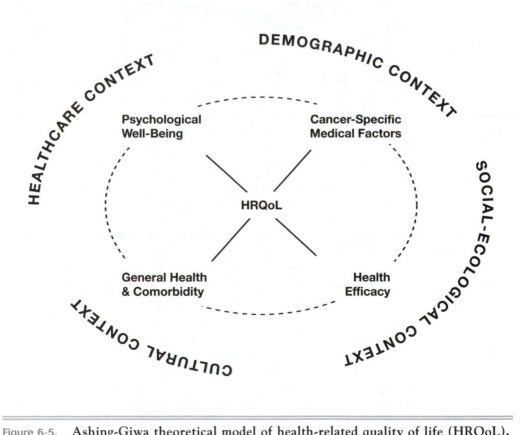

Figure 6-5.   **Ashing-Giwa theoretical model of health-related quality of life (HRQoL).**

Source: With kind permission from Springer Science+Business Media: Quality of Life Research, The contextual model of HRQoL: A paradigm for expanding the HRQoL framework, Vol. 14, 2005, 297–307, Ashing-Giwa, Figure 1.

factors (i.e., disease characteristics such as cancer characteristics and age at diagnosis), health efficacy (i.e., motivation), and psychological well-being (i.e., level of functioning).

The contextual model clarifies the relationship between macro- and individual-level contextual factors and HRQOL. The model is useful in planning research studies and hypothesizing relationships. However, two areas need to be revised. First, the definition of interconnectedness as an aspect of culture (i.e., the quality and pressure of family life and social relationships), and the domain of social well-being (i.e., ability to participate in family and network activities) partially overlap because both include elements of social relationships. Second, the individual-level contextual component of psychological well-being completely overlaps with the psychological well-being domain of HRQOL. Both are operationalized as depression and anxiety (Ashing-Giwa, 2005). The problem of conceptual and operational overlap between predictor and outcome variables raises the problem of circularity as illustrated in a study of breast cancer in four ethnic groups in which contextual predictors of HRQOL include psychological factors, while one of the HRQOL outcomes is emotional well-being (Ashing-Giwa, Tejero, Kim, Padilla, & Hellemann, 2007).

The Ashing-Giwa model offers a wide range of contextual macro and individual predictors of HRQOL, including culture. It also includes a fairly comprehensive definition of HRQOL that can accommodate diverse cultures and vary within ethnic groups and between individuals. Of importance is the distinction between ethnic and socio-economic status, and between socio-ecological and cultural factors. These distinctions promote a greater understanding of the unique influence of the various contextual predictors on HRQOL.

The Spilker (1996) and Ashing-Giwa (2005) models explicitly accommodate cultural determinants of HRQOL outcomes. However, the other models do not exclude cultural considerations. Ferrell and colleagues' (1991) model (Figure 6-3) suggests that the pain experience includes a physical and emotional component. Each may be affected by culture. Pain may be conceptualized as an integral part of the whole human response to life events and as central to quality of life or as only one aspect of life and, therefore, less central to life's quality. The Padilla and Grant (1985) framework reduces QOL responses to specific antecedents that may or may not be relevant across cultures. The Sprangers and Schwartz model (1999) (Figure 6-4) conceptualizes the disease experience as the trigger that starts an accommodation process resulting in a response shift. Culture is an important determinant of the impact of the catalyst. Culture also shapes expectations concerning the catalyst, the type of accommodation mechanisms to be used, the appraisal of QOL, and the nature of the response shift.

As investigators continue to develop their frameworks of HRQOL, including the authors of the models described here, there is a growing recognition of the influence of culture. Federal policy that requires the inclusion of women, minorities, and children in research supported by the US Public Health Service (National Institutes of Health, 2001, October) and US Military (Department of Defense, 2002, March) has played a very important role in the attention to cultural and ethnic factors in all research, including HRQOL studies, conducted in the United States.

Operational Definitions of Health-Related Quality of Life Across Cultures

Health-Related Quality of Life Questionnaires

Two types of HRQOL questionnaires are available for cross-cultural studies. One type of measure is developed in one language for use in a specific group. Because of interest by investigators, clinicians, or policy makers, the measure is later translated into other languages for use in a variety of cultures and countries around the globe. Examples of two questionnaires developed in the United States and translated for worldwide use are described here.

According to QualityMetric's home page, their most popular generic surveys of functional health and well-being for adults (SF-36v2 Health Survey and shorter versions SF-12v2 and SF-8) are available in 120 languages. In India alone, the SF-36v2 Health Survey is available in 12 languages from Bengali to Urdu including Indian English (QualityMetric, 2010). The three forms of the SF Health Survey measure the same health domains. Physical health is measured by physical functioning, role-physical, bodily pain, and general health domains. Mental health is measured by vitality, social functioning, role-emotional, and mental health domains. To simplify cross-language, cross-cultural, and other cross-group comparisons, scores are calibrated so that the average score is 50.

In 1991, the International Quality of Life Assessment (IQOLA) project was established to translate and validate the original SF-36 Health Survey. The IQOLA project established a process for developing conceptually equivalent and culturally appropriate translations following these steps (QualtyMetric, 2010, p. 1):

- "Multiple independent forward translations by consultants who live in-country and who are native speakers of the target language and bilingual in English
- Translators place emphasis on conceptual rather than literal equivalence, and strive for a reading level appropriate for the country (age 14 or lower)
- Reconciliation of the independent translations into one preliminary translation
- Backward translation of this form into English and evaluation of the backward translation for conceptual equivalence with the original survey by US researchers
- Debriefing interviews with lay people who are native speakers of the target language and living in-country to evaluate the clarity, common language usage, and conceptual equivalence of the translation
- Formatting and proofreading"

The second questionnaire, the Functional Assessment of Cancer Therapy General version (FACT-G), is a basic HRQOL scale that can be applied to any cancer patient. The FACT-G is the most popular measure of the Functional Assessment of Chronic Illness Therapy (FACIT) measurement system. This system includes general, cancer-specific, other disease-specific, symptom-specific, and treatment-specific measures of HRQOL domains (FACIT, 2010). Twenty-seven items of the FACT-G Version 4 measure four primary domains of well-being. These are physical, social/family, emotional, and functional well-being. Population norms are available for the United States and other countries. The FACT-G was first published in 1993 (Cella et al., 1993) and is now available in 53 languages from Afrikaans to Zulu. This, however, does not reflect the extent of the translations. For example, the Spanish version has forms for Puerto Rico, Mexico, and other Spanish language countries.

The FACT-G translation process includes seven steps that are similar to the Quality-Metric approach. The process is summarized here (Aaronson, 2005, page 416). For specific information on the translation and validation process, visit the FACIT Web site (www.FACIT.org).

- Forward translations from English to the target language by two bilingual speakers
- Reconciliation of the forward translations
- Back translation of reconciled version from the target language to English by one bilingual translator
- Independent reviews by three or four bilingual experts
- Review by a coordinating committee to produce one translated version
- Verification of spelling and grammar
- Pilot test of the translated questionnaire with patients in the target language

The second type of HRQOL cross-cultural questionnaire is one developed specifically for cross-cultural projects. From the beginning, the questionnaire is intended to be conceptually and psychometrically equivalent across cultures and languages represented by the experts participating in its development. Two examples are the WHOQOL-100 (WHOQOL Group, 1995, 1998), and the EQ-5D (EuroQol Group, 2010). Both measures were developed with processes (World Health Organization, 1993) similar to those described for the SF-36v2 and the FACT-G.

The WHOQOL-100 consists of 100 items that measure physical aspects (energy and fatigue, pain and discomfort, and sleep and rest); psychological aspects (bodily image and appearance, negative feelings, positive feelings, self-esteem, and thinking, learning, memory, and concentration); aspects of independence (mobility, activities of daily living, dependence on medical substances and medical aids, and work capacity); social aspects (personal relationships, social support, and sexual activity); environmental aspects (financial resources; freedom; physical safety and security; health and social care accessibility and quality; home environment; opportunities for acquiring new information and skills; participation in and opportunities for recreation/leisure; physical environment, which includes pollution, noise, traffic, and climate, and transportation); and spiritual aspects (religion, spirituality, and personal beliefs) of QOL. It also measures overall QOL and health with four additional items. A shorter 26-item version is also available, called the WHOQOL-BREF (World Health Organization, 2004).

The EQ-5D (EuroQol Group, 2010) was develop by the EuroQol Group for the specific purpose of having a standardized, nondisease-specific measure of health-related quality of life. Seven centers in England, Finland, the Netherlands, Norway, and Sweden were the original members. Current membership has expanded to countries in Eastern Europe, Canada, the United States, Africa, Asia, New Zealand, and other areas. The instrument measures five dimensions of HRQOL: mobility, self-care, usual activities, pain/discomfort, and anxiety/depression. Three responses are possible for each dimension (no problems, some or moderate problems, or extreme problems). The rating of one's current HRQOL state is done on a 20cm visual analogue vertical scale (worst imaginable health state at 0 to best imaginable health state at 100). With only five items and one visual analogue scale, it is a very brief measure.

From these four widely used measures, it is clear that across very diverse cultures, QOL as related to one's health status is defined by physical (including symptoms), functional (including a certain amount of independence such as self-care), and emotional (covering feelings like anxiety and depression) well-being. Social well-being was left out of the EQ-5D, but included in the other three questionnaires. The WHOQOL-100 is the most comprehensive measure of HRQOL because it incorporates elements of HRQOL not included in the other measures, such as self-esteem, sexual activity, physical safety and security, the ability to acquire new information and skills, and spirituality. For research purposes, the WHOQOL-100 provides better information for understanding how health influences QOL across cultural groups, and how health disparities specifically impact HRQOL.

These questionnaires also illustrate that measures subjected to an appropriate translation process from the original culture or language to another culture or language or purposefully developed cross-culturally, result in valid, reliable, and useful instruments. The global use of HRQOL questionnaires, such as those described above, are evidence that dimensions of well-being in the context of health resonate across language, national, and cultural boundaries.

Equivalence of QOL and HRQOL Across Cultures

The processes involved in the development of cross-culturally appropriate measures were described in the previous decade (Herdman, Fox-Rushby, & Badia, 1998). However, it is important to remember that three of the four questionnaires described in this chapter, excluding the WHOQOL-100, were developed primarily by investigators from Western cultures where health, well-being, individuality, and autonomy are linked. This may not be the case in non-Western cultures (Parker & Fox-Rushby, 1995). Studies about end-of-life care have shown that beliefs and values about life or about sustaining life are not universal (Blackhall et al., 1999; Kagawa-Singer & Blackhall, 2001). Research efforts over the last 20 years have yielded valid and reliable measures of QOL and HRQOL that can be used cross-culturally.

Cross-cultural studies of QOL and HRQOL can only be undertaken when researchers achieve equivalence of instruments to measure these constructs. The literature includes as many as 17 different types of equivalence, and each type is defined in various ways. The most common types of equivalence include conceptual, semantic, functional, technical, scalar/metric, and operational (Herdman, Fox-Rushby, & Badia, 1997). The least common forms of equivalence include criterion, content, item, cultural, language, meaning, construct operationalization, idiomatic, construct, measurement, and experiential (Herdman et al., 1997).

Fortunately, a streamlined model for assessing cross-cultural equivalence of questionnaires is available (Herdman et al., 1998). The assessment model follows a logical order to investigate cultural equivalence. The model also supports backtracking at any point to reinvestigate a previous type of equivalence.

Step 1. Conceptual equivalence: The domains of the concept in the source and target cultures, the emphasis on domains in these cultures, and the relationship between the domains are the same. The decision to adapt a questionnaire across cultures and the level of adaptation (complete, partial, not possible) depend on the degree of conceptual equivalence.

Step 2. Item equivalence: Items measure the same domain and are similarly relevant and acceptable in the source and target cultures. If conceptual equivalence is supported, then some level of adaptation is possible. The next step is to determine item equivalence. If the majority of items are suitable for use with only a few items unsuitable and these can be adapted or replaced, then semantic and functional equivalence should be investigated. If items can't be adapted or replaced, then adaptation ends.

Step 3. Semantic equivalence: The meaning of a word or phrase transfers across languages and cultures such that the word or phrase has the same effect on questionnaire respondents from the source and target cultures. Translated items should be investigated for functional equivalence.

Step 4. Operational equivalence: The format of the questionnaire including instructions and layout, and the procedures for scaling items, scoring, administering the questionnaire, etc. are similar and appropriate for the source and target cultures. A determination of operational equivalence next leads to an investigation of measurement equivalence and functional equivalence.

Step 5. Measurement equivalence: The different language or cultural versions of the questionnaire achieve acceptable psychometric properties of reliability and validity. Whether psychometric properties are the same or different, functional equivalence needs to be determined.

Step 6. Functional equivalence: ". . . the extent to which an instrument does what it is supposed to do equally well in two or more cultures . . . To be able to demonstrate functional equivalence, it is therefore necessary to be able to say, firstly, how the underlying trait is defined or conceptualized in the target culture, secondly, how well the instrument design reflects that underlying trait; and, finally, how the results obtained from a given instrument compare across cultures." (Herdman et al., 1998, p. 331)

These six types of equivalence are the basis for developing cross-cultural questionnaires. However, conceptual equivalence is the most important type and requires qualitative research to determine the domains of a construct in the target culture. The results of such research are the basis for determining whether an instrument can be adapted to the target culture.

These minimum requirements for cross-cultural equivalence of QOL and HRQOL instruments (Herdman et al., 1998) apply to questionnaires that are adapted or translated from the source to the target culture, meaning sequential development (Bullinger, Anderson, Cella, & Aaronson, 1995). These requirements for equivalence also apply when questionnaires develop parallelly or simultaneously (Bullinger et al., 1995). Parallel development occurs when a cross-cultural team participates in conceptualizing a measure, and develops new items or draws items from existing scales so that all items reflect the same conceptual domain in each culture. Simultaneous development occurs when an interactive strategy is used to develop a new instrument reflective of each participating culture's unique and common domains (Bullinger et al., 1995).

The approach taken by Hendricson and colleagues (Hendricson et al., 1989) in developing a Spanish version of the Arthritis Impact Measurement Scale for use in a South Texas population illustrates a strategy to investigate equivalence. For each item, the Spanish translation was printed along side the English version. This format provided a practical strategy to investigate conceptual, item, semantic, and operational equivalence (Herdman et al., 1998). It also made it easier for bicultural and bilingual focus groups to evaluate conceptual equivalence.

Issues in Cross-Cultural Research

Stable vs. Changeable Characteristics of QOL and HRQOL

Basic assumptions about QOL and HRQOL are that well-being is dynamic, not static, and that changes are reflected in assessments of our own or others' well-being. The notion that HRQOL consists of state (environmental) and trait (genetic) components has been advanced by Sprangers and Schwartz (2008). HRQOL can be affected by a person's emotional state, which, in turn, may be influenced by environmental characteristics and genetic predispositions (Sprangers et al., 2010). Understanding what and why HRQOL components may be changed can lead to learning how and when interventions will be successful in improving and maintaining desirable levels of well-being.

In advancing their state and trait constructs of HRQOL, Sprangers and Schwartz (2008) focus on happiness (the "what" component of HRQOL), adaptation and positive psychology research ("why" HRQOL is changeable), and genetic studies ("why" HRQOL is stable). Happiness is explained as a reflection of overall quality of life, therefore, a significant aspect of emotional well-being. The authors (Sprangers & Schwartz, 2008) explain the Hedonic Treadmill theory of adaptation (Brickman & Campbell, 1971) as one that holds that each person has a genetically based set-point for happiness. The set-point reflects stable personality traits that likely determine the upper and lower limits of happiness for an individual. Individuals adapt to new life circumstances, whether better or worse, and eventually arrive at a hedonically neutral state. The theory implies that the constant search for happiness is, in the long run, "futile" (Diener, Lucas, & Scollon, 2006).

However, the revised treadmill theory of adaptation (Diener et al., 2006), based on empirical work, offers a more optimistic view of people's ability to increase long-term happiness. Diener and colleagues (2006) proposed these revisions:

1. Set-points are not neutral. Despite some cultural variation between Inughuit, Amish, and Maasai, most people are generally happy, and not in a neutral hedonic state (Biswas-Diener, Vittersø, & Diener, 2005).

2. Apart from culture, set-points are also based on individual temperaments. Research shows that level of well-being is reasonably stable over time. In a 17-year study of Germans, Fujita and Diener (2005) found that 24% changed significantly from the first to the last five years of the study. This still left a majority of the sample relatively unchanged. Set-points are also partly genetic and thus heritable (Tellegen et al., 1988) as well as strongly correlated with personality (Diener & Lucas, 1999).

3. Aspects of happiness, meaning well-being, may have different set-points. Well-being is not a single, global concept with one set-point (Diener et al., 2006). For example, life satisfaction and unpleasant emotions may have different set-points within the same person and may move in the same or different directions and at different rates (Scollon & Diener, 2006). This characteristic of set-points was shown in a study of 42 countries around the world (Inglehart & Klingemann, 2000).

4. Set-points of happiness, meaning well-being, can change under certain circumstances. In their review of various waves of multicountry surveys of positive–negative effect balance and life satisfaction carried out by the European Values Study Group and World Values Survey Association (2005), Diener, Lucas, and Scollon (2006) reported that aspects of well-being do change and are affected by life circumstances. Another review of the results of subjective well-being (SWB) surveys across 55 nations (Diener, Diener, & Diener, 2009) revealed that high income, individualism, human rights, and societal equality correlated strongly with each other and with SWB. Of all the predictors of SWB, only individualism correlated consistently with the construct when other factors were controlled. Cultural homogeneity was not a good predictor of SWB. Levels of happiness can be stable, but can also change over the long term (Fujita & Diener, 2005).

5. The final revision asserted that individuals differ in their adaptation to events; while some change, others do not (Diener et al., 2006). Individuals whose happiness set-points change the most are those who experience events unlike their usual experiences (Oishi, Diener, Choi, Kim-Prieto, & Choi, 2007). For example, persons or cultures whose common experience is of positive life events respond to another positive event with little change in level of happiness than would persons or cultures that usually experience negative events.

These revised notions about adaptation support the propositions that QOL, defined as well-being, happiness, life satisfaction, or emotional states, is both an individual and a cultural characteristic, can change both in the short and long term, and is both a trait and a state.

Focusing on the Positive: Improving and Sustaining QOL and HRQOL

In their report, Sprangers and Schwartz (2008) uphold the notion that intentional activities can exert a significant impact on happiness. They base this idea on Lyubomirsky's model and meta-analysis of studies of happiness and success (Lyubomirsky, Sheldon, & Schkade, 2005). Lyubomirsky found that happiness is associated with and also precedes many successful outcomes, for example, success at work and school. In addition, happy people are more likely to engage in behaviors that promote success, such as getting along with others, helping others, and being a good organizational citizen. Lyubomirsky concluded that positive affect may be the cause of many desirable characteristics that are associated with happiness. Altruistic behavior can lead to happiness and is associated with health benefits (Post, 2007).

Heritable and Dispositional Characteristics of QOL and HRQOL

This chapter has emphasized the influence of culture, meaning the environment, on HRQOL. However, an overlooked factor is genetic predisposition. In proposing that HRQOL has state (environmental) and trait (genetic) components, Sprangers and Schwartz remind us that some aspects of HRQOL can be improved, while others resist change (Sprangers & Schwartz, 2008). A meta-analysis of twin studies showed that 31.6% of the variance in anxiety disorder was attributable to genetics in both males and females (Hettema, Neale, & Kendler, 2001). Twin studies also revealed familial aggregation in the case of major depression with additive genetic effects, meaning that heritability estimates reached 37% (Sullivan, Neale, & Kendler, 2000). A study of Swedish twins examined the correlations between perceived social support and depression or life satisfaction (Bergeman, Plomin, Pedersen, & McClearn, 1991). The absolute phenotypic correlations between perceived support and depression (0.20) and perceived support and life satisfaction (0.27) were small. However, a large part of the covariations of these correlations were due to common genetic influences (65% and 56% respectively). An important contribution to the state–trait notion of HRQOL are findings from the study by Sloan and Zhao (2006). These investigators hypothesized that variations in three specific folate genes would correlate with 494 cancer patients' QOL prior to any chemotherapy, because the target genes are involved in cellular stress response. Seven different markers were significantly related to fatigue. These and other findings underscore the importance of considering genetic contributions to HRQOL in addition to culture and other environmental predictors.

In light of support for the revised treadmill theory of happiness, for the influence of intentional, altruistic activities on happiness and the state–trait composition of quality of life, Sprangers and Schwartz recommend "...interventions that teach ways of refocusing one's perspective and priorities, and that these increases are sustained over time. Although this newfound flexibility is heartening, it is important to recognize the genetic or predetermined constraints that limit the extent to which HRQOL can be enhanced" (Sprangers & Schwartz, 2008). They point out that theories of HRQOL need to account for the fixed and changeable aspects of the construct. This means that future research needs to consider which aspects of a catalyst, an intervention or an adaptation mechanism, are likely to impact or not impact HRQOL.

Role of Acculturation

Acculturation means learning the beliefs, values, and standards of behavior of another cultural group to function comfortably in that group, typically the dominant culture, and, in the case of immigrants—the host culture. Assimilation means taking on the beliefs, values, and practices of the host culture and giving up those of one's own native culture. Individuals may acculturate to varying degrees without necessarily assimilating to the host culture. Acculturation can modify the significance of any of the variables listed in Table 6-2 that contribute to disparities in disease incidence and mortality between ethnic groups. A common conceptualization of acculturation comprises the domains of preferred language, self-identity, friendship choices that determine social boundaries, standards of acceptable behavior, generation since family immigration to the host country, country of origin, and attitudes (willingness to behave in certain ways) (Suinn, Rickard-Figueroa, Lew, & Vigil, 1987). Acculturation has also been defined generically by length of residence, age at arrival in the host country, and by media influence (Marin, Sabogal, Vann Oss-Marin, Otero-Sabogal, & Perez-Stable, 1987). However, these last are less important indicators of HRQOL. To these lists Alarcon and colleagues expanded on language proficiency including usage, and preferences, and added type of neighborhood (Alarcon et al., 1999). Measures of acculturation may be specifically determined by knowledge and practices concerning the traditions of a culture. For example, Hishinuma and colleagues measured Hawaiian acculturation as knowledge and practices about the Hawaiian way of life, valuation and maintenance of Hawaiian beliefs and non-Hawaiian beliefs, Hawaiian blood quantum, and specific cultural traditions using seven subscales (lifestyles, customs, activities, folklore, causes-locations, causes-access, and language proficiency) (Hishinuma et al., 2000).

Knowledge of acculturation and assimilation provides insight into health-seeking attitudes of ethnic groups, reasons for success or failure of prevention and treatment regimens, ways to best reach diverse ethnic groups with health-related messages, and strategies for opening access to health care for ethnic groups (Padilla & Perez, 1995). Acculturation is associated with HRQOL when demographic, medical, socioecologic, and healthcare access factors are controlled (Kim, Ashing-Giwa, Kagawa-Singer, & Tejero, 2006). However, large race or ethnic categories, such as "Asian American" commonly used in research, can mask the different effects of acculturation among ethnic subgroups such as Filipino, Korean, or Japanese. For example, Kim and colleagues found that Korean Americans reported poorer QOL than other Asian subgroups (Kim et al., 2006). It is important for cross-cultural studies to include a measure of acculturation.

As stated previously, people can acculturate without assimilating into the host culture. The ability to gain sufficient knowledge about a culture to transact easily within that culture does not necessarily mean that one gives up his or her original culture. In fact, an individual can belong to several cultural groups. An understanding of the influence of culture on HRQOL needs to consider ethnic affiliation as well as level of acculturation and assimilation into another, usually the host, culture.

For many years, operational definitions of acculturation reflected a linear, unidimensional construct. Measures of nativity, length of stay in the host country, and language use exemplify unidimensional definitions. More comprehensive views of acculturation consider multidimensional frameworks, reciprocal interactions between the individual and the environment, adoption of attitudes, values, customs, beliefs, and behaviors of another culture, food and music preferences, and other "acculturative processes" (Abraido-Lanza, Armbrister, Florez, & Aguirre, 2006). Abraido-Lanza and colleagues recommend that acculturation be represented as a latent variable with a number of indicators defining acculturation. In this way, components of acculturation can be identified as risk or protective factors for health problems and for HRQOL.

Validity and Reliability of Group Coding Schemes

Valid, reliabile, and consistent coding schemes to identify cultural and ethnic or racial groups is key to cross-cultural research. Unfortunately, broad categories are generally used resulting in mixtures of people within grouping codes. Inconsistent codes make it difficult to compare data across studies. The National Institutes of Health's Targeted/Planned Enrollment Table codes human subjects by ethnicity (Hispanic/Latino or Not Hispanic/Latino) and race (American Indian or Alaska Native, Asian, native Hawaiian or Other Pacific Islander, black or African American, and white) (US Department of Health and Human Services Public Health Service, Revised September 2004). However, the National Center for Health Statistics uses 10 racial categories: white, black, Indian (e.g., Aleut, Eskimoan, Mexican Indian, Red, Ute), Chinese, Japanese, Hawaiian, Filipino, Other Asian or Pacific Islander (e.g., Asian Indian, Thai, Cambodian), other entries, and not reported (National Center for Health Statistics, 1998 December). Government coding schemes have not kept pace with the widening diversity of race and ethnicity in the United States.

Race and ethnicity classification schemes are often unreliable. This is true for ethnicity data from hospitals (Riddle, 2005), infant birth and death information (Hahn, Mulinare, & Teutsch, 1992), and adult death information (Harwell et al., 2002; Kelly, Chu, Diaz, Leary, & Buehler, 1996). These errors result in inaccurate information about ethnic mortality and morbidity, and potentially inequitable distribution of diagnosis and treatment resources among groups.

Broad racial and ethnic categories and coding errors result in culturally invalid data. Lumping together as "black" new immigrants from Africa with descendents of African slaves or coding descendants of Spanish settlers, first generation Mexican citizens, and Puerto Ricans as "Latino" is detrimental to each of the groups. Each ethnic and cultural group holds some unique beliefs and values about quality of life. Coding schemes should be checked against self-identified cultural labels in determining the validity of the code.

Kaplan and Bennett describe challenges and provide guidelines concerning the use of race and ethnicity in biomedical publications (Kaplan & Bennett, 2003). The authors challenge writers and editors of biomedical publications to avoid stereotyping groups, and creating racial and ethnic divisions that threaten people's health. The guidelines offer constructive help to investigators to promote rigorous research and accurate language when using the constructs of "race" and "ethnicity" (Table 6-1).

Table 6-1.   **Challenges and Guidelines for Use of "Race" and "Ethnicity" in Biomedical Publications**

Challenge

Accounting for limitations in racial/ethnic data	• Constructs of race/ethnicity are complex and imprecise. • Race/ethnic identity is dynamic, not fixed and immutable, and not easily determined. • Categories of race/ethnicity lack standardization and are inconsistently applied across studies. Reliability and validity of racial/ethnic assignment can't be assumed. Admitting clerks, clinicians, and others may not be trained to provide accurate racial/ethnic codes. • Range and operational definition of race/ethnic categories differ across studies.
Distinguishing between race/ethnicity as risk factor or risk marker	• Race/ethnicity is a marker for risk of a particular disease or health problem if incidence or prevalence of the condition is greater in one's race/ethnic group compared to others. • Race/ethnicity is a risk factor when membership in the group increases the likelihood of developing the condition. However, race/ethnicity as risk factors are not well understood; a strong association doesn't infer causality.
Avoiding contributing to racial/ethnic divisions	• Avoid contributing to or reinforcing stereotypes and generalizations about groups or about differences between groups (e.g., all people of color are poor).

Guidelines

Race/ethnicity as a study variable	• Specify reason for its use.
Race/ethnicity data source	• Describe how subjects assigned to racial/ethnic categories. • Specify if self-reported race/ethnicity based on open-ended response or fixed categories.
Race/ethnicity and genetic variation	• Support any inference about genetic differences with evidence from rigorous gene studies. Differences within groups are usually greater than differences between groups.
Hypotheses and results concerning race/ethnicity	• Distinguish between race/ethnicity as a risk factor and race/ethnicity as a risk marker.
Interpretation of racial/ethnic differences	• Consider relevant factors: discrimination, racism, SES, environment, diet, nutrition, health beliefs and practices, country of birth, time in country of residence, etc. • Adjust for effects of SES and social class.
Descriptions of race/ethnic groups	• Do not use stigmatizing terms. • Do not use unscientific classification systems. • Do not suggest that race/ethnicity is an intrinsic attribute.

Source: Adapted from Kaplan and Bennett, 2003.

Table 6-2.   **Variables That Contribute to the Difference Between Ethnic Populations in Disease Incidence and Mortality**

Physiological and Biochemical Differences

Genetic differences	Consanguinity, mutation rates, genetic predisposition, or protective barriers
Environmental factors	Exposure to toxic elements, dietary influences
Exposure to infectious agents	

Socioeconomic Factors

Poverty	Differential access to medical diagnoses/treatments/procedures; work exposure to toxic elements; available and affordable healthy food in adequate quantities; educational base (knowledge of treatment, adherence, value of early detection); discrimination
Insurance	Under or uninsured
Costs of family and home care	Direct and indirect costs
Shifts from hospital to home for semiacute and long-term care	

Structural Aspects of the Healthcare System

Documentation	Errors of measurement; completeness of morbidity and mortality data; lack of completeness and detail in coding categories; lack of representativeness in ethnic samples
Availability issues	Lack of facilities within reasonable distances or that address cultural needs
Accessibility	(See *Socioeconomic Factors*)
Practitioner/patient interactions	Time restrictions in clinical encounters; clinic settings in which different doctors seen at each visit; focus only on chief complaint to detriment of other problems; institutional racism; insensitivity to needs/diseases of diverse ethnic groups

Cultural Factors for Patients and Practitioners

Misconceptions conceptions concerning culture	

Table 6-2. **continued**

Cultural Factors for Patients and Practitioners (continued)

Acculturation and assimilation variation	
Acceptability of recommendation	
Differential use of available facilities	
Culturally competent practitioners	
Attitudes, beliefs, behaviors about illness/specific diseases	Early detection; consequences of late diagnosis; treatment plans; role of healthcare practitioners; social stigma
Lifestyle differences in personal customs or habits	Reproductive nursing habits; sexual practices; smoking, alcohol, drug use, diet
Response to racism	

Source: Adapted from Kagawa-Singer, 1995, p. 110. Copyright 1995 W.B. Saunders.

Epidemiology and Prevalence of Disease in Relation to Cultural and Ethnic Diversity

Ethnic and racial groups exhibit differences in disease prevalence, incidence, mortality, and morbidity. It is, therefore, logical to examine cross-cultural differences in the epidemiology and prevalence of a physical or mental illness prior to assessing its impact on HRQOL. The four categories of variables that influence the distribution of cancer prevalence, incidence, mortality, and morbidity across different cultural and ethnic or racial groups discussed by Kagawa-Singer generalize to other diseases (Kagawa-Singer, 1995). The four categories are physiologic and biochemical, socioeconomic, healthcare system structure, and cultural factors. Specific sources of ethnic diversity within each of these factors are listed in Table 6-2. These major sources of variability are seldom independent of one another, but instead exercise an interactive effect on disease incidence and mortality in culturally/ethnically diverse populations (Kagawa-Singer, 1995). Consequently, they are also expected to exert an interactive influence on HRQOL. However, due to errors in racial and ethnic classification, investigators need to be cautious when using national databases in determining differences between ethnic groups in mortality, morbidity, socioeconomic indicators, and other variables (Hahn et al., 1992; Harwell et al., 2002; Kelly et al., 1996). Five major limitations in the use of national cancer databases also apply to other diseases. These limitations include racial mis-classification; undercounting due to sampling error; insufficient sample size of particular ethnic groups for statistical analyses; geographic uniqueness that precludes generalizations; and lack of uniformity in the operationalization of key variables (Kagawa-Singer, 1995).

CONCLUSION

Scientific evidence concerning culture, ethnic affiliation, and health underscores the unequal burden of disease endured by discriminated cultural groups, by ethnic minorities, and by socio-economically disadvantaged people. To illustrate, in the United States, the cancer incidence in women is highest among whites, followed by blacks, yet, the death rate is highest among blacks, then whites (US Cancer Statistics Working Group, 2010). Recognizing the impact of culture and health disparities on HRQOL for individuals and groups, this chapter drew from older and more recent literature to briefly review aspects of quality of life, health, and culture that are relevant to cross-cultural studies of HRQOL.

The WHOQOL definition of quality of life (WHOQOL Group, 1995) together with the Kagawa-Singer transcultural framework (Kagawa-Singer, 1988) of culture provide a broad, practical, descriptive, and prescriptive definition of quality of life, as related to health, that is likely to be valid in similar and diverse cultures. Several operational definition issues need to be considered in the study of HRQOL. These include the distinction between QOL and HRQOL, between determinants and dimensions of HRQOL, the selection of appropriate predictors of HRQOL outcomes, the recognition of response shift in HRQOL measures, and the distinction between macro and individual levels of HRQOL predictors. Investigators should be especially aware of the contextual influence of culture on HRQOL and the difference between culture, ethnicity, and race. Questionnaires used in cross-cultural research need to pass tests of equivalence across cultural boundaries. Investigators need to be aware that HRQOL consists of state and trait components and that level of acculturation is usually an important factor in health beliefs and practices. Nations are increasingly characterized by cultural and ethnic diversity. In 2008 Hispanics and non-White groups made up 34.4% of the US population (US Census Bureau, 2010, April 22). Cross-cultural studies can provide important information about the effectiveness and efficacy of interventions to improve or sustain HRQOL.

REFERENCES

Abraido-Lanza, A. F., Armbrister, A. N., Florez, K. R., & Aguirre, A. N. (2006). Toward a theory-driven model of acculturation in public health research. *Am J Public Health, 96*(8), 1342–1346.

Alarcon, G. S., Rodriguez, J. L., Benavides, G. J., Brooks, K., Kurusz, H., & Reveille, J. D., with LUMINA Study Group. (1999). Systemic lupus erythematosus in three ethnic groups. V. Acculturation, health-related attitudes and behaviors, and disease activity in Hispanic patients from the LUMINA cohort. Lupus in minority populations, nature versus nurture. *Arthritis Care and Research, 12*(4), 267–276.

Aaronson, N. K. (2005). Cross-cultural use of health-related quality of life assessments in clinical oncology. In J. Lipscomb, C. C. Gotay & C. Snyder (Eds.), *Outcomes assessment in cancer: Measures, methods, and applications* (pp. 406–424). Cambridge: Cambridge University Press.

Ashing-Giwa, K. T. (2005). The contextual model of HRQOL: A paradigm for expanding the HRQOL framework. *Quality of Life Research, 14*(2), 297–307.

Ashing-Giwa, K. T., Kagawa-Singer, M., Padilla, G. V., Tejero, J. S., Hsiao, E., Chhabra, R., et al. (2004). The impact of cervical cancer and dysplasia: A qualitative, multiethnic study. *Psychooncology, 13*(10), 709–728.

Ashing-Giwa, K. T., Padilla, G. V., Bohorquez, D. E., Tejero, J. S., Garcia, M., & Meyers, E. A. (2006). Survivorship: A qualitative investigation of Latinas diagnosed with cervical cancer. *J Psychosoc Oncol, 24*(4), 53–88.

Ashing-Giwa, K. T., Tejero, J. S., Kim, J., Padilla, G. V., & Hellemann, G. (2007). Examining predictive models of HRQOL in a population-based, multiethnic sample of women with breast carcinoma. *Qual Life Res, 16*(3), 413–42.

Bergeman, C.S., Plomin, R., Pedersen, N.L., McClearn, G.E. (1991). Genetic mediation of the relationship between social support and psychological well-being. *Psychol Aging, 6*(4), 640–646.

Berzon, R. A., & Shumaker, S. A. (1995). Preface. In S. A. Shumaker & R. A. Berzon (Eds.), *The international assessment of health-related quality of life: Theory, translation, measurement and analysis* (pp. v–vi). Oxford: Rapid Communication.

Biswas-Diener, R., Vitterso, J., & Diener, E. (2005). Most people are pretty happy, but there is cultural variation: The Inughuit, the Amish, and the Maasai. *Journal of Happiness Studies, 6*, 205–226.

Blackhall, L. J., Frank, G., Murphy, S. T., Michel, V., Palmer, J. M., & Azen, S. P. (1999). Ethnicity and attitudes towards life sustaining technology. *Social Science and Medicine, 48*(12), 1779–1789.

Brady, M. J., Peterman, A. H., Fitchett, G., Mo, M., & Cella, D. (1999). A case for including spirituality in quality of life measurement in oncology. *Psycho-Oncology, 8*(5), 417–428.

Brickman, P., & Campbell, D. T. (1971). Hedonic relativism and planning the good society. In M. H. Appley (Ed.), *Adaptation level theory: A symposium* (pp. 287–302). New York, NY: Academic Press.

Bullinger, M., Anderson, R., Cella, D., & Aaronson, N. (1995). Developing and evaluating cross-cultural instruments from minimum requirements to optimal models. In S. A. Shumaker & R. A. Berzon (Eds.), *The international assessment of health-related quality of life: Theory, translation, measurement and analysis* (pp. 83–91). Oxford: Rapid Communication.

Cella, D. F., Tulsky, D. S., Gray, G., Sarafian, B., Linn, E., Bonomi, A., et al. (1993). The Functional Assessment of Cancer Therapy scale: Development and validation of the general measure. *Journal of Clinical Oncology, 11*(3), 570–579.

Center for Advanced Research on Language Acquisition. (2010, January 22). *What is culture: Definition.* Retrieved May 17, 2010, from http://www.carla.umn.edu/culture/definitions.html.

City of Hope Pain and Palliative Care Resource Center. (2010). *Research Instruments/Resources/Quality of Life Instruments.* Retrieved May 31, 2010, from http://prc.coh.org.

Department of Defense. (2002, 25 March). *Protection of human subjects and adherence to ethical standards in DoD supported research, 4.6. Inclusion of women and minorities in clinical research projects.* Retrieved May 31, 2010, from http://www.dtic.mil/whs/directives/corres/pdf/321602p.pdf.

Diener, E., Diener, M., & Diener, C. (2009). Factors predicting the subjective well-being of nations. In E. Diener (Ed.), *Culture and well-being: The collected works of Ed Diener* (1 ed., Vol. 38, pp. 43–70): Springer, Netherlands.

Diener, E., & Lucas, R. E. (1999). Personality and subjective well-being. In D. Kahneman, E. Diener, & N. Schwarz (Eds.), *Well-being: The foundations of a hedonic psychology* (pp. 213–229). New York, NY: Russell Sage Foundation.

Diener, E., Lucas, R. E., & Scollon, C. N. (2006). Beyond the hedonic treadmill: Revising the adaptation theory of well-being. *Am Psychol, 61*(4), 305–314.

Edmondson, D., Park, C. L., Blank, T. O., Fenster, J. R., & Mills, M. A. (2007). Deconstructing spiritual well-being: Existential well-being and HRQOL in cancer survivors. *Psychooncology, 1*(2), 161–169.

European Values Study Group, & World Values Survey Association. (2005). *European and World Values Surveys Integrated Data File, 1999–2002, Release I (2nd ICPSR version)* [Data file]. Ann Arbor, MI: Inter University Consortium for Political and Social Research.

EuroQol Group. (2010). *EQ-5D: A standardized instrument for use as a measure of health outcome*. Retrieved May 31, 2010, from http://www.euroqol.org/euroqol-group/about-us.html.

FACIT. (2010). *FACIT: Functional assessment of chronic illness therapy*. Retrieved February 12, 2011, from http://www.facit.org/.

Ferrell, B., Grant, M., Padilla, G., Vemuri, S., & Rhiner, M. (1991). The experience of pain and perceptions of quality of life: Validation of a conceptual model. *Hospice Journal, 7*(3), 9–24.

Ferrell, B. R., Grant, M., Funk, B., Otis-Green, S., & Garcia, N. (1998). Quality of life in breast cancer: Part II: Psychological and spiritual well-being. *Cancer Nurs, 21*(1), 1–9.

Fletcher, J. F. (1990). Four indicators of humanhood: The enquiry matures. In J. J. Walter & T. A. Shannon (Eds.), *Quality of life: The new medical dilemma* (pp. 11–17). Mahwah, New Jersey: Paulist Press.

Foster, M. W., & Sharp, R. R. (2004). Beyond race: Towards a whole-genome perspective on human populations and genetic variation. *Nat Rev Genet, 5*(10), 790–796.

Fujita, F., & Diener, E. (2005). Life satisfaction set point: Stability and change. *Journal of Personality and Social Psychology, 88*, 158–164.

Gill, T. M., & Feinstein, A. R. (1994). A critical appraisal of the quality of quality-of-life measurements. *Jama, 272*(8), 619–626.

Greeff, M., Uys, L. R., Wantland, D., Makoae, L., Chirwa, M., Dlamini, P., et al. (2010). Perceived HIV stigma and life satisfaction among persons living with HIV infection in five African countries: A longitudinal study. *Int J Nurs Stud, 47*(4), 475–486.

Hahn, R. A., Mulinare, J., & Teutsch, S. M. (1992). Inconsistencies in coding of race and ethnicity between birth and death in US infants: A new look at infant mortality, 1983 through 1985. *Jama, 267*(2), 259–263.

Harwell, T. S., Hansen, D., Moore, K. R., Jeanotte, D., Gohdes, D., & Helgerson, S. D. (2002). Accuracy of race coding on American Indian death certificates, Montana 1996–1998. *Public Health Rep, 117*(1), 44–49.

Hendricson, W. D., Russell, I. J., Prihoda, T. J., Jacobson, J. M., Rogan, A., Bishop, G. D., et al. (1989). Development and initial validation of a dual-language English-Spanish format for the Arthritis Impact Measurement Scales. *Arthritis and Rheumatology, 32*, 1153–1159.

Herdman, M., Fox-Rushby, J., & Badia, X. (1997). 'Equivalence' and the translation and adaptation of health-related quality of life questionnaires. *Qual Life Res, 6*(3), 237–247.

Herdman, M., Fox-Rushby, J., & Badia, X. (1998). A model of equivalence in the cultural adaptation of HRQOL instruments: The universalist approach. *Qual Life Res, 7*(4), 323–335.

Hettema, J. M., Neale, M. C., & Kendler, K. S. (2001). A review and meta-analysis of the genetic epidemiology of anxiety disorders. *Am J Psychiatry, 158*(10), 1568–1578.

Higuchi, K. (1985). *Quality of life in cancer patients and their psychological care*. Paper presented at the Quality of Life in Cancer Patients: A Current Topic in Cancer Treatment and Care. Proceedings of the Workshop on Quality of Life in Cancer Patients-Tokyo, Tokyo, Japan.

Hirschman, C., Alba, R., & Farley, R. (2000). The meaning and measurement of race in the U.S. census: Glimpses into the future. *Demography, 37*(3), 381–393.

Hishinuma, E. S., Andrade, N. N., Johnson, R. C., McArdle, J. J., Miyamoto, R. H., Nahulu, L. B., et al. (2000). Psychometric properties of the Hawaiian Culture Scale—Adolescent Version. *Psychological Assessment, 12*(2), 140–157.

Inglehart, R., & Klingemann, H. D. (2000). Genes, culture, democracy, and happiness. In E. Diener & E. M. Suh (Eds.), *Culture and subjective well-being* (pp. 165–184). Cambridge, MA: MIT Press.

Institute of Medicine. (2001). *Health and behavior: The interplay of biological, behavioral, and societal influences*. Washington D. C.: National Academy Press.

Juarez, G., Ferrell, B., & Borneman, T. (1998). Influence of culture on cancer pain management in Hispanic patients. *Cancer Pract*, 6(5), 262–269.

Kagawa-Singer, M. (1988). *Bamboo and oak: A comparative study of adaptation to cancer by Japanese-American and Anglo-American cancer patients*. Unpublished dissertation, University of California at Los Angeles, Los Angeles, CA.

Kagawa-Singer, M. (1993). Redefining health: Living with cancer. *Social Science and Medicine*, 37, 295–304.

Kagawa-Singer, M. (1995). Socioeconomic and cultural influences on cancer care of women. *Seminars in Oncology Nursing*, 11(2), 109–119.

Kagawa-Singer, M. (2000). Improving the validity and generalizability of studies with underserved U.S. populations expanding the research paradigm. *Annals of Epidemiology*, 10(8, Suppl.), S92–S103.

Kagawa-Singer, M. (2001). From genes to social science: Impact of the simplistic interpretation of race, ethnicity, and culture on cancer outcome. *Cancer*, 91(1, Suppl.), 226–232.

Kagawa-Singer, M. (2006). Population science is science only if you know the population. *J Cancer Educ*, 21(1, Suppl.), S22–S31.

Kagawa-Singer, M., & Blackhall, L. J. (2001). Negotiating cross-cultural issues at the end of life. *Journal of the American Medical Association*, 286(23), 2993–3001.

Kagawa-Singer, M., & Chung, R. (1994). A paradigm for culturally based care for minority populations. *Journal of Community Psychology*, 22(2), 192–208.

Kaplan, J. B., & Bennett, T. (2003). Use of race and ethnicity in biomedical publication. *Jama*, 289(20), 2709–2716.

Kelly, J. J., Chu, S. Y., Diaz, T., Leary, L. S., & Buehler, J. W., with the AIDS Mortality Project Group and The Supplement to HIV/AIDS Surveillance Project Group. (1996). Race/ethnicity misclassification of persons reported with AIDS. *Ethn Health*, 1(1), 87–94.

Kim, J., Ashing-Giwa, K. T., Kagawa-Singer, M., & Tejero, J. S. (2006). Breast cancer among Asian Americans: Is acculturation related to health-related quality of life? *Oncol Nurs Forum*, 33(6), E90–E99.

Kirkham, S. R., Pesut, B., Meyerhoff, H., & Sawatzky, R. (2004). Spiritual caregiving at the juncture of religion, culture, and state. *Can J Nurs Res*, 36(4), 148–169.

Larios, S. E., Davis, J. N., Gallo, L. C., Heinrich, J., & Talavera, G. (2009). Concerns about stigma, social support and quality of life in low-income HIV-positive Hispanics. *Ethnicity and Disease*, 19(1), 65–70.

Lipscomb, J., Gotay, C. C., & Snyder, C. (2005). *Outcomes assessment in cancer: Measures, methods, and applications*. Cambridge: Cambridge University Press.

Lyubomirsky, S., Sheldon, K. M., & Schkade, D. A. (2005). Pursuing happiness: The architecture of sustainable change. *Review of General Psychology*, 9, 111–131.

Marin, G., Sabogal, F., Vann Oss-Marin, B., Otero-Sabogal, R., & Perez-Stable, E. J. (1987). Development of a short acculturation scale for Hispanics. *Hispanic Journal of Behavioral Sciences*, 9, 183–199.

Montagu, A. (1962). *Culture and the evolution of man*. New York, NY: Oxford University Press.

Montagu, A. (1997). *Man's most dangerous myth: The fallacy of race* (6th ed.). Walnut Creek, CA: Alta Mira Press.

Moons, P., Van Deyk, K., Budts, W., & De Geest, S. (2004). Caliber of quality-of-life assessments in congenital heart disease: A plea for more conceptual and methodological rigor. *Arch Pediatr Adolesc Med*, 158(11), 1062–1069.

National Center for Health Statistics. (1998, December). *Instruction manual, part 3a: Classification and coding instructions for live birth records, 1999*. Retrieved August 19, 2007, from http://www.cdc.gov/nchs/data/dvs/3amanual.pdf.

National Institutes of Health. (2001, October). *Inclusion of women and minorities as participants in research involving human subjects—Policy implementation page (NIH Revitalization Act of 1993, PL 103-43, First signed into law June 10, 1993, last update October 2001)*. Retrieved May 31, 2010, from http://grants.nih.gov/grants/funding/women_min/guidelines_amended_10_2001.htm.

Oishi, S., Diener, E., Choi, D. W., Kim-Prieto, C., & Choi, I. (2007). The dynamics of daily events and well-being across cultures: When less is more. *J Pers Soc Psychol, 93*(4), 685–698.

Padilla, G. V., Ferrell, B., Grant, M. M., & Rhiner, M. (1990). Defining the content domain of quality of life for cancer patients with pain. *Cancer Nurs, 13*(2), 108–115.

Padilla, G. V., & Grant, M. M. (1985). Quality of life as a cancer nursing outcome variable. *ANS Adv Nurs Sci, 8*(1), 45–60.

Padilla, G. V., Grant, M. M., Ferrell, B. R., & Presant, C. (1996). Quality of life— Cancer. In B. Spilker (Ed.), *Quality of life and pharmacoeconomics in clinical trials* (2nd ed., pp. 301–308). New York, NY: Lippincott-Raven.

Padilla, G. V., & Perez, E. (1995). Minorities and arthritis. *Arthritis Care Res, 8*(4), 251–256.

Parker, M., & Fox-Rushby, J. A. (1995). International comparisons in health-related quality of life: Acquiescence in academia. In S. A. Shumaker & R. A. Berzon (Eds.), *The international assessment of health-related quality of life: Theory, translation, measurement and analysis* (pp. 153–154). Oxford: Rapid Communication.

Post, S. G. (2007). *Altruism & health: Perspectives from empirical research.* New York, NY: Oxford University Press.

QualityMetric. (2010). *What we do: Language translations.* Retrieved May 31, 2010, from http://www.quality metric.com/WhatWeDo/LanguageTranslations/tabid/213/Default.aspx.

Rapkin, B. D., & Schwartz, C. E. (2004). Toward a theoretical model of quality-of-life appraisal: Implications of findings from studies of response shift. *Health Qual Life Outcomes, 2*, 14.

Riddle, B. L. (2005). On the coding and reporting of race and ethnicity in New Hampshire for purposes of cancer reporting. *Ethn Dis, 15*(2), 324–331.

Royal, C. D., & Dunston, G. M. (2004). Changing the paradigm from 'race' to human genome variation. *Nat Genet, 36*(11, Suppl.), S5–S7.

Schwartz, C. E., & Sprangers, M. A. (1999). Methodological approaches for assessing response shift in longitudinal health-related quality-of-life research. *Soc Sci Med, 48*(11), 1531–1548.

Scollon, C. N., & Diener, E. (2006). Love, work, and changes in extraversion and neuroticism over time. *Journal of Personality and Social Psychology, 91*(6), 1152–1165.

Sein, U. T. (2002). Constitution of the world health organization and its evolution. *Regional Health Forum, 6*(1), 47–64.

Sherman, A. C., Simonton, S., Latif, U., & Bracy, L. (2010). Effects of global meaning and illness-specific meaning on health outcomes among breast cancer patients. *Journal of Behavioral Medicine* (May 26. [Epub ahead of print]).

Shumaker, S. A., & Naughton, M. J. (1995). The international assessment of health-related quality of life: A theoretical perspective. In S. A. Shumaker & R. A. Berzon (Eds.), *The international assessment of health-related quality of life: Theory, translation, measurement and analysis* (pp. 3–10). Oxford: Rapid Communication.

Sloan, J. A., & Zhao, C. X. (2006). Genetics and quality of life. *Curr Probl Cancer, 30*(6), 255–260.

Spector, R. (2004). *Cultural diversity in health and illness* (6th ed.). Upper Saddle River, NJ: Prentice Hall.

Spilker, B. (1996). Introduction. In B. Spilker (Ed.), *Quality of life and pharmacoeconomics in clinical trials* (pp. 1–10). New York, NY: Lippincott-Raven.

Sprangers, M. A., Bartels, M., Veenhoven, R., Baas, F., Martin, N. G., Mosing, M., et al. (2010). Which patient will feel down, which will be happy? The need to study the genetic disposition of emotional states. *Quality of Life Research*, [Epub ahead of print].

Sprangers, M. A., & Schwartz, C. E. (1999). Integrating response shift into health-related quality of life research: A theoretical model. *Soc Sci Med, 48*(11), 1507–1515.

Sprangers, M. A., & Schwartz, C. E. (2008). Reflections on changeability versus stability of health-related quality of life: Distinguishing between its environmental and genetic components. *Health Qual Life Outcomes, 6*, 89.

Stewart, A. L. (1992). Conceptual and methodologic issues in defining quality of life: State of the art. *Progress in Cardiovascular Nursing, 7*(1), 3–11.

Strickland, O. L. (1991, 1992). *Measures and instruments*. Paper presented at the Patient Outcomes Research: Examining the Effectiveness of Nursing Practice. Proceedings of the State of the Science Conference, National Center for Nursing Research.

Suinn, R. M., Rickard-Figueroa, K., Lew, S., & Vigil, P. (1987). The Suinn-Lew Asian self-identity accul-turaiton scale: An initial report. *Educational and Psychological Measurement, 47*, 401–407.

Sullivan, P. F., Neale, M. C., & Kendler, K. S. (2000). Genetic epidemiology of major depression: Review and meta-analysis. *Am J Psychiatry, 157*(10), 1552–1562.

Taylor, E. J. (2001). Spirituality, culture, and cancer care. *Semin Oncol Nurs, 17*(3), 197–205.

Tellegen, A., Lykken, D. T., Bouchard, T. J., Jr., Wilcox, K. J., Segal, N. L., & Rich, S. (1988). Personality similarity in twins reared apart and together. *J Pers Soc Psychol, 54*(6), 1031–1039.

US Cancer Statistics Working Group. (2010). *United States Cancer Statistics: 1999–2006 Incidence and Mortality*. Retrieved April 22, 2010, from http://www.cdc.gov/uscs.

US Census Bureau. (2010, April 22). *State and County Quick Facts: USA Quick Facts*. Retrieved June 1, 2010, from http://quickfacts.census.gov/qfd/states/00000.html.

US Department of Health and Human Services Public Health Service. (Revised 2004, September, Reis-sued 2006, April). *Application for a Public Health Service Grant PHS 398, Targeted/Planned Enrollment Table Format Page*. Retrieved February 12, 2011, from http://grants.nih.gov/grants/funding/phs398/enrollment.doc.

WHOQOL Group. (1995). The World Health Organization Quality of Life Assessment (WHOQOL): Position paper from the World Health Organization. *Social Science and Medicine, 41*(10), 1403–1409.

WHOQOL Group. (1998). The World Health Organization Quality of Life Assessment (WHOQOL): Development and general psychometric properties. *Social Science and Medicine, 46*(12), 1569–1585.

World Health Organization. (1946). *Preamble to the Constitution of the World Health Organization as adopted by the International Health Conference, New York, 19 June–22 July 1946; signed on 22 July 1946 by the representatives of 61 States and entered into force on 7 April 1948*. Retrieved from http://www.who.int/substance_abuse/research_tools/en/english_whoqol.pdf

World Health Organization. (1993). *WHOQOL Study Protocol: The development of the World Health Organization Quality of Life assessment instrument* (No. No. MNH/PSF/93.9). Geneva, Switzerland: Division of Mental Health, World Health Organization.

World Health Organization. (2004). WHO Quality of Life - BREF (WHOQOL-BREF) [Electronic version] from http://www.who.int/substance_abuse/research_tools/whoqolbref/en/

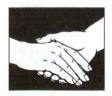

Chapter Seven

Health-Related Quality of Life in Children and Adolescents with Cancer

PAMELA S. HINDS • JOAN E. HAASE

Introduction

Cancer care for individual children and adolescents could further improve if the health-related quality of life (HRQOL) of these patients was carefully, accurately, and consistently solicited from them from diagnosis to cure, from diagnosis to living with recurrent disease, and from diagnosis to end of life. Well timed documentation of their HRQOL reports could help to determine the benefits and burdens of certain treatments and could be the determining factor when two treatments have similar clinical outcomes but different demands on the lives of the children and adolescents receiving each treatment. Health-related qualifty-of-life reports of these patients could also be the stimulus for focused attention on certain cancer-related symptoms and thus prompt improved symptom control. Incorporating HRQOL patient reports into care is credited with improving patient-to-clinician and family-to-clinician communication and care satisfaction. Further, HRQOL reports from survivors of childhood cancer can guide preventive care efforts related to late effects of treatment that they are experiencing. The clinical benefits of soliciting the HRQOL reports of pediatric oncology patients at any point in the care continuum are considerable. Fortunately, these clinical benefits are better matched now than in the past with conceptual and measurement advances related to HRQOL in pediatric oncology.

Significant advances have been made in the past several years in terms of defining, conceptualizing, and measuring health-related quality of life in children and adolescents with cancer. In addition, theory-driven, evidence-based interventions designed to improve the HRQOL of these children and adolescents have begun to be implemented and evaluated by nurses and others. Certain of these advances are uneven in that they occur in some patient groups (primarily in survivors of childhood cancer) but not in others (particularly not with patients at end of life). Most recently, measurement of HRQOL in children and adolescents with cancer has moved in a unique direction from administering cancer-specific instruments only to including generic measures developed using item response theory and designed to be applicable to children and adolescents experiencing various chronic illnesses. This change in instrumentation will allow comparisons of HRQOL scores reported by children and adolescents with cancer with scores reported by similar aged children and adolescents who are experiencing other illnesses such as sickle cell, obesity, and cystic fibrosis. We will very likely gain knowledge about the HRQOL in children and adolescents with cancer through these comparisons with the reports of children experiencing other illnesses. We address here the advances as well as the work that is in development. In this chapter we describe the current conceptual and empirical work on HRQOL, including instrumentation, in children and adolescents diagnosed with cancer; discuss the significance of HRQOL to nursing care, education, administration, and research; and make recommendations for future conceptual, research, and clinical work with HRQOL in children and adolescents.

The Concept of Health-Related Quality of Life in Pediatric Oncology: Can It Be Precisely Defined?

How accurately a concept is measured and evaluated is directly related to the clarity with which it is first defined (Knafl & Deatrick, 1993). Recent advances in defining HRQOL in children and adolescents with cancer include the purposeful inclusion of the child and adolescent perspectives (Cremeens, Eisert, & Blades, 2006; Hinds et al., 2004). In addition, longitudinal measurement of HRQOL and related concepts obtained from child, adolescent, and parent reports have begun to be completed with sufficiently large sample sizes. These advances will help to describe the mechanisms that foster HRQOL in children and adolescents and the relationship of HRQOL to other important concepts (e.g., coping and adaptation, well-being). In addition, these advances in definition will help to distinguish HRQOL in children and adolescents from their parents' quality of life and that of other family members during their treatment for cancer, or from one defined point in treatment to another. The research leading to these distinctions between HRQOL and related concepts will likely yield exciting and useful new knowledge about the cancer experience for children and adolescents. Research to clarify the conceptual overlap is moving forward through carefully planned programs by nurses and scientists working in collaboration with clinicians.

The conceptual challenges with HRQOL in pediatric oncology patients include the following needs:

1. Discover the meaning, importance, and characteristics of HRQOL for children and adolescents.
2. Use descriptive terms and clear language when defining and referring to HRQOL for these developmentally diverse age groups.
3. Determine whether, for the purposes of a complete description, this definition should reflect contextual differences such as diagnosis, prognosis, or point on the continuum of care for childhood cancer.

The urgency to discover the meaning and importance of HRQOL for children and adolescents makes obvious the need to ask them directly about their cancer experience and its effects on their feelings, thoughts, choices, decisions, and other health-related outcomes. Reports in the literature generally agree that the child or youth's view of his or her HRQOL should be solicited (Eiser, Cotter, Oades, Seamark & Smith, 1999; Bradlyn et al., 1995; Raphael, 1996), and that the child's ratings of his or her HRQOL should be considered the primary rating rather than that from a proxy (such as a parent or clinician) (Gong, Young, Dempster, Porepa, & Feldman, 2007; Sherifali & Pinelli, 2007). Further, a recently released report from the US Food and Drug Agency (FDA) included explicit language intended to provide guidance for researchers and clinicians related to soliciting self-reports from children and adolescents who are in clinical trials that could be used to support drug labeling. The clear language recommends the use of patient reports in pediatrics and *not* parent or clinician proxy reports (US Department of Health and Human Services, 2009). Creative efforts to directly obtain child and youth perspectives are being explored with some success (Cremeens et al., 2006; Haase, Heiney, Ruccione, & Stutzer, 1999; Hockenberry-Eaton & Hinds, 2000). In one such effort to solicit the views on quality of life of children and adolescents with cancer, 36 pediatric oncology cancer patients were asked to describe what made a good day for them during treatment, what made a bad day, and what they wanted to do now but could not because of treatment. Qualitative techniques were used to analyze the data and a definition of cancer-related quality of life for children and adolescents in active treatment resulted: "an overall sense of well-being based on being able to participate in usual activities; to interact with others and feel cared about; to cope with uncomfortable physical, emotional, and cognitive reactions; and to find meaning in the illness experience" (Hinds et al., 2004, p.767). Using the same methods, six dimensions were identified: symptoms, usual activities, social and family interactions, health status, mood, and meaning of being ill. A consensus definition formulated at a workshop sponsored by the American Cancer Society on the quality of life for pediatric oncology patients and derived from expert healthcare professionals was "the physical, social, and emotional functioning of the child, measured from the perspective of both the child and his/her family, and sensitive to changes that occur throughout development" (Nathan, Furlong, & Barr, 2004, p. 215). The definition from the patient perspective differs from that derived from the expert clinician and researcher panel particularly in regard to the meaning of illness dimension. This important difference in the definitions needs to be recognized and reflected in the care provided by the child's healthcare professionals. Although the two definitions differ, their shared emphasis is on seeking the patients' reports of their HRQOL.

Similar dimensions have been used to guide cancer-related HRQOL interviews or instrument studies with children and adolescents. Commonly used and alternate labels for the dimensions include symptoms (e.g., somatic distress or perceived effect on physical appearance), normal activities (e.g., school and physical functioning, cognitive functioning, or role function), social/family interactions (e.g., quality of interactions, peer rejection, parental behavior, or social and personal resources), and mood (psychological functioning and mood disturbances, manipulation of emotion or mental health). Other identified, but infrequently used, dimensions include communication, compliance, and disclosing behavior (Eiser et al., 1999; Nathan et al. 2004; Phipps, Dunavant, Jayawardene, & Srivastava, 1999; Varni, Limbers, & Burwinkle, 2007). Certain HRQOL conceptualizations are disease- or treatment-specific. For example, in one study involving pediatric and adult patients who had received treatment for a primary bone tumor, the HRQOL dimensions used to guide the HRQOL patient interviews were labeled as follows: effect on schooling, work, mobility, pain and body image, emotional well-being, and functional evaluation of reconstructive procedures (Eiser et al., 1997). In a second example, HRQOL of pediatric brain tumor patients was conceptualized as having the following dimensions: cognitive problems, pain and hurt, movement and balance, procedural anxiety, nausea, and worry (Palmer, Meekse, Katz, Burwinkle, & Varni, 2007). Although some differences are apparent in the disease-specific HRQOL studies, there is a growing consensus about the general dimensions of cancer-related pediatric HRQOL and the importance of directly soliciting the perspective of the pediatric oncology patient. A very important element remains to be further developed and that is a clinically useful means of interpreting the HRQOL data obtained that conveys the meanings and importance of any given dimension to pediatric patients and families and how the meaning or importance may change over the course of the illness and its treatment.

When family members or healthcare providers are asked to serve as proxy reporters for a child or adolescent's HRQOL information, there is increasing effort to compare their proxy perspectives for congruence with the child or adolescent's perspective (Levi & Drotar, 1999; Parsons, Barlow, Levy, Supran, & Kaplan, 1999; Phipps et al., 1999; Sherifali & Pinelli, 2007). This careful comparison is prompted by the concern that pediatric patients and their parents may define the patients' HRQOL differently, and that clinicians may define the patient's HRQOL differently from both the patient and the parent. Recent research reports support this concern with findings of children and adolescents basing their HRQOL reports on concrete and often single recalled examples as compared to their adult proxy reporters who base their ratings on multiple examples that span more than the immediate period (Davis et al. 2007; Eiser & Eiser, 2000). These and other research findings are serving as cautions in relying on parent proxy reports in place of the HRQOL reports of the child or adolescent; instead, the findings support continuing to solicit both perspectives (patient and parent). In a recent longitudinal study, parent and child and adolescent ratings of symptoms became more similar over a 10-day period (Hinds et al., 2007), indicating that with time and repeated opportunities to report, patient and parent ratings could become more similar. If this is supported in other longitudinal designs involving HRQOL, we could have more confidence in relying on parent reports of their ill child's HRQOL when their child's report is not available. Conducting more such comparison studies will help shed light on questions of how HRQOL experiences for patients are distinct from, or highly influenced by, those of the family. Comparison studies will also help to specifically identify the patient–proxy congruence or disagreement specific to each dimension of HRQOL and whether or how congruence or disagreement varies over the course of cancer treatment. An additional need is to determine how the developmental levels of both the child and family contribute to their unique and shared perceptions of HRQOL. Completing the conceptual work on the construct of HRQOL in pediatric oncology patients will necessarily involve soliciting comparisons of the perceptions of developmentally and culturally diverse patients and families. That knowledge will ultimately provide a basis for nursing and medical care of pediatric oncology patients and their families and will enable healthcare professionals to decide whether the patient or the family is the most effective target for a HRQOL intervention.

Completely and accurately defining HRQOL for children and adolescents with cancer as derived from its identified dimensions requires clear language. This requirement is especially important because of the present difficulty in conceptually distinguishing HRQOL from related, but different, concepts. Other terms historically used interchangeably with HRQOL for children and adolescents were well-being (Bradlyn et al., 1993; Czyzewski, Mariotto, Bartholomew, LeCompte, & Sockrider, 1994; Haase et al., 1999) and global health status (Barr et al., 1993; Feeny & Leiper, 1993). Some works neglect to conceptually define HRQOL and other apparently equivalent terms (Cadman, Goldsmith, Torrance, Boyle, & Furlong, 1986; Bradlyn et al., 1993; Czyzewski et al., 1994; see Table 7-1). Despite inherent difficulties with conceptual clarity and completeness, the definitions in the literature do have important similarities, including attributes of multidimensionality, subjectivity, dynamism, inclusivity, and comparison of past and current circumstances with desired future outcome. Differences in the specificity of each of the dimensions indicate the need to continue to refine these broad domains to capture the aspects most important to the child or adolescent and parent. The specific HRQOL dimensions valued most by children and adolescents as well as their parents are unique to each of them and are dependent on past experiences, current circumstances, and future hopes and expectations (Eiser & Morse, 2001). In addition, more precise specification of relationships among HRQOL-related concepts is needed as well as the testing of these relationships for their ability to predict clinical outcomes.

Conceptualizing about HRQOL dimensions is a cognitive tool that helps us first to organize our thoughts and knowledge about HRQOL in children and adolescents; conceptualizing about the dimensions also serves a practical function for nursing and healthcare interventions. For example, HRQOL may be reported by the parent or family member as quite high in the dimension of physical health, but low in psychological or spiritual health. Such a report would direct the healthcare assessment and subsequent intervention to the dimension of the lower score. Improvement in one or more dimensions of HRQOL may positively affect other dimensions. The available literature also helps to identify differences or disagreements in the conceptual work with HRQOL in pediatric patients. Differences in conceptual definitions include the extent to which objective aspects are included, the positive or negative slant reflected, the sense of time (past, present, or future) conveyed, and the extent to which context such as setting or culture influence quality of life (Table 7-1). Definitions or descriptions generated by nurses tend not to include the objective social aspects (e.g., socioeconomic status, neighborhood, or type of dwelling) that other disciplines include. Nurses' efforts to focus only on those aspects of HRQOL directly influenced by nursing care may account for this difference.

There remain important conceptual challenges in HRQOL research for children, adolescents, and their families. Both creative and systematic efforts to determine how pediatric oncology patients describe or define their HRQOL at differing points in treatment are needed, including how disease, treatment, patient and family characteristics, and even research methods influence their definitions. Triangulation of methods (qualitative and quantitative), sources (i.e., self-, parent-, healthcare provider reports), and research and clinicians are needed to continue our significant progress in understanding the HRQOL of children and adolescents experiencing cancer.

Table 7-1. **Definition and Dimensions of Quality of Life in Children and Adolescents**

Definition	Dimensions	Source
None offered	Sensory and communication ability, happiness, self-care ability, freedom from moderate to severe chronic pain or discomfort, learning and school ability, physical ability	Cadman, Goldsmith, Torrance, Boyle, & Furlong, 1986
Children's and adolescent's subjective and changeable sense of well-being, which reflects how closely their desires and hopes match what is actually happening, and their orientation toward the future, both their own and that of others.	Hopefulness, self-esteem/self-efficacy, symptom distress, adverse physical effects of treatment	Hinds, 1990, p. 285
The impact of illness and predicament of a biological disorder	Incidence, prevalence, physiological dysfunction, or mortality rate	Rosenbaum, Cadman, & Kerpalani, 1990, p. 207
A term describing the total existence of an individual or group, including the more positive aspects of health	External conditions, internal conditions, personal psychological conditions	Lindstrom & Kohler, 1991, p. 121
None offered	Mobility, physical activity, social activity	Bradlyn, Harris, Warner, Ritchey, & Zaboy, 1993, p. 250
"Quality of life is a multidimensional construct, incorporating both objective and subjective data, including (but not limited to) the social, physical, and emotional functioning of the child and, when indicated, his/her family. QOL measurement must be sensitive to changes that occur throughout development."	Social functioning, physical functioning, emotional functioning	Pediatric Oncology Group, 1993

Table 7-1. **continued**

Definition	Dimensions	Source
None offered	Physical symptoms and functionality in the areas of mobility, physical activity, and social activity	Czyzewski, Mariotto, Bartholomew, LeCompte, & Sockrider, 1994, p. 966
Personal opinions reflecting satisfaction with current circumstances, participation in activities and relations, and the opportunity to have control over one's life and to make choices	Satisfaction, well-being, social belonging, empowerment/control	Keith & Schalock, 1994, p. 84
The way in which individuals view their own health and the degree to which they are satisfied with it	None specified	Vivier, Bernier, & Starfield, 1994, p. 532
Impact of disease and treatment on self-perceptions of functioning	Core: physical, psychological, social Symptom: pain, nausea	Seid, Varni, Rode, & Katz, 1999, p. 72
Discrepancy between what the child can and would like to be able to do	Social, physical, actual self, ideal self	Eiser, Cotter, Oades, Seamark, & Smith, 1999, p. 87
Preference-based valuation of overall disability reported by each subject and reported in a single summary utility score	Global	Barr, Chalmers, DePauw, Furlong, Weitzman, & Feeny, 2000, p. 3281

Significance of Health-Related Quality of Life in Children and Adolescents Who Have Cancer

One research approach to HRQOL in children and adolescents with cancer is to consider HRQOL as an endpoint indicator, or a measure that could determine whether one treatment arm of a clinical trial is more demanding of or beneficial for a patient than another (Razzouk et al., 2006). Variables that influence or are components of HRQOL are studied by nurse researchers and others as process and outcome variables that are or could be influenced directly and indirectly by care (Hinds, 1990; Grant, Padilla, & Creimel, 1996; Stam, Grootenhuis, Brons, Caron, & Last, 2006). Using that research approach, HRQOL has implications for nursing care, education, administration, and research. Increasingly, there is an emphasis on viewing HRQOL more holistically by acknowledging a link between physical and psychosocial domains (Eiser & Morse, 2001; Varni et al., 2007). The nursing profession's acceptance of the clinical relevance of HRQOL is derived in good measure from the desire for knowledge and understanding of the care-related experiences of pediatric oncology patients (Hinds & Varricchio, 1996; King, Hinds, Dow, Schum, & Lee, 2002). Nurses want to use this knowledge to provide more sensitive care that is tailored to each child or adolescent, and they believe that HRQOL information can assist them in providing the most appropriate care interventions.

Incorporating HRQOL issues into all levels of formal nursing education is also an interest in nursing. Because of the nature of our discipline's work (giving sensitive, competent, individualized care that helps a care recipient to achieve the most positive health outcomes possible), most nursing curricula already contain certain philosophic and practice-based assumptions similar to, consistent with, or at least parallel to, those of HRQOL. A more formal, focused reflection of HRQOL also encourages nurses to view their care and research with patients as needing to reflect the following:

1. The interrelated aspects of the various dimensions of a child's or youth's being
2. Actual or at least possible change (situational or developmental) in any of the identified dimensions of the child's or youth's HRQOL and the quality of life of their family
3. The opinion or perception of the child or youth
4. The influencing context within which the child or youth lives and experiences health-related situations
5. The role of nursing care in facilitating HRQOL for children and adolescents as a way of promoting their health.

The administrative interest in HRQOL is twofold. First, nurse administrators are aware that nurses experience job-related meaning and satisfaction when they feel they have contributed to the HRQOL of their patients (Jones, 1990; Wakefield, Curry, Price, Mueller, & McCloskey, 1988). The importance to nurses of making a positive difference to pediatric oncology patients and their families is often reflected in the findings from nursing role satisfaction or meaning and function studies (Hinds, Quargnenti, Hickey, & Mangum, 1994; Olson et al., 1998; Steen, Burghen, Hinds, Srivastava, & Tong, 2003).

Second, nurse administrators want to justify the importance of HRQOL work by nurses in terms of patient and family outcomes, outcomes that may be difficult to define and quantify. How may quality-of-life care by nurses be figured into a patient acuity system? What is the cost of that kind of care or the lack of it?

Research interests are derived from the clinical, educational, and administrative questions and concerns in nursing. The significance here is the nursing profession's determination to carefully and completely determine (conceptually and empirically) the nature and characteristics of HRQOL for children and adolescents who are experiencing or have experienced cancer. Building on that work, the related intention of nurses is to independently or collaboratively develop and test care interventions designed to promote HRQOL in these children and youths, with systematic focus on the processes by which HRQOL is affected and the outcomes of those interventions. An additional research priority is to examine HRQOL as a correlate and a predictor of certain cancer-related clinical variables.

Conceptual Models of Health-Related Quality of Life in Children and Adolescents with Cancer

Several conceptual models and frameworks that may contribute to our understanding of HRQOL for children and adolescents are presented here. Function- and meaning-based models represent differing conceptual approaches to HRQOL. Function-based models primarily emphasize role functions (such as the ability to attend school and keep up with friends) as indicators of HRQOL, whereas meaning-based models rely on subjective reports of meaning (such as finding meaning in life or strengthening friendships as a result of having cancer). While meaning-based approaches recognize the importance of function, emphasis is placed on the interpretation and importance of that function as a primary indicator of HRQOL.

The Life-Span Development Framework provides a basis for understanding the dynamic nature of HRQOL within a context of universal and unique developmental experiences. In addition, four substantive models specific to HRQOL in pediatric oncology patients are described. These models offer descriptive detail about the process components and outcomes of HRQOL and together convey that in assessing HRQOL in pediatric oncology patients, a blend of function- and meaning-based conceptual approaches may be a more complete approach to assessing patients' HRQOL.

Function- and Meaning-Based Models

Function-based models dominate in HRQOL research in adult oncology (Costain, Hewison, & Howes, 1993). Function-based models are most often used to examine outcomes of treatments from a biomedical perspective of objectivity and reductionism. They emphasize goal setting to manage clinical concerns, toxicity of treatments, and role-related tasks or functions. In adult oncology, acceptance of the function-based models seems to be occurring without critical evaluation of the underlying assumptions of function as the basis for

HRQOL and without a clear definition of HRQOL and its dimensions. In particular, function-based models have not been examined for their congruence with the nursing profession's philosophic perspectives of holism or the expressed needs of children and adolescents.

Meaning-based models focus on the experience of the illness from the perspective of the child or adolescent or parent and incorporate a more holistic view. Meaning-based models view HRQOL as enabling patients to choose and realize their own goals through the exploration of meanings derived from the personal experiences of illness and its treatment. Meaning can also be derived from patients' understanding of their situation, autonomy, beliefs, choices, and relationships with others. These and other HRQOL models currently being used to guide research involving pediatric oncology patients and their families are primarily based on data from patients who are in active treatment. However, the preponderance of completed research involves survivors of childhood cancer, and the majority of these reported studies do not include the model or study framework used to guide the research (Ginsberg et al., 2004; Hoffman, Gosheger, Gebert, Jurgens, & Winkelmann, 2006; Koopman et al. 2005; Marchese, Ogle, Womer, Doromans & Ginsberg, 2004; Nagarajan et al., 2004; Shankar et al., 2005; Tabone et al., 2005). An important area for future development is the models that represent the transitions involved in HRQOL for children and adolescents as they move from active treatment to survivorship, from disease-free states to disease recurrence or second malignancy, or from treatment to end of life.

Several studies on pediatric oncology HRQOL include assertions of the importance of function-based models forming the minimum data set for HRQOL assessment (Eiser, 1997; Bradlyn & Pollock, 1996). For example, the guidelines for HRQOL research adopted in the past by one pediatric oncology cooperative group are derived in part from the definition of health offered by the World Health Organization (1947). The guidelines defined HRQOL as "a multidimensional construct . . . that includes, but is not limited to, social, physical, and emotional functioning of the child and, when indicated, his or her family" (Pediatric Oncology Group, 1993, p. 3). This definition appears to be holistic, but it emphasizes functioning, whether physical, psychological, or social. This emphasis is more behavioral than holistic in nature, in that how well a child or adolescent functions does not necessarily reveal the meaning, value, importance, or satisfaction that he or she derives from those functions. Two examples may help distinguish these important differences between function- and meaning-based models. The loss of hair for one adolescent may have an important negative effect on her HRQOL and, indeed, may negatively influence social functioning. For another adolescent, the meaning of hair loss may be minor and have very little influence on her evaluation of HRQOL. For a third, the loss of hair could conceivably have a positive effect on HRQOL, for example, if friends communicated their strong connectedness by shaving off their own hair or a bald head helped an adolescent convey a desired "attitude" and identity. When social function is assessed in terms of the child's or adolescent's ability to carry out typical social activities, often the assessment does not consider whether the activities are meaningful to him or her. Thus, when a child or adolescent is asked if he or she is able to continue with school activities, a "no" answer may be interpreted as increased isolation and an indicator of decreased HRQOL. Missing from this response is the meaning that staying at home has for the pediatric oncology patient, or the meaning that parents find in being able to provide care to their ill child at home in the manner they desire. Although such isolation is assumed to be unpleasant and burdensome, qualitative data from one study indicated that some children and families use the isolation as an opportunity to be together and strengthen family ties, and to focus on the strength of friendships that endure in spite of the isolation (Haase & Rostad, 1994). In that same study, one adolescent who was unable to attend school reported feeling cheated of an important time in high school, but another adolescent described positive outcomes from her home schooling. Both patients had a decrease in social functioning, but their experiences of the decrease differed because of the meaning attached to the change. Meaning is not likely to be assessed in traditionally function-based methods, and potentially misleading conclusions could be drawn about the HRQOL of pediatric oncology patients.

When meaning-based models are used with HRQOL research, functioning is considered within the greater context of the meaning of the cancer experience. The perceptions of the child and the family about the meaning of the altered functioning are the essential research data. Did the child and family consider the altered functioning to be a loss or an opportunity? Is the particular social activity that is being used as an indicator of HRQOL important to the child and family? These are the kinds of questions reflected in research that is guided by meaning-based models and would likely contribute substantially to efforts to develop conceptual completeness of HRQOL in pediatric oncology patients. In addition, interventions to enhance HRQOL would look very different if the emphasis was on helping a child make meaning from the experience, rather than improving function. For example, many of the expressive therapies, such as journaling, music therapy, or art, are focused on helping participants to form meaning, and improvement in function often follows. Further, emphasis on either function or meaning in isolation sets up an artificial dichotomy, and such a dichotomy is not reflective of child and adolescent experiences.

The Life-Span Development Framework

An additional conceptual approach that may be valuable in HRQOL work with children and adolescents with cancer is the Life-Span Developmental Framework. This framework "seeks to determine the historical and contemporary influences on development as well as the quantitative and qualitative aspects of (child) and adolescent responses to illness" (Weekes, 1991, p. 42). The following are important principles of life-span development:

1. Development is change that has an underlying temporal and logical order that results in systematic and progressive alterations in organization.
2. Developmental changes arise from a combination of influences (e.g., biological, psychological, social, historical, or evolutionary).
3. The person and environment or context are embedded in, and interact to influence, each other.
4. Developmental factors are normative age-graded (e.g., children typically begin walking between 12 and 16 months), normative history- or experienced-graded (e.g.,

school-age children in the United States whose first exposure to terrorism was the September 11, 2001, attacks on New York and Washington, DC), and nonnormative universal occurrences (e.g., illness) (Baltes, 1979; Lerner, 1986).

The life-span perspective recognizes the nonnormative aspects of developmental change that can be caused by the cancer experience and assumes that treatment effects are not identical for all people and will change over time.

This framework is particularly helpful when evaluating the importance of differences in meaning from a developmental perspective. The following example about the characteristics of pain (i.e., cause, source, intensity, and management) may help to illustrate these differences and their clinical importance. An adult may experience and interpret the characteristics of pain as pressure from a tumor (cause and source) that is quite painful (intensity) but manageable with morphine sulphate (management). Children of a certain developmental perspective experience and interpret pain as "I did something for which I am being punished (cause) by powerful adults (source) who do things that cause more pain (intensity) from which I must escape or withdraw" (management).

Substantive Models for Quality of Life in Pediatric Oncology Patients

Although the construct of pediatric HRQOL is not yet thoroughly defined, factors that influence it are now being identified. Hinds (1990) used a combined deductive and inductive approach to develop a model of environmental sources of influences. The assumptions underlying this model are that HRQOL in children and adolescents with cancer is sensitive to input from external others; highly changeable due to daily events and chronic problems; and tempered by personality styles, cognitive abilities, and expectations and desires. The three levels of environment that may directly influence HRQOL (Figure 7-1) are as follows:

- The internal environment, which represents factors of the child or adolescent such as feelings about self
- The immediate environment, which includes factors of significant others such as family members and healthcare providers and their ability to deal with the demands of the illness
- The institutional environment, or factors of the greater social system such as financial support from the public for cancer care and research.

Additional examples of the components of each level of environment are shown in Figure 7-1. Two other methods of assessing HRQOL in adolescents exist that also propose interrelated multilevel influences on adolescents' health behavior (Lindstrom, 1994; Raphael, 1996), although the focus of those models is healthy adolescents.

A second substantive model that identifies factors that influence the HRQOL of adolescents with cancer is the Adolescent Resilience Model (ARM) (Corey, Hase, Azzouz, & Monahan, 2008; Haase et al., 1999) (Figure 7-2). This model, also developed from both deductive and inductive methods, helps to distinguish the influencing factors from the

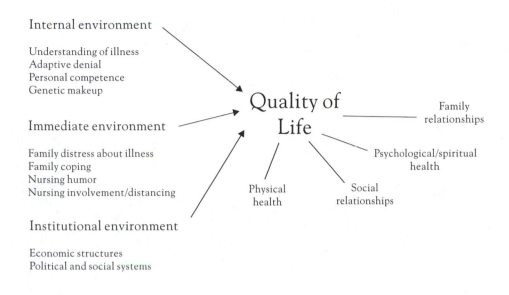

Internal environment

Understanding of illness
Adaptive denial
Personal competence
Genetic makeup

Immediate environment

Family distress about illness
Family coping
Nursing humor
Nursing involvement/distancing

Institutional environment

Economic structures
Political and social systems

Quality of
Life

Family
relationships

Psychological/spiritual
health

Physical
health

Social
relationships

Figure 7-1.   Quality-of-life model depicting the direct influence of three levels of
environment.

actual dimensions of HRQOL. The initial work in developing the ARM was a phenome-nological study of courage in chronically ill adolescents. Since the initial study, the ARM has been tested and refined in two samples of adolescents ($n = 73$; $n = 130$) with chronic illness or cancer. The model is currently being examined longitudinally and with an inter-vention targeting both process and outcome variables. The model indicates that individual (patient-specific), family, and social characteristics directly influence how the adolescent responds to an illness experience. That response, in turn, influences the adolescent's resilience to the experience. Ultimately, the adolescent's resilience directly influences his or her HRQOL (the greater the adolescent's resilience, the greater the HRQOL). As sub-stantive models are developed, it will be important to consider their applicability across diverse cultures. A recent effort to examine the Adolescent Resilience Model for applica-bility in Taiwan led to conclusions that the model and measurements would need to be adapted—again, because certain meanings are not the same across cultures. For example, in the ARM fatalism is considered a less than positive coping strategy. However, in a study of experiences of Taiwanese adolescent survivors of brain tumors fatalism is considered to be a positive process that indicates acceptance of the current situation as a way to help ancestors and to pave the way for the afterlife (Chen, Chen, & Haase, in press).

The third substantive model is the Self-Sustaining Model (Figure 7-3), which was developed inductively with adolescents who had cancer (Hinds & Martin, 1988; Ishibashi

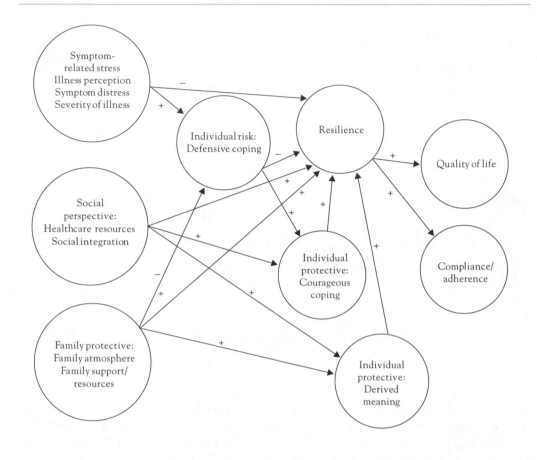

Figure 7-2. **Depiction of the adolescent resilience model (ARM).**

et al., 2010). The model was developed to convey how adolescents help themselves to achieve and maintain hopefulness during their cancer experience. The assumptions under-lying the model were that hopefulness is crucial for adolescents with cancer because it helps them cope with a life-threatening illness, and that adolescents' ability to help themselves feel hopeful is a developmentally important accomplishment for them. The model was comprised of four sequential phases representing adolescents' efforts to comfort themselves during health-threatened periods by using certain behavioral and cognitive strategies (labeled "Self-Care Strategies" in Figure 7-3). Their efforts result in a sense of personal competence in resolving health threats. The model has been further developed and tested in a recent study of 78 adolescents newly diagnosed with cancer. Correlation findings pro-vide moderate to strong support for all of the theorized linkages in the model (Hinds, 1995; Hinds et al., 2000). The study findings for this model represent a test of the internal envi-ronment on selected dimensions of HRQOL.

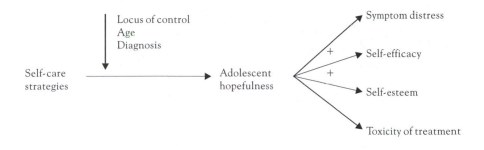

Figure 7-3.   **Self-sustaining model of adolescents with cancer.**

None of the previously described models has been applied to dying children and adolescents. The fourth substantive model is based on a combination of inductive and deductive research studies and depicts HRQOL in pediatric oncology patients who are dying (see Figure 7-4). In this recently developed model, the underlying premises are that the focus is jointly on the child or adolescent and his or her family, and that HRQOL is likely the ultimate outcome of interest in end-of-life care (Bradlyn, Varni, & Hinds, 2003; Nuss, Hinds, & LaFond, 2005). Because the formal study of HRQOL at end of life for children, adolescents, and their families has only recently begun, we do not yet know what exact type and number of dimensions might best represent these patients and their families. Dying children and adolescents commonly and repeatedly express intense concerns about the well-being of their family members (Hinds, Oakes, & Furman, 2001; Hinds et al., 2005), as do family members about the dying child. This mutual concern is the basis for the joint focus in this model on the dying child and on his family. The presence of symptoms that are inadequately managed adversely affects the patients' and family members' HRQOL (Hinds, Bradshaw, Oakes, & Pritchard, 2003). Other sources of influence include the parents' satisfaction with their ability to be "good parents" to their dying child, the ability of the family to maintain some degree of normalcy, and the influence of child development and culture (Goh, Lum, Chan, Baker, & Chong, 1999; Rushton, 1994; Hinds et al., 2001; Hinds et al., 2009). Both research findings and clinical observations suggest that a model of HRQOL at end of life for a child or adolescent and his family needs to reflect fluidity of the clinical situation. An example of such fluidity in a HRQOL model is the recently developed Individualized Care Planning and Coordination Model used in the clinical care of children and adolescents who are at end of life following intensive curative efforts (Baker, Barfield, Hinds, & Kane, 2007). This model incorporates strategies that include regularly reviewing child and family goals for care and hopes for self and for others.

Because they provide additional information about validity and generalizability, the conceptual and empirical similarities and differences among these substantive models are the focus of much interest. Careful comparison among the factors identified in each model

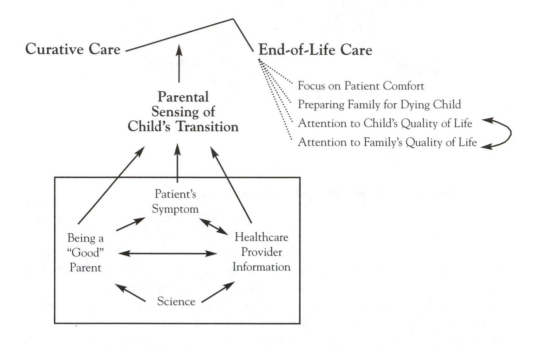

Figure 7-4. Model of quality of life at end of life that emphasizes the dual focus on the dying child or adolescent and his family.

helps to distinguish influencing factors from the outcome of HRQOL itself (and its components). Factors sometimes measured elsewhere as indicators of HRQOL are viewed in these models as contributing to, but not equating with, HRQOL in children and adolescents with cancer. The same comparison of the four substantive models also helps to identify the complex, multidimensional nature of the factors that influence HRQOL.

Measuring Health-Related Quality of Life in Children and Adolescents with Cancer

Because of ongoing conceptual work, there is no single universally accepted way to measure the HRQOL of children and adolescents including those with cancer. Measurement issues include self-report in the pediatric oncology population; shifting standards of comparison during the cancer care experience; the use of proxy reporters; the developmental, clinical, and cultural sensitivity of available measures; and the recent development and testing of a core set of instruments intended to facilitate patient-reported HRQOL using standardized measures that are not unique to a single disease or time point in treatment.

Researchers began measuring HRQOL in pediatric oncology patients and their parents despite unfinished conceptual work because of pressing clinical research and care demands. Certainly there are risks secondary to moving to measurement when steps to ensure conceptual clarity are incomplete. Risks include that incomplete, incorrect, or misleading data could result from the use of such instruments and the findings could be interpreted as indicating that HRQOL is not relevant to clinical trials in pediatric oncology. Additionally, such findings could become the basis for clinical interventions that are ill-informed and unlikely to accurately explain outcomes of the interventions. One recent review indicated that many studies found no differences in outcomes of child cancer survivors, compared with healthy children. Yet, this same review strongly criticized the instruments used in most of the studies reported (Eiser, Hill, & Vance, 2000).

Self-Report Measures

Measures, including open-ended or structured interviews as well as single-item to multidimensional instruments, that solicit subjective reports directly from children and adolescents help to ensure that their perspectives are considered. Multiple instruments exist for evaluating one or more dimensions of HRQOL, but few are derived from the perspective of the child or adolescent. A variety of self-report HRQOL instruments have been reported as valid and reliable in children as young as 5; however, appropriate measures for children younger than 4 or 5 years of age have not been developed. This lack of developmentally appropriate instruments is attributed to the rapid physical, emotional, cognitive, and social advances made by preschool-aged children (Nathan et al., 2004). Children as young as 5 years and adolescents are typically willing and able to respond to developmentally appropriate interview questions or questionnaires. However, they may provide incomplete responses if they lose interest or find the questions irrelevant or difficult to understand (Hinds, Quargnenti, & Wentz, 1992). Formatting differences by child's age or cognitive abilities may also influence the level of participation by children and adolescents with cancer. For example, in age-specific HRQOL instruments, children 8 years of age and older complete items by responding to a 5-point range of options, while children 5 to 7 years of age respond to a 3-point range (Varni et al., 2007).

Because of the need to have sensitive and developmentally appropriate HRQOL instruments, a serious commitment to developing such measures for children and adolescents with cancer must begin with careful qualitative efforts to learn the pediatric perspective. Instruments developed in this manner will reflect language and ideas understood by the child or adolescent and are more likely to result in greater receptiveness and increased participation (including fewer unanswered items) from the pediatric patient. For example, in a study by Haase and Rostad (1994), adolescents with cancer completed a lengthy interview about their cancer experience. Interview questions such as "In what way have your friendships changed since your diagnosis?" and "What helps you to get through treatments?" directly solicited the adolescents' perspectives and were positively received by the participants. The researchers received comments of appreciation from some adolescents, who expressed relief at being asked about what was important to them. An additional factor that contributes to the sensitivity of an HRQOL instrument is its administration. Allowing a latency age child or an adolescent to independently complete a self-report instrument when clinically possible acknowledges his or her competence. However, the same instrument's content, language, and response format may need to be adapted for a younger child to ensure valid responses. Greater efforts should also be made to develop technologically accessible measures.

Quite recently, a patient-reported outcomes (PRO) measurement initiative supported by the National Institutes of Health (NIH) has developed multiple indicators of pediatric HRQOL based on item response theory. The initiative, Patient-Reported Outcomes Measurement Information System (PROMIS) is a cooperative network established as part of the NIH Roadmap for Medical Research. Using a variety of strategies, including focus groups and review of items from established pediatric instruments, researchers in the PROMIS network have identified domains of HRQOL and are creating and evaluating item banks to quantify symptoms and care outcomes (Castel et al., 2008; DeWalt, Rothrock, Young, & Stone, 2007; Walsh, Irwin, Meier, Varni, & DeWalt, 2008). The item banks are considered public domain and are available in computerized adaptive test form. The pediatric PROMIS domains include physical functioning, fatigue, pain, emotional distress, and social health. Within these domains, measures exist for anxiety, depression, fatigue, pain, peer relationships, anger, cognitive functioning, and physical functioning. Current efforts include development of other measures, including a pediatric sleep quality measure.

Use of Proxy Reports for Patients' HRQOL

Certainly the standard for measuring HRQOL in pediatric oncology patients needs to be the patient's self-report, but because of the likelihood of clinical situations in which the child or adolescent with cancer will decline or be unable to provide a self-report, the use of proxy reports will remain an important source of information about the patients' HRQOL (Hinds et al., 2007; Varni et al., 2007). Consistent involvement, beginning early in treatment, in providing HRQOL ratings on behalf of the ill child may help proxy raters to become more sensitive reporters (Hinds et al., 2007). However, this possibility has not yet been documented. Research reports indicate that patients and their parent proxy reporters tend to have higher agreement on observable, objective dimensions of HRQOL than on the more subjective dimensions (Eiser & Morse, 2001). The same discordance has been reported between parent proxies and well children (Davis et al., 2007). Agreement between pediatric oncology patients and parent proxies is influenced by age with more disagreement occurring with adolescents than with younger children (Chang & Yeh, 2005) and by the parents' own levels of distress and HRQOL (Eiser & Eiser, 2000; Eiser, Eiser, & Stride, 2005). The HRQOL instrument used may also be a source of influence with instruments having more objective items rather than subjective items, which can achieve higher agreement levels (Sung et al., 2004).

Shifting Standards of Comparison

Usefulness in a repeated-measures design implies that the measure is able to capture real change in the dimensions of HRQOL, and is brief enough that the child or adolescent will not object to completing it more than once during his or her cancer experience. Of concern here is the ability of the measure to determine whether the standard of comparison used by the child or adolescent changes over time. Hinds (1995) observed that adolescents based their subjective reports on a shifting standard of comparison. For example, newly diagnosed adolescents would provide ratings that compared present perceptions with those they had prior to diagnosis or any symptoms being noticed. Three months later, those same adolescents provided ratings that compared their present perceptions with what they imagined to be the experience of other patients who had a more serious health condition. Such a shift is theorized to be because of adaptation to the illness experience and thus represents a true change in how the pediatric patient perceives his or her HRQOL (Nathan et al., 2004). A similar shift has been noted in mothers of children being treated for a bone tumor and was attributed to their shift from problem-solving coping to emotion-focused coping (Earle, Eiser, & Grimer, 2005). This shift may be somewhat addressed in longitudinal study designs by including a fixed standard of comparison in the directions for the measure, or by asking patients one or more interview questions to establish their standard of comparison prior to having them rate their HRQOL.

Developmental Sensitivity of the Measures

A concern with HRQOL measures that are used over time with pediatric oncology patients is the developmental appropriateness of the measures. For example, the Rand questionnaires and the PedsQL instruments designed to measure HRQOL in pediatric patients, including pediatric oncology patients, have age-specific forms. The Rand questionnaires are available in the following age groups: 0 through 4 years, 5 through 13 years, and 14 years and older. Each differs in content and format. The PedsQL generic and cancer modules are available in parent report forms for 2-to-4 year-old children, and patient and parent report forms for 5 to 7 years, 8 to 12 years, and 13 to 18 years (Varni, Burwinkle, Katz, Meeske, & Dickinson, 2002). When these questionnaires are used over time with pediatric oncology patients, it is possible that more than 3 years may exist between the patient's diagnosis and the gathering of post-treatment HRQOL scores. Differences between these scores and those obtained at diagnosis may reflect true change in HRQOL measure or change in the value or expectations of the respondent to specific HRQOL dimensions. The measurement challenge here is to accurately determine change in HRQOL reports or scores when the patient moves to another age or developmental group with different desires and needs. One of the benefits of the pediatric PROMIS measures is that the same items are used for 8 to 17 year olds and thus no change in measure form is necessary.

Clinical Sensitivity of Measures

Another concern is the need for measures that detect clinically significant changes in HRQOL. For example, certain symptoms experienced early in treatment can persist at similar rates throughout treatment but may be rated differently by the patient because of adaptation over time or increasing weariness secondary to treatment over time. Efforts are now underway to identify the minimally clinically important difference in pediatric HRQOL scores for children experiencing chronic illnesses.

Cultural Sensitivity of Measures

The cultural meanings associated with illness need to be reflected in measures of HRQOL for children and adolescents (Leininger, 1994; Marshall, 1990; Sartorius, 1987). Cultural concepts of collective rather than individualistic goal setting, acceptance of "what is" rather than prevention or cure, and time as passages of life rather than a linear progression are several of the distinguishing features that will need to be incorporated in culturally sensitive measures of quality of life. Indeed, even perspectives on such concepts as pain and suffering need to be studied within cultural contexts. For example, a qualitative theme identified in a group of Middle Eastern children from a strategy they use to deal with pain was labeled "learning to suffer well," but the predominate Western cultural perspective is to "alleviate suffering" (Voigtman, 2002).

Purpose of Measurement: Statistical or Clinical Significance

The issue of clinical versus statistical significance addresses the change in score of a particular quality-of-life measure (e.g., outcome indicator in a clinical trial or an indicator for clinical management) that would be considered important. The degree to which a measure is statistically significant is important when HRQOL data are being collected, for example, to help determine the effect of a particular therapy on children. In contrast, measures need to have high clinical significance when the information gathered is to be used in decision making for one particular child. The scores and the size of the change in the scores over time would be weighed differently in these two situations.

General Guidelines for Measuring Quality of Life in Children and Adolescents

The following general principles of measurement may help clarify the issues that need to be addressed when measuring quality of life:

1. The purpose of the study needs to be explicit, to guide decisions about which dimensions of quality of life to measure and which methods and measures to use. For example, comparing patients' functional status in two arms of a clinical trial differs considerably from describing their quality-of-life trajectories throughout their cancer experience. Consequently, different study purposes lead to the incorporation of different designs and measures.

2. Selection of measures needs to be based on a clearly identified theoretical or conceptual model in which quality of life and other included concepts are defined, model assumptions are specified, relationships are described and are logically congruent, and a developmental perspective is incorporated. Without careful stipulation, we will be unable to build a coherent body of knowledge about HRQOL in children and adolescents. Equally serious, we could waste costly resources in studies that lack these characteristics.

3. In its current definition, HRQOL appears to be a latent variable, one that cannot be directly measured (Aaronson et al., 1987; Rudin, Martinson, & Gillis, 1988). Therefore, multiple measures or indicators of HRQOL are necessary. However, the quality of studies reported in the literature using multiple measures has been evaluated as poor (Eiser, 2001). This is likely a reflection of the lack of a sound theoretical perspective in selection of instruments, and caution is advised in design of such studies as they often require a larger sample.

4. Concept analysis work and inductive development of concepts and measures need to continue, particularly when the components of a proposed model are unclear. The sources of influence and the components of HRQOL seem similar or related. Efforts to better identify the antecedents and consequences of quality of life in children and adolescents and the critical attributes of this concept need to continue.

5. Conceptualizations of HRQOL and their underlying assumptions should be examined for cultural relevance, especially when measures based on these conceptualizations are to be used in different cultures.

Measures Used to Index HRQOL in Children and Adolescents

The number of generic and disease-specific HRQOL measures for children and adolescents is rapidly increasing, with over 40 instruments reported in the literature in various stages of development and testing (Eiser & Morse, 2001). Self-report measures are being used with children as young as 5 years of age (Varni, Seid, & Rode, 1999) as indicators of HRQOL dimensions in children and adolescents, but there continues to be a limited number of child-report measures and a larger number of parent proxy instruments. For many instruments, evidence of reliability as either stability or internal consistency is preliminary and only a few measures have sustained evidence of validity (Eiser & Morse, 2001).

The number of dimensions studied in any instrument ranges from 1 to 17 (Eiser & Morse, 2001). Most instruments include the components of HRQOL identified by the World Health Organization. Some instruments more clearly reflect the pediatric experience as indicated by the child-centered measurement approach or the domains represented. For example, Eiser's Perceived Illness Experience measures three unique domains reflective of child and adolescent concerns, which are disclosure, appearance, and peer rejection (Eiser, Havermans, Craft, & Kernahan, 1995).

Measurement approaches have varied, with one approach involving disease-specific instruments and another approach combining disease-specific with generic HRQOL instruments. Examples of generic HRQOL forms include the Health Utilities Index Mark (HUI2 and HUI3), as well as the Child Health Questionnaire (Feeny et al., 1992; Landgraf, Abetz, & Ware, 1996) and the pediatric PROMIS measures. An example of a modular approach of combining disease-specific and generic instruments in one study would be the Pediatric Quality of Life Inventory (PedsQL v.4.0) and the Pediatric Quality of Life Cancer Mondule (PedsQL v.3.0) (Varni et al., 2002).

Recommendations for Future Conceptual, Research, and Clinical Work with Health-Related Quality of Life in Children and Adolescents

Future conceptual work needs to focus on reports solicited directly from children and adolescents that describe their definition and perception of HRQOL during the cancer experience. This focus will entail careful qualitative work to completely capture their language, meaning, and the importance they place on quality of life. This conceptual work will be most beneficial if completed across the continuum of cancer care (from diagnosis to long-term survivorship or terminal care), so that the actual trajectory of HRQOL is documented. In addition, the conceptual work must include the perspectives of children and adolescents of different ages, and these perspectives should be analyzed for any differences associated with age or developmental level.

Conceptual work with parents needs to focus on their definition and experience of their quality of life (as parents and as a family) throughout the cancer care continuum. Their definition and experience of their diagnosed child's HRQOL also should be addressed; the comparison of their perspectives may lead to a better understanding of these two experiences. Conceptual models particular to HRQOL in children and adolescents should then be developed more fully.

Measures based on the conceptual work described earlier need to be developed. Those measures must be tested in multiple studies that have different purposes (e.g., clinical trials and clinical intervention studies). The resulting HRQOL scores should be examined for differences related to age, diagnosis, point on the care continuum, and other disease or patient variables. In addition, scores on HRQOL measures as reported by the patient, parent, and healthcare provider will need to be compared, and sources of agreement or difference identified and explained. Intervention studies that include measures of HRQOL prior to and following a nursing care intervention also should be completed. Finally, studies that measure the meaning of quality-of-life work for nurses in terms of their role meaning and satisfaction are necessary.

Even though the conceptual and research work with HRQOL in children and adolescents with cancer is incomplete, nurses will continue to incorporate such issues in their daily care of these patients. The following guidelines are offered to help nurses design general questions for assessing the HRQOL in the child or adolescent. Questions should be modified to ensure that they are developmentally appropriate for patients of different ages. Use the same general question over time and patients will help nurses recognize usual and unexpected responses. Questions that work best clinically include a built-in standard of comparison—for example, "When you think back on how things were for you during your first chemotherapy session, how are things going for you right now?" More specific questions designed to elicit the child or adolescent's perception of each of the dimensions of HRQOL might follow. Nurses will obtain a more comparable assessment standard if each patient is asked the same set of questions at key times throughout the cancer experience.

Nurses need to determine in advance the purpose of the clinical assessment of the child's HRQOL. Is it a general assessment question, an issue-specific question, or a protocol- or treatment-driven question? The purpose of the assessment will give direction to the manner in which the questions posed to the child are varied. Nurses can also provide valuable clinical observations by documenting the following: the responses offered by the child or adolescent, the exact intervention initiated by the nurse, and the patient outcomes of that intervention. These anecdotal reports will contribute to the future clinical care efforts for that child or adolescent, while also helping to build conceptual models of quality of life for children and adolescents with cancer.

Finally, the clinical benefit to children and adolescents of providing their HRQOL perspectives to healthcare providers needs to be documented. The time and effort that they and their parents give to providing these perspectives needs to have a likelihood of benefit for them. As noted by leaders in the Division of Cancer Prevention at the National Cancer Institute in the United States, the added research value of including HRQOL instruments in cancer clinical trials needs to be firmly established to justify their continued inclusion in such trials (Buchanan, O'Mara, Kelaghan, & Minasian, 2005).

CONCLUSION

The definition of HRQOL from the perspective of the child or adolescent with cancer is receiving renewed attention. Because of their considerable interest in this construct, nurses are likely to expend the efforts necessary for completely defining quality of life and identifying its attributes. As a result, HRQOL assessments derived from sound empirical research will become standard in the nursing care of children and adolescents with cancer.

REFERENCES

Aaronson, N., Bakker, W., Stewart, A., van Dam, F., van Zandwijk, N., Yarnold, J., et al. (1987). Multidimensional approach to the measurement of quality of life in lung cancer clinical trials. In N. K. Aaronson & J. Beckman (Eds.), *The quality of life of cancer patients.* New York, NY: Raven Press.

Baker, J. N, Barfield, R., Hinds, P. S., & Kane, J. R. (2007). A model to facilitate decision making in pediatric stem cell transplantation: The Individualized Care Planning and Coordination Model. *Biology of Blood and Marrow Transplantation, 13*(3), 245–254.

Baltes, P. B. (1979). Life-span developmental psychology: Some converging observations on history and theory. In P. B. Baltes & O. G. Brim (Eds.), *Life-span development and behavior* (pp. 225–279). San Diego, CA: Academic Press.

Barr, R. D., Chalmers, D., De Pauw, S., Furlong, W., Weitzman, S., Feeny, D. (2000). Health-related quality of life in survivors of Wilms' tumor and advanced neuroblastoma: A cross-sectional study. *Journal of Clinical Oncology, 18,* 3280–3287.

Barr, R. D., Furlong, W., Dawson, S., Whitton, A. C., Strautmanis, I., Pai, M., et al. (1993). An assessment of global health status in survivors of acute lymphoblastic leukemia in childhood. *The American Journal of Pediatric Hematology/Oncology, 15*(4), 284–290.

Bradlyn, A. S., Harris, C. V., Warner, J. E., Ritchey, A. K., & Zaboy, K. (1993). An investigation of the validity of the quality of well-being scale with pediatric oncology patients. *Health Psychology, 12*(3), 246–250.

Bradlyn, A. S., & Pollock, B. H. (1996). *Quality of life research in the Pediatric Oncology Group: 1991–1995*. Morgantown, WV: Department of Behavioral Medicine and Psychiatry, Robert C. Byrd Health Sciences Center.

Bradlyn, A. S., & Pollock, B. H. (1996). Quality-of-life research in the Pediatric Oncology Group: 1991–1995[Monograph]. *Journal of the National Cancer Institute, 20,* 49–53.

Bradlyn, A. S., Ritchey A. K., Harris, C. V., Moore, A. K., O'Brien, R. T., Parsons, S. K., et al. (1995). *Quality of life research in pediatric oncology: Research methods and barriers.* Morgantown, WV: Department of Behavioral Medicine and Psychiatry, Robert C. Byrd Health Sciences Center.

Bradlyn, A., Varni, J., & Hinds, P. (2003). Assessing health-related quality of life in end-of-life care for children and adolescents. In M. Field & R. Behrman (Eds.), *Care of dying children and their families.* Institute of Medicine, Washington, DC.

Buchanan, D. R., O'Mara, A. M., Kelaghan, J. W., & Minasian, L. M. (2005). Quality-of-life in the symptom management trials of the National Cancer Institute-supported Community Clinical Oncology Program. *Journal of Clinical Oncology, 23*(3), 591–598.

Cadman, D., Goldsmith, C., Torrance, G. W., Boyle, B. H., & Furlong, W. (1986). *Development of a health status index for Ontario children.* Final report to the Ontario Ministry of Health on research grant DM 648 (00633). Hamilton, Ontario: McMaster University.

Castel, L. D., Williams, K. A., Bosworth, H. B., Eisen, S. V., Hahn, E. A., Irwin, D. E., et al. (2008). Content validty in the PROMIS social-health domain: A qualitative analysis of focus-group data. *Quality of Life Research, 17*(5), 737–749.

Chang, P. C, Yeh, C. H. (2005). Agreement between child self-report and parent proxy-report to evaluate quality of life in children with cancer. *Psycho-Oncology, 14,* 125–134.

Chen, C. M. Chen, Y.C., & Haase, J. E. (2008). Games of lives in surviving childhood brain tumors. *Western Journal of Nursing Research, 30*(4), 435–457.

Corey, A. L., Haase, J. E., Azzouz, F., & Monahan, P. O. (2008). Social support and symptom distress in adolescents/young adults with cancer. *Journal of Pediatric Hematology/Oncology Nurses, 25*(5), 275–284.

Costain, K., Hewison, J., & Howes, M. (1993). Comparison of a function-based model and a meaning-based model of quality of life in oncology: Multidimensionality examined. *Journal of Psychosocial Oncology, 11*(4), 17–37.

Cremeens, J., Eiser, C., & Blades, M. (2006). A qualitative investigation of school-aged children's answers to items from a generic quality of life measure. *Child: Care, Health and Development, 33*(1), 83–89.

Czyzewski, D. I., Mariotto, M. J., Bartholomew, L. K., LeCompte, S. H., & Sockrider, M. M. (1994). Measurement of quality of well-being in a child and adolescent cystic fibrosis population. *Medical Care, 32*(9), 965–972.

Davis, E., Nicolas, C., Waters, E., Cook, K., Gibbs, L., Gosch, A., et al. (2007). Parent-proxy and child self-reported health-related quality of life: Using qualitative methods to explain the discordance. *Quality of Life Research, 16*(5), 863–871.

DeWalt, D., Rothrock, N., Young, S. & Stone, A. (2007). Evaluation of item candidates: The PROMIS qualitative item review. *Medical Care, 45,* 512–521.

Earle, E. A., Eiser, C., Grimer, R. (2005). 'He never liked sport anyway'—Mother's views of young people coping with a bone tumour in the lower limb. *Sarcoma, 9*(1/2), 7–13.

Eiser, C. (1997). Children's quality of life measures. *Archives of Disease in Childhood, 77*(4), 350–354.

Eiser, C. (2001). The measurement of quality of life in children: Past and future perspectives. *Journal of Developmental & Behavioral Pediatrics, 22*(4), 248–256.

Eiser, C., Cool, P., Grimer, R. J., Carter, S. R., Cotter, I. M., Ellis, A. J., et al. (1997). Quality of life in children following treatment for a malignant primary bone tumour around the knee. *Sarcoma, 1,* 39–45.

Eiser, C., Cotter, I., Oades, P., Seamark, D., & Smith, R. (1999). Health-related quality-of-life measures for children. *International Journal of Cancer Suppl.*, *12*, 87–90.

Eiser, C., & Eiser, J. R. (2000). Social comparisons and quality of life among survivors of childhood cancer and their mothers. *Psychology and Health*, *15*, 435–450.

Eiser, C., Eiser, J. R., & Stride, C. B. (2005). Quality of life in children newly diagnosed with cancer and their mothers. *Health and Quality of Life Outcomes*, *3*(29). Retrieved on April 26, 2007 from http://www.hqlo.com/content/3/1/29.

Eiser, C., Havermans, T., Craft, A., & Kernahan, J. (1995). Development of a measure to assess the perceived illness experience after treatment for cancer. *Archives of Disease in Childhood*, *72*, 302–307.

Eiser, C., Hill, J. J., & Vance, Y. H. (2000). Examining the psychological consequences of surviving childhood cancer: Systematic review as a research method in pediatric psychology. *Journal of Pediatric Psychology*, *25*(6), 449–460.

Eiser, C., & Morse, R. (2001). Quality-of-life measures in chronic diseases of childhood. *Health Technology Assessment*, *5*(4),1–110.

Feeny, D., Furlong, W., Barr, R., Torrance, G. W., Rosenbaum, P., & Weitzman, S. (1992). A comprehensive multiattribute system for classifying the health status of survivors of childhood cancer. *Journal of Clinical Oncology*, *10*(6), 923–928.

Feeny, D., & Leiper, A. (1993). The comprehensive assessment of health status in survivors of childhood cancer: Application to high-risk acute lymphoblastic leukaemia, *British Journal of Cancer*, *67*(5), 1047–1052.

Ginsberg, J. P., Cnaan, A., Zhao, H., Clark, B. J., Paridon, S. M., Chin, A. J., et al. (2004). Using health-related quality of life measures to predict cardiac function in survivors exposed to anthracyclines. *Journal of Clinical Oncology*, *22*(15), 3149–3155.

Goh, A. Y., Lum, L. C., Chan, P. W., Baker, F., & Chong, B. O. (1999). Withdrawal and limitation of life support in pediatric intensive care. *Archives of the Disabled Child*, *80*, 424–428.

Gong, G. W., Young, N. L., Dempster, H., Porepa, M., & Feldman, B. M. (2007). The Quality of My Life questionnaire: The minimal clinically important difference for pediatric rheumatology patients. *Journal of Rheumatology*, *34*(3), 581–587.

Grant, M., Padilla, G., & Creimel, E. (1996). Survivorship and quality of life issues. In R. McCorkle, M. Grant, M. Frank-Stromborg, & S. Baird (Eds.), *Cancer nursing: A comprehensive textbook* (pp. 1312–1321). Philadelphia, PA: W. B. Saunders.

Haase, J. E., Heiney S. P., Ruccione, K. S., & Stutzer, C. (1999). Research triangulation to derive meaning-based quality-of-life theory: Adolescent resilience model and instrument development. *International Journal of Cancer—Supplement*, *12*, 125–131.

Haase, J., & Rostad, M. (1994). Experiences of completing cancer treatments: Child and adolescent perspectives. *Oncology Nursing Forum*, *21*, 1483–1492.

Hinds, P. S., Gattuso, J. S., Fletcher, A., Baker, E., Coleman, B., Jackson, T., et al. (2004). Quality of life as conveyed by pediatric patients with cancer. *Quality of Life Research*, *13*, 761–772.

Hinds, P., Quargnenti, A., & Wentz, T. (1992). Measuring symptom distress in adolescents with cancer. *Journal of Pediatric Oncology Nursing*, *9*, 84–86.

Hinds, P. S. (1990). Quality of life in children and adolescents with cancer. *Seminars in Oncology Nursing*, *6*, 285–291.

Hinds, P. S. (1995). *Self-care outcomes in adolescents with cancer.* Final report to the National Cancer Institute on research grant 1 R01 CA 48432. Memphis, TN: St. Jude Children's Research Hospital.

Hinds, P., Bradshaw, G., Oakes, L., & Pritchard, M. (2003). Children and their rights in life and death situations. In R. Kastenbaum (Ed.), *Encyclopedia of Death and Dying.* New York, NY: Macmillan Reference Publishers.

Hinds, P. S., Brandon, J., Allen, C., Hijiya, N., Newsome, R., & Kane, J. (2007). Patient-reported outcomes in end-of-life research in pediatric oncology. *Journal of Pediatric Psychology*, *32*(9), 1079–1088.

Hinds, P. S., Hockenberry, M. J., Gattuso, J. S., Srivastave, D. K., Tong, X., Jones, H., et al. (2007). Dexamethasone alters sleep and fatigue in pediatric patients with acute lymphoblastic leukemia. *Cancer, 110*(10), 2321–2330.

Hinds, P. S., & Martin, J. (1988). Self-care outcomes in adolescents with cancer. *Nursing Research, 37*(6), 336–340.

Hinds, P., Oakes, L., Drew, D., Fouladi, M., Spunt, S., Church, C., Furman, C. (2005). End-of-life care preferences of pediatric patients with cancer. *Journal of Clinical Oncology, 23*(36), 9146–9154.

Hinds, P. S., Oakes, L., & Furman, W. (2001). End-of-life decision making in pediatric oncology. In B. R. Ferrell & N. Coyle (Eds.), *Textbook of Palliative Nursing* (pp. 450–460). New York, NY: Oxford University Press.

Hinds, P. S., Oakes, L., Furman, W., Quargnenti, A., Olson, M. S., Foppiano, P., et al. (2001). End-of-life decision making by adolescents, parents, and healthcare providers in pediatric oncology. *Cancer Nursing, 24*, 122–136.

Hinds, P. S., Oakes, L. L., Hicks, J., Powell, B., Srivastava, D. K., Spunt, S. L., et al. (2009). "Trying to be a good parent" as defined by interviews with parents who made end-of-life decisions for their children. *Journal of Clinical Oncology, 27*(35), 5979–5985.

Hinds, P., Quargnenti, A., Bush, A., Fairclough, D., Betcher, D., Rissmiller, G., et al. (2000). An evaluation of the impact of a self-care coping intervention on psychological and clinical outcomes in adolescents with newly diagnosed cancer. *European Journal of Oncology Nursing, 4*(1),6–17.

Hinds, P. S., Quargnenti, A. G., Hickey, S. S., & Mangum, G. H. (1994). A comparison of the stress-response sequence in new and experienced pediatric oncology nurses. *Cancer Nursing, 17*(1), 61–71.

Hinds, P. S., & Varricchio, C. G. (1996). Quality of life: The nursing perspective. In B. Spilker (Ed.), *Quality of life and pharmacoeconomics in clinical trials* (2nd ed.) (pp. 529–533). Philadelphia, PA: Lippincott-Raven.

Hockenberry-Eaton, M., & Hinds, P. S. (2000). Fatigue in children and adolescents with cancer: Evolution of a program of study. *Seminars in Oncology Nursing, 16*(4), 261–272.

Hoffman, C., Gosheger, G., Gebert, C., Jurgens, H., & Winkelmann, W. (2006). Functional results and quality of life after treatment of pelvic sarcomas involving the acetabulum. *Journal of Bone and Joint Surgery, 88A*(3), 575–582.

Ishibashi, A., Ueda, R., Kawano, Y., Nakayama, H., Matsuzaki, A., & Matsumura, T. (2010). How to improve resilience in adolescents with cancer in Japan. *Journal of Pediatric Hematology/Oncology Nursing, 27*(2), 73–93.

Jones, C. (1990). Staff nurse turnover costs: Part II: Measurement and results. *Journal of Nursing Administration, 20*(5), 27–32.

Keith, K., & Schalock, R. (1994). The measurement of quality of life in adolescence: The quality of life questionnaire. *The American Journal of Family Therapy, 22*(1), 83–87.

King, C., Hinds, P. S., Dow, K., Schum, L., & Lee, C. (2002). The nurses relationship-based perceptions of patient quality of life. *Oncology Nursing Forum, 29*(10), E118–E126.

Knafl, K., & Deatrick, J. (1993). Knowledge synthesis and concept development in nursing. In B. Rodgers & K. Knafl (Eds.), *Concept development in nursing: Foundations, techniques and applications* (pp. 35–50). Philadelphia, PA: W. B. Saunders.

Koopman, H. M., Koetsier, J. A., Taminiau, A. H. M., Hijnen, K. E., Bresters, D., & Egeler, R. M. (2005). Health-related quality of life and coping strategies of children after treatment of a malignant bone tumor: A 5-year follow-up study. *Pediatric Blood and Cancer, 45*, 694–699.

Landgraf, J. M., Abetz, L., Ware, J. L. (1996). The CHQ: A User's Manual (2nd Printing), Boston, MA: The Health Institute.

Leininger, M. (1994). Quality of life from a transcultural nursing perspective. *Nursing Science Quarterly, 7*, 22–28.

Lerner, R. M. (1986). *Concepts and theories of human development* (2nd ed.). New York, NY: Random House.

Levi, R. B., & Drotar, D. (1999). Health-related quality of life in childhood cancer: Discrepancy in parent-child reports. *International Journal of Cancer—Supplement, 12*, 58–64.

Lindstrom, B. (1994). *The essence of existence: On the quality of life of children in the Nordic countries.* Goteborg, Sweden: Nordic School of Public Health.

Lindstrom, B., & Kohler, L. (1991). Youth, disability, and quality of life. *Pediatrician, 18*, 121–128.

Marchese, V. G., Ogle, S., Womer, R. B., Dormans, J., & Ginsberg, J. P. (2004). An examination of outcome measures to assess functional mobility in childhood survivors of osteosarcoma. *Pediatric Blood and Cancer, 42*, 41–45.

Marshall, P. (1990). Cultural influences on perceived quality of life. *Seminars in Oncology Nursing, 6*, 278–284.

Nagarajan, R., Clohisy, D. R., Neglia, J. P., Yasui, Y., Mitby, P. A., Sklar, C., et al. (2004). Function and quality-of-life of survivors of pelvic and lower extremity osteosarcoma and Ewing's sarcoma: The Childhood Cancer Survivor Study. *British Journal of Cancer, 91*, 1858–1865.

Nathan, P. C., Furlong, W., & Barr, R. D. (2004). Challenges to the measurement of health-related quality of life in children receiving cancer therapy. *Pediatric Blood and Cancer, 434*, 215–223.

Nuss, S., Hinds, P. S., & LaFond, D. (2005). Collaborative clinical research on end-of-life care in pediatric oncology. *Seminars in Oncology Nursing, 21*, 125–134.

Olson, M. S., Hinds, P. S., Euell, K., Quargnenti, A., Milligan, M., Foppiano, P., et al. (1998). Peak and nadir experiences and their consequences described by pediatric oncology nurses. *Journal of Pediatric Oncology Nursing, 15*(1), 13–24.

Palmer, S. N., Meeske, K. A., Katz, E. R., Burwinkle, T. M., & Varni, J. W. (2007). The PedsQL Brain Tumor Module: Initial reliability and validity. *Pediatric Blood and Cancer, 49*(3), 287–293.

Parsons, S. K., Barlow, S. E., Levy, S. L., Supran, S. E., & Kaplan, H. (1999). Health-related quality of life in pediatric bone marrow transplant survivors: According to whom? *International Journal of Cancer-Supplement, 12*, 46–51.

Pediatric Oncology Group, Quality of Life Subcommittee. (1993). Guidelines for incorporating quality of life measures into clinical trials. Unpublished manuscript.

Phipps, S., Dunavant, M., Jayawardene, D., & Srivastava, D. (1999). Assessment of health-related quality of life in acute in-patient settings: Use of the BASES instrument in children undergoing bone marrow transplantation. *International Journal of Cancer—Supplement, 12*, 18–24.

Raphael, D. (1996). Quality of life and adolescent health. In R. Renwick, I. Brown, & M. Nagre (Eds.), *Quality of life in health promotion and rehability: Conceptual approaches, issues and applications* (pp. 307–324). Thousand Oaks, CA: Sage.

Razzouk B., Hord, J., Hockenberry, M., Hinds, P. S., Feusner, J., Williams, D., et al. (2006). Double-blind, placebo-controlled study of quality-of-life, hematologic end points, and safety of weekly epoetin alfa in children with cancer receiving myelosuppressive chemotherapy. *Journal of Clinical Oncology, 24*, 3583–3589.

Rosenbaum, P., Cadman, D., & Kerpalani, H. (1990). Pediatrics: Assessing quality of life. In B. Spilker (Ed.), Quality of life assessments in clinical trials (pp. 205–215). New York, NY: Raven Press.

Rudin, M., Martinson, I., & Gillis, C. (1988). Measurement of psychosocial concerns of adolescents with cancer. *Cancer Nursing, 11*, 144–149.

Rushton, C. (1994). Moral decision making by parents of infants who have life-threatening congenital disorders. Unpublished doctoral dissertation, School of Nursing, Catholic University of America, Washington, DC.

Sartorius, N. (1987). Cross-cultural comparisons of data abot quality of life: A sample of issues. In N. K. Aaronson & J. Beckman (Eds.), *The quality of life of cancer patients.* New York, NY: Raven Press.

Seid, M., Varni J. W., Rode, C. A., Katz, E. R. (1999). The Pediatric Cancer Quality of Life Inventory: a modular approach to measuring health-related quality of life in children with cancer. *International Journal of Cancer, Supplement, 12*, 71–76.

Shankar, S., Robison, L., Jenney M. E. M., Rockwood, T. H., Wu, E., Feusner, J., et al. (2005). Health-related quality of life in young survivors of childhood cancer using the Minneapolis-Manchester Quality of Life-Youth Form. *Pediatrics, 115*, 435–442.

Sherifali, D., & Pinelli, J. (2007). Parent as proxy reporting: Implications and recommendations for quality of life research. *Journal of Family Nursing, 13*(1), 83–98.

Stam, H., Grootenhuis, M. A., Brons, P. P. T., Caron, H. N., Last, B. F. (2006). Health-related quality of life in children and emotional reactions of parents following completion of cancer treatment. *Pediatric Blood and Cancer, 47*, 312–319.

Steen, B., Burghen, E., Hinds, P. S., Srivastava, D. K., & Tong, X. (2003). The development and testing of the Role-Related Meaning Scale for Staff in Pediatric Oncology. *Cancer Nursing, 26*(3), 187–194.

Sung, L., Young, N. L., Greenberg, M. L., McLimont, M., Samanta, T., Wong, J., et al. (2004). Health-related quality of life (HRQOL) scores reported from parents and their children with chronic illness differend depending on utility elicitation method. *Journal of Clinical Epidemiology, 57*, 1161–1166.

Tabone, M. D., Rodary, C., Oberlin, O., Gentet, J. C., Pacquement, H., & Kalifa, C. (2005). Quality of life of patients treated during childhood for a bone tumor: Assessment by the child health questionnaire. *Pediatric Blood and Cancer, 45*, 207–211.

US Department of Health and Human Services, Food and Drug Administration. (2009). Guidance for industry patient-reported outcome measures: Use in medical product development to support labeling claims. Rockville, MD, Author.

Varni, J. W., Burwinkle, T. M., Katz, E. R., Meeske, K., & Dickinson, P. (2002). The PedsQL in pediatric cancer: Reliability and validity of the Pediatric Quality of Life Inventory Generic Core Scales, Multidimensional Fatigue Scale, and Cancer Module. *Cancer, 94*, 2090–2106.

Varni, J. W., Limbers, C., & Burwinkle, T. M. (2007). Literature review: Health-related quality of life measurement in pediatric oncology: Hearing the voices of children. *Journal of Pediatric Psychology*, 1–13.

Varni, J. M., Seid M., & Rode, C. (1999). The PedsQL: Measurement model for the pediatric quality of life inventory. *Medical Care, 37*(2), 126–139.

Voigtman, J. (2002). *Learning to Suffer: Pain Response in a Community of Saudi Arab Children with Sickle Cell Disease*. Unpublished doctoral dissertation, University of Arizona.

Wakefield, D., Curry, J., Price, J., Mueller, C., & McCloskey, J. (1988). Differences in unit outcomes: Job satisfaction, organizational commitment, and turnover among hospital nursing department employees. *Western Journal of Nursing Research, 10*(1), 98–105.

Walsh, T. R., Irwin, D. E., Meier, A., Varni, J. W., & DeWalt, D. A. (2008). The use of focus groups in the development of the PROMIS pediatrics item bank. *Quality of Life Research Journal, 17*(5), 725–735.

Weekes, D. (1991). Application of the life-span developmental perspective to nursing research with adolescents. *Journal of Pediatric Nursing, 6*, 38–48.

World Health Organization. (1947). The Constitution of the World Health Organization. *WHO Chronicle*.

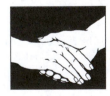

Research

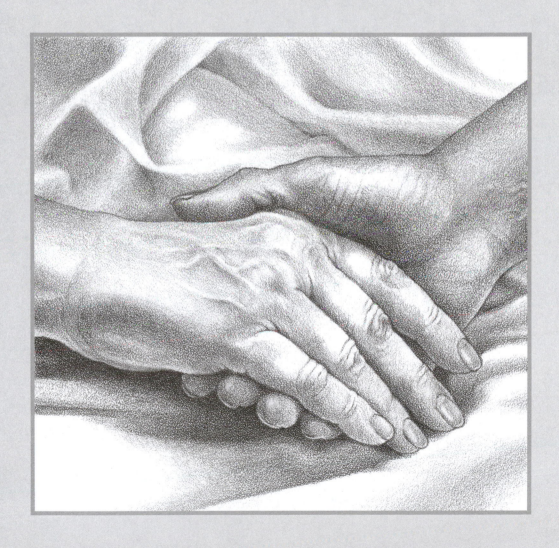

Chapter Eight

Quality of Life: Methodological and Measurement Issues

MEL R. HABERMAN • NIGEL E. BUSH

Introduction

The construct of quality of life (QOL) offers oncology nursing an organizing framework for describing the caring behaviors of nurses. The QOL paradigm for practice is holistic and acknowledges important outcomes of care, such as physical mobility, adherence to treatment, self-care behaviors, psychosocial and cognitive functioning, symptom management, and spirituality. Oncology nurses systematically incorporate QOL outcomes into standards of care, guidelines for practice, and care pathways. Moreover, QOL outcomes are valuable to all members of the multidisciplinary cancer team and appear to be relevant whether the goal of therapy is cure or palliation and comfort (Donnelly, Rybicki, & Walsh, 2001; Groenvold, 1999; McCahill et al., 2002; McMillan & Weitzner, 2000; Seow et al., 2009). Quality-of-life issues are particularly important to the treatment choices of persons with cancer when two cancer therapies are expected to yield similar life expectancy but the toxicities of one treatment are significantly greater than the other (Bottomley, 2002; Cella, 2009). With the increasing sophistication of information and decision aids available on the Internet, persons with cancer now routinely ask their physicians and nurses questions about how various treatment options will affect their quality of life (Detmar & Aaronson, 1998; Mark, Johnson, Fortner, & Ryan, 2008).

Oncology nurses are challenged more than ever to conduct research and to build a systematic knowledge base for evidence-based practice. The purpose of this chapter is to describe some of the conceptual and methodological issues that influence the design of QOL studies in an effort to promote QOL research. The chapter focuses on measurement issues pertaining to research conducted on adults rather than those pertaining to children (Barrera, D'Agostino, Gammon, Spencer, & Baruchel, 2005; Hinds, Burghen, Haase, & Phillips, 2006; Matza, Swensen, Flood, Secnik, & Leidy, 2004; Nathan, Furlong, & Barr, 2004), adolescents (Chang & Yeh, 2005; Ravens-Sieberer et al., 2006), or families (Lewis & Zahlis, 1997).

Conceptual Issues That Guide QOL Measurement

Multidimensional Nature of QOL

Healthcare researchers agree QOL is a multidimensional construct (Cella, 2001; Donnelly et al., 2001; Gotay & Muraoka, 1998; King et al., 1997). However, because no specific definition of QOL is widely accepted among researchers, many investigators implicitly have defined the concept by the way they measure it (Ganz, 1994; Holzner et al., 2001; (McCabe, Begley, Collier, & McCann, 2008). This convention is contrary to typical methods of quantitative science, where measurement is based on clearly defined concepts. Moreover, investigators have often neglected to base their measurement operations on an explanatory model of QOL (Sousa, 1999). For instance, if spirituality is identified by the researcher as an important conceptual dimension of QOL after cancer diagnosis, the QOL questionnaire selected for a study must have items that measure the construct of spirituality.

There is some consensus among health researchers regarding the minimum components to include when measuring QOL. Quality-of-life measurement can be enhanced by including a minimum of four dimensions, plus global measures of perceived health status and QOL (Aaronson, 1990; Bush, Donaldson, Haberman, Dacanay, & Sullivan, 2000; Bush, Haberman, Donaldson, & Sullivan, 1995; Ganz, 1994; Moinpour, Hayden, Thompson, Feigl, & Metch, 1990; Velikova, Stark, & Selby, 1999). These four dimensions include physical functioning, emotional and psychological functioning, social functioning, and disease- or treatment-related symptoms. Table 8-1 identifies some of the components of each dimension of QOL.

In addition to the core set of QOL indicators listed in Table 8-1, other health-related issues may be of interest to nurse scientists when measuring QOL. Some of these additional facets of QOL include vocational and insurance discrimination, the stigma of cancer, financial well-being, the demands or hardships of cancer survivorship, and physical growth and cognitive development following childhood cancer. When designing a QOL study, investigators must determine what they mean by QOL and specify the dimensions to be measured (Gill & Feinstein, 1994; Montazeri, Gillis, & McEwen, 1996; McCabe et al., 2008). Some situational or disease characteristics of QOL may be time-limited and available for measurement only at specific stages of cancer survivorship (Epstein, 2000). For instance, the disruptions caused by cancer recurrence would not be expected to influence QOL until the actual recurrence of disease.

QOL as a Research Outcome

QOL outcomes now are an integral component of many cancer clinical trials. In 1990, the National Cancer Institute (NCI) held a landmark workshop to identify guidelines for systematically assessing QOL outcomes (Nayfield, Ganz, Moinpour, Cella, & Hailey, 1992; Nayfield, Hailey, & McCabe, 1991). Several American, Canadian, and international cooperative research groups have standardized the measurement of QOL endpoints in Phase III clinical trials (de Haes et al., 2000; Lee & Chi, 2000; Moinpour et al., 1990; Osoba, Dancey, Zee, Myles, & Pater, 1996).

Table 8-1. **Dimensions of Quality of Life**

Physical Functioning

Activities of daily living

Physical mobility, independence, and ability to exercise

Ability to perform work, school, and recreation activities

Self-care and personal hygiene activities

Nutrition and dietary management activities

Psychological Functioning

Mood states: depression, anxiety, anger, joy

Cognitive or mental status: orientation, memory, concentration, attention, perception, thinking, alertness, confusion

Perceptions of well-being: life satisfaction, happiness, positive attitude, life outlook, morale, meaning and purpose, inner peace, personal success, perceived control, hope

Spirituality, self-transcendent experiences, altruism

Self-esteem, body image, self-worth, self-mastery, self-efficacy

Social Role Functioning

Sexual functioning, intimacy, and warmth

Managing interpersonal, family, work, and school relationships

Managing relationships with healthcare providers

Negotiating healthcare organizations and bureaucracies

Participating in support groups or volunteer activities

Disease- and Treatment-Related Symptoms

Fatigue and energy levels

Physical stamina, strength, and endurance

Nausea, vomiting, diarrhea, constipation

Mucositis, dysphagia, dyspnea

Taste changes, pain, infections, dermatitis

Sleep alterations and rest

All regimen-related toxicities or side effects of therapy

Health-related QOL outcomes (Table 8-1) can be used in the following ways: to predict survival rates; document the transition from symptom impairment to complete recovery; compare the results of different types of therapy for the same disease; establish norms of morbidity among diverse cultural groups and populations of cancer survivors; document quality indicators of care for the purpose of improving care delivery, satisfaction with care, and therapeutic outcomes; compare the efficacy of traditional and complementary therapies; screen persons at risk of developing psychosocial morbidity; track symptom clusters that linger after the end of active therapy; and compare the incidence and severity of regimen-related toxicities among therapies that have similar disease outcomes but different toxicities (Aaronson, 1990; Bush et al., 2000; Clinch & Schipper, 1993; Ganz, 1994; Shapiro et al., 2001).

Lack of a Gold Standard for Measurement

Health researchers have yet to reach agreement on a gold standard, or best method, of measuring QOL (Cella & Tulsky, 1990; King et al., 1997; McCabe et al., 2008). There is simply no perfect way to measure QOL given the current state of the science and the complex nature of the construct. Systematic advances in QOL measurement will occur in tandem with finding answers to other unresolved issues. The science of QOL measurement will progress as QOL conceptual models advance to theoretical frameworks; as definitions of QOL emerge from empirical qualitative and quantitative research; and as the effect of QOL-related health disparities on cancer prevention, screening, treatment, and survivorship is better understood.

Because the majority of health-related QOL (HRQOL) questionnaires were developed in nonminority and well-educated groups, researchers continue to examine whether these questionnaires are equivalent conceptually and methodologically across diverse racial, ethnic, geographic, age, and gender populations (Ashing-Giwa & Kagawa-Singer, 2006; Baker, Jodrey, Zabora, Douglas, & Fernandez-Kelly, 1996; Stewart & Napoles-Springer, 2000). In the absence of establishing universal consensus on the ideal way to measure QOL, researchers should strive to define QOL clearly and to establish boundaries on a suitable conceptual framework (Sousa, 1999). In addition, investigators should establish the relevance of QOL measurement across the continuum of therapy (Testa, 2000). For instance, how does QOL vary across the continuum of care for breast cancer from the time of initial surgery, chemoradiotherapy, and adjuvant therapy to the later emergence of either disease remission, recurrent, or metastatic disease?

Quantitative and Qualitative Measurement

Quantitative Measurement
A variety of methods exist for measuring QOL. Each method provides a different vantage point and type of outcome data. One method of QOL measurement is the use of standardized, fixed-item, or forced-choice questionnaires (Testa, 2000; Velikova et al., 1999). Some examples of this type of QOL instrument include the 30-item European Organization for

Table 8-2. **Design and Measurement Issues for QOL Research**

- Describe the specific aims, purpose, and significance of the study.
- Provide a conceptual definition and theoretical framework for QOL.
- Link the theoretical framework to health-related QOL outcomes.
- Select a research design (i.e., descriptive or intervention trial).
- Select methods for data collection (i.e., qualitative and/or quantitative).
- Select a single QOL instrument or battery of questionnaires.
- Select a comprehensive, multidimensional assessment strategy.
- Select either generic or cancer-specific instruments.
- Examine the reliability and validity of all questionnaires.
- Match the QOL measures with the ethnic diversity of the study.
- Obtain data at a single time point or on multiple occasions.
- Identify the appropriate time for obtaining baseline measurement.
- Standardize measurement procedures across sites and treatment groups.
- Obtain data from the perspective of the person with cancer.
- Evaluate the strengths and limitations of data obtained by self-report.
- Minimize responder burden and sources of measurement error.
- Conduct a pilot study of procedures and pretest of the instruments.
- Select a sampling plan and identify study entry and exclusion criteria.
- Identify a sampling plan and estimate sample size if making comparisons between or among groups.
- Establish scoring procedures for all instruments.
- Develop an analysis plan for all forms of raw data.
- Conduct a data audit trail to monitor the reliability of all data operations.
- Ensure the self-determination and protection of human participants.
- Monitor the informed consent process and the ethical conduct of the study.
- Establish a data safety and monitoring board if conducting a Phase III clinical trial.

Research and Treatment of Cancer Questionnaire (EORTC QLQ-30), Quality of Life Questionnaire (Aaronson et al., 1993; Fayers & Bottomley, 2002; Scott et al., 2009), and the Functional Assessment of Chronic Illness Therapy (FACIT) or Functional Assessment of Cancer Therapy (FACT-G) (Cella, Bullinger, Scott, & Barofsky, 2002; Cella et al., 1993; FACIT, 2009; Webster, Cella, & Yost, 2003).

There are several advantages to using standardized questionnaires. Standardized tools typically have known reliability and validity—every participant is asked the same set of items; the questionnaires are often easy to administer and complete; the statistical analysis is generally straightforward; and results can be compared across studies using the same instruments. However, because fixed-item questionnaires limit responses only to the items on the questionnaire, many aspects of QOL may be overlooked. For instance, if the questionnaire focuses on physical functioning and activities of daily living, participants will not be asked to identify problems related to social, emotional, or cognitive functioning.

Qualitative Measurement

Qualitative inquiry is another form of systematic measurement. Selecting a qualitative method may be as simple as including a few open-ended questions at the end of a forced-choice questionnaire or conducting a short, semi-structured interview. Examples of open-ended questions include, "How would you describe your quality of life today?" and "How does your quality of life today compare with your quality of life before cancer?" Additional qualitative methods include participant observation, storytelling, written diaries, interviewing key informants, focus groups, and the systematic examination of archived records and artifacts. Although the use of written diaries may provide chronological, narrative-based log of symptoms or health behaviors, some investigators report participant noncompliance with paper diaries (Stone, Shiffman, Schwartz, Broderick, & Hufford, 2002).

More formal and methodologically rigorous approaches to qualitative inquiry include ethnography, phenomenology, grounded theory, and hermeneutics (Haberman, 1995; Haberman, & Lewis, 1990). Each of these formal approaches is based on unique worldviews and philosophical stances, as well as specific strategies for sampling, data collection, analysis, and write-up. Although rigorous forms of qualitative inquiry can provide a rich source of empirical data, these methodologies are labor-intensive and require advanced research preparation to learn and administer.

Mixed Methods

It is becoming common for investigators to use multiple types of data collection in one study, a strategy known as methodological triangulation (Mitchell, 1986). In mixed methods research, one or more self-report, standardized instruments are administered in combination with a semi-structured interview or set of open-ended questions. For instance, in a mailed survey to long-term cancer survivors, Hassey-Dow and colleagues (Dow, Ferrell, Haberman, & Eaton, 1999) combined open-ended questions and standardized QOL questionnaires to obtain a multidimensional perspective of QOL. Instrument development research often uses a mixed method approach to psychometric evaluation. Respondents may be asked to complete both a forced-choice questionnaire that is under development and a brief set of open-ended items on the same topic. The open-ended data can be analyzed to generate a pool of new items for inclusion in the questionnaire, or responder feedback can be solicited on the wording and clarity of existing items. Gill and Feinstein (1994) suggest all QOL standardized questionnaires should be augmented with additional open-ended items that ask the client to identify missing factors.

It is clear the analysis plan will be different for qualitative data collection than for quantitative. Simple forms of qualitative data can be analyzed using standard content analysis or thematic analysis (Denzin & Lincoln, 2005). Data obtained from the more sophisticated approaches to qualitative inquiry should be analyzed according to the methods developed for those specific approaches.

Unidimensional, Multidimensional, Modular, and Global Assessment of QOL

Unidimensional Assessment

Historically, QOL measurement included the use of unidimensional, single-item scales, such as a simple, five-point rating scale to measure fatigue or pain intensity. The use of unidimensional scales as the only single-item measure of QOL in a study is falling into disuse in favor of a more comprehensive assessment. In fact, some QOL proponents argue unidimensional scales should not even be considered as QOL outcomes because they fail to provide a multidimensional assessment (Cella & Tulsky, 1990; Osoba, 1994; Varricchio, 2006), while other investigators still find value for global, single-item outcome measures when used in mixed methods research (McCabe et al., 2008). The Karnofsky Performance Scale (KPS) (1949), completed by clinicians or other proxies, is a popular single-item scale measuring physical functioning. Regrettably, some clinical researchers still consider it an adequate measure of QOL. Studies have shown this scale suffers from poor interrater reliability and that clinician-based ratings of QOL universally correlate poorly with ratings provided by clients themselves (Aaronson, 1990; Osoba, 1994).

Multidimensional Assessment

Health-related quality of life is a complex phenomenon representing many intertwining facets of life that, by definition, are all attributed to cancer or a specific health condition. Instruments that provide a comprehensive assessment of QOL are the current recommended standard. One option for multidimensional assessment is to choose several instruments, each of which measures only a single domain or component of QOL. For example, one would select one questionnaire to measure symptom side effects, another to assess cognitive functioning, and a third to evaluate mood states. Another option is to select a single multidimensional instrument designed to measure many domains or components of QOL. Multidimensional questionnaires vary greatly in the content measured; consequently, it may be impossible to compare results across studies unless the identical questionnaire is used. Because multidimensional instruments are limited in focus, investigators often combine measures, adding one or more single-domain instrument to supplement the information obtained from a multidimensional scale (Mast, 1995). For instance, Bush and colleagues (2000) combined the EORTC-QLQ-C30 multidimensional questionnaire with the Profile of Mood States and other standardized instruments to assess QOL after marrow and stem cell transplantation. Jalowiec (1990) observed it is exceptionally difficult for any single multidimensional instrument to identify the entire constellation of life changes that occur with a life-threatening illness such as cancer.

A battery approach combines several types of measures to obtain a comprehensive assessment of QOL, for example, unidimensional scales and a combination of single-domain and multidimensional instruments (Ganz, 1994; McCabe et al., 2008). Investigators can select a single scale or battery of questionnaires based on the specific aims of the study, characteristics of the client population, and desired study endpoints (Grant, Padilla, Ferrell, & Rhiner, 1990). Selecting a battery of instruments for a comprehensive assessment of QOL creates its own special problems. Investigators must evaluate the equivalency of response formats to determine whether the different formats will confuse respondents. For example, one questionnaire may use a five-point Likert-type scale, while another may use a 100-mm visual analog scale. Or, different response options on various questionnaires may use completely different adjectives to rate the items, contributing to confusion, or perhaps erroneous data, if the participant does not read the rating scale carefully. Other aspects to evaluate when using a battery of several questionnaires include the clarity of the instructions and the equivalency of the time period used to frame responses. One questionnaire may ask participants to recall events that occurred during the past week and another during the past month. Researchers must examine the content of different questionnaires on an item-by-item basis, while also examining the instruments' reliability, validity, and scoring instructions, as well as the time needed to complete the entire battery, and the potential for substantial responder burden. Padilla and colleagues (Padilla, Frank-Stromborg, & Koresawa, 2004) cautioned that multiple operationalism, or the use of several standardized questionnaires, may not always be practical or even possible.

Modular Assessment
Another recent trend in QOL measurement is the modular assessment approach. A modular-type questionnaire is composed of two main sections: a core set of general items, which are applicable to many types of cancer, and a disease- or treatment-specific module (Aaronson, Bullinger, & Ahmedzai, 1988; King, 2006; Scott et al., 2009; Varricchio, 2006). The core items are useful for comparing results across different cancer populations. However, due to their general nature, the core items may fail to capture disease- or treatment-specific issues, such as symptom side effects specific to surgical resection for colon cancer. Modules have been developed for the late complications of bone marrow transplantation (Bush et al., 2000; Bush et al., 1995); lung cancer (Aaronson et al., 1993); and for 64 other types of cancer, including breast, prostate, head and neck, and pancreatic cancer (Cella, 2001; Cella et al., 1993; FACIT, 2009).

Global Scales to Measure QOL or Health Status
Another current trend in QOL assessment is to use a single-item indicator that measures global perceptions of QOL or health status. Global scales should not be confused with the single-item, unidimensional scales described previously, such as the Karnofsky Performance Status Index. A typical global indicator may ask the person with cancer, "How would you rate your overall quality of life today?" or "How would you rate your overall health today?" Global items may be scaled using a 100-mm visual analog scale, in which responses range from 0 (worst imaginable QOL or health) to 100 (best imaginable QOL or health). Likert-type scales with response options ranging from 1 (poor QOL or health) to 5 (excellent QOL or health) also are common.

A global scale is sensitive enough to reflect the different values and preferences of clients (Gill & Feinstein, 1994). Global items are useful for making comparisons between treatment types and evaluating changes across time because they represent the summation of many factors that are often difficult to quantify (Bernhard, Sullivan, Hurny, Coates, & Rudenstam, 2001). Oftentimes, QOL studies use different batteries of QOL instruments, but the same global measure of health status or QOL, making it relatively easy to compare global ratings across studies. Because global ratings reflect a common-sense alternative or complementary approach to QOL measurement, some authors recommend the use of two global ratings in all studies: one that asks about non-illness QOL and another that asks about health-related QOL (Gill & Feinstein, 1994).

Generic and Cancer-Specific Instruments

Generic Instruments

A distinction can be made between generic and cancer-specific questionnaires (Varricchio, 2006; Velikova et al., 1999). Generic instruments measure health functioning across a wide variety of chronic illnesses and cancers and provide a common database for comparing results, allocating resources, and developing health policy (Aaronson, 1990). Some examples of generic instruments include the Demands of Illness Inventory (Haberman, Woods, & Packard, 1990), the Sickness Impact Profile (Bergner, Bobbitt, Carter, & Gilson, 1981), the Medical Outcome Study Short Form General Health Survey (Stewart, Hays, & Ware, 1988), and the Functional Assessment of Chronic Illness Therapy (FACIT-G) by Cella and colleagues (Cella et al., 1993; FACIT, 2009). The FACIT-G is a general QOL scale, which can be used to measure QOL in other situations besides oncology, including heart disease, chronic obstructive pulmonary disease, renal disease, arthritis, or AIDS. Many generic instruments are lengthy, research-oriented, and difficult to score, making them of little use for routine clinical assessment. Although generic measures are used commonly in QOL research, they may not identify issues unique to the cancer experience.

Cancer-Specific Instruments

Cancer-specific instruments are designed to focus on the QOL of various populations of persons with cancer. A cancer-specific measure must identify differences between treatments or types of cancer, for example, the differences in symptoms experienced by people with leukemia undergoing primary chemotherapy versus people undergoing blood cell transplantation.

The nonequivalence of cancer-specific questionnaires may make it difficult, if not impossible, to compare results across studies. Some cancer-specific tools are applicable to a single type of cancer, while others are more general and pertain to a variety of cancers and therapies. For instance, the Breast Cancer Chemotherapy Questionnaire (Levine et al., 1988) and the Body Image and Relationship Scale (Hormes et al., 2008) are limited to QOL issues associated with breast cancer, while the Cancer Rehabilitation Evaluation System (CARES) is applicable to virtually all types of cancer (Ganz, Rofessart, Polinsky, Schag, & Heinrich, 1986; Schag, Ganz, & Heinrich, 1991, 2006). Table 8-3 lists many of the most commonly used generic and cancer-specific QOL questionnaires. The reliability and validity of many of these questionnaires are described in several sources (Frank-Stromborg & Olsen, 2004; Omery & Dean, 2004; Padilla et al., 2004).

Table 8-3. **QOL Questionnaires**

Generic Questionnaires

The Beck Depression Inventory (BDI)

The Crumbaugh Purpose-in-Life Test (PIL)

Demands of Illness Inventory (DOII)

Functional Assessment of Cancer Therapy-General Scale (FACT-G)

Global Adjustment to Illness Scale

Hospital Anxiety and Depression Scale (HADS)

The Lewis Psychological Coherence Scale

The McCorkle & Young Symptom Distress Scale

The McGill Pain Full or Short-Form Questionnaire

The McMaster Health Index Questionnaire

Medical Outcome Study Short-Form General Health Survey (MOS)

The Norbeck Social Support Scale

The Nottingham Health Profile

Profile of Mood States (POMS)

Psychosocial Adjustment to Medical Illness (PAIS)

Quality of Life Index by Padilla et al. (QLI)

Quality of Life Index by Spitzer et al. (QL-Index)

The Rosenberg Self-Esteem Scale

Sickness Impact Profile (SIP)

The Spielberger State-Trait Anxiety Inventory (STAI)

The Ware Health Perceptions Questionnaire

Cancer-Specific Questionnaires

Breast Cancer Chemotherapy Questionnaire

The Bush Bone Marrow Transplant Symptom Inventory

Cancer Rehabilitation Evaluation System (CARES)

City of Hope, Quality of Life: Bone Marrow Transplant

Demands of Bone Marrow Transplant Inventory (DBMT)

Demands of Breast Cancer Inventory

European Organization for Research and Treatment of Cancer Quality of Life Questionnaire (EORTC-QLQ-C30); modules for breast cancer (EORTC-QLQ-BR23), lung cancer (EORTC-QLQ-LC13), and head and neck cancer (EORTC-QLQ-H&N35)

Functional Assessment of Cancer Therapy Scale (FACT-G), modules for most types of cancer

Functional Living Index: Cancer (FLIC)

Table 8-3.   **continued**

Cancer-Specific Questionnaires (continued)

Linear Analog Self-Assessment (LASA): Breast Cancer

Quality Adjusted Time Without Symptoms or Toxicity (Q-TWIST)

Quality of Life Index: Cancer Version, by Ferrans and Powers

The Rotterdam Symptom Checklist (QOL after breast cancer)

Southwest Oncology Group Quality of Life Questionnaire

Time Without Symptoms or Toxicity (TWIST)

Reliability and Validity of Measurement

Reliability refers to the reproducibility of data from one measurement occasion to another. Common forms of reliability are test–retest, internal consistency, alternate forms, and interrater reliability (Haberman, 1995). Validity provides some assurance that the questionnaire actually measures what it claims to measure, such as physical functioning, regimen-related toxicities, or fatigue (Haberman, 1994). Establishing validity is a cumulative process occurring over several research studies. The most popular types of validity are content or face validity, construct, and criterion-related validity, which include both predictive and concurrent validity. A comprehensive discussion of reliability and validity is available in several excellent references (Cella & Tulsky, 1990; Frank-Stromborg & Olsen, 2004; Grant et al., 1990).

Quality-of-life researchers continue to experience a dilemma when selecting instruments. Instruments with good reliability and validity are often designed for research purposes and may lack face validity and clinical relevance (Gill & Feinstein, 1994; King, 2006). Consequently, investigators often resort to developing a new QOL questionnaire pertinent to their clinical population, but with untested reliability and validity (Cella & Tulsky, 1990). The current trend is to use existing tools with established psychometric properties rather than develop another generation of new QOL questionnaires (Grant, 1995; King, 2006; King et al., 1997; Varricchio, 2006). Virtually all of the latest generation of QOL questionnaires have published reliability and validity estimates or these data can be obtained directly from the author(s) of the instrument.

Additional Measurement Issues

Consideration must be given to several other measurement issues when designing a QOL study. The design and methodological issues now being discussed include using a single-measurement occasion or repeated measures design, obtaining a meaningful baseline measurement, standardizing data collection procedures, and using self-report data. Other issues discussed include the potential for responder burden, methods for scoring QOL questionnaires, the need to pilot procedures and pretest instruments, and factors that influence the selection of study eligibility. Also described are treatment effectiveness designs, statistical power, clinical significance, and options for statistical analysis.

Single or Repeated Measurements

Investigators must determine whether the data will be collected at one point in time or on multiple occasions. A cross-sectional design that gathers data on a single occasion is economical, places little burden on research participants, and often results in less missing data than a repeated measures design. While cross-sectional designs provide a static, snapshot view, they do not capture the dynamic changes in QOL that occur over time.

Serial or repeated measurement presents many challenges for QOL research design, analysis, and interpretation (Gotay, Korn, McCabe, Moore, & Cheson, 1992; Hollen, Gralla, & Rittenberg, 2004). Some of the methodological issues pertaining to a QOL instrument's sensitivity and responsiveness to detecting changes in clinical status over time are described by Epstein (2000) and Hyland (2003). The advantage of using a repeated measures design is that QOL outcomes can be examined longitudinally for fluctuations over time. Because QOL data are time dependent, QOL data cannot be recovered once lost or retrieved at some later time if initially overlooked (Clinch & Schipper, 1993; Gotay et al., 1992), which highlights the advantage of serial measurement. For instance, Sadetsky and colleagues (Sadetsky, Hubbard, Carroll, & Satariano, 2009) reported several domains of QOL (physical functioning, vitality, social functioning, general health) obtained from serial measurement were associated significantly with longer survival over the entire course of disease in a large sample of localized prostate cancer patients.

Some disadvantages of serial measurement include that it is both labor-intensive and prone to measurement error. If a questionnaire has poor reliability, for example, any unreliability of measurement that occurs at the first measurement occasion will be magnified across subsequent measurement occasions. When using a serial measurement design, data collection intervals must be chosen carefully so the effects of the treatment delivery schedule and anticipated changes in the client's QOL are captured (Gotay et al., 1992). A fixed schedule of data collection that is not linked to disease- or therapy-specific issues is unlikely to yield useful information (Epstein, 2000; Gotay et al., 1992; Moinpour et al., 1989). For instance, if the research goal is to document the effects of lymphedema following full mastectomy for breast cancer, select at least one measurement occasion when the effects of lymphedema are most evident clinically. In an effort to standardize the serial collection of QOL data in clinical trials, the Southwest Oncology Group recommends obtaining data on a minimum of three occasions: a baseline measurement prior to the initiation of therapy, a second measurement occurring sometime during the course of active treatment when symptoms are at their maximum intensity, and a final measurement at some point after the conclusion of therapy (Moinpour et al., 1989).

Other measurement challenges occur with the use of repeated measures designs. Prospective, longitudinal designs are prone to higher attrition rates than cross-sectional designs. Research participants may become bored when asked to complete the same questionnaires repeatedly. Moreover, individuals may move geographically and be lost to contact, become too sick to participate in the study, or die while enrolled in a study spanning over months or years. Strategies for minimizing study attrition include the use of one data collector who can establish a relationship with the participant by making telephone calls or sending postcard reminders to study participants prior to data collection occasions, and collecting data in the participant's home or through regularly scheduled clinic visits (Haberman, Bush, Young, & Sullivan, 1993).

Another potential problem with longitudinal data collection is response shift. Response shift is the change in the meaning of self-reported QOL scores resulting from changes in internal expectations and values of QOL rather than a valid change in health status (Rapkin & Schwartz, 2004). Response shift may occur in repeated measures studies when the observed clinical state of participants appears to disagree with their QOL assessment scores (Oort, Visser, & Sprangers, 2009; Varricchio, 2006). For instance, a person nearing the end of life may report high QOL during an office visit in an attempt to convey a sense of hope despite severe disabilities and low scores on a QOL questionnaire. Sprangers and colleagues (Sprangers, Moinpour, Moynihan, Patrick, & Revicki, 2002) developed an extensive checklist to aid clinicians in assessing meaningful changes in QOL over time.

Baseline Measurement

Identifying when to obtain entry-level or baseline data is a long standing measurement issue not amenable to an easy solution (Clinch & Schipper, 1993; Gotay et al., 1992; Sprangers et al., 2002). Quality-of-life studies generally use participants as their own internal controls, and normative baseline data often are unavailable. The data obtained at the first data point must provide the anchor, or point of comparison, for all subsequent measurement (Bush et al., 2000; Clinch & Schipper, 1993).

The most meaningful baseline data point occurs prior to onset and diagnosis of cancer. A precancerous baseline generally is impractical, if not impossible, to obtain unless data are available from prospective, long-range cancer prevention trials or studies of healthy people spanning many decades. An example of this latter type of study is the Nurses' Health Study (Harvard, 2008), which collected information on health, disease morbidity, and causes of death from 238,000 nurses since 1976. Many factors must be considered when selecting a baseline measurement occasion such as the following: the emotional turmoil and life stressors that often accompany initial diagnosis and cancer therapy; the timing of surgery and cycles of chemotherapy, radiation, and hormonal therapy; the intensity and duration of treatment side effects; and future patterns of disease remission, progression, and relapse. Selecting the first data point often is an ethical dilemma. Investigators must attempt to balance the need to obtain meaningful baseline data with the realities of clinical care and the need to protect the privacy, self-determination, and well-being of participants.

Standardized Data Collection Procedures

It is imperative data be collected systematically and consistently. For example, if the study has two groups or arms (experimental and treatment as usual), it is essential to collect the data at the identical time point in each arm of the study. Additionally, the consistency of data collection is critical if more than one person gathers the data or if data collection takes place at several research sites. Training sessions are needed to ensure everyone involved with data collection can practice the full range of data gathering procedures and receive constructive feedback from the investigator on protocol breaches. Data collectors should undergo repeated training until a high degree of interrater reliability is achieved, usually 85% agreement. Moreover, all procedures must be monitored for the entire duration of the study to ensure continuing adherence to the established data collection protocol and to identify the need for retraining sessions.

Another strategy for standardizing data collection is the use of an audit trail. An audit trail is a systematic method of monitoring the reliability of data collection, management, and entry activities. Audit trails are one important component of monitoring the scientific integrity of clinical research. An audit trail may include routine examination of all questionnaires and data collection sheets for missing or incorrect data entry. An audit may be required by the funding agency to track the data across the entire study protocol. This includes data abstracted from the medical record and recorded on a data collection sheet, data entered into computer files, and data used for analysis. Additionally, data extracted from the medical record and forced into categories, such as ratings of low, medium, and high nausea, must be audited by comparing the categorized ratings with the original raw data. Data entered into a statistical software program for data storage and management must be checked for accuracy to identify any errors in data entry. Similarly, transcribed interview data should be compared with original audiotape recordings to check for reliable transcription.

Use of Self-Report Data

It is acknowledged widely that QOL data should be gathered from the perspective of the person with cancer, rather than from healthcare professionals, caregivers, or family member proxies (Bush et al., 1995; King, 2006; King et al., 1997). Assessment of QOL by an observer will be biased by the observer's internal standards of what constitutes a desirable QOL (Osoba, 1994). Gill and Feinstein (1994) noted QOL assessment is "aimed at the wrong target unless individual patients are given the opportunity to express their individual opinions and reactions" (p. 624). Evidence exists that self-report QOL data obtained from oncology patients is consistent with QOL-related information found in the patient's medical record (Velikova et al., 2001).

Self-report is the only direct method for obtaining appropriate information on variables such as the meaning of illness, the burden of therapy, deficits in functioning, and symptom distress. There are exceptions to this viewpoint; when the purpose of the study is to compare different perspectives of QOL, or to investigate the QOL of children who are too young to complete questionnaires designed for adults, or when the health status of the client is waning, data must be obtained from family members, caregivers, parents of young children, or healthcare providers.

Investigators must evaluate the limitations of self-report data, namely, missing or inconsistent responses, misunderstood directions, or barriers due to language differences and cultural diversity (Cella & Tulsky, 1990). Other major limitations of self-assessment data include the effects of social desirability, lack of truthfulness, and a poor memory for recalling distant events (Polit & Beck, 2008). Because it is difficult to obtain a reliable retrospective account of life events, the time frame for questionnaire responses should be limited to the past one or two weeks (Bush et al., 1995; Cella & Tulsky, 1990). Any time frame greater than this results in response biases due to memory loss, distortion, and the selective recall of events.

Responder Burden

Investigators should try to minimize the burden placed on research participants, clinical staff, and institutional resources, although many respondents in QOL studies view their participation as therapeutic rather than burdensome (Bush et al., 1995). Respondents generally are relieved and gratified when researchers are willing to listen to their personal stories and document deficits in QOL.

Responder burden can be reduced in many ways. Generally speaking, the use of a single instrument or short packet of questionnaires is better than administering a taxing battery of tools. Some investigators compile a large packet of instruments because they fear they will miss a critical variable. However, large batteries of standardized tools often are redundant by measuring the same thing and are subject to random measurement error from fatigue, boredom, or frustration. In an effort to ease responder burden and to test the feasibility of using new technology, some investigators have turned to computer-administered questionnaires for QOL assessment (Fortner, Okon, Schwartzberg, Tauer, & Houts, 2003; King, 2006). Velikova and colleagues (1999) found good reliability, data quality, and acceptance when cancer patients were given QOL tools both by paper and pencil, and by automated computer touch-screen. Similarly, Bush and colleagues (2005) found that online, daily home self-assessment of QOL was embraced readily by hematopoietic stem cell transplant recipients, who found online data collection easy to use, reliable, understandable, and convenient. Compliance was good and compared favorably with less frequent, conventional paper-and-pencil QOL data gathering.

Fatigue or irritability that occurs during data collection can lead to measurement error, missing data, or study attrition (Bernhard et al., 1998; Polit & Beck, 2008). Investigators should watch for disease- and treatment-related symptoms that may contribute to measurement error or responder burden, such as disease progression, periods of active therapy, nausea, fatigue, mental confusion, or insomnia. Moreover, longitudinal or serial assessment requires more effort from participants than data collection at a single time point, particularly if there are time-dependent changes in the respondents' health, (e.g., disease progression, regimen-related toxicities, disease relapse, a dying life course). In general, participants are more likely to decline initial participation in the study or drop out early if they are experiencing active symptoms. In designing a study, researchers should estimate the magnitude of attrition and either intentionally oversample or have a plan for the systematic replacement of study participants. For instance, if 10% attrition is anticipated, the study can oversample by initially enrolling an additional 10% of participants.

When QOL data are gathered during active treatment, responder burden can be kept within reasonable limits by staggering the administration of instruments. For instance, the full battery of questionnaires can be administered at baseline, a smaller subset can be given during active therapy, and the full packet can be given once again at the conclusion of therapy. The data selected for exclusion during active therapy will result in a nonequivalent data set; some questionnaires will not be completed during every measurement occasion. Investigators must decide which facets of QOL are of core interest and give priority to collecting this minimum data set at all data points. The minimum set of core data can be used to make statistical comparisons across all time points, while the data collected at baseline and again at the conclusion of therapy provide comparisons at only two time points.

Pilot and Pretesting

Whenever possible, investigators should pilot the data collection procedures and pretest the questionnaires. A rigorous pilot study can identify problems with obtaining informed consent, recruiting and retaining participants, and collecting data at multiple study sites. A pilot test also can identify sources of measurement error, the total time needed to complete a packet of questionnaires or interview, the potential for missing data, and potential rates of attrition. A pretest provides information on questionnaire selection and construction, such as the clarity of items and instructions and the possible offensiveness of some questions.

Scoring QOL Questionnaires

Most multidimensional standardized instruments include a scoring manual, which identifies the items in each QOL domain or subscale, the possible range of scores for the subscales and instrument as a whole, the items that are reverse-scored, the weighing of items, and more.

Researchers handle the weight given to individual QOL items or subscales on a multidimensional questionnaire in different ways. Some investigators advocate a summing of scores to obtain a total score for the entire instrument, while others argue in favor of reporting only the separate subscale scores (Edwards, 1970). For instance, if a questionnaire has a spirituality, emotional functioning, and symptom subscale, the investigator most likely would choose to report the scores for each of the three subscales. Summing scores to obtain an aggregate score assumes that all domains of QOL are weighted equally and contribute equally to the overall QOL score. However, the number of items in a subscale can lead to the over- or under-emphasis of specific domains of QOL, if some dimensions have a greater or fewer amount of questions, respectively (Clinch & Schipper, 1993). In this case, a total obtained by summing the individual items is weighted implicitly by the number of items that compose each subscale or dimension of QOL. For example, if a physical-functioning subscale has 15 items and a body-image subscale has only 5 items, then the total subscale scores can give the false impression that physical functioning is a more important component of QOL than body image. Moreover, two people may have the same total score on the instrument, but one person may have poor physical functioning and excellent body image while the other person may have just the opposite pattern of scores.

From both the conceptual and psychometric perspectives, it is more informative to report QOL scores on an item-by-item or subscale-by-subscale basis than to aggregate the results into a single composite score (Bush et al., 1995; Edwards, 1970; Gill & Feinstein, 1994; Haberman, 1995; Osoba, 1994). Summing subscale scores on a multidimensional questionnaire is akin to mixing apples and oranges, resulting in a summary statistic that is conceptually meaningless (Edwards, 1970; Haberman, 1995). Aggregate scores reduce the many facets of QOL to a single, summary statistic that provides no information about the effects of individual items or subscale scores on QOL. In an effort to clarify how people weigh the individual facets of their lives, Ferrans and Powers (1985, 1992) developed a QOL index that asks respondents not only to rate the frequency or occurrence of individual items, but also to weight each item for its relative importance. Gill and Feinstein (1994) advocated that all QOL studies should obtain ratings of both the severity and perceived importance of a problem.

Entry Criteria

Inclusion and exclusion criteria place parameters on the selection of a research sample. Common inclusion criteria include the type of cancer, treatments, disease staging, age, gender, racial/ethnic background, ability to read and write English or another language, cognitive or mental status, and ratings of Karnofsky Performance Status (Karnofsky & Burchenal, 1949) or Eastern Cooperative Oncology Group Performance Status (2006). Entry criteria, as a form of design control, attempt to maximize the sample's homogeneity and minimize the effects of confounding factors that may potentially result in type II statistical error (i.e., false negative). The factors selected as inclusion criteria can be used as covariates in the analysis to examine, for instance, how different ethnicities may affect the outcome variable of QOL.

If a selected entry characteristic is expected to be correlated with the study's QOL outcomes, it should be stratified and statistically controlled, either as an independent variable or covariate (Cella & Tulsky, 1990). For example, several studies have found an inverse relationship between the variable "age at the time of bone marrow transplant" and long-term QOL; the higher the age, the poorer the QOL (Andrykowski, Henslee, & Farrall, 1989; Bush et al., 1995). Age can be used to stratify the sample when testing for group differences in QOL outcomes. Conversely, if there is no reason to suspect an entry characteristic is associated in some fashion with the study's QOL endpoints, then participants should not be excluded from the study based on that specific inclusion characteristic (Cella & Tulsky, 1990).

Clinical Trial or Treatment Effectiveness Designs

Clinical trial studies often are called treatment effectiveness or experimental intervention trials. For example, a nursing study may use a randomized, controlled clinical trial design to test whether a new exercise regimen for cancer-related fatigue improves the QOL outcome of physical functioning more than the existing standard of care that provides a brochure to cancer survivors on the benefits of exercise.

Clinical trial designs have several key characteristics: the random selection and/or assignment of participants to an experimental and control condition; an intervention administered in the experimental group, but not the control condition; the application of design strategies that control for threats to internal validity and integrity of the intervention protocol; and the measurement of selected QOL-dependent variables (Haberman,

1995; Lipsey, 1990; Meinert & Tonascia, 1986; Wang & Bakhai, 2006). Conducting statistical tests to determine whether a significant difference exists between the means of the experimental and treatment-as-usual groups on each QOL-dependent measure is a central feature of clinical trial research designs (Lipsey, 1990). An evaluation of the quality of 159 randomized, controlled clinical trials conducted between 1990 and 2004 found health-related QOL studies were more robust and supported clinical decision-making better than earlier studies (Efficace et al., 2007).

Statistical Power, Statistical Analysis Plan, and Clinical Significance

The concept of statistical power is an important part of statistical analysis. Statistical power is the probability a statistically significant difference will be detected, given that a treatment or experimental effect really exists (Lipsey, 1990; Meinert & Tonascia, 1986). It is determined by four factors: alpha level, effect size, sample size, and statistical analysis plan. Alpha level is the probability that the null hypothesis of "no difference" is rejected when, in fact, it is actually true. In other words, the investigator concludes, falsely, that a difference exists between two treatments when, in fact, it does not—a false positive (Haberman, 1995). Investigators strive to minimize this type of erroneous conclusion by selecting a stringent alpha or p-value such as $p = 0.05$. A larger alpha makes statistical significance easier to attain than a smaller alpha.

Effect size is the second factor that influences statistical power and is the magnitude of response or the degree to which there is a real, prespecified difference between the therapeutic conditions (Lipsey, 1990; Meinert & Tonascia, 1986). Lipsey (1990) noted the larger the effect size produced by the new therapy, the more likely statistical significance will be attained and the greater the statistical power. A recent meta-analysis (King et al., in press) provides evidence-based effect sizes for a commonly used, cancer-specific, quality-of-life questionnaire, the Functional Assessment of Cancer Therapy-General Version.

The third factor influencing statistical power is sample size. Because sampling error is greater for small samples and virtually negligible for very large samples, the size of the sample affects the probability of making erroneous statistical conclusions and, consequently, the statistical power (Lipsey, 1990). Selecting a sufficiently large sample is critical when conducting a nursing intervention or clinical trial research. Sample size estimation informs the investigator of the exact number of participants needed to detect a statistical difference between the experimental and control condition, if the hypothesized therapeutic effect actually exists (Haberman, 1995). Typically, the investigator selects the desired parameters and then refers to a chart or table to ascertain the required sample size. The criterion for statistical power usually is set between 0.80 and 0.95. Alpha usually is set at $p = 0.05$ and a suitable effect size ranges from low (0.20), to moderate (0.50), to high (0.80). Several references provide charts and, if necessary, additional statistical techniques that precisely calculate the estimated sample size needed (Cohen, 1988; Julious, Campbell, Walker, George, & Machin, 2000; Lipsey, 1990). Software is also available to determine sample size estimates and to conduct power analysis (Biostat, 1986; Dupont & Plummer, 1990).

The analysis plan is the last factor that affects statistical power. Various statistical tests will result in different levels of power when used for the same data set. Descriptive analysis, the most basic type of summary analysis, examines how QOL variables are distributed based on properties of symmetry, peakedness, central tendency, and dispersion (Polit & Beck, 2008). Descriptive statistics include frequencies; the mean, median, and mode; standard deviations; ranges; and skewness.

At a higher level of analysis, QOL variables can be examined for their degree of association. Variables are said to be associated to the extent that they covary. If two variables are highly interrelated, then one variable is a good predictor of the other. Some examples of measures of association include the bivariate regression coefficient, chi-square, Pearson product-moment correlation, point-biserial r, Spearman's *rho*, and Kendall's *tau* (Polit & Beck, 2008).

Hypothesis testing and tests of significance are other types of analyses commonly used in QOL research. A hypothesis is a predictive statement of a relationship between two variables. Hypothesis testing involves some type of statistical comparison for differences within or between two or more groups. For instance, the mean values on a QOL questionnaire can be compared for women receiving an individualized in-home exercise intervention versus a group intervention at an exercise facility in order to determine which intervention results in a higher QOL. The researcher asks the question "Is the difference between the two methods of exercise statistically significant?" In addition to determining whether there is a statistically significant difference within or between groups, measures of association can be added to examine the magnitude of the relationship. Depending on the level of data (nominal, ordinal, interval, or ratio-level data) the types of statistical tests most commonly used to examine the magnitude of the association between or among groups are the chi-square, analysis of variance (ANOVA), Fisher's test, Kruskal-Wallis test, McNemar test, t-test, repeated-measures ANOVA, and the Wilcoxon test (Polit & Beck, 2008).

Causal analysis is the highest form of statistical analysis. Causal modeling is used when the investigator is trying to explain, predict, or control for the effect of one or more independent variables on a single QOL-dependent variable. More complex types of causal modeling may add some intervening or mediating variables into the path analysis. For example, the technique of multivariate causal analysis examines the effects of a set of selected variables on the dependent variable while controlling for other intervening variables statistically (Nuamah, Cooley, Fawcett, & McCorkle, 1999). Examples of causal analysis techniques are analysis of covariance, canonical correlation, discriminant analysis, regression analysis, path analysis, LISREL, stratified analysis, and log-linear model testing.

Clinical Significance

In recent years, researchers have focused increasingly on the clinical importance or significance of QOL scores (Cella et al., 2002; Frost, Bonomi, Ferrans, Wong, & Hays, 2002; Guyatt, Osoba, Wu, Wyrwich, & Norman, 2002; Hurst & Bolton, 2004; Sloan, Aaronson, Cappelleri, Fairclough, & Varricchio, 2002; Sloan et al., 2002). Although it may be relatively simple to determine the statistical significance of changes in QOL, placing the magnitude of these changes in a context meaningful for health professionals has not been so easy. McCabe and associates (2008) advocate for the use of mixed methods research to interpret the difference between statistical and clinical significance. Two methods of assessing clinical significance have become popular thus far, namely anchor-based methods and distribution-based methods.

Anchor-based methods examine the relationship between scores on a QOL measure and some independent (anchor) measure. Some anchor-based methods are based on population. For example, a change in a QOL physical functioning score might be related to another measurement, that of mobility (anchor). If 32.1% of patients who have a physical functioning score of 40 can walk a single block, and 49.7% who score 50 can walk a single block, then a difference in the physical functioning score of 40–50 means a 17.6% increase in the ability to walk a single block.

Other anchor-based methods concentrate on the individual and the minimally important difference (MID) in a change of score. A minimally important difference specifies the threshold in QOL scores between a trivial and important change. Specifically, the MID establishes the smallest change in QOL scores that patients themselves consider, on average, to be important, and then estimates the proportion of patients who have achieved that MID. For example, a researcher might have patients rate how much they feel better or worse on various QOL dimensions since they last completed the QOL questionnaire. The degree of change in that better or worse score is related to the actual change in the corresponding QOL questionnaire score. So a change in physical functioning score over time of 5–10 points might be correlated with "a little better," 10–20 = "moderately better," and over 20 = "very much better."

An alternative to anchor-based methods is the distribution-based method that examines the underlying distribution of results to determine the significance, or size, of an effect. Standard deviation (SD) is employed commonly as the measure of distribution. An effect size might be expressed as the SD between patients in the treatment group compared to the SD of a control group at baseline, or the SD of change that an individual experienced over time. Cohen (1988) suggested guidelines for MID using 0.2–0.5 SDs to represent small change or MID, 0.5–0.8 SDs to correspond to a moderate change, and > 0.8 SDs to describe a large change. Therefore, with a 0.3 SD difference between a treatment and control group, one might expect a small improvement in QOL with treatment.

Directions for Future Research

The current state of the science of QOL measurement calls for a comprehensive, multidimensional assessment of health-related cancer outcomes, gathered from the perspective of the person with cancer, and with minimal burden to the respondent. Investigators may choose from a variety of generic or cancer-specific QOL questionnaires that report excellent reliability and validity.

Investigators are encouraged to use multiple methods of data collection, depending on the endpoints of interest and available resources. Data gathered from qualitative inquiry may augment or serve as a substitute for data obtained by standardized questionnaires. Qualitative inquiry offers an explanatory richness that is unattainable from quantitative approaches. Cancer survivors can tell their stories in their own words and give voice to the personal meaning of QOL through qualitative methods (DeSanto-Madeya, Bauer-Wu, & Gross, 2007; Dow et al., 1999).

Although nurse scientists now have many tools for documenting the QOL endpoints of nursing care, there remains a need to develop QOL tools suitable for routine clinical assessment of cancer survivors (Detmar, Aaronson, Wever, Muller, & Schornagel, 2000; King, 2006; King et al., 1997). To aid the collection of clinically relevant outcome data, Klee and colleagues (Klee, King, Machin, & Hansen, 2000) developed a clinical model for the routine assessment of QOL in persons receiving chemotherapy. Moreover, Detmar and Aaronson (1998) found routine QOL assessments in an outpatient oncology setting stimulated physicians to discuss specific issues related to the QOL of their patients. In addition, Grunfeld (2009) reported good patient satisfaction and quality-of-life outcomes following nurse-led follow-up after breast cancer surgery. Despite the desire by many clinicians to fold QOL evaluation into daily practice, more research is needed on several fronts, to examine the competing expectations that exist between patients and clinicians as to who should initiate the discussion of QOL issues (Detmar et al., 2000). Research is also needed regarding the challenges faced by clinicians in interpreting QOL scores (Santana et al., 2009); the assessment by nurses of the devastating impact of psychological distress on quality of life (Pasacreta, Kenefick, & McCorkle, 2008); the barriers and facilitators to the growing use of computer-assisted, Web-based QOL symptom assessment in oncology clinics (Cantrell & Lupinacci, 2007; Mark et al., 2008); the design of nursing interventions so oncology nurses can affect the QOL of persons with cancer positively (King, 2006); and the use of QOL measurement to obtain baseline data in intensive care units for later comparison with a follow-up evaluation after discharge from the hospital (Hofhuis et al., 2009).

Grant (1995) indicated QOL research is needed to examine the cost efficacy of different models of cancer care delivery, such as managed care or case management, and the efficacy of nursing therapeutics from a holistic view of cancer survivorship. Ramsey and colleagues (in press) developed a conceptual model to guide research on the economic value of using patient navigators in oncology clinics. Research also is needed to determine whether some facets of QOL are trait-like and prone to stability or state-like and predisposed to fluctuations and instability. Research is also needed to determine whether QOL questionnaires correlate with measures of state–trait anxiety (Den Oudsten, Van Heck, Van der Steeg, Roukema, & De Vries, 2009).

Osoba (1994) identified several future research issues that are relevant today. He noted that studies are needed to find better methods for selecting the most appropriate QOL instrument for a given situation and to distinguish the effects of disease from the outcomes of therapy. Osoba (1994) also commented that instrumentation research is needed to examine how to assign weights to the various domains of QOL, as well as to identify which finding is more relevant, a statistically significant difference in QOL or a difference that is meaningful to the person with cancer. Fitzsimmons and colleagues (2009) concluded from a review of 31 health-related QOL studies that most QOL tools ignore the needs of older persons with cancer and Lewis and Zahlis (1997) noted that QOL, in the context of family functioning, requires further testing with regard to the feasibility of delivering family-focused care in a variety of clinical venues.

Recent initiatives call for an active public health research agenda to determine the effects of ovarian cancer on QOL and quality care (Trivers, Stewart, Peipins, Rim, & White, 2009), for trials to examine clinically usable decision aids to assist patients undergoing external beam radiotherapy in selecting treatment options that result in the least burden to QOL (Valdagni, Rancati, & Fiorino, 2009), and for studies to develop QOL indicators for cancer end-of-life care (Seow et al., 2009). Researchers are being challenged on several fronts: to rethink chemoprevention trials because preventing breast cancer is more effective than treatment and more beneficial to QOL and economic concerns (Blaha et al., 2009); to chart a new landscape for research on cancer survivors' health-related outcomes and care (Pollack, Rowland, Crammer, & Stefanek, 2009); and to link psychosocial functioning and behavior modification to both the biology of cancer and stress to achieve a reduction in cancer recurrence and benefit survival (Stefanek, Palmer, Thombs, & Coyne, 2009). Ganz and Goodwin (2007) address the methodological issues raised by the Food and Drug Administration's guidelines for the use of patient-reported outcomes and call for increased research on the relationships among symptoms, symptom clusters, health-related quality of life, and other outcome measures.

CONCLUSION

In summary, oncology nurses are positioned strategically in the healthcare system to advance evidence-based practice by the infusion of rigorous QOL research findings in daily practice, to augment the extant research base on QOL, and to resolve many of the design and methodological challenges that confront QOL researchers.

REFERENCES

Aaronson, N. K. (1990). Quality of life research in cancer clinical trials: A need for common rules and language. *Oncology (Williston Park)*, 4(5), 59–66; discussion 70.

Aaronson, N. K., Ahmedzai, S., Bergman, B., Bullinger, M., Cull, A., Duez, N. J., et al. (1993). The European Organization for Research and Treatment of Cancer QLQ-C30: A quality-of-life instrument for use in international clinical trials in oncology. *Journal of National Cancer Institute*, 85(5), 365–376.

Aaronson, N. K., Bullinger, M., & Ahmedzai, S. (1988). A modular approach to quality-of-life assessment in cancer clinical trials. *Recent Results in Cancer Research*, 111, 231–249.

Andrykowski, M. A., Henslee, P. J., & Farrall, M. G. (1989). Physical and psychosocial functioning of adult survivors of allogeneic bone marrow transplantation. *Bone Marrow Transplant*, 4(1), 75–81.

Ashing-Giwa, K., & Kagawa-Singer, M. (2006). Infusing culture into oncology research on quality of life. *Oncology Nursing Forum*, 33(1, Suppl.), 31–36.

Baker, F., Jodrey, D., Zabora, J., Douglas, C., & Fernandez-Kelly, P. (1996). Empirically selected instruments for measuring quality-of-life dimensions in culturally diverse populations. *Journal of National Cancer Institute Monographs*, (20), 39–47.

Barrera, M., D'Agostino, N., Gammon, J., Spencer, L., & Baruchel, S. (2005). Health-related quality of life and enrollment in phase I trials in children with incurable cancer. *Palliative and Support Care*, 3(3), 191–196.

Bergner, M., Bobbitt, R. A., Carter, W. B., & Gilson, B. S. (1981). The Sickness Impact Profile: Development and final revision of a health status measure. *Medical Care, 19*(8), 787–805.

Bernhard, J., Cella, D. F., Coates, A. S., Fallowfield, L., Ganz, P. A., Moinpour, C. M., et al. (1998). Missing quality of life data in cancer clinical trials: Serious problems and challenges. *Statistics in Medicine, 17*(5–7), 517–532.

Bernhard, J., Sullivan, M., Hurny, C., Coates, A. S., & Rudenstam, C. M. (2001). Clinical relevance of single item quality of life indicators in cancer clinical trials. *British Journal of Cancer, 84*(9), 1156–1165.

Biostat. (1986). *Statistical power analysis.* Retrieved October 24, 2009, from http://www.power-analysis.com/home.htm

Blaha, P., Dubsky, P., Fitzal, F., Bachleitner-Hofmann, T., Jakesz, R., Gnant, M., et al. (2009). Breast cancer chemoprevention: A vision not yet realized. *European Journal of Cancer Care (English), 18*(5), 438–446.

Bottomley, A. (2002). The cancer patient and quality of life. *Oncologist, 7*(2), 120–125.

Bush, N., Donaldson, G., Moinpour, C., Haberman, M., Milliken, D., Markle, V., et al. (2005). Development, feasibility and compliance of a web-based system for very frequent QOL and symptom home self-assessment after hematopoietic stem cell transplantation. *Quality of Life Research, 14*(1), 77–93.

Bush, N. E., Donaldson, G. W., Haberman, M. H., Dacanay, R., & Sullivan, K. M. (2000). Conditional and unconditional estimation of multidimensional quality of life after hematopoietic stem cell transplantation: A longitudinal follow-up of 415 patients. *Biology of Blood and Marrow Transplantation, 6*(5A), 576–591.

Bush, N. E., Haberman, M., Donaldson, G., & Sullivan, K. M. (1995). Quality of life of 125 adults surviving 6–18 years after bone marrow transplantation. *Social Sciences & Medicine, 40*(4), 479–490.

Cantrell, M. A., & Lupinacci, P. (2007). Methodological issues in online data collection. *Journal of Advanced Nursing, 60*(5), 544–549.

Cella, D. (2009). Quality of life in patients with metastatic renal cell carcinoma: The importance of patient-reported outcomes. *Cancer Treatment Reviews, 35*(8), 733–737.

Cella, D., Bullinger, M., Scott, C., & Barofsky, I. (2002). Group vs individual approaches to understanding the clinical significance of differences or changes in quality of life. *Mayo Clinic Proceedings, 77*(4), 384–392.

Cella, D. F. (2001). Quality of life measurement in oncology. In A. Baum & B. L. Andersen (Eds.), *Psychosocial interventions for cancer* (pp. 57–76). Washington, DC: American Psychological Association.

Cella, D. F., & Tulsky, D. S. (1990). Measuring quality of life today: Methodological aspects. *Oncology (Williston Park), 4*(5), 29–38; discussion 69.

Cella, D. F., Tulsky, D. S., Gray, G., Sarafian, B., Linn, E., Bonomi, A., et al. (1993). The Functional Assessment of Cancer Therapy scale: Development and validation of the general measure. *Journal of Clinocal Oncology, 11*(3), 570–579.

Chang, P. C., & Yeh, C. H. (2005). Agreement between child self-report and parent proxy-report to evaluate quality of life in children with cancer. *Psycho-oncology, 14*(2), 125–134.

Clinch, J. J., & Schipper, H. (1993). Quality of life assessment in palliative care. In D. Doyle, G. Hanks, & N. MacDonald (Eds.), *Oxford textbook of palliative medicine* (pp. 61–70). Oxford, UK: Oxford University Press.

Cohen, J. (1988). *Statistical power analysis for the behavioral sciences.* Hillsdale, NJ: Lawrence Erlbaum Associates.

de Haes, J., Curran, D., Young, T., Bottomley, A., Flechtner, H., Aaronson, N., et al. (2000). Quality of life evaluation in oncological clinical trials: The EORTC model. The EORTC Quality of Life Study Group. *European Journal of Cancer, 36*(7), 821–825.

Den Oudsten, B. L., Van Heck, G. L., Van der Steeg, A. F., Roukema, J. A., & De Vries, J. (2009). The WHOQOL-100 has good psychometric properties in breast cancer patients. *Journal of Clinical Epidemiology, 62*(2), 195–205.

Denzin, N. K., & Lincoln, Y.S. (Ed.). (2005). *The Sage Handbook of Qualitative Research* (3rd ed.). Thousand Oaks, CA: Sage Publications.

DeSanto-Madeya, S., Bauer-Wu, S., & Gross, A. (2007). Activities of daily living in women with advanced breast cancer. *Oncology Nursing Forum, 34*(4), 841–846.

Detmar, S. B., & Aaronson, N. K. (1998). Quality of life assessment in daily clinical oncology practice: A feasibility study. *European Journal of Cancer, 34*(8), 1181–1186.

Detmar, S. B., Aaronson, N. K., Wever, L. D., Muller, M., & Schornagel, J. H. (2000). How are you feeling? Who wants to know? Patients' and oncologists' preferences for discussing health-related quality-of-life issues. *Journal of Clinical Oncology, 18*(18), 3295–3301.

Donnelly, S., Rybicki, L., & Walsh, D. (2001). Quality of life measurement in the palliative management of advanced cancer. *Supportive Care in Cancer, 9*(5), 361–365.

Dow, K. H., Ferrell, B. R., Haberman, M. R., & Eaton, L. (1999). The meaning of quality of life in cancer survivorship. *Oncology Nursing Forum, 26*(3), 519–528.

Dupont, W. D., & Plummer, W. D. (1990). *Power and sample size (PS version 3.0.12)*. Retrieved October 24, 2009, from http://biostat.mc.vanderbilt.edu/wiki/Main/PowerSampleSize.

Eastern Cooperative Oncology Group. (2006). *ECOG performance status*. Retrieved October 24, 2009, from http://ecog.dfci.harvard.edu/general/perf_stat.html.

Edwards, A. L. (1970). *The measurement of personality traits by scales and inventories*. New York, NY: Holt, Rhinehart and Winston.

Efficace, F., Osoba, D., Gotay, C., Sprangers, M., Coens, C., & Bottomley, A. (2007). Has the quality of health-related quality of life reporting in cancer clinical trials improved over time? Towards bridging the gap with clinical decision making. *Annals of Oncology, 18*(4), 775–781.

Epstein, R. S. (2000). Responsiveness in quality-of-life assessment: Nomenclature, determinants, and clinical applications. *Medical Care, 38*(9, Suppl.), II91–94.

FACIT. (2009). *Functional assessment of chronic illness*. Retrieved October 19, 2009, from http://www.facit.org/.

Fayers, P., & Bottomley, A. (2002). Quality of life research within the EORTC-the EORTC QLQ-C30. European Organisation for Research and Treatment of Cancer. *European Journal of Cancer, 38*(Suppl. 4), S125–S133.

Ferrans, C. E., & Powers, M. J. (1985). Quality of life index: Development and psychometric properties. *ANS Advances in Nursing Science, 8*(1), 15–24.

Ferrans, C. E., & Powers, M. J. (1992). Psychometric assessment of the Quality of Life Index. *Research in Nursing & Health, 15*(1), 29–38.

Fitzsimmons, D., Gilbert, J., Howse, F., Young, T., Arraras, J. I., Bredart, A., et al. (2009). A systematic review of the use and validation of health-related quality of life instruments in older cancer patients. *European Journal of Cancer, 45*(1), 19–32.

Fortner, B., Okon, T., Schwartzberg, L., Tauer, K., & Houts, A. C. (2003). The Cancer Care Monitor: Psychometric content evaluation and pilot testing of a computer administered system for symptom screening and quality of life in adult cancer patients. *Journal of Pain and Symptom Management, 26*(6), 1077–1092.

Frank-Stromborg, M., & Olsen, S. J. (Eds.). (2004). *Instruments for clinical health-care research* (3rd ed.). Sudbury, MA: Jones and Bartlett.

Frost, M. H., Bonomi, A. E., Ferrans, C. E., Wong, G. Y., & Hays, R. D. (2002). Patient, clinician, and population perspectives on determining the clinical significance of quality-of-life scores. *Mayo Clinic Proceedings, 77*(5), 488–494.

Ganz, P. A. (1994). Quality of life and the patient with cancer: Individual and policy implications. *Cancer, 74*(4, Suppl.), 1445–1452.

Ganz, P. A., & Goodwin, P. J. (2007). Health-related quality of life measurement in symptom management trials. *Journal of the National Cancer Institute Monographs, 37*, 47–52.

Ganz, P. A., Rofessart, J., Polinsky, M. L., Schag, C. C., & Heinrich, R. L. (1986). A comprehensive approach to the assessment of cancer patients' rehabilitation needs: The cancer inventory of problem situations and a companion interview. *Journal of Psychosocial Oncology, 4*(3), 27–42.

Gill, T. M., & Feinstein, A. R. (1994). A critical appraisal of the quality of quality-of-life measurements. *The Journal of the American Medical Association, 272*(8), 619–626.

Gotay, C. C., Korn, E. L., McCabe, M. S., Moore, T. D., & Cheson, B. D. (1992). Quality-of-life assessment in cancer treatment protocols: Research issues in protocol development. *Journal of the National Cancer Institute, 84*(8), 575–579.

Gotay, C. C., & Muraoka, M. Y. (1998). Quality of life in long-term survivors of adult-onset cancers. *Journal of the National Cancer Institute, 90*(9), 656–667.

Grant, M. (1995). Quality of life research: Where we are, where we need to go. *Nurse Investigator, 2*(1), 1–2.

Grant, M., Padilla, G. V., Ferrell, B. R., & Rhiner, M. (1990). Assessment of quality of life with a single instrument. *Seminars in Oncology Nursing, 6*(4), 260–270.

Groenvold, M. (1999). Methodological issues in the assessment of health-related quality of life in palliative care trials. *Acta Anaesthesiologica Scandinavica, 43*(9), 948–953.

Grunfeld, E. (2009). Optimizing follow-up after breast cancer treatment. *Current Opinion in Obstetrics and Gynecology, 21*(1), 92–96.

Guyatt, G. H., Osoba, D., Wu, A. W., Wyrwich, K. W., & Norman, G. R. (2002). Methods to explain the clinical significance of health status measures. *Mayo Clinic Proceedings, 77*(4), 371–383.

Haberman, M. (1994). Quality of life outcomes for oncology nursing. In P. T. Rieger (Ed.), *Fighting fatigue: Resolving issues for the cancer patient* (pp. 30–36). Beachwood, OH: Pro Ed.

Haberman, M. (1995). Nursing research. In P. C. Buchsel & M. B. Whedon (Eds.), *Bone marrow transplantation: Administrative and clinical strategies* (pp. 365–402). Sudbury, MA: Jones and Bartlett.

Haberman, M., Bush, N., Young, K., & Sullivan, K. M. (1993). Quality of life of adult long-term survivors of bone marrow transplantation: A qualitative analysis of narrative data. *Oncology Nursing Forum, 20*(10), 1545–1553.

Haberman, M. R., & Lewis, F. M. (1990). Selection of research designs. Section I: Qualitative paradigms. In M. M. Grant & G. V. Padilla (Eds.), *Cancer nursing research: A practical approach* (pp. 77–83). Norwalk, CT: Appleton and Lange.

Haberman, M. R., Woods, N. F., & Packard, N. J. (1990). Demands of chronic illness: Reliability and validity assessment of a demands-of-illness inventory. *Holistic Nurse Practitioner, 5*(1), 25–35.

Harvard University. (2008). *Nurses' Health Study.* Retrieved October 20, 2009, from http://www.channing.harvard.edu/nhs/.

Hinds, P. S., Burghen, E. A., Haase, J. E., & Phillips, C. R. (2006). Advances in defining, conceptualizing, and measuring quality of life in pediatric patients with cancer. *Oncology Nursing Forum, 33*(1, Suppl.), 23–29.

Hofhuis, J. G., van Stel, H. F., Schrijvers, A. J., Rommes, J. H., Bakker, J., & Spronk, P. E. (2009). Health-related quality of life in critically ill patients: How to score and what is the clinical impact? *Current Opinion in Critical Care, 15*(5), 425–430.

Hollen, P. J., Gralla, R. J., & Rittenberg, C. N. (2004). Quality of life as a clinical trial endpoint: Determining the appropriate interval for repeated assessments in patients with advanced lung cancer. *Supportive Care in Cancer, 12*(11), 767–773.

Holzner, B., Kemmler, G., Sperner-Unterweger, B., Kopp, M., Dunser, M., Margreiter, R., et al. (2001). Quality of life measurement in oncology—a matter of the assessment instrument? *European Journal of Cancer, 37*(18), 2349–2356.

Hormes, J. M., Lytle, L. A., Gross, C. R., Ahmed, R. L., Troxel, A. B., & Schmitz, K. H. (2008). The body image and relationships scale: Development and validation of a measure of body image in female breast cancer survivors. *Journal of Clinical Oncology, 26*(8), 1269–1274.

Hurst, H., & Bolton, J. (2004). Assessing the clinical significance of change scores recorded on subjective outcome measures. *Journal of Manipulative and Physiological Therapeutics, 27*(1), 26–35.

Hyland, M. E. (2003). A brief guide to the selection of quality of life instrument. *Health and Quality of Life Outcomes, 1*, 24.

Jalowiec, A. (1990). Issues in using multiple measures of quality of life. *Seminars in Oncology Nursing, 6*(4), 271–277.

Julious, S. A., Campbell, M. J., Walker, S. J., George, S. L., & Machin, D. (2000). Sample sizes for cancer trials where health related quality of life is the primary outcome. *British Journal of Cancer, 83*(7), 959–963.

Karnofsky, D. S., & Burchenal, J. H. (1949). The clinical evaluation of chemotherapeutic agents in cancer. In C. M. MacLeod (Ed.), *Evaluation of chemotherapeutic agents.* New York, NY: Columbia University Press.

King, C. R. (2006). Advances in how clinical nurses can evaluate and improve quality of life for individuals with cancer. *Oncology Nursing Forum, 33*(1, Suppl.), 5–12.

King, C. R., Haberman, M., Berry, D. L., Bush, N., Butler, L., Dow, K. H., et al. (1997). Quality of life and the cancer experience: The state-of-the-knowledge. *Oncology Nursing Forum, 24*(1), 27–41.

King, M. T., Stockler, M. R., Cella, D. F., Osoba, D., Eton, D. T., Thompson, J., et al. (in press). Meta-analysis provides evidence-based effect sizes for a cancer-specific quality-of-life questionnaire, the FACT-G. *Journal of Clinical Epidemiology.*

Klee, M. C., King, M. T., Machin, D., & Hansen, H. H. (2000). A clinical model for quality of life assessment in cancer patients receiving chemotherapy. *Annals of Oncology, 11*(1), 23–30.

Lee, C. W., & Chi, K. N. (2000). The standard of reporting of health-related quality of life in clinical cancer trials. *Journal of Clinical Epidemiology, 53*(5), 451–458.

Levine, M. N., Guyatt, G. H., Gent, M., De Pauw, S., Goodyear, M. D., Hryniuk, W. M., et al. (1988). Quality of life in stage II breast cancer: An instrument for clinical trials. *Journal of Clinical Oncology, 6*(12), 1798–1810.

Lewis, F. M., & Zahlis, E. H. (1997). The nurse as coach: A conceptual framework for clinical practice. *Oncol Nurs Forum, 24*(10), 1695–1702.

Lipsey, M. W. (1990). *Design sensitivity: Statistical power for experimental research.* Newbury Park, CA: Sage.

Mark, T. L., Johnson, G., Fortner, B., & Ryan, K. (2008). The benefits and challenges of using computer-assisted symptom assessments in oncology clinics: Results of a qualitative assessment. *Technololy in Cancer Research and Treatment, 7*(5), 401–406.

Mast, M. E. (1995). Definition and measurement of quality of life in oncology nursing research: Review and theoretical implications. *Oncology Nursing Forum, 22*(6), 957–964.

Matza, L. S., Swensen, A. R., Flood, E. M., Secnik, K., & Leidy, N. K. (2004). Assessment of health-related quality of life in children: A review of conceptual, methodological, and regulatory issues. *Value Health, 7*(1), 79–92.

McCabe, C., Begley, C., Collier, S., & McCann, S. (2008). Methodological issues related to assessing and measuring quality of life in patients with cancer: Implications for patient care. *European Journal of Cancer Care (English), 17*(1), 56–64.

McCahill, L. E., Krouse, R., Chu, D., Juarez, G., Uman, G. C., Ferrell, B., et al. (2002). Indications and use of palliative surgery-results of Society of Surgical Oncology survey. *Annals of Surgical Oncology, 9*(1), 104–112.

McMillan, S. C., & Weitzner, M. (2000). How problematic are various aspects of quality of life in patients with cancer at the end of life? *Oncology Nursing Forum, 27*(5), 817–823.

Meinert, C. L., & Tonascia, S. (1986). *Clinical trials: Design, conduct, and analysis.* New York, NY: Oxford University Press.

Mitchell, E. S. (1986). Multiple triangulation: A methodology for nursing science. *ANS: Advances in Nursing Science, 8*(3), 18–26.

Moinpour, C. M., Feigl, P., Metch, B., Hayden, K. A., Meyskens, F. L., Jr., & Crowley, J. (1989). Quality of life end points in cancer clinical trials: Review and recommendations. *Journal of National Cancer Institute, 81*(7), 485–495.

Moinpour, C. M., Hayden, K. A., Thompson, I. M., Feigl, P., & Metch, B. (1990). Quality of life assessment in Southwest Oncology Group trials. *Oncology (Williston Park), 4*(5), 79–84, 89; discussion 104.

Montazeri, A., Gillis, C. R., & McEwen, J. (1996). Measuring quality of life in oncology: Is it worthwhile? I. Meaning, purposes and controversies. *European Journal of Cancer Care (English), 5*(3), 159–167.

Nathan, P. C., Furlong, W., & Barr, R. D. (2004). Challenges to the measurement of health-related quality of life in children receiving cancer therapy. *Pediatric Blood & Cancer, 43*(3), 215–223.

Nayfield, S. G., Ganz, P. A., Moinpour, C. M., Cella, D. F., & Hailey, B. J. (1992). Report from a National Cancer Institute (USA) workshop on quality of life assessment in cancer clinical trials. *Quality of Life Research, 1*(3), 203–210.

Nayfield, S. G., Hailey, B. J., & McCabe, M. (1991). *Quality of life assessment in cancer clinical trials.* Report of the workshop on quality of life research in cancer clinical trials in Bethesda, MD.

Nuamah, I. F., Cooley, M. E., Fawcett, J., & McCorkle, R. (1999). Testing a theory for health-related quality of life in cancer patients: A structural equation approach. *Research in Nursing & Health, 22*(3), 231–242.

Omery, A. K., & Dean, H. (2004). Multiple instruments for measuring quality of life. In M. Frank-Stromborg & S. Olsen (Eds.), *Instruments for clinical health-care research* (3rd ed., pp. 150–163). Sudbury, MA: Jones and Bartlett.

Oort, F. J., Visser, M. R., & Sprangers, M. A. (2009). Formal definitions of measurement bias and explanation bias clarify measurement and conceptual perspectives on response shift. *Journal of Clinical Epidemiology, 62*(11), 1126–1137.

Osoba, D. (1994). Lessons learned from measuring health-related quality of life in oncology. *Journal of Clinical Oncology, 12*(3), 608–616.

Osoba, D., Dancey, J., Zee, B., Myles, J., & Pater, J. (1996). Health-related quality-of-life studies of the National Cancer Institute of Canada Clinical Trials Group. *Journal of National Cancer Institute Monographs, 20,* 107–111.

Padilla, G., Frank-Stromborg, M., & Koresawa, S. (2004). Single instruments for measuring quality of life. In M. Frank-Stromborg & S. Olsen (Eds.), *Instruments for clinical health-care research* (3rd ed., pp. 128–149). Sudbury, MA: Jones and Bartlett.

Pasacreta, J. V., Kenefick, A. L., & McCorkle, R. (2008). Managing distress in oncology patients: Description of an innovative online educational program for nurses. *Cancer Nursing, 31*(6), 485–490.

Polit, D. F., & Beck, C. T. (2008). *Nursing research: Creating and assessing evidence for nursing practice* (8th ed.). Philadelphia, PA: Wolters Kluwer, Lippincott, Williams and Wilkins.

Pollack, L. A., Rowland, J. H., Crammer, C., & Stefanek, M. (2009). Introduction: Charting the landscape of cancer survivors' health-related outcomes and care. *Cancer, 115*(18, Suppl.), 4265–4269.

Ramsey, S., Whitley, E., Mears, V. W., McKoy, J. M., Everhart, R. M., Caswell, R. J., et al. (in press). Evaluating the cost-effectiveness of cancer patient navigation programs: Conceptual and practical issues. *Cancer.*

Rapkin, B. D., & Schwartz, C. E. (2004). Toward a theoretical model of quality-of-life appraisal: Implications of findings from studies of response shift. *Health and Quality of Life Outcomes, 2,* 14.

Ravens-Sieberer, U., Erhart, M., Wille, N., Wetzel, R., Nickel, J., & Bullinger, M. (2006). Generic health-related quality-of-life assessment in children and adolescents: Methodological considerations. *Pharmacoeconomics, 24*(12), 1199–1220.

Sadetsky, N., Hubbard, A., Carroll, P. R., & Satariano, W. (2009). Predictive value of serial measurements of quality of life on all-cause mortality in prostate cancer patients: Data from CaPSURE (cancer of the prostate strategic urologic research endeavor) database. *Quality of Life Research, 18*(8), 1019–1027.

Santana, M. J., Au, H. J., Dharma-Wardene, M., Hewitt, J. D., Dupere, D., Hanson, J., et al. (2009). Health-related quality of life measures in routine clinical care: Can FACT-fatigue help to assess the management of fatigue in cancer patients? *International Journal of Technology Assessment in Health Care, 25*(1), 90–96.

Schag, C. A., Ganz, P. A., & Heinrich, R. L. (1991). Cancer Rehabilitation Evaluation System–short form (CARES-SF): A cancer specific rehabilitation and quality of life instrument. *Cancer, 68*(6), 1406–1413.

Schag, C. A., Ganz, P. A., & Heinrich, R. L. (2006). Cancer rehabilitation evaluation system-short form (CARES-SF): A cancer specific rehabilitation and quality of life instrument. *Cancer, 68*(6), 1406–1413.

Scott, N. W., Fayers, P. M., Aaronson, N. K., Bottomley, A., de Graeff, A., Groenvold, M., et al. (2009). Differential item functioning (DIF) in the EORTC QLQ-C30: A comparison of baseline, on-treatment and off-treatment data. *Quality of Life Research, 18*(3), 381–388.

Seow, H., Snyder, C. F., Shugarman, L. R., Mularski, R. A., Kutner, J. S., Lorenz, K. A., et al. (2009). Developing quality indicators for cancer end-of-life care: Proceedings from a national symposium. *Cancer, 115*(17), 3820–3829.

Shapiro, S. L., Lopez, A. M., Schwartz, G. E., Bootzin, R., Figueredo, A. J., Braden, C. J., et al. (2001). Quality of life and breast cancer: Relationship to psychosocial variables. *Journal of Clinical Psychology, 57*(4), 501–519.

Sloan, J. A., Aaronson, N., Cappelleri, J. C., Fairclough, D. L., & Varricchio, C. (2002). Assessing the clinical significance of single items relative to summated scores. *Mayo Clinic Proceedings, 77*(5), 479–487.

Sloan, J. A., Cella, D., Frost, M., Guyatt, G. H., Sprangers, M., & Symonds, T. (2002). Assessing clinical significance in measuring oncology patient quality of life: Introduction to the symposium, content overview, and definition of terms. *Mayo Clinic Proceedings, 77*(4), 367–370.

Sousa, K. H. (1999). Description of a health-related quality of life conceptual model. *Outcomes Management for Nursing Practice, 3*(2), 78–82.

Sprangers, M. A., Moinpour, C. M., Moynihan, T. J., Patrick, D. L., & Revicki, D. A. (2002). Assessing meaningful change in quality of life over time: A users' guide for clinicians. *Mayo Clinic Proceedings, 77*(6), 561–571.

Stefanek, M. E., Palmer, S. C., Thombs, B. D., & Coyne, J. C. (2009). Finding what is not there: Unwarranted claims of an effect of psychosocial intervention on recurrence and survival. *Cancer.*

Stewart, A. L., Hays, R. D., & Ware, J. E., Jr. (1988). The MOS short-form general health survey: Reliability and validity in a patient population. *Medical Care, 26*(7), 724–735.

Stewart, A. L., & Napoles-Springer, A. (2000). Health-related quality-of-life assessments in diverse population groups in the United States. *Medical Care, 38*(9, Suppl.), II102–124.

Stone, A. A., Shiffman, S., Schwartz, J. E., Broderick, J. E., & Hufford, M. R. (2002). Patient non-compliance with paper diaries. *British Medical Journal, 324*(7347), 1193–1194.

Testa, M. A. (2000). Interpretation of quality-of-life outcomes: Issues that affect magnitude and meaning. *Medical Care, 38*(9, Suppl.), II166–174.

Trivers, K. F., Stewart, S. L., Peipins, L., Rim, S. H., & White, M. C. (2009). Expanding the public health research agenda for ovarian cancer. *Journal of Womens Health (Larchmt), 18*(9), 1425–1433.

Valdagni, R., Rancati, T., & Fiorino, C. (2009). Predictive models of toxicity with external radiotherapy for prostate cancer: Clinical issues. *Cancer, 115*(13, Suppl.), 3141–3149.

Varricchio, C. G. (2006). Measurement issues in quality-of-life assessments. *Oncology Nursing Forum, 33*(1, Suppl.), 13–21.

Velikova, G., Stark, D., & Selby, P. (1999). Quality of life instruments in oncology. *European Journal of Cancer, 35*(11), 1571–1580.

Velikova, G., Wright, E. P., Smith, A. B., Cull, A., Gould, A., Forman, D., et al. (1999). Automated collection of quality-of-life data: A comparison of paper and computer touch-screen questionnaires. *Journal of Clinical Oncology, 17*(3), 998–1007.

Velikova, G., Wright, P., Smith, A. B., Stark, D., Perren, T., Brown, J., et al. (2001). Self-reported quality of life of individual cancer patients: Concordance of results with disease course and medical records. *Journal of Clinical Oncology, 19*(7), 2064–2073.

Wang, D., & Bakhai, A. (2006). *Clinical trials: A practical guide to design, analysis and reporting* (1st ed.). London, UK: Remedica Publishing.

Webster, K., Cella, D., & Yost, K. (2003). The Functional Assessment of Chronic Illness Therapy (FACIT) Measurement System: Properties, applications, and interpretation. *Health and Quality of Life Outcomes, 1*, 79.

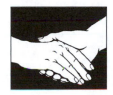

Chapter Nine

Quality of Life and Symptoms

TAMI BORNEMAN • DENICE ECONOMOU

Introduction

Several major organizations have been instrumental in initiating and promoting better pain and symptom management, as well as end-of-life care, for patients with advanced diseases (Institute of Medicine, 2003; National Comprehensive Cancer Network, 2009a; Oncology Nursing Society, 2010). The Committee on Quality Health Care in America suggested specific efforts be made to identify and intervene with factors that adversely affect health-related quality of life (HRQOL) (World Health Organization, 2002). In addition, the National Comprehensive Cancer Network (NCCN) recommends implementing methods for routine assessment and detection of distressing symptoms for cancer patients (National Comprehensive Cancer Network, 2009b).

A number of factors have been identified as affecting the physical well-being of the patient with cancer. Many of these factors are associated with the disease itself, while others are associated with the various treatments for the disease (Barsevick, 2007; Cella, Chang, Lai, & Webster, 2002). A major component of physical well-being is the area of symptom control, and when symptoms go undetected or untreated, they adversely affect the patients' HRQOL. Many cancer patients experience more than one symptom. In fact, those with advanced cancer have more symptoms, which often occur in clusters (Armstrong, 2003; Barsevick, 2007; Cooley, Short, & Moriarty, 2002). Armstrong (2003) suggests symptoms are guideposts for oncology nursing practice. The role of the nurse, in conjunction with the physician, in providing symptom management is "directly linked to the identification of symptoms through ongoing and systematic assessments" (p. 469). Clinical practice guidelines that only address a single symptom in isolation fail to account for concurrent symptoms and will be less than effective (Dodd, Miaskowski, & Paul, 2001; Holland & Chertkov, 2001).

Symptoms and symptom clusters have been identified as affecting HRQOL (Cella et al., 2002; Esper & Heidrich, 2005; Fleishman, 2004; Le et al., 2003; Miaskowski et al., 2006). Common symptoms include appetite disturbance, nausea, vomiting, constipation, pain, fatigue, dysphagia, sleep deprivation, weight loss, and sometimes anxiety and depression (Cella et al., 2003; Fu, LeMone, & McDaniel, 2004; Lacasse & Beck, 2007; Stark et al., 2002). Additionally, cancer patients often have comorbidities resulting in symptoms specific to that condition, further affecting the patient's function and HRQOL (Gift, 2007; Given, Given, Sikorskii, & Hadar, 2007; Read et al., 2004). This chapter highlights how HRQOL is affected by symptoms and symptom clusters, clinical issues in managing symptoms, barriers to symptom management, and research issues.

Effect of Symptoms on Quality of Life

The major domains of quality of life (QOL) include physical well-being, psychological well-being, social concerns, and spiritual well-being (Figure 9-1) (Ferrell, Dow, Leigh, Ly, & Gulasekaram, 1995). Although these domains can be isolated and discussed as separate entities, a dynamic interaction exists among them. Disturbances in physical status and the occurrence of physical symptoms related to disease and/or treatment processes have a direct and profound effect on all aspects of QOL (Leo et al., 2010; Nagula et al., 2010; Wong et al., 2009). Physical concerns such as uncontrolled symptoms or decreased function affect psychological well-being by creating tremendous anxiety, depression, and frustration in the client (Fox & Lyon, 2006; Leo et al., 2010; Stark et al., 2002).

Physical symptoms pose a direct threat to the client's social concerns, as any limitation in the physical well-being of the client is almost certain to create a domino effect on family

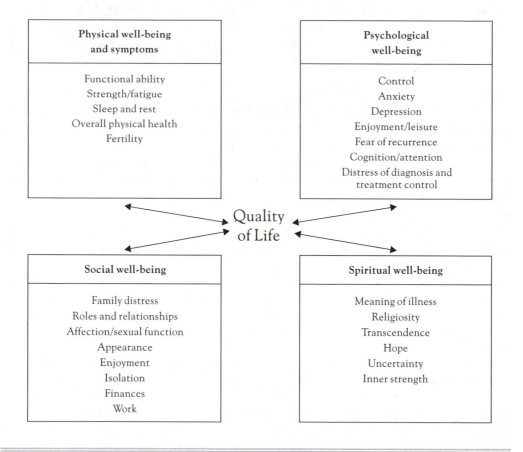

Figure 9-1. **Quality-of-life model applied to cancer survivors.**
Source: Ferrell, Hassey Dow et al., 1995. Used with permission of Oncology Nursing Press.

and friends who must assume care activities or symptom management duties (Dumont et al., 2006; Ferrell & Whitlatch, 2007; Leo et al., 2010; Lewis, 2004; Nagula et al., 2010; Zabora & Loscalzo, 2007). Physical well-being has a direct effect on spirituality as well. Studies have documented that declining physical status creates an increased awareness of personal mortality and often heightens the individual's spiritual needs (Bussing, Fischer, Ostermann, & Matthiessen, 2008; Bussing et al., 2009; Mako, Galek, & Poppito, 2006; Skalla & McCoy, 2006). Clients struggle with the meaning of illness and issues of religiosity as they confront the deterioration of the body and multiple symptoms (Holt et al., 2009; Woll, Hinshaw, & Pawlik, 2008). Figure 9-1 illustrates the dynamic process of the effect of physical well-being on other dimensions of QOL.

Symptom Management Defined

The term "symptom" comes from the Greek language meaning accident or misfortune and can be defined as a departure from normal function that is noticed by the patient (Merriam Webster, 2011). Dodd and colleagues (2001) define symptom as a "subjective experience reflecting the bio-psycho-social functioning, sensations, or cognition of an individual" (p. 466). Symptom management is defined as self-monitoring, self-care, self-regulation, self-management, or self-treatment (Dodd, Janson, et al. 2001).

One of the first researchers in oncology nursing to focus on symptoms was Jeanne Quint Benoliel (1963). Early in her research career, Dr. Benoliel focused on clients with breast cancer and recognized the importance of symptoms and QOL concerns. At that time, it was believed individuals with breast cancer were content just to have survived, even if there were serious side effects from the radical mastectomy. Dr. Benoliel's research revealed many ongoing symptoms of breast cancer and treatment that influenced QOL. Benoliel pioneered oncology nursing research in the area of physical symptoms, as well as in the area of psychosocial effects of cancer and its treatment. She also advocated scientifically sound nursing practice.

In 1987, Rhodes and Watson edited an edition of *Seminars in Oncology Nursing* that focused on symptom distress (Rhodes & Watson, 1987). This volume of the journal examined, defined, and discussed symptom occurrence and symptom distress and explored a broad spectrum of symptoms including fatigue, insomnia, depression, anxiety, nausea, vomiting, anorexia, elimination problems, and breathing difficulty. The authors emphasized that symptoms should be defined in terms of frequency, duration, and severity and that each of these aspects may require a different measurement or scale. More recently, the focus of research has expanded to include symptom clusters in order to better understand their multiple complexities from disease and treatment (Barsevick, 2007). The editors of *Seminars in Oncology Nursing* published an entire edition on symptom clusters (Yarbro, 2007).

Equally important is the need to define symptom distress. Rhodes and Watson (1987) define symptom distress as the "physical or mental anguish or suffering that results from the experience of symptom occurrence" (p. 242). Symptom distress has been distinguished previously in the work of Johnson (1973), who in the 1960s differentiated the amount of pain clients were experiencing from the distresses associated with the pain. In her work on decreasing distress following surgery, diagnostic tests, and other potentially painful clinical experiences, Johnson asked clients to rate not only the pain or discomfort they were experiencing, but also the associated distress. The concept of symptom distress was refined further by Cella and others into a model in which multiple factors and subdomains contribute to the broad categories of physical, mental, and social well-being (Gershon et al., 2003).

The importance of symptom distress is that it is directly related to the effect of symptoms on the client and, thus, on QOL (Boehmke, 2004; Bultz & Holland, 2006; Fu et al., 2004; Larsen, Nordstrom, Ljungman, & Gardulf, 2004; Leo et al., 2010; Nagula et al., 2010; Vitek, Rosenzweig, & Stollings, 2007; Wong et al., 2009). Symptom distress is also what causes the client to seek medical help for the diagnosis of disease or for relief. Symptom distress, when alleviated, may promote recovery in the client. Alleviating symptom distress may also allow the chronically ill client to maintain function and improve QOL. So important is the management of distress that the National Comprehensive Cancer Network (NCCN) developed the first set of standards and clinical practice guidelines in 1998, with the latest version in 2009 (National Comprehensive Cancer Network, 2009b). They define distress as a "multifactorial unpleasant emotional experience of a psychological (cognitive, behavioral, emotional), social, and/or spiritual nature that may interfere with the ability to cope effectively with cancer, its physical symptoms, and its treatment. Distress extends along a continuum, ranging from common normal feelings of vulnerability, sadness, and fears to problems that can become disabling, such as depression, anxiety, panic, social isolation, and existential and spiritual crisis" (p. DIS-2).

Clinical Issues in Symptom Management and QOL

Nurses have the ability to positively affect the QOL of patients with cancer (King, 2006). Understanding the dimensions of quality of life and the importance of the nurse–patient relationship is the basis for making the difference. Managing the symptoms patients experience in a judicious and effective way is the guideline for research-based interventions. The clinical goal is focused on reducing the intensity and distress of symptoms while preserving QOL. Depression is an example of a symptom experienced by 50% of cancer patients (Winell & Roth, 2005). Risk factors that contribute to the experience of depression include functional disability, loss of spouse, uncontrolled pain, lack of emotional support, advanced illness, poor physical condition life stressors or losses, and previous history. Depression can magnify other side effects associated with cancer and treatment regimens, increase the negative impact of side effects, and decrease quality of life (Badger, Braden, & Mishel, 2001).

Symptoms, then, are subjective phenomena that indicate a departure from normal functioning, sensation, or appearance and are frequently used to diagnose disease (Ferrell, Grant, Chan, Ahn, & Ferrell, 1995). Subjective responses are difficult to compare in a quantitative manner. Tools to measure responses pose an additional problem that requires careful consideration. Defining the intensity of the symptom from the distress a patient may be feeling requires careful consideration. Work is needed on both symptom alleviation and control (Barsevick et al., 2006; Fox & Lyon, 2006).

Identifying the key symptoms cancer patients experience and the relationship those symptoms have for the overall understanding of the cancer experience has been the focus of much research. In July 2002, the State of the Science Conference on Symptom Management in Cancer: Pain, Fatigue, and Depression, supported by the National Institutes of Health, identified methods to improve the research in symptom management. Specific recommendations that should be used in clinical assessment of symptoms were identified (Institute of Medicine, 2003). These recommendations have helped organize and guide research in this area. Providing rational strategies for the relief of symptoms such as pain, fatigue, and depression is important and has been the basis for the research using symptom clusters. Symptom clusters are defined as two or more symptoms that occur together and are related to each other (Kim, McGuire, Tulman, & Barsevick, 2005; Miaskowski et al., 2006). They may or may not share the same etiology and include both the subjective report of the symptom as well as the objective signs. In a study done by Fox and Lyon (2006), they attempted to examine the multiple symptoms experienced by lung cancer survivors and their relationship to QOL. They found there might be a synergistic effect between depression and fatigue and patient outcomes that included QOL. Depression and fatigue were significantly related, and this cluster explained 29% of the variance in the lung cancer subgroup. This study identified the significance in this case as fatigue, pain, and depression that are subjective in nature and are many times underdiagnosed in these patients (Fox & Lyon, 2006).

Another area of symptom research and the cascade effect it plays on patients' experience of QOL includes pain, sleep disturbance, and fatigue. These responses are seen frequently in the form of physical or psychological symptoms. Beck, Dudley and Barsevick (2005) looked at these three symptoms and attempted to describe the relationship of them to one another. They determined, based on their findings, that in a specific group of patients with cancer and multiple primary diagnoses, pain influenced fatigue directly and affected sleep indirectly. The outcome was important in helping nurses begin prioritizing interventions in an effort to relieve multiple symptoms, improve patient outcomes, and improve QOL (Beck, Dudley, & Barsevick, 2005).

Cancer-related fatigue is experienced by a large number of cancer patients and is associated with feelings of distress and depression, and affects quality of life (Morrow, 2007). According to the NCCN, fatigue guidelines suggest cancer-related fatigue is more distressing and severe then normal fatigue and does not improve with rest in the manner non-cancer-related fatigue would improve. Fatigue is more distressing to patients than pain, nausea, vomiting, or depression (National Comprehensive Cancer Network, 2009a). The definition of fatigue, according to the NCCN Fatigue Guidelines Committee is "a distressing, persistent, subjective sense of tiredness or exhaustion related to cancer or cancer treatment that is not proportional to recent activity and interferes with functioning" (p. FT-1). Fatigue is an example of a multidimensional symptom that affects multiple dimensions of the patients' life (Beck, Dudley, & Barsevick, 2005; Hofman, Ryan, Figueroa-Moseley, Jean-Pierre, & Morrow, 2007). Fatigue-like pain can be described from the dimensions of the City of Hope Quality of Life Model as physical, psychological, social, and spiritual discomfort. This multidimensional approach describes the physical component as lack of energy, inability to complete activities of daily living (ADLs), or lack of energy for leisure activities. This also includes mechanisms underlying cancer-related fatigue like serotonin dysregulation, metabolic effects related to the hypothalamic-pituitary-adrenal axis response, or muscle metabolism leading to peripheral fatigue and loss of muscle capacity (Evans & Lambert, 2007; Ryan et al., 2007). The psychological component includes the depressed mood experienced by some, effects on cognitive abilities, ability to focus attention, and distress. The sociocultural response includes effect on social life and family needs, work and home roles, and isolation. The spiritual component includes the meaning of illness, religious activities, loss of hope, or loss of inner strength (Hofman et al., 2007).

Understanding the cascade effect of one symptom upon another and the patients' response to symptoms has clinical significance for understanding these relationships and will allow nurses to focus on relieving the primary symptom, reducing or relieving the next symptom, and ultimately helping with all the symptoms in the cluster. Beck and colleagues (Beck, Dudley, & Barsevick, 2005) recognized that the common sense relationship between pain, fatigue, and sleep disturbance could lead to the clinical management strategy of improving sleep by improving pain management, which then could lead to decreased fatigue. Nurses play a significant role in identifying and improving the symptoms and alleviating the suffering that affects the patients' experience of quality of life (King, 2006).

The challenge of managing symptoms has become more difficult as patients survive longer with their cancers and deal with increasing symptoms and side effects associated with their treatment and disease over time (Ganz, 2006; Rowland, Hewitt, & Ganz, 2006). Managing symptoms is an important QOL concern in all cancer care settings. This includes hospitals, outpatient cancer centers, physician offices, hospice, and home care. The home care setting requires extensive attention to symptoms across the trajectory of care by the patient, the nurse, and, frequently, the family caregiver. Research in this area emphasizes the importance of symptom control to family caregivers. Symptoms are the major source of family concern. The presence of uncontrolled symptoms affects QOL for both the patient and family caregiver (Ferrell & Borneman, 1999, 2000; Osta & Bruera, 2009; Payne & Hudson, 2009; Zabora & Loscalzo, 2007).

Nurses depend on patients and family caregivers to provide an understanding of the intensity of symptoms the patient experiences. McMillan and Moody (2003) compared the symptom ratings for pain, dyspnea, and constipation between patients and their family caregiver. The results proved that caregivers significantly overestimated symptom intensity for all three of the symptoms (p =.000). It is essential for oncology nurses to educate both patient and caregiver in how to assess their patients' symptoms (Kim et al., 2005; McMillan & Moody, 2003). The presence of uncontrolled symptoms affects QOL for both the patient and family caregiver (King, 2006; Morrow, 2007). Learning to identify appropriate strategies to deal with multiple symptoms will decrease the burden for patients and their families and provide better patient outcomes (Gapstur, 2007).

Additional aspects of symptom management that underline its importance is its effect on healthcare costs. For example, in a study done by Curt and colleagues (2000), 75% of the participants needed to change their positions in response to fatigue. Seventy-seven percent also lost at least one day at work as a result of fatigue (Curt et al., 2000; Kim, 2007). The actual costs of fatigue to society are difficult to estimate. Improving fatigue also increases productive time and decreases the need to employ help to maintain a patient's lifestyle (Hofman et al., 2007). In this manner, cost savings could be a benefit to both the business community as well as the individual patient.

New trends in symptom management include the use of advanced practice nurses (APN). Advanced practice nurses have advanced training in symptom management and advanced degrees such as clinical nurse specialist (CNS) or nurse practitioner (NP). New models for care may provide a more cost effective approach to intensive symptom management (Meier & Beresford, 2006). This level of nurse has the potential to do third-party billing, which may offer a method of recouping portions of their salary and overhead costs while providing palliative care (Meier & Beresford, 2006). Cancer survivorship care and follow-up is becoming increasingly more managed in NP-run follow-up care clinics. Nurses are leaders in symptom management and continue to provide the bulk of that care to patients and families.

Barriers to Symptom Management

One of the most essential aspects to treating symptoms is an accurate systematic symptom assessment, but one seldom is implemented (Cella et al., 2003; Osta & Bruera, 2009). Up until the past decade, standard symptom and HRQOL tools were long and cumbersome, and therefore not well suited for integration into clinical practice. As a result, there is a gap in provider knowledge of, familiarity with, and perceived usefulness of available instruments used to conduct standard assessments (Bezjak et al., 2001; Carlson, Speca, Hagen, & Taenzer, 2001; Osta & Bruera, 2009; Velikova et al., 2001).

Adding to this challenge is a lack of good communication. "Communication is the foundation from which assessments are ascertained, goals of care are developed, and relationships are established" (Dahlin & Giansiracusa, 2006, p. 67). Kirk, Kirk, and Kristjanson (2004) interviewed 35 patient-family dyads and two patients regarding the disclosure process and satisfaction with information sharing during the course of illness. Many participants were dissatisfied with the communication process. The six following attributes were identified for effectively communicating information:

1. Playing it straight (being honest and direct when providing information)
2. Making it clear (providing information in understandable terms)
3. Showing you care (expressing verbal/nonverbal messages with compassion and empathy)
4. Giving time (allowing enough time for discussion of information)
5. Pacing information (being sensitive to the quantity and rate of information needed for assimilation)
6. Staying the course (conveying assurance they will not be abandoned during the illness progression) (Kirk, Kirk, & Kristjanson, 2004).

Keep in mind these barriers occur within the context of reduced time for face-to-face patient care, as the healthcare environment continues to reward shorter clinic and consultation time (Institute of Medicine, 2003; Yarnall, Pollak, Ostbye, Krause, & Michener, 2003).

Another important barrier is a lack of adequate instrumentation to measure symptoms and symptom distress (Boehmke, 2004; Higginson & Addington-Hall, 2004). Nursing scientists have begun to address this problem area through the development of texts, workshops, presentations, and publications focusing on instrumentation (Frank-Stromborg & Olsen, 2004; Higginson & Addington-Hall, 2004). However, much remains to be done to develop instruments that are valid, reliable, sensitive, and easy to use clinically. Davis and Cella (2002) identified several factors for routine assessment (Chang et al., 2002; Davis & Cella, 2002). First, there needs to be a set of measures from which to choose. The tool needs to be brief and easy to administer, complete, score, and interpret. Second, the tool needs to provide clinical relevance and if possible, present the results in a format that facilitates and guides interventions. Buy-in from both healthcare providers and patients is important for routine assessment to be effectively implemented (Chang et al., 2002; Velikova et al., 2004). If the availability of these assessment tools is lacking, scientific evidence on the effect of interventions for clinical management will be difficult to demonstrate.

Research Issues in Symptom Management and QOL

Research related to symptoms and symptom clusters requires establishment of a model to help understand the complex relationships of the symptoms as well as conceptualization, design, measurement, and analytic issues in the study design (Barsevick, Dudley, & Beck, 2006). Research to understand additional factors contributing to multiple symptoms, for example the "alternative mechanisms" between pain and fatigue, is also needed (Beck, Dudley, & Barsevick, 2005). Research in symptom management must be held to the same rigorous standards as clinical trials evaluating the effectiveness of cancer treatment regimens (Varricchio & Sloan, 2002). Sloan and Varricchio (2001) suggest self-reported measures of symptom severity or the symptoms' effect on QOL be equated to biologic markers of tumor progression. This would mean clinically meaningful change or clinically significant change endpoints would be established prior to starting the study. The authors also stress the importance of presenting complete data with supportive assumptions to allow the reader to judge the quality of the findings. Cella and colleagues (2003) attempted to identify the symptoms cancer patients receiving chemotherapy experience by level of importance, as decided on by physicians and nurses from 17 National Comprehensive Cancer Network (NCCN) institutions (Cella et al., 2003). These symptoms were prioritized across tumor sites, and the most important symptoms were described depending on disease. These symptoms will then be evaluated in the second step of the study by patients in these disease populations for agreement. They describe the need to use a multidimensional tool to measure QOL and the Functional Assessment of Cancer Therapy (FACT). These tools will be modified, with detailed, tumor-specific symptom assessments added to the general questionnaire. The hope is that by using individualized disease-specific tools on their own rather than within large questionnaires, the results will be more acceptable and appropriate to guide chemotherapy decisions. Choosing treatment based on disease-specific symptoms and the treatment's ability to relieve those symptoms would be the goal of this study. The ability to understand the symptoms that are associated with a specific disease would allow nurses to assess patients comprehensively for all symptoms known to be related to the disease. This would then decrease the undertreatment of symptoms due to incomplete assessment and improve patient outcomes, such as QOL (Cella et al., 2003).

Computerized systems have been used to improve the communication and management of symptoms and symptom clusters of cancer patients (Ruland, White, Stevens, Fanciullo, & Khilani, 2003). In this study, Creating better Health Outcomes by Improving Communication about Patients' Experiences (CHOICEs) used electronic monitoring to allow patients to report symptoms and preferences during outpatient clinic visits. This study looked at cancer-specific symptoms using a comprehensive patient assessment tool on a touch-pad tablet computer. The tool was linked also to Web pages using Java servlets to support education and could be tailored to a subject's previous responses (Ruland et al., 2003). This study represents one example of future areas where research in symptom management strategies can help to improve patient-centered care. This technology allows for the multiple symptom evaluation necessary to further work in symptom clusters and effects on QOL. Certainly in the area of cancer-related fatigue, this approach would be most helpful. Evaluating the multiple assessment tools and comparing unidimensional tools or independent multiple-item tools could be streamlined using computer-assisted versions.

Efforts need to be made to understand potential gender differences in the experience of symptoms and their effect on the patients' QOL. Cultural relevance of different symptoms must also be examined. In a study looking at Chinese patients newly diagnosed with gastrointestinal cancer, researchers found depression, symptom distress, and social support accounted for 44% of HRQOL, while financial difficulty and symptom distress accounted for 20% of the total global QOL (Yan & Sellick, 2004). Financial concerns may have more of an effect on the male cancer patient who is the primary financial provider for his family.

The assessment tools used to measure QOL in relation to symptom management are best evaluated using a multidimensional assessment like the QLQ-C30, which incorporates five functional scales (physical, role, cognition, emotional, and social) and nine symptom scales (fatigue, pain, nausea/vomiting, dyspnea, insomnia, loss of appetite, constipation, diarrhea, and financial problems) (Gupta, Lis, & Grutsch, 2007). Validating the relationship between relieving a specific symptom and that relief being responsible for the improvement in QOL ratings requires continued research and explanation of the hypothetical relationships (Buchanan, O'Mara, Kelaghan, & Minasian, 2005; Jean-Pierre et al., 2007). The Memorial Symptoms Assessment Scale (MSAS) and the Functional Living Index for Cancer (FLIC) both measure QOL. Health-related quality of life is also rated with the Cancer Rehabilitation Evaluation System-Short Form (CARES-SF), which makes 59 statements relating to common problems experienced by the cancer patient and scores these across each of the five domains. Cancer Rehabilitation Evaluation System-Short Form also is sensitive to cancer site, stage of disease, performance status, treatment modality, and tumor response and has been used in culturally different cancer populations (Yan & Sellick, 2004).

There are at least two important dimensions in the assessment of symptoms and function. Research has shown it is very helpful to assess not only the intensity of symptoms, but also the distress associated with them. For example, in measuring pain, the patient is asked first, "How much pain do you have?" in order to assess intensity on a scale of 0 to 10, with 0 being no pain and 10 being severe pain. This indicates the intensity of the pain. The patient then is asked, "How distressing is the pain to you?" This technique enables the patient to express how bothersome or distressing a particular symptom may be. This technique also assists healthcare professionals to appreciate the importance of individual problems of the patient. For example, patients may rate their fatigue as fairly mild but describe it as extremely distressing because it limits them from participating in important activities (Ruland et al., 2003).

The second measurement issue relates to the timing of physical well-being assessments. Many of the symptoms patients experience are, in fact, intermittent problems. It may be misleading sometimes to ask a patient a simple question such as, "Do you have any nausea?" Patients may be inclined to report their status only at that moment, rather than providing a sense of their usual patterns or their problems over recent days or weeks. It is important for the clinician or researcher to establish the time frame of the measurement. Scales that measure a symptom over time are important to be able to measure the intensity of, as well as the length of time, this symptom is experienced. Rather than asking questions requiring a simple yes or no, more precise measures (i.e., 0 to 10 ordinal scales or visual analog scales) enable nurses to measure changes in a particular symptom over time or to evaluate the effectiveness of a nursing intervention.

Table 9-1 presents examples of symptom items in eight frequently used QOL instruments. Symptom items commonly are included in these instruments. Many symptoms, such as pain and nausea, are universal items, while assessment of other symptoms varies across instruments. Understanding the multiple aspects of measuring cancer-related fatigue alone is daunting (Jean-Pierre et al., 2007). Consider the challenge of fatigue and its multiple physical and psychological factors that may also be related to other medical and psychological conditions—how do you differentiate them from one another?

Applying qualitative research methods can provide a mechanism for understanding the patient's experience of symptoms and physical status in a way not achievable through quantitative scales or methods. Most of the nursing studies conducted at the City of Hope Medical Center combine quantitative and qualitative methods to obtain the most complete descriptions of QOL from cancer patients.

Future research must focus on intervention studies related to the management of symptoms and symptom clusters. This will allow nurses to manage patients using evidence-based approaches that are aimed at reducing symptoms and alleviating distress.

CONCLUSION

Symptom management remains a critical mandate for oncology nurses. Failure to manage symptoms adequately has a direct and profound influence on the QOL of our patients and their families. Effective assessment of patients' symptoms offers the potential of guiding

Table 9-1. **Examples of Symptom Items in Select QOL Tools**

Physical	CARES	FLIC	FACT-G	QOL-BMT	QOL-BR	SDS
Pain	X	X	X	X	X	X
Nausea/Vomiting	X	X	X	X	X	X
Fatigue	X		X	X	X	X
Function Ability	X	X	X			
Weight Changes	X				X	
Sleep Differences	X		X	X	X	X
Bowel/Bladder	X			X	X	X
Appetite	X			X	X	X
Concentration	X			X	X	X
Memory	X			X	X	
Vision				X		
Skin Changes				X		
Bleeding Problems				X		
Mouth Dryness				X		
Hearing Loss				X		
Ringing in Ears				X		
SOB/Breathing Difficulty				X		X
Fertility/Menopausal Symptoms				X	X	
State of Health/ Perceived Wellness		X	X	X	X	
Cough						
Strength	X			X		
Anxiety	X		X	X	X	
Depression	X	X		X	X	
Fear of Metastases	X			X	X	
Fear of Recurrence	X			X	X	
Fear of Second Cancer				X	X	
Sexual Function	X	X	X	X	X	

CARES—Cancer Rehabilitation Evaluation System (Schag, Heinrich, Aadland, & Ganz, 1990).
FLIC—Functional Living Index of Cancer (Schipper, Clinch, McMurray, & Levitt, 1984).
FACT-G—Functional Assessment of Cancer Therapy-General Version (Cella et al., 1993).
QOL-BMT—Quality of Life, Bone Marrow Transplant Version, City of Hope (Grant, Ferrell, Schmidt, Fonbuena, Niland, & Forman, 1992).
QOL-BR—Quality of Life, Breast Version, City of Hope (Ferrell, Hassey Dow, & Grant, 1995).
SDS—Symptom Distress Scale (McCorkle & Young, 1978).

treatment decisions to improve patient outcomes and QOL. Cancer involves physical and psychological symptoms in response to the disease and treatment. As with many aspects of cancer care, nursing interventions in symptom management also have a profound influence on family members whose experiences are greatly influenced by the symptoms they observe in those they love.

Understanding symptoms and symptom clusters associated with specific diseases will play a role in the future of health care. Applying information gained on multiple disease types and treatment response will guide healthcare professionals in effective and efficient symptom management practice. Oncology nursing has helped humanize the experience of cancer by addressing symptom management as a primary component of care. Research must continue in the study of symptom clusters and how that information will improve symptom distress and QOL. Quality of life and its relationship to symptom burden remains a multivariable concept and a difficult one to understand, but uncovering this information is imperative for nursing interventions to be effective, time efficient, and cost saving (Gapstur, 2007). These issues are increasingly crucial as we face a future of uncertainty related to healthcare provision in our country.

ACKNOWLEDGMENT

We would like to acknowledge the work Dr. Betty Ferrell and Dr. Marcia Grant have done on this subject for first and second editions. We thank them for their continued support of this project.

REFERENCES

Armstrong, T. S. (2003). Symptoms experience: A concept analysis. *Oncology Nursing Forum, 30*(4), 601–606.

Badger, T. A., Braden, C. J., & Mishel, M. H. (2001). Depression burden, self-help interventions, and side effect experience in women receiving treatment for breast cancer. *Oncology Nursing Forum, 28*(3), 567–574.

Barsevick, A. M. (2007). The concept of symptom cluster. *Seminars in Oncology Nursing, 23*(2), 89–98.

Barsevick, A. M., Dudley, W. N., & Beck, S. L. (2006). Cancer-related fatigue, depressive symptoms, and functional status: A mediation model. *Nursing Research, 55*(5), 366–372.

Beck, S. L., Dudley, W. N., & Barsevick, A. (2005). Pain, sleep disturbance, and fatigue in patients with cancer: Using a mediation model to test a symptom cluster. *Oncology Nursing Forum, 32*(3), 542.

Benoliel, J. (1963). Impact of mastectomy. *American Journal of Nursing, 63*, 88–92.

Bezjak, A., Ng, P., Skeel, R., Depetrillo, A. D., Comis, R., & Taylor, K. M. (2001). Oncologists' use of quality of life information: Results of a survey of Eastern Cooperative Oncology Group physicians. *Quality of Life Research, 10*(1), 1–13.

Boehmke, M. M. (2004). Measurement of symptom distress in women with early-stage breast cancer. *Cancer Nursing, 27*(2), 144–152.

Buchanan, D. R., O'Mara, A. M., Kelaghan, J. W., & Minasian, L. M. (2005). Quality-of-life assessment in the symptom management trials of the National Cancer Institute-supported Community Clinical Oncology Program. *Journal of Clinical Oncology, 23*(3), 591–598.

Bultz, B., & Holland, J. (2006). Emotional distress in patients with cancer: The sixth vital sign. *Community Oncology, 3*(5), 311–314.

Bussing, A., Fischer, J., Ostermann, T., & Matthiessen, P. F. (2008). Reliance on God's help, depression and fatigue in female cancer patients. *International Journal of Psychiatry and Medicine, 38*(3), 357–372.

Bussing, A., Michalsen, A., Balzat, H. J., Grunther, R. A., Ostermann, T., Neugebauer, E. A., et al. (2009). Are spirituality and religiosity resources for patients with chronic pain conditions? *Pain Medicine, 10*(2), 327–339.

Carlson, L. E., Speca, M., Hagen, N., & Taenzer, P. (2001). Computerized quality-of-life screening in a cancer pain clinic. *Journal of Palliative Care, 17*(1), 46–52.

Cella, D., Chang, C. H., Lai, J. S., & Webster, K. (2002). Advances in quality of life measurements in oncology patients. *Seminars in Oncology, 29*(3, Suppl. 8), 60–68.

Cella, D., Paul, D., Yount, S., Winn, R., Chang, C. H., Banik, D., et al. (2003). What are the most important symptom targets when treating advanced cancer? A survey of providers in the National Comprehensive Cancer Network (NCCN). *Cancer Investigation, 21*(4), 526–535.

Chang, C. H., Cella, D., Fernandez, O., Luque, G., de Castro, P., de Andres, C., et al. (2002). Quality of life in multiple sclerosis patients in Spain. *Multiple Sclerosis, 8*(6), 527–531.

Cooley, M. E., Short, T. H., & Moriarty, H. J. (2002). Patterns of symptom distress in adults receiving treatment for lung cancer. *Journal of Palliative Care, 18*(3), 150–159.

Curt, G. A., Breitbart, W., Cella, D., Groopman, J. E., Horning, S. J., Itri, L. M., et al. (2000). Impact of cancer-related fatigue on the lives of patients: New findings from the Fatigue Coalition. *Oncologist, 5*(5), 353–360.

Dahlin, C., & Giansiracusa, D. (2006). Communication in palliative care. In B. Ferrell & N. Coyle (Eds.), *Textbook of palliative nursing.* (2nd ed., pp. 67–93). New York, NY: Oxford University Press.

Davis, K., & Cella, D. (2002). Assessing quality of life in oncology clinical practice: A review of barriers and critical success factors. *The Journal of Clinical Outcomes Management, 9*(6), 327–332.

Dodd, M., Janson, S., Facione, N., Faucett, J., Froelicher, E. S., Humphreys, J., et al. (2001). Advancing the science of symptom management. *Journal of Advanced Nursing, 33*(5), 668–676.

Dodd, M. J., Miaskowski, C., & Paul, S. M. (2001). Symptom clusters and their effect on the functional status of patients with cancer. *Oncology Nursing Forum, 28*(3), 465–470.

Dumont, S., Turgeon, J., Allard, P., Gagnon, P., Charbonneau, C., & Vezina, L. (2006). Caring for a loved one with advanced cancer: Determinants of psychological distress in family caregivers. *Journal of Palliative Medicine, 9*(4), 912–921.

Esper, P., & Heidrich, D. (2005). Symptom clusters in advanced illness. *Seminars in Oncology Nursing, 21*(1), 20–28.

Evans, W. J., & Lambert, C. P. (2007). Physiological basis of fatigue. *American Journal of Physical Medicine and Rehabilitation, 86*(1, Suppl.), S29–S46.

Ferrell, B., & Borneman, T. (1999). Hospice home management of pain and symptoms. *Primary Care & Cancer, 19*(7), 8–10.

Ferrell, B., & Borneman, T. (2000). Maintaining quality of life in the home. *Principles and Practice of Supportive Oncology Updates, 3*(5), 1–8.

Ferrell, B., & Whitlatch, B. (2007). Home care and caregivers. In A. Berger, J. Shuster, & J. Von Roenn (Eds.), *Principles and practice of palliative care and supportive oncology* (3rd ed., pp. 615–622). Philadelphia, PA: Lippincott, Williams, & Wilkins.

Ferrell, B. R., Dow, K. H., Leigh, S., Ly, J., & Gulasekaram, P. (1995). Quality of life in long-term cancer survivors. *Oncology Nursing Forum, 22*(6), 915–922.

Ferrell, B. R., Grant, M., Chan, J., Ahn, C., & Ferrell, B. A. (1995). The impact of cancer pain education on family caregivers of elderly patients. *Oncology Nursing Forum, 22*(8), 1211–1218.

Fleishman, S. B. (2004). Treatment of symptom clusters: Pain, depression, and fatigue. *Journal of the National Cancer Institute Monographs, 32*, 119–123.

Fox, S. W., & Lyon, D. E. (2006). Symptom clusters and quality of life in survivors of lung cancer. *Oncology Nursing Forum, 33*(5), 931–936.

Frank-Stromborg, M., & Olsen, S. J. (2004). *Instruments for clinical health-care research* (3rd ed.). Sudbury, MA: Jones and Bartlett Publishers.

Fu, M. R., LeMone, P., & McDaniel, R. W. (2004). An integrated approach to an analysis of symptom management in patients with cancer. *Oncology Nursing. Forum, 31*(1), 65–70.

Ganz, P. A. (2006). Monitoring the physical health of cancer survivors: A survivorship-focused medical history. *Journal of Clinical Oncology, 24*(32), 5105–5111.

Gapstur, R. L. (2007). Symptom burden: A concept analysis and implications for oncology nurses. *Oncology Nursing Forum, 34*(3), 673–680.

Gershon, R., Cella, D., Dineen, K., Rosenbloom, S., Peterman, A., & Lai, J. S. (2003). Item response theory and health related quality of life in cancer. *Pharmacoeconomics and Outcomes Research, 3*(6), 783–791.

Gift, A. G. (2007). Symptom clusters related to specific cancers. *Seminars in Oncology Nursing, 23*(2), 136–141.

Given, B. A., Given, C. W., Sikorskii, A., & Hadar, N. (2007). Symptom clusters and physical function for patients receiving chemotherapy. *Seminars in Oncology Nursing, 23*(2), 121–126.

Grant, M., Ferrell, B., Schmidt, G.M., Fonbuena, P., Niland, J. C., Forman, S. J. (1992). Measurement of quality of life in bone marrow transplantation survivors. *Quality of Life Research, 1*(6), 375–384.

Gupta, D., Lis, C. G., & Grutsch, J. F. (2007). The relationship between cancer-related fatigue and patient satisfaction with quality of life in cancer. *Journal of Pain and Symptom Management, 34*(1), 40–47.

Higginson, I., & Addington-Hall, J. (2004). The epidemiology of death and symptoms. In D. Doyle, G. Hanks, N. Cherny, & S. K. Calman (Eds.), *Oxford textbook of palliative medicine* (pp. 14–22). New York, NY: Oxford University Press.

Hofman, M., Ryan, J. L., Figueroa-Moseley, C. D., Jean-Pierre, P., & Morrow, G. R. (2007). Cancer-related fatigue: The scale of the problem. *Oncologist, 12*(Suppl. 1), 4–10.

Holland, J., & Chertkov, L. (2001). Clinical practice guidelines for the management of psychosocial and physical symptoms of cancer. In K. M. Foley & H. Gerband (Eds.), *Improving palliative care for cancer*. Washington, DC: National Academy Press.

Holt, C. L., Caplan, L., Schulz, E., Blake, V., Southward, P., Buckner, A., et al. (2009). Role of religion in cancer coping among African Americans: A qualitative examination. *Journal of Psychosocial Oncology, 27*(2), 248–273.

Institute of Medicine. (2003). *Improving palliative care: We take better care of people with cancer*. Washington, DC: National Academy of Science.

Jean-Pierre, P., Figueroa-Moseley, C. D., Kohli, S., Fiscella, K., Palesh, O. G., & Morrow, G. R. (2007). Assessment of cancer-related fatigue: Implications for clinical diagnosis and treatment. *Oncologist, 12*(Suppl. 1), 11–21.

Johnson, J. E. (1973). Effects of accurate expectations about sensations on the sensory and distress components of pain. *Journal of Personality and Social Psychology, 27*(2), 261–275.

Kim, H. J., McGuire, D. B., Tulman, L., & Barsevick, A. M. (2005). Symptom clusters: Concept analysis and clinical implications for cancer nursing. *Cancer Nursing, 28*(4), 270–282; quiz 283–274.

Kim, P. (2007). Cost of cancer care: The patient perspective. *Journal of Clinical Oncology, 25*(2), 228–232.

King, C. R. (2006). Advances in how clinical nurses can evaluate and improve quality of life for individuals with cancer. *Oncology Nursing Forum, 33*(1, Suppl.), 5–12.

Kirk, P., Kirk, I., & Kristjanson, L. J. (2004). What do patients receiving palliative care for cancer and their families want to be told? A Canadian and Australian qualitative study. *British Medical Journal, 328*(7452), 1343.

Lacasse, C., & Beck, S. L. (2007). Clinical assessment of symptom clusters. *Seminars in Oncology Nursing, 23*(2), 106–112.

Larsen, J., Nordstrom, G., Ljungman, P., & Gardulf, A. (2004). Symptom occurrence, symptom intensity, and symptom distress in patients undergoing high-dose chemotherapy with stem-cell transplantation. *Cancer Nursing, 27*(1), 55–64.

Le, T., Leis, A., Pahwa, P., Wright, K., Ali, K., & Reeder, B. (2003). Quality-of-life issues in patients with ovarian cancer and their caregivers: A review. *Obstetrical and Gynecological Survey*, *58*(11), 749–758.

Leo, F., Scanagatta, P., Vannucci, F., Brambilla, D., Radice, D., & Spaggiari, L. (2010). Impaired quality of life after pseumonectomy: Who is at risk? *The Journal of Thoracic and Cardiovascular Surgery*, *139*(1), 49–52.

Lewis, F. M. (2004). Shifting perspectives: Family-focused oncology nursing research. *Oncology Nursing Forum*, *31*(2), 288–292.

Mako, C., Galek, K., & Poppito, S. R. (2006). Spiritual pain among patients with advanced cancer in palliative care. *Journal of Palliative Medicine*, *9*(5), 1106–1113.

McCorkle, R., Young, K. (1978). Development of a symptom distress scale. *Cancer Nursing*, *1*(5), 373–378.

McMillan, S. C., & Moody, L. E. (2003). Hospice patient and caregiver congruence in reporting patients' symptom intensity. *Cancer Nursing*, *26*(2), 113–118.

Meier, D. E., & Beresford, L. (2006). Billing for palliative care: An essential cost of doing business. *Journal of Palliative Medicine*, *9*(2), 250–257.

Merriam Webster. (2011). *Symptom*. Retrieved March 31, 2011, from http://www.merriam-webster.com/dictionary/symptom

Miaskowski, C., Cooper, B. A., Paul, S. M., Dodd, M., Lee, K., Aouizerat, B. E., et al. (2006). Subgroups of patients with cancer with different symptom experiences and quality-of-life outcomes: A cluster analysis. *Oncology Nursing Forum*, *33*(5), E79–E89.

Morrow, G. R. (2007). Cancer-related fatigue: Causes, consequences, and management. *Oncologist*, *12*(Suppl. 1), 1–3.

Nagula, S., Ishill, N., Nash, C., Markowitz, A., Schattner, M., Temple, L., et al. (2010). Quality of life and symptom control after stent placement or surgical palliation of malignant colorectal obstruction. *Journal of the American College of Surgeons*, *210*(1), 45–53.

National Comprehensive Cancer Network. (2009a). *Cancer-related fatigue*. Retrieved January 18, 2010 from National Comprehensive Cancer Network, volume 1, 2009, http://www.nccn.org/professionals/physician_gls/PDF/fatigue.pdf.

National Comprehensive Cancer Network. (2009b). *Distress management*. Retrieved January 18, 2010, from National Comprehensive Cancer Network, volume 1, 2009, http://www.nccn.org/professionals/physician_gls/PDF/distress.pdf.

Oncology Nursing Society (2010). Oncology Nursing Society and Association of Oncology Social Work Joint Position on Palliative and End-of-Life Care. Retrieved December 15, 2010, from http://www.ons.org/publications/media/ons/docs/positions/endoflife.pdf

Osta, B., & Bruera, E. (2009). Symptom research. In D. Walsh (Ed.), *Palliative medicine*, (pp. 161–165). Philadelphia, PA: Saunders Elsevier.

Payne, S., & Hudson, P. (2009). Assessing the family and caregivers. In D. Walsh (Ed.), *Palliative medicine*. (pp. 320–325). Philadelphia, PA: Saunders Elsevier.

Read, W. L., Tierney, R. M., Page, N. C., Costas, I., Govindan, R., Spitznagel, E. L., et al. (2004). Differential prognostic impact of comorbidity. *Journal of Clinical Oncology*, *22*(15), 3099–3103.

Rhodes, V. A., & Watson, P. M. (1987). Symptom distress—the concept: Past and present. *Seminars in Oncology Nursing*, *3*(4), 242–247.

Rowland, J. H., Hewitt, M., & Ganz, P. A. (2006). Cancer survivorship: A new challenge in delivering quality cancer care. *Journal of Clinical Oncology*, *24*(32), 5101–5104.

Ruland, C. M., White, T., Stevens, M., Fanciullo, G., & Khilani, S. M. (2003). Effects of a computerized system to support shared decision making in symptom management of cancer patients: Preliminary results. *Journal of the American Medical Informatics Association*, *10*(6), 573–579.

Ryan, J. L., Carroll, J. K., Ryan, E. P., Mustian, K. M., Fiscella, K., & Morrow, G. R. (2007). Mechanisms of cancer-related fatigue. *Oncologist*, *12*(Suppl. 1), 22–34.

Schag, C. A., Heinrich, R., Aadland, R. L., Ganz, P. A. (1990). Assessing problems of cancer problem situations. *Health Psychology, 9*(1), 83–102.

Schipper, H., Clinch, J., McMurray, A., Levitt, M. (1984). Measuring the quality of life of cancer patients: the Functional Living Index-Cancer: development and validation. *Journal of Clinical Oncology, 2*(5), 472–83.

Skalla, K., & McCoy, J. P. (2006). Spiritual assessment of patients with cancer: The moral authority, vocational, aesthetic, social, and transcendent model. *Oncology Nursing Forum, 33*(4), 745–751.

Sloan, J. A., & Varricchio, C. (2001). Quality of life endpoints in prostate chemoprevention trials. *Urology, 57*(4, Suppl. 1), 235–240.

Stark, D., Kiely, M., Smith, A., Velikova, G., House, A., & Selby, P. (2002). Anxiety disorders in cancer patients: Their nature, associations, and relation to quality of life. *Journal of Clinical Oncology, 20*(14), 3137–3148.

Varricchio, C. G., & Sloan, J. A. (2002). The need for and characteristics of randomized, phase III trials to evaluate symptom management in patients with cancer. *Journal of the National Cancer Institute, 94*(16), 1184–1185.

Velikova, G., Booth, L., Smith, A. B., Brown, P. M., Lynch, P., Brown, J. M., et al. (2004). Measuring quality of life in routine oncology practice improves communication and patient well-being: A randomized controlled trial. *Journal of Clinical Oncology, 22*(4), 714–724.

Velikova, G., Wright, P., Smith, A. B., Stark, D., Perren, T., Brown, J., et al. (2001). Self-reported quality of life of individual cancer patients: Concordance of results with disease course and medical records. *Journal of Clinical Oncology, 19*(7), 2064–2073.

Vitek, L., Rosenzweig, M. Q., & Stollings, S. (2007). Distress in patients with cancer: Definition, assessment, and suggested interventions. *Clinical Journal of Oncology Nursing, 11*(3), 413–418.

Winell, J., & Roth, A. J. (2005). Psychiatric assessment and symptom management in elderly cancer patients. *Oncology (Williston Park), 19*(11), 1479–1490; discussion 1492, 1497, 1501–1477.

Woll, M. L., Hinshaw, D. B., & Pawlik, T. M. (2008). Spirituality and religion in the care of surgical oncology patients with life-threatening or advanced illnesses. *Annals of Surgical Oncology, 15*(11), 3048–3057.

Wong, J., Hird, A., SZhang, L., Tsao, M., Sinclair, E., Barnes, E., et al. (2009). Symptoms and quality of life in cancer patients with brain metastases following palliative radiotherapy. *International Journal of Radiation Oncology, Biology and Physics, 75*(4), 1125–1131.

World Health Organization. (2002). *National cancer control programme: Policies and managerial guidelines* (2nd ed.). Geneva: World Health Organization.

Yan, H., & Sellick, K. (2004). Symptoms, psychological distress, social support, and quality of life of Chinese patients newly diagnosed with gastrointestinal cancer. *Cancer Nursing, 27*(5), 389–399.

Yarbro, C. H. (2007). Symptom clusters. *Seminars in Oncology Nursing, 23*(2).

Yarnall, K. S., Pollak, K. I., Ostbye, T., Krause, K. M., & Michener, J. L. (2003). Primary care: Is there enough time for prevention? *American Journal of Public Health, 93*(4), 635–641.

Zabora, J. R., & Loscalzo, M. J. (2007). Psychosocial consequences of advanced cancer. In A. Berger, J. Shuster, & J. Von Roenn (Eds.), *Principles and practice of palliative care and supportive oncology* (3rd ed., pp. 593–604). Philadelphia, PA: Lippincott Williams & Wilkins.

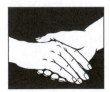

Chapter Ten

Quality of Life of Family Caregivers of Cancer Patients

BONNIE TESCHENDORF • CAROL ESTWING FERRANS

Introduction and Demographics of Family Caregivers of Cancer Patients

Providing support is frequently a spontaneous response when a family member is diagnosed with cancer, yet it involves a vaguely defined commitment. At the outset, family members rally to offer emotional support and encouragement. Later, the role can extend beyond soothing frayed nerves, evolving into operational duties such as driving to clinical appointments, recording or reciting medical history, waiting during care delivery, and finally, participating in personal care. These events occur with some regularity, yet, the importance of caregiving in cancer is not widely understood, and caregivers rarely comprehend the implications for their own health outcomes.

Studies have consistently shown that women make up the majority of family caregivers of cancer patients, as with other disease groups. (Barrett, 2004; Cameron, Franche, Cheung, & Stewart, 2002; Emanuel et al., 1999; Hileman, Lackey, & Hassanein, 1992). A recent study of 1666 family caregivers found that 78.9% were women (Kim, Kashy, Spillers, & Evans, 2009). The spouse is usually the primary caregiver, followed by daughters, sons, or other related persons. Neighbors and friends are enlisted to help with impersonal tasks. Children (under 18 years of age) also provide substantial caregiving, especially when the disease process is chronic. This can be true for many types of cancer. Teenagers, in particular, may be caregivers for elderly grandparents during after school hours. These caregivers are often unacknowledged as important members of the caring network, yet they could be supplying care that is essential to the well-being and even survival of the patient (Young Caregivers in the United States, 2005). Young caregivers frequently assume duties such as household chores and personal assistance. While they may become expert at performing the tasks, their contributions diminish the time available for personal pursuits and scholarly activities. Some teenagers report feeling that they have a lot of responsibility compared to their contemporaries. The academic performance and perceptions of role overload of young caregivers should be monitored by parents and members of the healthcare team. Altered self-esteem, changing aspirations for the future, and poor performance should be adequate indicators of the need for duty relief.

Most cancer patients are over the age of 65 at diagnosis, and the spouse, the most common family caregiver, is often unemployed at the time of the diagnosis. However, for other spouses or family caregivers the freedom to assist may be restrained by other commitments. National surveys have shown that many family caregivers work outside the home; few have other unpaid help to care for the patient (Barrett, 2004). Employed women often try to find other resources to augment their caregiving, because they may not wish to, or may be unable to, forfeit their income and time to provide these services. The primary caregiver usually manages the bulk of responsibilities, which could include paying bills, scheduling appointments, and assisting with personal care. Of course, not every patient requires help throughout the disease continuum, but many require assistance for specific tasks.

The pilot caregiver module of the Behavioral Risk Factor Surveillance System reported that approximately 12% of the study participants in the state of North Carolina cared for a family member with cancer (Andresen, 2006). If these estimates were extrapolated for the nation we could expect to find over 4.3 million cancer family caregivers actively providing care within the United States at any given time.

Becoming a Family Caregiver

Caregivers may become involved in their role without much forethought. Some self-select and decide they are the logical person to provide care, while others have little choice in the matter and are assigned by other family members or by assumptions of healthcare professionals. Choice does make a difference in how caregivers view their role and in how they execute their duties. Some derive pleasure from helping, while others resent the work and can harbor feelings of bitterness. The responsibilities may not suit all persons as some duties can be onerous or unappealing (Teschendorf, Schwartz, Ferrans, O'Mara, & Sloan, 2007). In fact, research has shown that the caregiver's *perception* of the burden of caregiving, combined with his or her confidence in caregiving, has more impact on the caregiver's quality of life than the actual demands of the care itself (Tang, Li, & Chen, 2008).

People provide care based both on their relationship to the patient and their capacity to provide specific services. Litwak (1985) demonstrated the specificity of service delivery in his seminal work in aging, a principle that holds true for family caregiving as well; people provide service for which they are emotionally and physically prepared and when they know the service will be acceptable to the care recipient (Litwak, 1985). For example, family members who are adept at financial issues may provide help with accounting and banking, whereas others in the family may provide personal care and meal preparation.

Social theorists have attempted to explain family ties as part of a learned and shared value system. Attachments among kinship groups and the social integration within the web of the family unit are elements that contribute to the bonds that tie people to helping roles during illness and hardship. Emotional support is learned in this social context. Families provide examples of caring behavior and supportive interactions for children who reenact similar actions in later life. Bowlby (1969) introduced the idea of attachment theory, which suggests that kin provide a ring of protection or a sort of home base. During illness this secure base offers the patient the advantage of affectional bonds linking him to others who can meet his needs. Family members are often a key to the success of caregivers as well. Many of the difficulties that family caregivers encounter require affirmation of satisfactory decision making and reciprocity for assistance.

As people move through the life course, they continually add to the number of people in their social network and new members offer relevant sources of information, strength, and reinforcement. The expanding membership of the network is referred to as a *convoy* of social support (Antonucci & Akiyama, 1987). This means that some people could be the same age as the patient while others could be older or younger, a distinct advantage for an ill or disabled person. People of different ages and talents may enlist help unique to their own reference group. A convoy exists both for the patient and the family caregiver, often with differing membership for each. The cancer caregiver must be able to recruit resources in order to effectively provide the required care while retaining personal physical and emotional health.

Cultural groups differ regarding the expectations they have of the family member's obligation to provide care. For example, in Taiwan it is generally expected that family members, particularly children, will provide care in conformance to the Confucian ideal of filial piety (Tang et al., 2008). As a result, family caregivers provide care for 90% of dependent and chronically ill patients in Taiwan, as compared to an estimated 75% in the United States (Tang et al., 2008). The toll of care on the family can be significant, however. In a prospective, longitudinal study of 167 family caregivers in Taiwan, Tang and colleagues found that their quality of life deteriorated significantly as the patient's death approached (Tang et al., 2008). Similarly, depression was found to be prevalent among Korean family caregivers ($n = 310$); 67% had high depression scores, and 35% had very high depression scores. In this study, the perceived burden of care was the best predictor of depression (Rhee et al., 2008).

The Concept of Social Support

The classical literature describes social support as one of the primary methods that networks of people, bound by relationship, common values, and experience, influence the physical and mental health status of one another (Sarason, Sarason, & Pierce, 1990). The ways in which this happens stretch across many types of exchanges and constitute a rich interweaving of life experiences. Support can be measured as that which is received, that which is perceived to be available, or that which is given. All of these perspectives collectively represent the scope of a transaction offering and receiving help of some kind. In the case of the caregivers discussed in this chapter, the perspective is that of support given and the caregiver's personal reaction to its provision.

Caregiver Health Status and Models of Social Exchange

Caregiver personal health status changes and quality of life now form an intriguing line of new inquiry. Berkman and Glass (2000) proposed a model of upstream and downstream factors that influence the impact of social networks on the health status of a care recipient. The model could also be useful when considering the effect of caregiving on the caregiver's personal health status. At the macro level are the environmental factors, such as culture, policy, and socioeconomic factors in society. At the next level, the mezzo level, the social network factors, such as structure, number of social ties, reciprocity, and intimacy, influence the social mechanisms of supportive interactions. The third level, micro issues, includes those elements usually measured as social support: types of support available, social engagement, and social influence. The last portion of the model, at the downstream portal, depicts factors that impact health status through various pathways. The model is useful as it organizes a broad array of influences that should be considered when explaining outcomes of the social exchange. This expanded scope could enhance the potency and usefulness of findings.

A descriptive study of cancer caregivers found that primary personal health status concerns centered on emotional health, overload of responsibilities leading to fatigue, and lack of time for reflection, contemplation, and personal thought processes (Teschendorf et al., 2007.) Application of these concepts fits well into the downstream depiction of social network exchange and the effect on the caregiver's health.

Quality of Life of the Family Caregiver

The impact on the family caregiver's quality of life varies widely, based on the unique elements and demands of the caregiving situation. In this discussion we address the manner in which the illness of one person affects the quality of life of a family member who assumes the role of caregiver. Even though they are participating in a shared experience, healthcare providers need to clearly differentiate between the quality of life of the care recipient and that of the family caregiver. Perceived and self-reported outcomes of health care are now well developed for the person with cancer, but it is not as clear how the illness experience changes the lives of family members attending that patient. Quality of life for a caregiver may be especially affected by the shared illness experience with an oncology patient, as we have learned that caregivers also may become ill as a consequence of the work of caregiving (Schulz & Beach, 1999).

Conceptualizations of health-related quality of life (HRQOL) vary in scope, and Ferrans has categorized these definitions into three groups (Ferrans, 2005). The first group is comprised of HRQOL definitions that are quite specific with a narrow focus on dysfunction (e.g., sexual dysfunction) resulting from an illness and its treatment, and which are essentially negative in nature. The second category is comprised of somewhat broader definitions in that they focus on the negative impact of illness on other aspects of life, such as on a marital relationship. The third and broadest set of HRQOL definitions are those that include all aspects of an individual's life in the presence of an illness. These are the most comprehensive in that they explicitly include positive effects as well as the negative effects encompassed by the previous two categories. An example is the definition provided by Padilla and colleagues, who state that quality of life was a "personal, evaluative statement summarizing the positivity or negativity of attributes that characterize one's psychological, physical, social, and spiritual well-being at a point in time when health, illness, and treatment conditions are relevant" (Padilla, Grant, Ferrell, & Presant, 1996, p. 301). For example, some of the positive effects of caregiving, such as a sense of satisfaction and strengthening of relationships, would be considered as fitting into the third category of definitions of quality of life. It is this third category of HRQOL definitions that we recommend for characterizing the effect of caregiving on the caregiver's quality of life.

The factors that alter caregivers' assessment of their own quality of life are affected by their interpretation of the importance of illness events and of the change imposed in their own lives. If, for example, the person notes a dramatic redistribution in use of family income, he or she may perceive a change in personal quality of life. If he or she is overwhelmed by new information and tasks to perform, there may also be a report of diminished quality of life. Most importantly, the work of caregiving may alter the health status of the caregiver him or herself. In each case, it is the comparator that is important. The individual uses recall of a previous state and reports the outcome based on the comparison (Fayers & Machin, 2001; Rothman, Beltran, Cappelleri, Lipscomb, & Teschendorf, 2006).

The Diverse Roles of a Family Caregiver

Families provide a broad range of care tasks, such as physical care, transportation, symptom management, communication, and locating community services (Hinds, 1985; McDonald, Stetz, & Compton, 1996; Oberst, Thomas, Gass, & Ward, 1989). Several responsibilities gain importance at specific intervals. For example, transportation may be critical during treatment whereas personal care becomes important during advanced cancer. In addition to the delivery of direct care, family caregivers are caught up in the acquisition of information related to the disease and the requirements of treatment. Transitions in care and advancing illness may step up the pace and character of responsibilities, forcing families to include paid services if they are unable or unwilling to provide the care (Stetz & Brown, 1997; Stetz & Brown, 2004).

Seventy percent of caregivers report that their role is difficult (The National Profile of Caregivers in Canada, 2002). There are many reasons for this, partially because of the lack of preparation, but also due to the endless nature of the work with a progression of escalating responsibilities. Caregivers may feel overwhelmed by the responsibility, unappreciated by others, and may experience little time for themselves (Teschendorf et al., 2007). Terminology such as *caregiver burden* depicts the role as one with layers of responsibility and undesirable requirements of effort expended on behalf of another person (Given, Given, Strommel, Collins, King, & Franklin, 1992; Zarit, Reever, & Bach-Peterson, 1980). Yet, not all caregivers find the role to be burdensome, suggesting that the role can affirm personal values (Teschendorf et al., 2007). For those caregivers of patients diagnosed in late-stage cancer with functional decline, there may be extra responsibilities. The loss of physical function imposes more strain on the caregiver as resources for assistance must be assessed, help arranged, and overall care managed. The caregiver's time commitments may preclude regular work attendance or attention to other family commitments. Children may receive less parental guidance, and household duties may be delayed. Family caregivers are usually involved in medical decision making while providing emotional support to the patient. These caregivers are also exposed to the suffering of the patient, and in turn experience personal suffering as a result of their observations of severe illness (Hinds, 1985; Schulz, 2006; Tang et al., 2008). The caregivers become so engaged in the responsibilities of managing the care for their ill relative, as well as other life commitments, that they may not perceive decrements in personal quality of life until much later.

Advanced cancer escalates the commitment of a family caregiver and requires more comprehensive care tasks. Caring at the end of life can be particularly difficult as personal feelings of distress heighten, and emotional and physical overload may increase, particularly in isolated caregivers (Soothill et al., 2001). Most family caregivers manage the burden of their multiple demands, but approximately one third report significant distress, especially when caring for someone near the end of life (Weitzner, McMillan, & Jacobsen, 1999). At this juncture, the relationship of caregiver distress, demands of care, and physical function of the patient become paramount; caregiver distress increases as the patient's functional status diminishes and the caregiver burden increases (Dumont et al., 2006; Tang et al., 2008).

A Caregiver's Ability to Cope and Retain Quality of Life

Four major features of the caregiving experience directly affect a family caregiver's adjustment to the caregiver role, coping capacity, and ultimately their perception of quality of life when engaged in advanced cancer care: (1) high caregiving demands; (2) loss of caregiver physical health; (3) psychological distress of the caregiver; and (4) interference with other life roles. Most caregiver's lives are affected by each of these factors, and the work of designing effective educational interventions to address these topics is in its infancy. Part of the difficulty lies in the fact that individual caregiving situations and the needs of caregivers are quite varied, depending on the configuration of the family unit, age range, educational level, and general health status of caregivers prior to the time they commence caregiving.

High Caregiving Demands

The care situation itself imposes both physical and emotional challenges that most caregivers are under-prepared to manage (Glajchen, 2004). The high intensity of care and overtaxed support systems can strain caregivers and influence their health status (Barrett, 2004). The demand of caregiving is increased by patient characteristics such as functional disability, cognitive impairment, multiple unrelieved symptoms, and prolonged duration of the caregiving situation (Given & Sherwood, 2006). Strategies useful in helping to resolve or reduce caregiver demands include obtaining technical information, enhancing problem-solving skills, and maintaining physical stamina. Studies have found that educational approaches are effective in reducing caregiver anxiety and perceived life disruption, and improving caregiver self-acceptance, competence, and satisfaction (Salmon, Kwak, Acquaviva, Brandt, & Egan, 2005), while others have improved coping and enhanced confidence and problem solving (Cameron, Shin, Williams, & Stewart, 2004). Reduction in the perception of high demands may be as simple as learning to perform tasks more efficiently, for example, by using correct body mechanics to move a patient. Asking for help should not be perceived as an admission of diminished mastery of care skills but rather an attempt to attain new skill levels as physical care demands increase.

Loss of Caregiver Physical Health

Caregivers frequently ignore their personal health issues and focus their energy on attending to the patient's needs (Grunfeld et al., 2004). Loss of sleep and intense attention to care demands may induce feelings in the family caregiver of being overwhelmed or threaten their perceived competence and mastery over caring tasks (Coristine, Crooks, Grunfeld, Stonebridge, & Christie, 2003). Declining caregiver health status is highly correlated with demanding care tasks accompanied by altered patient behavioral changes, inability to eat, or inability to move independently. The intensity of care, the complexity of care, and the range of diverse tasks that are involved in the care of a very ill person may serve to overwhelm some family members and influence their personal health status. Caregivers often fail to arrange for personal preventive health care (e.g., mammograms) in deference to their commitment to caregiving. They may later be surprised and distressed to learn that they are also ill.

Psychological Distress of the Caregiver

Caregivers who experience combined high physical and emotional demands are particularly at risk of psychological distress; caregivers with low education levels are especially at risk of such distress (Barrett, 2004; Cameron et al., 2002; Alptekin, Gonullu, Yucel, & Yaris, 2009). Caregiver coping ability is influenced by observing the physical decline of the patient and dealing with the patient's suffering (Haley, 2003; Tang et al., 2008). The observation of suffering and the resulting anguish have been observed to be two of the most difficult aspects of being a family caregiver (Schulz, 2006). Caregivers have been found to experience decrements in quality of life (physical, psychological, social, and spiritual domains) that mirror that of the patient (Juarez, Ferrell, Uman, Podnos & Wagman, 2008; Northouse et al., 2007; Janda et al., 2007; Kim, Wellisch, & Spillers, 2008). Caregivers can even experience burden, anxiety, and depression to a greater degree than their ill family member (Grunfeld et al., 2004; Rhee et al., 2008). High burden of care can erode optimism and exhaust personal reserve over time.

Interference with Other Life Roles

Caregivers may miss work or work irregular hours when providing care at the end of life (Grunfeld et al., 2004). Younger caregivers may be stressed by the loss of their own productivity as they modify work schedules to care for a family member (Spillers, Wellisch, Kim, Matthews, & Baker, 2008). Additionally, out-of-pocket expenses may require reallocation of household funds, making it difficult to maintain usual activities (Haley, 2003). Finally, caregivers often limit their social interactions with others outside their family as they focus efforts on providing care to the ill family member, resulting in a decrement in their quality of life (Alptekin et al., 2009), and increasing the potential difficulty for reestablishing relationships later.

Learning to Perform Caregiving Tasks

The amount of time a caregiver spends each day or week with caregiving tasks varies by the stage of the ill family member's cancer at diagnosis; the treatment, symptoms, and side effect profiles; the functional status of the patient both prediagnosis and posttreatment; and, finally, the interval of the disease and treatment continuum. In a population-based study, female caregivers spent 50% more time providing care than male caregivers (Feinberg, 2003). Cancer caregivers may find that the intensity of caregiving peaks at specific time intervals in the disease trajectory. Caregiving may be less demanding early in the course of treatment, but during a relapse or at the end of life caregiving may become time and energy consuming as personal care tasks and use of technical equipment increase. The visiting nurse is essential as a teacher to help families organize and understand the work of caring for the patient and maintaining the equipment.

Mastery of the skills required to competently provide care to cancer patients is a serious dilemma for family caregivers. Discovering their needs and finding ways to enhance their skill level are addressed in a later section of this chapter. Most caregivers have little or no preparation for the tasks they perform, and although they may observe a procedure performed in the clinic, they may be unable to competently repeat the performance or display an understanding of the rationale for its use. Caregivers desire to offer competent care, but they rarely have access to the few courses or other resources related to caregiving tasks. In a report from the National Center on Caregiving/Family Caregiver Alliance, findings state that 38% of caregivers do not know how to change bandages or dressings; nearly 20% were never taught to operate the medical equipment in the home; and 16% indicate they do not know how to manage a drug and dosing schedule (Feinberg, 2003).

Professional staff often provide instruction and emotional support for family caregivers within their busy clinic schedules. Referrals to home care agencies may be beneficial in some situations, especially when more technical service delivery is required at the home. Resources on the Web are viable sources for families, yet few clinics distribute a list of reliable and relevant Web sites. (See Appendix A on page 241 for suggested books, materials, and Web sites for family caregiving assistance.)

Impact of Caregiving on Quality of Life

Early in the disease course (during diagnosis and initial treatment), few caregivers notice a change in their own quality of life. It is their schedule that is dramatically modified, causing them to alter their expectations for time, patience, and communication patterns. They may be required to obtain information, quickly become familiar with the disease, assist in decision making about the next steps in care plans, and provide assurance to the patient. The realization that they have become a family caregiver may not occur to them initially. The work of the caregiver in this phase of care is far less physically demanding, but it is essential and can be very emotionally taxing. Emotional strain during this period is usually related to the lack of familiarity with medical terminology, procedures, and the inability to predict the future.

As caregiving demands increase, their effects can extend into all domains of life, as identified by Ferrans (1996). For caregivers of patients with advanced cancer, the percentage of caregivers with high psychological distress has been found to be two to three times higher than in the general population (Dumont et al., 2006). Consistently across studies, caregiver strain and distress are key factors contributing to poor physical health for caregivers. Twenty-seven percent of the variance in health status has been explained by caregiver burden and stress alone (Sanford, Jounhson, & Townsend-Rocchiccioli, 2005). In a prospective population-based study, strained caregivers had significantly higher levels of depressive symptoms and anxiety, and lower levels of perceived health, compared with age and gender matched controls who were not caregivers (Schulz & Beach, 1999). In fact, caregivers with spousal loss were 63% more likely to die within 4 years than noncaregivers, even after adjusting for sociodemographic factors and comorbidities. A major factor attributed to the increased mortality was the caregivers' neglect of their own health needs. As compared with controls, they were less likely to get enough rest in general, to rest when they were sick, or have time to exercise. In addition, sleep disturbances, fatigue, backache, and headache are common problems experienced by caregivers (Sanford et al., 2005).

Social and economic domains are also affected by caregiving. Lifestyle interference has been found to be a unique correlate of emotional distress in caregivers (depression, tension, and mood disturbance), regardless of the amount of care provided (Cameron et al., 2002). When caregiving activities interfere with participation in valued activities and interests, such as work, recreation, and social outings, caregivers experience increased emotional distress (Cameron et al., 2002). The loss of personal freedom and time to sustain their other relationships can diminish a caregiver's perceived and self-reported quality of life. Conflict over the dual roles of caregiving and employment may produce feelings of guilt and worry about financial concerns (Teschendorf et al., 2007). Moreover, the economic impact of caregiving to a family can be considerable. In addition to lost hours from work, it has been estimated that the cost of informal caregiving for cancer patients translates to an average annual cost of over $1 billion nationally (Hayman et al., 2001).

Family relationships are particularly vulnerable to the strains of caregiving. Caregivers have reported feelings of guilt and inadequacy due to the inability to attend to the needs of other family members while providing care for one person (Teschendorf et al., 2007). Guilt compromises caregivers physically as well as psychologically, as shown by a study of 635 family caregivers of cancer patients (Spillers et al., 2008). In this study, guilt was associated with poorer physical, mental, and social functioning, in addition to greater psychological distress. Caregivers are often required to provide emotional support for the care recipient by keeping peace and providing an upbeat atmosphere, while receiving minimal personal reinforcement from other family members (Teschendorf et al., 2007). As some family members abdicate their responsibility for helping, additional physical care demands fall on the primary caregiver, resulting in anger and resentment (Teschendorf et al., 2007). This can produce high levels of distress, particularly for younger women who receive insufficient tangible and emotional support from others with caregiving tasks (Dumont et al., 2006; Spillers et al., 2008).

Despite the hardships, most caregivers express few regrets about the experience even if caring is more difficult than anticipated (Coristine et al., 2003; Teschendorf, Ferrans, O'Mara, Schwartz, & Sloan, 2005). Caregivers have reported an increased emotional closeness with the care recipient, as well as personal meaning and growth (Teschendorf et al., 2007). For some, caregiving provides an important opportunity to repay someone for taking care of them in the past (Teschendorf et al., 2005; Teschendorf et al., 2007). Reflection frequently enables new perspectives, shedding light on the positive aspects of providing life-sustaining help. Furthermore, caregivers who may have thought their role was difficult at the time they provided care often shift their assessment once the tasks are completed and care is no longer required. At this point, they may reflect on the positive value added to their own life experience.

Responding to Articulated Needs of Caregivers

Unmet needs of family caregivers have a direct, negative effect on the quality of care they deliver, which was clearly demonstrated in a study of 1662 cancer patients at the end of life (Park et al., 2009). Health professionals must listen carefully to the needs articulated by caregivers at all stages of the illness experience as their stories shape the very nature of successful health care and the design of interventions to resolve their problems. It has been said that caregivers do not know what they need to know; this holds true as each phase of care commences (Rabow, Hauser, & Adams, 2004). Families often have no knowledge of the disease process, the treatment course outcomes, and the ramifications for everyday life of the patient. The literature suggests that family caregivers want help for specific problems and have a strong desire to understand the medical issues.

The needs of caregivers, sometimes described as problems without clear solutions, usually focus on three key elements: information, emotional or psychological support, and instrumental support (Coleman, Avis, & Turin, 1990; Hileman et al., 1992). The most important and regularly reported item is information. This includes information about the disease, treatment, and the available sources for adequate services. Families vary in the way they utilize information and people to meet the needs of the patient. Capturing key information, for example, is often managed by one individual, not necessarily the primary caregiver. Information is often disseminated through multiple sources and modes. Content available through the Internet is not customized or tailored to address the specific needs of the individual patient or family and may actually interfere with dialogue with healthcare providers. Healthcare providers must ask questions that elicit topics essential for the caregiver to succeed at the point of care. Families want to know about effective treatments, symptoms and the underlying reasons for them, expectations for the future, and ways to enhance care management. New information needs to unfold gradually with questions about relapse, chances of a second tumor, strategies to reassure the patient, and ways to reduce personal stress (Hileman et al., 1992).

Providing for the psychosocial needs of caregivers is critically important, because if unmet, these needs are strong predictors of poor mental health, not only during the time of diagnosis and treatment, but for years afterward (Kim, Kashy, Spillers, & Evans, 2009). Caregiver concerns about their own emotional equilibrium often increase as they provide emotional reassurance and support decisions (Northouse, 1984; Stetz, 1989). These efforts require learning new approaches for self assurance. The emotional strain may diminish the effectiveness of caregiver functioning; for example, long periods of illness and metastatic disease may induce increasing caregiver distress (Coristine et al., 2003). Caregivers who perceive accessible support experience a buffering of the negative aspects of caregiving, helping them adjust to daily demands (Kornblith et al., 2001). Reassurance regarding the future is important as caregivers find the course of cancer treatment to be highly unpredictable (Osse, Vernooij-Dassen, Schlade, & Grol, 2006). Interventions designed to help caregivers manage their emotional distress, find meaning in the caregiving experience, and promote supportive family relationships can contribute to improved quality of life, even years after the caregiving period is over (Kim et al., 2009).

The caregiver role requires learning new ways to deliver tangible help to perform tasks during initial diagnosis and as treatment ends (Brown & Stetz, 1999; Hileman et al., 1992). The need for instrumental assistance is most evident during recurrence or at the end of life when functional changes may impose more personal care tasks, and require learning about medical procedures, medications, and responses to various treatments. Caregivers may assume responsibility for reporting symptoms, need for medication changes, or other sequelae of treatment and disease (Anderson, Shapiro, Farrar, Crespin, & Wells-DiGregorio, 2005).

Each phase of care introduces new concerns for both the patient and caregiver. Problems must be overcome, perceived deficiencies of information must be addressed, and skill or emotional coping capacity must be sustained or enhanced. Identification of family caregiver needs is the foundation for the development of targeted interventions to alleviate role stress. Important questions remain about how to create effective sources of assistance that are acceptable to families. Several caregiver needs and primary concerns are highlighted (Feinberg, 2003; Osse et al., 2006; Teschendorf et al., 2005) in Figure 10-1.

Glajchen (2004) pointed out the importance of assessing caregiver needs prior to offers of an intervention. Part of the assessment question is based on who must complete the process, a professional who can then provide referral and advice or a family caregiver who can self-assess and independently find resources. The variation in age, personal competence, and the degree of care recipient all need to play into the response to these questions. Caregivers with the highest demand to provide complex care will very likely need to be formally assessed by a healthcare professional, whereas those who have less demanding roles may be able to self-assess. All family caregivers should be encouraged to self-refer to a healthcare provider when they recognize that they are beginning to feel overwhelmed or stressed.

Caregivers desire information to satisfy specific needs:

- Information on what to expect through stages of the cancer disease trajectory
- Information that is arranged and easily identified by stage of disease
- Information on how to access and negotiate the healthcare system
- Information on how to obtain reliable and factual information (Internet sources)
- Information on what to expect for normal reactions to cancer during the illness
- Information on warning signs that spell trouble for relapse of the cancer or symptoms

Other support needs identified by caregivers:

- Learning about coping strategies that are most effective; discovering coping strategies that work for other people
- How to address children's needs; multigenerational households must address the caregiving scope of responsibilities.
- How to improve family communication in order to increase support for all

Figure 10-1. **Caregiver primary concerns.**
Source: Based on: Teschendorf et al., 2006; Osse et al., 2006

Assessment of Caregiver Needs, Quality of Life, and the Impact of Service Delivery

Caregiver Assessment

Understanding the needs of caregivers is critical to providing any healthcare or health status assessment. Once the needs are pinpointed, goals must be developed either by the professional staff or by the caregiver. Following a logical progression, strategies to meet the needs and satisfy the goals are part of the planning process, and, finally, to refer to effective interventions. Using validated instruments is important to ascertain the effectiveness and credibility of the service provision and evaluation of outcomes.

Questions arise as to whether we can easily identify those who are in distress. It has been estimated that only about 17% of cancer caregivers are in distress, and some caregivers are unaware of the vulnerabilities that lead to a distressed state (The National Profile of Caregivers in Canada, 2002). Studies have shown that distress and depression increase with the burden of care, and this burden changes over time (Rhee et al., 2008; Tang et al., 2008). Posing practical questions that may drive an algorithm for decision making, with tools appropriate for the use of a family member, could assist caregivers to identify not only their problems and needs but perhaps some solutions. This sort of project would have practical application that could assist large numbers of caregivers.

Shultz (2006) identified linkages between transitions in the health status of an ill family member and distress in the family caregiver in a large study of caregivers. For example, family caregivers do not get relief from their distress when the ill family member is placed in a nursing home, because they continue to provide emotional support and some physical care. Only when the ill family member dies do family caregivers report being relieved of responsibilities and having an improvement in their own health status.

There are limited tools, few online resources, and a lack of understanding among clinicians regarding the ways in which support for the caregiver may impact the health status of the patient. Components of a comprehensive caregiver assessment could be done by professional staff if the needed resources were available. A comprehensive list of these elements was assembled by the Family Caregiver Alliance following a "think tank" meeting in 2005 (Feinberg, 2005). The resulting recommendations appear in their entirety in Table 10-1 (Family Caregiver Alliance, 2006).

Table 10-1. **Elements of Caregiver Assessment**

	Components for Assessment
Environmental context	• Caregiver relationship to care recipient • Physical environment • Household members—number • Financial status, economic issues • Quality of family relationships • Duration of caregiving • Employment status of primary caregiver • Network assessment • Social support available
Caregiver's perception of health, symptoms, and functional status of care recipient	• Activities of daily living and assistance required • Instrumental activities of daily living • Psychosocial needs • Medical tests, procedures required
Caregiver/recipient values and preferences	• Caregiver ability to assume care • Care recipient willingness to receive care • Perceived filial obligation to provide care • Culturally based norms • Preferences for scheduling and delivery of care • Communication capabilities/exchange
Caregiver personal health status and well-being	• Self-reported health • Past medical conditions, disability • Depression, mental health history • Degree of optimism • Life satisfaction • Self-assessed quality of life

continues

Table 10-1. **Elements of Caregiver Assessment (continued)**

	Components for Assessment
Consequences of caregiving	• Perceived challenges/difficulties • Social isolation/connectedness • Work strain, perceived burden of care • Financial strain • Family relationship strain • Perceived benefits • Satisfaction of helping family member • Developing new skills and competencies
Skills/abilities/knowledge to provide care recipient with needed care	• Caregiving confidence, competencies, mastery • Knowledge of medical care tasks
Potential resources for caregiver	• Helping network and perceived social support • Coping strategies • Information sources • Financial resources • Community resources and services

Source: Adapted from Feinberg, 2005.

Measurement of Caregiver Quality of Life

In addition to questions about the best method for assessing the needs of cancer caregivers, questions also remain about measuring the effect of caregiving on the quality of life of the family caregiver, and the effect of services provided to assist the caregivers. Caregivers have been shown to be capable of self-assessment of their health status and quality of life (Teschendorf, Ferrans, Moinpour, O'Mara, Schwartz, & Sloan, in preparation; Teschendorf et al., 2007;), using a new prototype instrument for caregivers. (See Appendix B: Caregiver QOL Self-Assessment Scale on page 241.) Several other instruments have been developed based on clinical and community research (Berg-Weger, Rubio, & Tebb, 2000; Deeken, Taylor, Mangan, Yabroff, & Ingham, 2003; Weitzner, Jacobsen, Wagner, & Friedland, 1999; Given et al., 1992; Weitzner & McMillan, 1999). Quality-of-life outcome assessment tools and some needs assessment tools are shown in Table 10-2. These instruments were developed for research purposes and are not readily accessible to caregivers either for reference or for use as a personal log of well-being. Several of the instruments could be adapted for caregiver self-report and could be placed into a Web site designed for family caregivers. The original purpose of the instrument shown in Appendix B was to enable caregivers to track their own quality-of-life changes in a Web-based tool. Caregivers who participated in the development phase supported the concept and indicated a desire to track their own well-being.

Table 10-2. Caregiver Quality-of-Life Assessment Scales and Self-Reported Outcomes

Instrument	Publication	Domain/Primary Purpose	Psychometrics
Caregiver Self-Assessment Questionnaire	Health risks of caregiving. (2003, November). *AMA News*. Editorial.	A series of questions are listed with possible dichotomous responses (*yes* or *no*). The final two questions require that the person rate stress and personal health status on a scale of one to ten. A comment section follows. The instrument was developed by a professional committee for use in physician's office practices. Intended for use with many diseases but not specific to cancer.	Minimal psychometric information available at this time. Developed instrument based on selected questions of other instruments, then tested with focus groups. Later used the instrument with 100 caregivers of persons with various diseases. Used correlations and factor analysis.
Caregiver Quality-of-Life Scale—Cancer	Weitzner, M. A., Jacobsen, P. B., Wagner, H., & Friedland, J. (1999). The Caregiver Quality of Life Index-Cancer (CQOLC) scale: Development and validation of an instrument to measure quality of life of the family caregiver of patients with cancer. *Quality of Life Research, 8*, 55–63. Weitzner, M. A., & McMillan, S. C. (1999). The Caregiver Quality of Life Index-Cancer (CQOLC) scale: Revalidation in a home hospice setting. *J Palliative Care, 15*(2), 13–20.	The instrument was developed for research, but the author speculates that it could also be used clinically. It has 35 items with Likert response categories ranging from zero (not at all) to four (very much). Domains included in the scale are burden, disruptiveness, positive adaptation, and financial concerns. Scoring procedures are provided.	Reliability: Internal consistency high alpha coefficients ranging form 0.73 to 0.90. Test–retest coefficients are also high ranging from 0.82 to 0.94. Convergent validity was tested using the SF-36. Significance was found for all of the domains with mental composite score on the SF-36. Positive adaptation was not significant.

continues

Table 10-2. Caregiver Quality-of-Life Assessment Scales and Self-Reported Outcomes (continued)

Instrument	Publication	Domain/Primary Purpose	Psychometrics
The Caregiver Reaction Assessment (CRA)	Given, C. W., Given, B., Strommel, M., Collins, C., King, S., & Franklin, S. (1992). The caregiver reaction assessment (CRA) for caregivers to persons with chronic physical and mental impairment. *Research in Nursing & Health, 15,* 271–283 Nijboer, C., Triemstra, M., et al. (1999). Measuring both negative and positive reactions to giving care to cancer patients: Psychometric qualities of the Caregiver Reaction Assessment. *Social Science & Medicine, 48,* 1259–1269.	Instrument is from author B. Given. It is a 24-item instrument designed to measure reactions of people caring for older people with variety of illnesses. The authors hoped to advance research into caregiver burden by refining the measures and comparing across illnesses. The instrument measures both negative and positive aspects of caregiving within five domains: caregiver esteem, lack of family support, impact on finances, impact on schedule, and impact on personal health. Rating scale is a 5-point scale (strongly agree to strongly disagree). The instrument is not cancer specific but has been used with families of cancer patients.	Reliability: Internal consistency measured by Cronbach's alpha was high across all of the domains (0.80 to 0.90). Scales show stability over time as the instrument was tested at 6 and 12 months. Validity: Content validity tested using comparative items from other scales and subjected to exploratory and confirmatory analysis. Construct validity was supported through comparison with CES-D and ADL scales. Clinical relevance: the instrument has been used effectively with people with Alzheimer's disease, several physical impairments, and cancer. Authors suggest that instrument could be used in face-to-face interview format, as a telephone interview, or self-administered. It has also been translated into Dutch.

Table 10-2. continued

Instrument	Publication	Domain/Primary Purpose	Psychometrics
Caregiver Assistance Scale and Caregiver Impact Scale	Cameron, J. I., Franche, R. L., Cheung, A. M., & Stewart, D. E. (2002). Lifestyle interference and emotional distress in family caregivers of advanced cancer patients. *Cancer*, 94(2), 521–527.	Instruments attached to article with correspondence with author. The Caregiver Assistance instrument measures the amount of assistance the caregiver provides to the recipient. Numeric ratings range from zero (none) to six (a lot). Domains include instrumental, IADL and ADL elements, emotional support, communication, health monitoring, and medication management. The Caregiving Impact Scale measures the degree to which the caregiving responsibilities interfere with personal aspects of life. Domains are covered by specific questions about personal health, diet, employment, household work, recreation, finances, relationship to spouse, sex life, other social relations, religious expression, and civic involvement. A 7-point Likert scale was used with ratings ranging from zero (not at all) to six (very much).	Small group (n = 44) of family caregivers participated in a single structured quantitative interview to develop the instrument. The Caregiver Assistance instrument was developed for use in this study and has not been validated elsewhere. The Caregiving Impact Scale was a modification of the Illness Intrusiveness Rating Scale by Devins (1983). Although the instruments have some appeal, evidence of strong psychometric properties are absent and thus author would eliminate these instruments from the list of potentially adoptable instruments. The authors discuss the limitations of the study and pose the idea that anticipatory grief could correlate with emotional distress, but it was not measured.

continues

Table 10-2. Caregiver Quality-of-Life Assessment Scales and Self-Reported Outcomes (continued)

Instrument	Publication	Domain/Primary Purpose	Psychometrics
Home Caregiver Need Survey	Hileman, J. W., & Lackey, N. R. (1990). Self-identified needs of patients with cancer at home and their home caregivers: A descriptive study. *Oncology Nursing Forum, 17*(6), 907–913. Hileman, J. W., Lackey, N. R., & Hassanein, R. S. (1992). Identifying the needs of home caregivers of patients with cancer. *Oncology Nursing Forum, 19*(5), 771–777.	90-item instrument: This is a five-page needs survey instrument that assesses each need in two ways: how important the need is at the moment, and how satisfied the respondent is at the present. Domains include: information needs, household needs, patient care needs, personal needs, spiritual needs, and psychological needs. Most important needs for caregivers were informational and psychological. Designed for use in the clinic and for research. *The instrument is most suited to measure caregiver needs, not QOL.*	Small sample was used to develop instrument (*n* = 30), qualitative methods used to identify themes and domains. A second study used 492 home caregivers to establish validity of the instrument. Principle factor analysis used to determine need categories; focus on the "importance" scores as they were viewed as most stable. Correlations demonstrated that when patient activity level decreased, a caregiver's psychological, personal, and household needs increased. Internal consistency using Cronbach's alpha demonstrated high coefficients (0.96 to 0.87).
Appraisal of Caregiving Scale	Oberst, M. T., Thomas, S. E., Gass, K. A., & Ward, S. E. (1989). Caregiving demands and appraisal of stress among family caregivers. *Cancer Nursing, 12*(4), 209–215.	The instrument was developed using 47 family members of people receiving radiotherapy. The scale is a 72-item self-report scale designed to measure the caregiver's perception of the intensity of the caregiving experience. It includes five domains. Topics of the domains focus on caregiver tasks, relationships, interpersonal support, lifestyle, emotional/	The authors established face validity using six clinical experts. Internal consistency ratings using Cronbach's alpha demonstrated high coefficients (0.77 to 0.91). The correlations were displayed for illness variables and caregiver variables and demonstrated little significance. Caregiver load scales were presented as means with SD; the highest load was for

Table 10-2. continued

Instrument	Publication	Domain/Primary Purpose	Psychometrics
		physical health, and impact on the person. Response on 5-point scale (very true to very untrue). *Instrument is focused on the instrumental tasks and may not be appropriate for QOL.*	transportation followed by emotional support.
Caregiver Well-Being Scale	Berg-Weger, M., Rubio, D. M., & Tebb, S. S. (2000). The caregiver well-being scale revisited. *Health & Social Work, 25*(4), 255–263. Tebb, S. S. (1995). An aid to empowerment: A caregiver well-being scale. *Health & Social Work, 20,* 87–92.	Scale development used a small (n = 144) sample size to use the instrument in a second round of data collection. The initial development was done by Tebb in 1995. Scale combines the ideas of Maslow's hierarchy of needs and caregiver tasks. May be useful for clinical pre-intervention screening. Scale has 45 items. Instrument developed for clinical use, covers caregiver needs and activities involved in the caregiving role. Domains of the activities form include time for self/leisure, maintenance of functions outside the home, available family support, household maintenance, and household tasks. Responses use a 5-point scale rated as *never* to *almost always*. *Instrument may not be suitable for some domains of caregiver QOL.*	Authors speculate on the usefulness of the scale. It lacks comprehensive validation. Reliability was stated as 0.94 and the criterion and construct validity were reported to be within acceptable limits. Authors used factor analysis for basic needs (BN) and activities of living (AOL). Construct validity was demonstrated by the study authors through convergent and discriminant validity testing.

continues

Table 10-2. Caregiver Quality-of-Life Assessment Scales and Self-Reported Outcomes (continued)

Instrument	Publication	Domain/Primary Purpose	Psychometrics
FAMCARE Scale	Kristjanson, L. J. (1993). Validity and reliability testing of the FAMCARE scale: Measuring family satisfaction with advanced cancer care. *Social Science & Medicine, 36*(5), 693–701.	Scale designed to measure family satisfaction with advanced cancer care. Four subscales are included: information giving, availability of care, psychosocial care, and physical patient care. Scale uses a Likert response ranging from *very satisfied* to *very dissatisfied*. Focus on satisfaction. *Instrument not suitable for measuring caregiver QOL.*	Internal cocsistency measured using Cronbach's alpha with coefficients of 0.93. Test–retest correlation of 0.91 and satisfactory criterion validity. Cluster analysis suggests four subdimensions.
Inventory of Needs (FIN)	Kristjanson, L. J., Atwood, J. A., & Degner, L. F. (1995). Validity and reliability of the family inventory of needs: Measuring the care needs of families of advanced cancer patients. *J Nursing Mgt, 3*(2), 109–126.	Ratings from zero to ten of how important the item is to the respondent, and whether the need was met or unmet. This is a 20-item instrument with focus on needs. *Instrument not suitable for measuring caregiver QOL.*	Cronbach's alpha for internal consistency was 0.80: construct validity tested with principal component analysis. Construct validity assessed with predictive modeling in regression analyses.

Currently, there are no instruments developed specifically to assess the impact of providing services to assist caregivers. A model to guide potential service delivery for family caregivers would include information on the effect of the following: economic stressors (e.g., loss of income, diminished savings); emotional stressors (e.g., anticipatory grief, depression, exhaustion, frustration); social costs of caregiving (e.g., loss of relationships, loss of social contact, altered family support); physical care and impact on personal health (e.g., exhaustion, injury, lack of respite care).

Self-Care for Caregivers

There are a number of options available for caregivers to obtain help in maintaining their own health status. E-health interventions are being developed but may lack an evidence base at this point. Several Web sites provide information about the caregiving process and link to other sites with resources. (See Appendix A on page 241 for suggested Web sites for family caregiving assistance.) Support groups in the community setting are diverse and not universally available for any of the usual approaches (e.g., telephone, face-to-face, Web-based). The Wellness Community, a nonprofit organization that provides free education and support services to people with cancer and their families runs a variety of support groups and should be explored as one possible source.

Social support for family and friends of the ill person could be encouraged through information dissemination at community and hospital resource centers. Books, written information, and verbal guidance could also be made available to encourage families to distribute the workload of caregiving over several people rather than reliance on one person. Distribution of tasks can be done using a match-up of task list and availability of family or friends for each of the tasks. Learning to delegate to other members of the family or social network is an important skill. Developing tools to match the task to the person will be helpful. The task list has been advocated because it is one method for each family member to visualize the work needed for the care of a patient and sign up for those components that best match individual skills (Foley, 2004).

Maintenance of caregiver personal health status is one key to a lasting relationship with the care recipient and the remaining family. Exercise and health promotion programs should also be encouraged through the use of a task list. Family members could take turns providing care, releasing the primary caregiver from duty and giving time for exercise. The ability to distribute work over the entire family unit spares the primary caregiver effort and feelings of guilt by offering opportunities to address other personal issues such as health care or social exchange. Caregivers who maintain annual appointments with their physicians for surveillance and monitoring of health status as well as regular dental visits for cleaning and check-ups have an easier time retaining their health over time.

Learning through formal education processes to alleviate caregiver needs is an ideal goal. Classes in caregiving methods could be offered through home care agencies similar to home health aide training. Financing for such a class remains undetermined, but there is expertise available to conduct the effort. An experimental program is underway in Vermont to pay informal or family caregivers who assist in keeping older persons on Medicaid at home. It appears to be a cost-effective model in the first year, however it is highly reliant on rural family networks for implementation (Basler, 2006).

A survey of caregivers identified solutions to caregiver problems based on responses to a series of preference-based questions (Naiditch, 2006). The highest ranking topics that caregivers said they would very likely use included the following: an expert to call 24 hours a day at a toll-free number to talk about stress and other caregiving issues, so that the caregiver does not feel alone (35%); a mobile health service that comes to the caregiver's neighborhood, with services such as blood tests, blood pressure monitoring, flu shots, or eye exams (33%); and someone who helps the caregiver identify tasks that other family members or friends could perform and thus save some time for the primary caregiver (19%). Apparently families are already aware of their priorities for help with the work of providing care, the professionals need only listen to their ideas and develop ways to meet the needs.

Educational Intervention Research to Support Family Caregivers

Interest in the development of caregiver educational interventions is growing, and with it expanding anticipation of finding effective interventions that can alleviate stress on caregivers (McMillan, 2005). Interventions reported since 2000 have used recommendations gleaned from earlier research. The interventions thought to have the greatest effect target learning and skill development (Grahn & Danielson, 1996; Harding et al., 2004; Harding & Higginson, 2003; Keefe et al., 2005; Nijboer, Tempelaar, Triemstar, van den Bos, & Sanderman, 2001).

The following discussion addresses a small number of reported education interventions. Two themes dominate educational interventions: learning new skills and developing psychological support. Nursing interventions designed to provide opportunities to learn new information are often aimed at proficiency applied to caring skills though education, counseling, and palliative care (Pasacreta & McCorkle, 2000). Psycho-educational interventions attempt to influence behavior; they provide information based on a social-cognitive theory to modify thinking or cognitive patterns, behaviors, and coping strategies. Several interventions in this discussion address the intent to modify behavior, increase knowledge, and improve self-efficacy and problem solving (Grahn & Danielson, 1996).

Information helps to diminish the patient's feeling of inadequacy when knowledge is deficient (Fawzy, 1995). Reinforcing knowledge is thought to be a viable intervention strategy to address caregiver insecurity and fear. Gagnon (2002) utilized the idea to design a caregiver educational intervention delivered by nurses in Canadian palliative care settings. Although the study did not randomize caregivers, a comparison group was used. The intervention group reported being better prepared to make care decisions with the information they received.

Educational programs for family caregivers have also improved the technical competence of caregivers and increased their confidence in performing caregiving tasks (Pascreta, Barg, Nuamah, & McCorkle, 2000). Giarelli and colleagues (2003) intervened with wives of men with prostate cancer who were unprepared for the caregiver role. The intervention offered phased in components of post-operative management information as well as some guidance for emotional adaptation. Although there was not a statistical difference in the groups, wives in the intervention group rated their information preparedness higher over time than did wives in the control group. In another brief problem-solving intervention using a pre–post test design, improved confidence and problem solving were demonstrated following a home care intervention that included a written guide and telephone follow-up (Cameron et al., 2004).

Psycho-educational interventions were shown in a meta-analysis to be effective in increasing knowledge and abilities, especially when directing the intervention at very specific outcomes of knowledge change (Sorensen, Pinquart, & Duberstein, 2002). Sorenson and other investigators concluded that interventions can succeed in increasing caregiver's perceived well-being, knowledge, and ability to perform care tasks, especially if the outcomes are focused on a single and very specific domain such as well-being, satisfaction, or knowledge. (Bultz, Speca, Brasher, Geggie, & Page, 2000; Kozachik et al., 2001; Ostroff, Ross, Steinglass, Ronis-Tobin, & Singh, 2004; Sorensen et al., 2002). Studies, especially those involving end-of-life care, often have problems with accrual, retention, or attrition (Kozachik et al., 2001; Ostroff et al., 2004; Kurtz et al., 2005;); dose and exposure issues (Ostroff et al., 2004); lack of clear patient-reported outcomes; and measures of effectiveness (Kozachik et al., 2001). As intervention research matures, it would be beneficial to identify which interventions work best for specific groups of caregivers or for intervals in the caregiver's career.

There is mounting evidence that educational interventions are effective in certain situations to decrease distress, improve problem-solving skills, improve care provided by family caregivers, and improve the well-being of families. Promising results are exemplified by a few studies using randomized designs discussed in this section, and also discussed in a comprehensive review (Northouse, 2005).

Although findings are inconsistent from one type of intervention to another, there is demonstrated positive change in many outcomes. Caregivers responded to a multi-faceted intervention with core content designed to inform and support during the recurrence of cancer (Northouse, Kershaw, Mood, & Schafenacher, 2005). The intervention was designed to enhance family involvement and support feelings of optimism while improving coping. The intervention group decreased their negative appraisal, including less hopelessness at 3 months, but gains were lost by 6 months. The time interval covered by the study included periods of changing health status for patients, perhaps explaining the loss of gains in appraisal. The investigators suggested that future studies needed to consider dose response for psycho-social interventions and include outcome measures that are sensitive to more subtle changes.

A randomized controlled trial designed to improve coping skills through a training course for caregivers reported modest success (McMillan et al., 2006). The study aimed to improve caregiver quality of life and mastery with an intervention delivering expert information on problems the patient experienced. The information provided a rationale for treatment, and although effective in improving quality of life and decreasing the burden of caring for symptoms, mastery was not affected. The study results are encouraging because they verified that caregivers are able to absorb and use new information, even in the stress of a hospice setting.

Many intervention studies focus on improving caregiver skills and problem solving, yet others focus on mental health outcomes. A feasibility study designed as a psycho-educational intervention for partners of breast cancer patients resulted in diminished mood disturbance, greater confidence, and improved caregiving communication among participants (Bultz et al., 2000). Some interventions designed to modify depressive episodes have not had positive results (Kozachik et al., 2001; Ostroff et al., 2004) while others report minimal changes (Kurtz et al., 2005). Selection of more targeted outcome measures is important as new studies are designed. Although the majority of new interventions will undoubtedly focus on the primary caregiver, it will be increasingly important to consider the effect of caregiving on the entire family unit. The financial and social implications of caregiving work extend well beyond the primary caregiver; omission of other family members could skew acceptance and effectiveness of future programs.

Health Policy and Implications for Future Caregiving in Oncology

Several advocacy groups are working to improve the lives of cancer caregivers, and the strides they make each year capture the attention of lawmakers. One relatively new focus is to increase the attention of healthcare professionals on caregiver assessment, caregiver health needs, and the effect on the overall health status of the patient. Another effort is to improve the access of caregiver reimbursement, making it possible for some families to provide care without the concomitant loss of personal income. There was considerable interest generated at the federal level in 2006 as evidenced by the proclamation by President Bush (see Appendix C on page 246). Although there is as yet no substantive change in policy, service delivery, or reimbursement for caregiving, it is important that these issues have risen to a level of recognition or awareness, which is the first step in policy agenda change.

CONCLUSION

Few would argue that family caregivers do not need more help, but the issues are not easily resolved. Family assistance can be expensive and, short of new allocations for this purpose, the healthcare system is highly reliant on the good will of individual caregivers, family, friends, and neighbors. New demonstration projects related to service delivery have emerged in the form of navigator programs, guiding families to resources. When there are no community resources and families are distant, these programs may be insufficient. New ideas for rewarding individuals with time and the capacity to provide care will emerge once we learn more about the effectiveness of specific interventions and the situations in which they work best. While we await future solutions it will be important to continue to fund family caregiver research, especially intervention research and new program development, with detailed evaluation.

REFERENCES

Alptekin, S., Gonullu, G., Yucel, I., & Yaris, F. (2009). Characteristics and quality of life analysis of caregivers of cancer patients [Epub ahead of print]. *Medical Oncology*.

Anderson, B. L., Shapiro, C. L., Farrar, W. B., Crespin, T., & Wells-DiGregorio, S. (2005). Psychological responses to cancer recurrence: A controlled prospective study. *Cancer, 104*(7), 1540–1547.

Andresen, E., (2006, September). Caregiver health as a public health issue. *Proceedings of Public Health of Caregiving*. Washington, DC: The Urban Institute.

Antonucci, T., & Akiyama, H. (1987). Social networks in adult life and a preliminary examination of the convoy model. *Journal of Gerontology, 42*, 519–527.

Barrett, L. (2004). *Caregiving in the United States*. Washington, DC: AARP & National Alliance for Caregiving.

Basler, B. (2006, December). Vermont's Caregiving Program Spells Success. *AARP Bulletin*.

Berg-Weger, M., Rubio, D. M., & Tebb, S. S., (2000). The caregiver well-being scale revisited. *Health & Social Work, 25*(4), 255–263.

Berkman, L. F., & Glass, T. (2000). Social integration, social networks, social support, and health. In L. F. Berkman & I. Kawachi (Eds.). *Social Epidemiology*. New York, NY: Oxford University Press.

Bowlby, J. (1969). Attachment and loss. *Attachment* (Vol. 1). London: Hogarth Press.

Brown, M. A., & Stetz, K. (1999). The labor of caregiving: A theoretical model of caregiving during potentially fatal illness. *Qualitative Health Research, 9*(2), 182–197.

Bultz, B. D., Speca, M., Brasher, P. M., Geggie, P. H., & Page, S. A. (2000). A randomized controlled trial of a brief psycho-educational support group for partners of early stage breast cancer patients. *Psycho-oncology, 9*(4), 303–313.

Cameron, J. I., Franche, R. L., Cheung, A. M., & Stewart, D. E. (2002). Lifestyle interference and emotional distress in family caregivers of advanced cancer patients. *Cancer, 94*(2), 521–527.

Cameron, J. I., Shin, J. L., Williams, D., & Stewart, D. E., (2004). A brief problem solving intervention for family caregivers to individuals with advanced cancer. *Journal of Psychosomatic Research, 57*(2), 137–143.

Coleman, S. B., Avis, J. M., & Turin, M. (1990). The study of the role of gender in family therapy training. *Family Process, 29*(4), 365–374.

Coristine, M., Crooks, D., Grunfeld, E., Stonebridge, C., & Christie, A. (2003). Caregiving for women with advanced breast cancer. *Psycho-oncology, 12*, 709–719.

Deeken, J. F., Taylor, K. L., Mangan, B. S., Yabroff, K. R., & Ingham, J. M. (2003). Care for the caregivers: A review of self-reported instruments developed to measure the burden, needs, and quality of life of informal caregivers. *Journal of Pain & Symptom Management, 26*(4), 922–953.

Dumont, S., Turgeon, J., Allard, P., Gagnon, P., Charbonneau, C., & Vezina, L. (2006). Caring for a loved one with advanced cancer: Determinants of psychological distress in family caregivers. *Journal of Palliative Medicine, 9*(4), 912–921.

Emanuel, E. J., Fairclough, D.L., Slutsman, J., Alpert, H., Baldwin, D., & Emanuel, L.I., (1999). Assistance from family members, friends, paid care givers, and volunteers in the care of terminally ill patients. *New England Journal of Medicine, 341*(13), 956–963.

Family Caregiver Alliance. (2006). *Caregivers count too! A toolkit to help practitioners assess the needs of family caregivers*. San Francisco, CA: Author.

Fawzy, F. L. (1995). A short-term psychoeducational intervention for patients newly diagnosed with cancer. *Supportive Care in Cancer, 3*(4), 235–238.

Fayers, P. M, & Machin, D. (2001). Clinical interpretation. *Quality of life: Assessment, analysis, and interpretation*. New York, NY: John Wiley & Sons.

Feinberg, L. F. (2003). *Family caregiving and public policy: Principles for change*. San Francisco, CA: National Center on Caregiving/Family Caregiver Alliance.

Feinberg, L. F. (2005, September). Fundamental principles for caregiver assessment. Proceedings of National Consensus Development Conference for Caregiver Assessment. San Francisco, CA: Family Caregiver Alliance.

Ferrans, C. E. (1996). Development of a conceptual model of quality of life. *Scholarly Inquiry for Nursing Practice, 10*(3), 293–304.

Ferrans, C. E., (2005). Definitions and conceptual models of quality of life. In J. Lipscomb, C. Gotay, & C. Snyder (Eds.), *Outcomes assessment in cancer: Measures, methods, and applications.* New York, NY: Cambridge University Press.

Foley, K., (Ed.) Back, A., Bruera, E., Coyle, N., Loscalzo, M. J., Shuster, J. L., Teschendorf, B., et al. (2004). *When the Focus is on Care: Palliative Care and Cancer.* Atlanta, GA: American Cancer Society.

Gagnon, P. (2002). Delirium in advanced cancer: A psychoeducational intervention for family caregivers. *Journal of Palliative Care, 18*(4), 253–261.

Given, C. W., Given, B., Strommel, M., Collins, C., King, S., & Franklin, S. (1992). The caregiver reaction assessment (CRA) for caregivers to persons with chronic physical and mental impairment. *Research in Nursing & Health, 15,* 271–283.

Given, B., & Sherwood, P. (2006). Family care for the older person with cancer. *Seminars in Oncology Nursing, 22*(1), 43–50.

Giarelli, E., McCorkle, R., & Monturo, C. (2003). Caring for a spouse after prostate surgery: The preparedness needs of wives. *Journal of Family Nursing, 9*(4), 453–485.

Glajchen, M. (2004). The emerging role and needs of family caregivers in cancer care. *Journal of Supportive Oncology, 2*(2), 145–155.

Grahn, G., & Danielson, M. (1996). Coping with the cancer experience, II: Evaluating an education and support program for cancer patients and their significant others. *European Journal of Cancer Care, 5*(3), 182–187.

Grunfeld, E., Coyle, D., Whelan, T., Clinch, J., Reyno, L., Earle, C. C., et al. (2004). Family caregiver burden: Results of a longitudinal study of breast cancer patients and their principal caregivers. *CMAJ, 170* (12, 1811–1812).

Haley, W. E. (2003). Family caregivers of elderly patients with cancer: Understanding and minimizing the burden of care. *Journal of Supportive Care, 1*(4, Suppl. 2), 25–29.

Harding, R., & Higginson, I. J. (2003). What is the best way to help caregivers? A systematic literature review of interventions and their effectiveness. *Palliative Medicine, 17*(1), 63–74.

Harding, R., Higginson, I. J., Leam, C., Donaldson, N., Pearce, A., & George, R. (2004). Evaluation of a short-term group intervention for informal carers of patients attending a home palliative care service. *Journal of Pain Symptom Management, 27*(5), 396–408.

Hayman, J., Langa, K., Kabeto, M., Katz, S., Demonner, S., Chernew, M., et al. (2001). Estimating the costs of informal caregiving for elderly patients with cancer. *Journal of Clinical Oncology, 19*(13), 3219–3225.

Hileman, J. W., Lackey, N. R., & Hassanein, R. S. (1992). Identifying the needs of home caregivers of patients with cancer. *Oncology Nursing Forum, 19*(5), 771–777.

Hinds, C. (1985). The needs of families who care for patients with cancer at home: Are we meeting them? *Journal in Advanced Nursing, 10*(6), 575–581.

Janda, M., Stenginga, S., Langbecker, D., Dunn, J., Walker, D., & Eakin, E. (2007). Quality of life among patients with a brain tumor and their careers. *Journal of Psychosomatic Research, 63,* 617–623.

Juarez, G., Ferrell, B., Uman, G., Podnos, Y., & Wagman, L. (2008). Distress and quality of life concerns of family caregivers of patients undergoing palliative surgery. *Cancer Nursing, 31*(1), 2–10.

Keefe, F. J., Ahles, T. A., Sutton, L., Dalton, J., Baucom, D., & Pope, M. S. (2005). Partner-guided cancer pain management at the end of life: A preliminary study. *Journal of Pain Symptom Management, 29*(3), 263–272.

Kim, Y., Kashy, D., Spillers, R., & Evans, T. (2009). Needs assessment of family caregivers of cancer survivors: Three cohorts comparison [Epub ahead of print]. *Psycho-Oncology.*

Kim, Y., Wellisch, D., & Spillers, R. (2008). Effects of psychological distress on quality of life of adult daughters and their mothers with cancer. *Psycho-Oncology, 17*, 1129–1136.

Kornblith, A. B., Herndon, J. E., Zuckerman, E., Viscoli, C. M., Horwitz, R. I., & Cooper, M. R. (2001). Social support as a buffer to the psychological impact of stressful life events in women with breast cancer. *Cancer, 91*(2), 443–454.

Kozachik, S. L., Given, C. W., Given, B. A., Pierce, S. J., Azzouz, F., & Rawl, S. M. (2001). Improving depressive symptoms among caregivers of patients with cancer: Results of a randomized clinical trial. *Oncology Nursing Forum, 28*(7), 1149–1157.

Kurtz, M. E., Kurtz, J. C., Given, C. W., & Given, B. (2005). A randomized, controlled trial of a patient/caregiver symptom control intervention: Effects on depressive symptomology of caregivers of cancer patients. *Journal of Pain Symptom Management, 30*(2), 112–122.

Litwak, E., (1985). *Helping the elderly: The complimentary roles of informal networks and formal systems.* New York, NY: Gilford Press.

McDonald, J. C., Stetz, K. M., & Compton, K. (1996). Educational interventions for family caregivers during marrow transplantation. *Oncology Nursing Forum, 23*(9), 1432–1439.

McMillan, S. C. (2005). Interventions to facilitate family caregiving at the end of life. *Journal of Palliative Medicine, 1*(Suppl.), 132–139.

McMillan, S. C., Small, B. J., Weitzner, M., Schonwetter, R., & Tittle, M. (2006). Impact of coping skills intervention with family caregivers of hospice patients with cancer. *Cancer, 106*(1), 214–222.

Naiditch, L. (2006). Caregivers in Decline: A close-up look at caregivers whose health is affected by caregiving. Proceedings of the *Caregiver Health as a Public Health Issue.* Washington, DC: Evercare & National Alliance for Caregiving.

The National Profile of Caregivers in Canada. (2002). [Decima research]. Unpublished raw data.

Nijboer, C., Tempelaar, R., Triemstar, M., van den Bos, G. A., & Sanderman, R. (2001). The role of social and psychologic resources in caregiving of cancer patients. *Cancer, 91*(5), 1029–1039.

Northouse, L. (1984). The impact of cancer on the family. *International Journal Psychiatry Medicine, 14*, 215–242.

Northouse, L. (2005). Helping families of patients with cancer. *Oncology Nursing Forum, 32*(4), 743–750.

Northouse, L., Kershaw, T., Mood, D., & Schafenacher, A. (2005). Effects of a family intervention on the quality of life of women with recurrent breast cancer and their family caregivers. *Psycho-oncology, 14*, 478–491.

Northouse, L., Mood, D., Montie, J., Ssandler, H., Forman, J., Jussain, M., et al. (2007). Living with prostate cancer: Patients' and spouses' psychosocial status and quality of life. *Journal of Clinical Oncology, 25*, 4171–4177.

Oberst, M. T., Thomas, S. E., Gass, K. A., & Ward, S. E. (1989). Caregiving demands and appraisal of stress among family caregivers. *Cancer Nursing, 12*, 209–215.

Osse, B. H., Vernooij-Dassen, M. J., Schlade, E., & Grol, R. P. (2006). Problems experiences by the informal caregivers of cancer patients and their needs for support. *Cancer Nursing, 29*(5), 378–388.

Ostroff, J., Ross, S., Steinglass, P., Ronis-Tobin, V., & Singh, B. (2004). Interest in and barriers to participation in multiple family groups among head and neck cancer survivors and their primary family members. *Family Process, 43*(2), 195–208.

Padilla G., Grant., M., Ferrell, B., & Presant (1996). Quality of life – cancer. In B. Spilker (Ed.), *Quality of life and pharmacoeconomics in clinical trials* (2nd ed., pp. 301–308). Philadelphia, PA: Lippincott-Raven.

Park, S., Kim, Y., Kim, S., Choi, J., Lim, H., Choi, Y., et al. (2009). Impact of caregivers' unmet needs for supportive care on quality of terminal cancer care delivered and caregivers' workforce performance [Epud ahead of print]. *Supportive Care in Cancer.*

Pasacreta, J. V., Barg, F., Nuamah, I., & McCorkle, R. (2000). Participant characteristics before and 4 months after attendance at a family caregiver cancer education program. *Cancer Nursing, 23*(4), 295–303.

Pasacreta, J. V., & McCorkle, R. (2000). Cancer care: Impact of interventions on caregiver outcomes. *Annual Review Nursing Research, 18,* 127–148.

Rabow, M. W., Hauser, J. M., & Adams, J. (2004). Supporting family caregivers at the end of life: "They don't know what they don't know". *JAMA, 291*(4), 483–491.

Rhee, Y., Yun, Y., Park, S., Shin, D., Lee, K., Yoo, H., et al. (2008). Depression in family caregivers of cancer patients: The feeling of burden as a predictor of depression. *Journal of Clinical Oncology, 26,* 5890–5895.

Rothman, M., Beltran, P., Cappelleri, J., Lipscomb, J., & Teschendorf, B. (2006, February). *Patient reported outcomes: The concept.* Paper presented at FDA Guidance on Patient Reported Outcomes: Discussion, Dissemination, and Operationalization at the Mayo Clinic, Chantilly, VA.

Salmon, J. R., Kwak, J., Acquaviva, K. D., Brandt, K., & Egan, K. A. (2005). Transformative aspects of caregiving at life's end. *Journal of Pain & Symptom Management, 29*(2), 121–129.

Sanford, J., Jounhson, A., & Townsend-Rocchiccioli, J. (2005). The health status of rural caregivers. *Journal of Gerontological Nursing, 31*(4), 25–31.

Sarason, B. R., Sarason, I. G., Pierce, G. R., (1990). *Social Support: An Interactional View.* New York, NY: John Wiley & Sons.

Schulz, R. (2006). Caregiver Health as a Public Health Issue, conference proceedings. *Research On Caregiver Health.* Washington, DC: The Urban Institute.

Schulz, R., & Beach, S. R. (1999). Caregiving as a risk factor for mortality: The caregiver health effects study. *Journal of the American Medical Association, 282*(23), 2215–2219.

Soothill, K., Morris, S. M., Harman, J. C., Francis, B., Thomas, C., & McIllmurray, M. B. (2001). Informal carers of cancer patients: What are their unmet psychosocial needs? *Health & Social Care in the Community, 6,* 464–475.

Sorensen, S., Pinquart, M., & Duberstein, P. (2002). How effective are interventions with caregivers? An updated meta-analysis. *Gerontologist, 42*(3), 356–372.

Spillers, R., Wellisch, D., Kim, Y., Mattews, A., & Baker, F. (2008). Family caregivers and quilt in the context of cancer care. *Psychosomatics, 49*(6), 511–519.

Stetz, K. (1989). The relationship among background characteristics, purpose in life, and caregiving demands on perceived health of spouse caregivers. *School Inquiry in Nursing Practice, 3*(2), 133–153.

Stetz, K. M., & Brown, M. A. (1997). Taking care: Caregiving to persons with cancer and AIDS. *Cancer Nursing, 20*(1), 12–22.

Stetz, K.M., & Brown, M.A. (2004). Physical and psychosocial health in family caregiving: A comparison of AIDS and cancer caregivers. *Public Health Nursing, 21* (6), 533-540.

Tang, S., Li, C., & Chen, C. (2008). Trajectory and determinants of the quality of life of family caregivers of terminally ill cancer patients in Taiwan. *Quality of Life Research, 17,* 387–395.

Teschendorf, B., Ferrans, C. E., O'Mara, A., Schwartz, C., & Sloan, J. (2005, October). *Challenges of Informal Cancer Caregivers.* Proceedings of ISOQOL, San Francisco, CA.

Teschendorf, B., Ferrans, C., Moinpour, C., O'Mara, A., Schwartz, C., & Sloan, J. (in preparation). *Development of a caregiver self-assessment scale.* Manuscript in preparation.

Teschendorf, B., Schwartz, C., Ferrans, C., O'Mara, A., & Sloan, J. (2007). Caregiver role stress: When families become providers. *Cancer Control, 14*(2), 1–7.

Weitzner, M. A., Jacobsen, P. B., Wagner, H., & Friedland, J. (1999). The Caregiver Quality of Life Index-Cancer (CQOLC) scale: Development and validation of an instrument to measure quality of life of the family caregiver of patients with cancer. *Quality of Life Research, 8,* 55–63.

Weitzner, M. A., & McMillan, S. C. (1999). The Caregiver Quality of Life Index-Cancer (CQOLC) Scale: Revalidation in a home hospice setting. *Journal of Palliative Care, 15*(2), 13–20.

Weitzner, M. A., McMillan, S. C., & Jacobsen, P. B. (1999). Family caregiver quality of life: Differences between curative and palliative cancer treatment settings. *Journal of Pain & Symptom Management, 17*(6), 418–428.

Zarit, S. H., Reever, K. E., & Bach-Peterson, J. (1980). Relatives of the impaired elderly: Correlates of feelings of burden. *Gerontologist, 20,* 649–655.

Appendix A: Caregiver Resources

Family Caregiver Alliance
http://www.caregiver.org/
Montgomery St, Ste 1100
San Francisco, CA 94104
phone: (415) 434.3388
(800) 445.8106
fax: (415) 434.3508
info@caregiver.org
A resource for information on caregiving.

National Family Caregivers Association
http://www.nfcacares.org/
Suzanne Mintz, President/Co-founder
Washington, DC
Web site has caregiver statistics and general information with citations from the literature.

Share the Care
http://www.sharethecare.org/
Quoted from the Web site:
"*ShareTheCaregiving*™*, Inc.* is a 501c3 not-for-profit organization dedicated to educating
the public, health professionals and clergy about group caregiving as a proven option for
meeting the needs of the seriously ill or dying, those in rehabilitiation, the elderly in
need of assistance and their caregivers. ShareTheCaregiving™ uses a widely adopted
group caregiving model known as SHARE THE CARE.
The SHARE THE CARE model provides a road map on how to take a group of ordinary
individuals (comprised of friends, relatives, neighbors, coworkers, and acquaintances)
and turn them into a 'caregiver family' to provide individuals and families with the help
they need to meet the daily challenges of caregiving."

CarePages
http://www.carepages.com/
A fully integrated service, CarePages demonstrates care for all needs, both emotional and
physical. The service provides a connection between healthcare providers and the large
and growing groups of their consumers: patients, caregivers, and their friends and family
members.
CarePages allows patient families to easily communicate with relatives and friends, share
health updates and photos and exchange supportive messages via a free, private Web site.

- Patient families can share news, without repeated telephone calls.
- Families stay close by sharing captioned photos.
- Loved ones send words of encouragement and support.
- Privacy controls enable patient families to manage visitors.
- CarePage visitors can recognize staff for excellent care.

Caregiver.Com
http://www.caregiver.com/
A magazine for caregivers

National Family Caregiver Support Program
http://www.aoa.gov/aoaroot/aoa_programs/hcltc/caregiver/index.aspx
Administration on Aging
Department of Health & Human Services
Washington, DC
Fact sheets, resources for staying healthy.

Women's Health.gov
http://www.womenshealth.gov/
Department of Health & Human Services
Washington, DC
Caregiver stress resource

Caregiver Guide
http://www.nia.nih.gov/Alzheimers/Publications/caregiverguide.htm
National Institutes of Health,
National Institute on Aging
Department of Health & Human Services
Washington, DC

Healthy Caregiver
http://www.healthycaregiver.com/
Online publication online

Caregiver's Homecare Companion
http://www.caregivershome.com/
Articles on special topics, links to Harvard publications.

Books:

Foley, K. M. (Ed.). (2005). *When the focus is on care: Palliative care and cancer.* Atlanta, GA: American Cancer Society.

Jacobs, B. J. (2006). *The emotional survival guide for caregivers.* New York, NY: Guilford Press.

McLeod, B. W. (1999). *Caregiving: The spiritual journey of love, loss, and renewal.* New York, NY: John Wiley.

Mintz, S. (2002). *Love, honor and value: A family caregiver speaks out about the choices and challenges of caregiving.* Herndon, VA: Capital Books.

Appendix B: Caregiver Quality of Life Self-Assessment Scale

© 2010 Bonnie Teschendorf, Carol Ferrans, Jeff Sloan, Carolyn Schwartx, Carol Moinpour

The caregiver role for a person with cancer is important. When responding to the following questions think about your caregiving experience over the last week. Respond to each question based on a "best estimate" of the impact of the occurrence or event.

Check the response category that best describes how caregiving has influenced you.

Social Relationships

	Almost Never	A Little	Half the Time	Most of the Time	Almost Always
1. I feel I cannot leave my relative alone.	[ ]	[ ]	[ ]	[ ]	[ ]
2. I get what I need from my family and friends.	[ ]	[ ]	[ ]	[ ]	[ ]
3. I feel cut off from other people.	[ ]	[ ]	[ ]	[ ]	[ ]
4. I feel a loss of privacy.	[ ]	[ ]	[ ]	[ ]	[ ]
5. Caregiving for ____ puts a strain on my relationship with him/ her.	[ ]	[ ]	[ ]	[ ]	[ ]

Economic Situation

	Almost Never	A Little	Half the Time	Most of the Time	Almost Always
1. Caregiving has put a financial strain on us.	[ ]	[ ]	[ ]	[ ]	[ ]
2. I worry about medical expenses.	[ ]	[ ]	[ ]	[ ]	[ ]
3. There is enough money to meet our needs.	[ ]	[ ]	[ ]	[ ]	[ ]

Emotional/Psychological Reactions

	Almost Never	A Little	Half the Time	Most of the Time	Almost Always
1. I resent having to take care of _____.	[ ]	[ ]	[ ]	[ ]	[ ]
2. Caring for _____ makes me feel good.	[ ]	[ ]	[ ]	[ ]	[ ]
3. I feel overwhelmed.	[ ]	[ ]	[ ]	[ ]	[ ]
4. I feel calm and peaceful.	[ ]	[ ]	[ ]	[ ]	[ ]
5. It upsets me to see what is happening to _____.	[ ]	[ ]	[ ]	[ ]	[ ]
6. I feel sad.	[ ]	[ ]	[ ]	[ ]	[ ]
7. I have trouble keeping my mind on what I am doing.	[ ]	[ ]	[ ]	[ ]	[ ]
8. I feel confined by caregiving.	[ ]	[ ]	[ ]	[ ]	[ ]
9. I worry about the future.	[ ]	[ ]	[ ]	[ ]	[ ]

Physical Reactions

	Almost Never	A Little	Half the Time	Most of the Time	Almost Always
1. I am taking care of my own health.	[ ]	[ ]	[ ]	[ ]	[ ]
2. I get enough sleep.	[ ]	[ ]	[ ]	[ ]	[ ]
3. I am tired.	[ ]	[ ]	[ ]	[ ]	[ ]
4. I have enough physical strength to take care of _____.	[ ]	[ ]	[ ]	[ ]	[ ]
5. I am eating regular meals (e.g. sitting down, balanced diet, no fast food).	[ ]	[ ]	[ ]	[ ]	[ ]
6. I take care of my own needs last.	[ ]	[ ]	[ ]	[ ]	[ ]

Spiritual Issues

	Almost Never	A Little	Half the Time	Most of the Time	Almost Always
1. My personal beliefs give me the strength to face difficulties.	[ ]	[ ]	[ ]	[ ]	[ ]

Overall Personal Health and Quality of Life

	Better	About the Same	Worse
1. Since I began providing care for ____, my quality of life is:	[ ]	[ ]	[ ]
2. My current personal health is ____ than this time last year.	[ ]	[ ]	[ ]

	Poor	Fair	Satisfactory	Very Good	Excellent
3. I would rate my overall quality of life as:	[ ]	[ ]	[ ]	[ ]	[ ]

Thank you for completing this assessment.

Additional information for Investigators:
RELIABILITY DATA (n=37 caregivers)

Scale	Cronbach Alpha
Total instrument	.89
Social subscale	.65
Economic subscale	.82
Psychological subscale	.69
Physical subscale	.88

Appendix C: Caregiver Month Proclamation (November 2006)

National Family Caregivers Month, 2006

A Proclamation by the President of the United States of America

Our country is blessed to have millions of compassionate citizens who bring love and support to family members and friends who are chronically ill, elderly, or disabled. During National Family Caregivers Month, we recognize these kind individuals who give of their hearts, resources, and energy to assist loved ones in need.

Family caregivers exemplify the true spirit of compassion by providing support to their loved ones and assisting with their everyday activities and special needs. These selfless people must often make great personal sacrifices to maintain the care and support their family and friends require. Their assistance provides those who may be ill, aging, or disabled an opportunity to stay in familiar surroundings and remain a part of their community.

My Administration is committed to supporting family caregivers and their vital role in our Nation's communities. The National Family Caregiver Support Program continues to provide information, counseling, and services and encourages cooperation among agencies and other providers that work with caregivers. These efforts assist caregivers and help ensure that all Americans receive the care they need.

As we observe National Family Caregivers Month, we honor family caregivers who take time out of their lives to improve the lives of family and friends. Their efforts demonstrate the best of the American spirit.

NOW, THEREFORE, I, GEORGE W. BUSH, President of the United States of America, by virtue of the authority vested in me by the Constitution and laws of the United States, do hereby proclaim November 2006 as National Family Caregivers Month. I encourage all Americans to honor the selfless service of caregivers who support their loved ones in need.

IN WITNESS WHEREOF, I have hereunto set my hand this thirtieth day of October, in the year of our Lord two thousand six, and of the Independence of the United States of America the two hundred and thirty-first.

—GEORGE W. BUSH

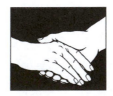

The Design, Conduct, and Analysis of HRQOL Studies: A Statistician's Perspective

Diane L. Fairclough

Introduction

Effective research about health-related quality of life (HRQOL) can contribute to improvements in therapy, patient care management, and treatment decision making. Poorly designed research can create the misconception that HRQOL research is not valuable, wastes resources, and creates unnecessary burdens for patients and their families. Poor quality HRQOL research often lacks a well defined research question and leaves unanswered the questions of real clinical interest. Given that HRQOL research does require resources, careful thought should be given as to whether the research can be implemented effectively in a particular setting. The two questions to address before implementing a study are "Is there a focused research question?" and "Is there the potential for changing clinical practice based on the study results?" If the answers are no, the investigator should reconsider implementing the study. If the answers are yes, the investigator should plan the design, conduct, and analysis of the study carefully. Without careful thought to these issues, the study may ultimately fail to provide investigators with the information needed to answer the relevant questions. Planning prior to implementing a study includes selection of the appropriate instruments for the assessment of HRQOL, the timing of the assessments, procedures for administration, decisions concerning follow-up of subjects, and analysis plans.

An HRQOL measure ought not to be selected for inclusion in a study without careful thought concerning the analytic methods necessary to interpret the results correctly. One of the major challenges is the analysis of longitudinal studies with non-randomly missing data. Unlike many laboratory or diagnostic measures usually obtained in clinical trials, missing HRQOL measures are more likely to occur in a patient who is experiencing greater morbidity due to the disease or its treatment. Analysis of the complete cases only or even the available data is likely to result in biased estimates of HRQOL. Another analytic issue is how to combine information on the quality and quantity of life. Without careful consideration of the study objectives and the corresponding analytic plan prior to initiating HRQOL research, the research objectives may not be achieved.

One of the best examples of an HRQOL study that contributed to changes in clinical practice was conducted by Sugarbaker and colleagues (Sugarbaker, Barofsky, Rosenberg, &

Gianola, 1982) comparing two therapeutic approaches for soft-tissue sarcoma. The initial study compared two therapeutic options. The first was limb-sparing surgery followed by radiation therapy. The second treatment approach was full amputation of the affected limb. The investigator hypothesized that sparing a limb, as opposed to amputating it, offers a quality-of-life advantage. As a result of the study, the hypothesis was rejected; subjects receiving the limb-sparing procedures reported limitations in mobility and sexual functioning. These observations were confirmed with physical assessments of mobility and endocrine function. As a result of these studies, radiation therapy was modified and physical rehabilitation was added to the limb-sparing therapeutic approach (Hicks, Lampert, Gerber, Glastein, & Danoff, 1985). The study included several desirable characteristics: a well defined hypothesis, investigators willing to modify therapy based on these results, and follow-up research founded on the rejected hypothesis.

Design

Well Defined Research Question

The most important step in the design of a HRQOL study is to develop a carefully defined and focused research question. An objective like "To compare HRQOL in patients treated with regimen A versus regimen B" provides no guidance concerning the selection of the HRQOL instrument, timing of assessments, or the analysis. Vague objectives leave important questions unanswered, such as "Is the investigator interested in the short-term impact or the long-term effect of the treatment on the patients HRQOL?" or "Is the population of interest only those subjects who respond to the therapy or is it all patients who are started on that therapy?" Consider an example of patients with cancer. The design of a study to answer questions about differences in HRQOL in long-term survivors will be quite different from a study designed to compare HRQOL for those same patients while being treated on two different regimens. Not only would the schedule for the assessments be different, the appropriate instruments for assessing differences would not be the same for the two differently designed studies. In the cases of the survivors, one would look for an HRQOL instrument that focused on the aspects of general living. In the question concerning the immediate effect of therapy on HRQOL, the instrument should contain questions about aspects of HRQOL affected by the disease and its treatment. Examples of focused questions include the following:

- Does palliative care, initiated after a specific end-of-life care decision, delay the decline in HRQOL for patients with advanced refractory cancer?
- Are there long-term differences 5 years after therapy in HRQOL between cancer patients treated for the same disease with surgery versus radiotherapy?
- Does the use of "colony stimulating factor" therapy improve HRQOL by reducing anemia-related fatigue during therapy?

Selection of HRQOL Instruments

There is not one HRQOL instrument that is the best for all studies. Even when considering studies where all the subjects have the same disease, other factors may influence which

HRQOL instrument is considered the best. The choice of instrument depends on the objectives of the study, the target population, the disease, and its treatment. Choice will be influenced by whether comparisons are being made between diseases, stages of disease, short- and long-term outcomes, or between patients with and without disease. Studies including economic analyses may require different instruments as well.

HRQOL instruments vary in several aspects. The first distinguishing feature is the content, or whether the questions are disease-specific. Generic instruments contain items regarding general aspects of physical, functional, emotional, and social well-being appropriate to patients with any disease or without active disease. This type of instrument would be most appropriate for long-term cancer survivors or when making comparisons between healthy individuals or patients with other diseases. The second group of HRQOL instruments is disease- or treatment-specific. These instruments are designed to be sensitive to differences in HRQOL among patients who have active disease and/or are receiving therapy.

The second distinguishing characteristic is the nature of the instrument and its intended use. There are two general types of health-related quality-of-life measures: health status assessments and patient preference assessments, which differ in their method of construction. These two forms of assessments were developed as a result of the differences between the two perspectives of psychometrics and econometrics. The majority of instruments are developed in a manner typical of psychometric research. These instruments sometimes are referred to as health status measures and are designed to measure the relative HRQOL between patients or within a patient over time. Thus, these instruments are appropriate in studies where the focus is the comparison of groups of individuals or identifying change over time within a group of individuals. In the health status assessment measures, multiple aspects of the patient's perceived well-being are self-assessed and a score is derived from the responses on a series of questions. This score reflects the patient's *relative* HRQOL as compared to other patients and to the HRQOL of the same patient at other times. The measures range from a single global question of asking patients to rate their current quality of life to a series of questions about specific aspects of their daily life during a recent period of time. Measures generally take 5 to 10 minutes to complete. Examples include the Functional Living Index-Cancer (FLIC) (Schipper, 1990), EORTC QLQ-C30 (Groenvold, Klee, Sprangers, & Aaronson, 1997), and the Functional Assessment of Cancer Therapy (FACT) (Cella et al., 1993). These instruments may consist of multiple questions, which are combined to compute a single score, or a single more global question. An example of a couple of questions from a multiple-item questionnaire might go as follows:

During the past week...	Not at all	A little	Moderately	A lot	All the time
How much were you bothered by hair loss?	0	1	2	3	4
How much were you bothered by nausea or vomiting?	0	1	2	3	4

A single global question might look like the following:

During the past week, how would you rate your overall quality of life?

0	100
Very poor	Excellent

The scores developed from these instruments often (but not always) range from 0 to 100 where higher scores indicate better HRQOL.

The second group of instruments has been developed in a manner typical of econometric research. These instruments sometimes are referred to as preference measures (Yabroff, Linas, & Schulman, 1996) or utilities. They are designed to relate the quality of life with the quantity of life and are used most commonly in studies where there is a concurrent economic analysis. These preference assessment measures are used to evaluate the trade off between the quality and quantity of life. Values of utilities are always between 0 and 1, with 0 generally associated with death and 1 with perfect health. Traditionally, the scores were determined by methods such as Time-Trade-Offs (TTO) (McNeil, Weichselbaum, & Pauker, 1981) and Standard Gamble (Torrance, Thomas, & Sackett, 1971) that require the respondent to make choices between alternative outcomes in the presence of uncertainty about the outcomes. This assessment method of utility scores is difficult to implement in clinical trials as assessment requires the presence of a trained interviewer or specialized computer program. Multi-attribute assessments (Feeny et al., 1992; Weeks, 1992) such as the Health Utilities Index (HUI) are alternatives that attempt to overcome the difficulties of obtaining utility scores. Because of these resource requirements, these approaches generally are too time- and resource-intensive to use in a large clinical trial. Multi-attribute assessment measures combine the advantages of self-assessment with the conceptual advantages of utility scores. Utilities have traditionally been used in the calculation of quality-adjusted life years for cost-effectiveness analyses and more recently in analytic approaches, such as Q-TWiST (Goldhirsch, Gelber, Simes, Glasziou, & Coates, 1989; Glasziou, Simes, & Gelber, 1990).

Finally, HRQOL instruments differ according to the content of the questions. Among health status measures, there is considerable range in the content of the questions. Some instruments focus more on the perceived impact of the disease and therapy (e.g., How much are you bothered by hair loss?), while others focus on the frequency and severity of symptoms (e.g., How *often* do you experience pain?). These instruments are designed primarily to compare groups of patients receiving different treatments or to identify change over time within groups of patients. As a result, these instruments have most often been used in clinical trials to facilitate the comparisons of therapeutic regimens. In some instruments, the subject is asked to evaluate the frequency and severity of symptoms or limitations. An example would be "How often have you had pain?" where the responses range from "Not at all" to "All the time." In other instruments, the questions may focus more on the impact of symptoms and the extent to which they have interfered with daily living, such as "Did pain interfere with your daily activities?" where the responses range from "Not at all" to "Very much." Generally, the frequency and severity of symptoms such as pain will be related closely to the impact of symptoms and the extent to which they have interfered with daily activities and the conclusions based on either scale will be the same.

The investigator should look closely at the questions before selecting a particular HRQOL instrument for a research study. The disease-specific assessment would provide the most sensitive measure of the differences between treatment regimens. In contrast, the generic measure would facilitate comparisons across more diverse populations of patients. Finally, the inclusion of a measure linked to preferences would expedite the computation of utility scores, providing information for cost-effectiveness and cost-utility analyses.

Schedule of Assessments

As with all the other aspects of research study design, the schedule of assessments depends on the research question. Does the question focus on acute or long-term impact of disease and its treatment? The frequency of assessments will depend on the rate of progression or recession of the medical condition. In a rapidly progressing disease, more frequent assessment will be required. Similarly, in a disease that responds quickly to treatment, more frequent assessment may be necessary to capture the changes in HRQOL. However, it should be recognized that HRQOL does not change from hour to hour and rarely from day to day, making it inappropriate to assess HRQOL on a daily or more frequent basis. Most HRQOL assessments ask respondents to describe their HRQOL over the last week or month and assessments should be no more frequent than the period of time referenced in the questionnaire. Balancing against the need to capture important changes is the need to minimize the patient burden of completing the questionnaire.

Some practical issues occur in the timing of assessments. The timing of baseline assessments is critical to the interpretation of the overall study results. Ideally, assessments should occur not only before an individual starts to receive the intervention, but also prior to their knowledge of their treatment assignments. Depending on how subjects feel about the particular treatment to which they were assigned randomly, the reported HRQOL scores may increase or decrease relative to what would have been reported prior to randomization. For example, subjects may become more optimistic if they have been assigned to the new innovative therapy. If the different treatments have different profiles of side effects, patient may begin to anticipate these differences. Several investigators in studies have noted these types of differences in HRQOL scores where some patients were evaluated after they were randomized (Brooks et al., 1998).

When a patient is undergoing therapy, the timing of assessments may be affected by the schedule of therapy. When therapy is given on a daily basis, the exact timing of assessment is not an issue. But some therapy is cyclic. A typical 3-week cycle of chemotherapy might consist of 1 to 7 days of toxic therapy, followed by approximately 2 weeks of recovery with no treatment. Depending on the particular drug, the most acute toxicity effects on HRQOL likely will occur sometime during that first week. However, typically HRQOL assessments are scheduled just prior to the beginning of the next cycle of therapy, several weeks after the worst side effects are experienced. This choice for the timing of assessments corresponds with the patient's availability and may underestimate the effect of acute toxicity on the patient's HRQOL. This may be reasonable in settings where the treatment is associated with a high probability of remission of the cancer, as these patients are willing to tolerate considerable acute non-life-threatening toxicities when there is a reasonable chance of cure. It may be more questionable in conditions where the therapy is palliative and the duration of life is much more limited. Challenges in the timing of assessments may become more difficult when the schedule of therapy differs among arms. In rare cases, the choice of a particular schedule of assessments could favor one therapy over another and should be considered critically before implementing the research.

If the treatment regimens have a fixed length of duration, but are of different durations, the timing of assessments at the end of therapy may be a challenge. Patients often anticipate the end of therapy and may minimize their perception of the impact of side effects. Depending on the nature of the research question, it is important to make sure that the final assessment occurs while the patients are on therapy are of equal time prior to the end of therapy.

An additional issue is whether to continue HRQOL assessment after the end of therapy. The issue is important particularly as it is common for a patient to discontinue therapy due to noncompliance with therapy, increased toxicity, or progression or regression of disease symptoms. When HRQOL assessments are limited to those patients who respond to therapy with minimal side effects, the subsequent analyses rarely answer the relevant questions about the HRQOL of individuals who are started on a particular therapy. For example, concern about HRQOL differs from the evaluation of acute toxicities associated with a particular drug or therapeutic regimen. In the latter case, the focus is on the acute toxicities associated with the regimen and these are more clearly identified when the observations are on those patients receiving the therapy. The concept of HRQOL includes both positive and negative benefits of being placed on a particular treatment regimen, possibly in contrast to another regimen. For example, if the consequences of failing a particular therapy are negative, such as rapid progression of disease symptoms, psychological distress, or placement on a more toxic therapy, the negative impact may be reflected in the individual's HRQOL scores. Continuing assessment of HRQOL in a patient who fails or succeeds with a particular therapy is critical if the results are to reflect an unbiased assessment of HRQOL.

The final issue is how long to measure HRQOL. The answer is related closely to the objectives of the research. The research objectives, and thus the duration of HRQOL assessment, must reflect the nature of the disease and the therapies under investigation. In addition, the investigators should consider the expected loss to follow-up among the individuals in the study. For example, if there is significant loss to follow-up due to mortality, it may not make sense to collect HRQOL assessments past the point where 50% of the subjects are expected to survive, unless there is a preplanned analytic strategy to use that information to answer a specific research objective.

Respondents

Health-related quality of life can be assessed from different perspectives, including the individual patient or a surrogate for the patient, who could be a healthcare professional, or an informal or family caregiver. When and where possible, the patient should be the primary source of information. There are, however, settings where gathering surrogate information may be necessary. This is especially true for very young children or for adults who are no longer able to complete self-assessments because of cognitive difficulties. While surrogate respondents generally provide a biased estimate of the patient's quality of life (Slevin et al., 1990; Slevin, Plant, Lynch, Drinkwater, & Gregory, 1988; Loprinzi et al., 1994), assessments by surrogate respondents may be used in analytic strategies to partially overcome the loss of information about HRQOL when the patients themselves are no longer able to complete self-assessments.

In economic analyses, the value of a specific health state as measured by utilities also may be assessed for different perspectives using different respondents to define these values. There is debate concerning whether the general public, who theoretically take on the burden of healthcare costs, or whether the patients, who are experiencing those health states, should set those values.

Sample Size

The primary objectives and related hypotheses determine the number of subjects necessary to complete HRQOL assessments to ensure the HRQOL study aims are achieved. The first step in determining sample size is the definition of the primary and secondary endpoints. In most studies, there will be multiple HRQOL scales measuring overall HRQOL, as well as individual domains. If multiple scales are included in the primary endpoints, the design phase of the study should include some strategies for handling multiple endpoints (Zhang, Quan, Ng, & Stepanavage, 1997). In longitudinal studies, the definition of the primary endpoint also involves specifying a specific time point or summary measure.

The second step in the determination of sample size is specifying "the smallest meaningful difference" in the primary HRQOL endpoint that the study should have sufficient power to detect. In some settings this may be determined from previous studies of similar patients where clinically relevant differences in HRQOL scores have been estimated. Where there is little or no previous experiences, investigators may want to indicate small, medium, or large effect sizes as defined by Cohen (1998).

If the study is longitudinal, the third step is obtaining estimates of the rates of loss to follow-up and the correlation of these measures over time. If estimates of loss to follow-up for HRQOL assessment from previous HRQOL studies in a similar population of subjects are not available, rates may be estimated partially from other loss to follow-up from other clinical data. However, because measurement of HRQOL is based on self-assessment and is not included in clinical routines, loss to follow-up for HRQOL assessments generally will be greater than that for clinical endpoints. HRQOL measurements of overall HRQOL or major domains (e.g., functional well-being) generally are moderately correlated over time

($rho = 0.3$ to 0.8). Instruments designed to measure symptom assessments (e.g., nausea and vomiting) may be more variable over time and thus less correlated. In the calculation of the sample size requirements, taking the lower limit of the expected correlation will result in a conservative estimate of sample size.

Finally, it is not unexpected that sample size requirements for the HRQOL component of a clinical investigation differ from the sample size requirements for other clinical endpoints of response. In many cases, the sample size requirement for the HRQOL component will be less than for the clinical endpoints. In this case, the investigator should consider strategies to reduce the HRQOL assessment burden, including limiting the HRQOL investigation to a subset of individuals. In some cases, the sample size requirements for the HRQOL component will be larger than for the other endpoints. In this case, the investigator must decide whether the HRQOL objectives are important enough to justify increasing the number of subjects in the study. If not, the HRQOL component should be dropped or the objectives revised.

Conduct of HRQOL Studies

In high quality research, methods of assessing HRQOL must be specified clearly in the study protocol. Education and training of research personnel is critical to the success of the study (Fairclough & Cella, 1996). Vehicles for education include the protocol (with strong justifications for the HRQOL assessments), symposia, video, and written materials. Videos may be valuable as a training vehicle for both research staff and for patients. Although there are often face-to-face training sessions at the initiation of a study, research personnel may change over time. Training tapes directed toward research personnel can deal with procedures in more detail than is possible in the protocol.

The first component is identifying and training research personnel in when, where, and how to administer HRQOL questionnaires. Training in the "when" addresses how the timing of administration can influence an individual's response to the questionnaire. Thus, it is important to administer the questionnaire before (not after) patients undergo any uncomfortable procedures, or before they receive information concerning the results of randomized treatment assignment or disease progression. Training in the "where" demonstrates to the research personnel how important it will be to identify a quiet place where the subject will not be interrupted. Training focused on the "how" illustrated that subjects should always be asked if they will complete the questionnaire and also be allowed to refuse to complete the questionnaire. Training should include providing positive ways of approaching the patient. For example, instead of referring to participation as burdensome (e.g., "We have a lot of forms that you'll need to fill out"), the HRQOL assessment can be placed in a positive light (Cella, Skeel, & Bonomi, 1993). For example, research personnel could say, "We want to know more about the quality of life of people as they go through this treatment and the only way to know is to ask you. In order to do this, we ask that you complete this brief questionnaire. It usually takes about (X) minutes." It is strongly recommended that family or friends *not* be allowed to assist the patient. It may be very difficult for the patient to answer the questions honestly in the presence of family and friends. If the subject cannot read the questionnaire or needs help recording the responses, a neutral individual (generally a research nurse) should be available.

Research personnel should not take the responsibility for determining whether subjects are too ill to complete the questionnaire, but allow subjects to make that assessment for themselves. Hopwood and colleagues (1998) noted that, in three trials for lung and head and neck cancer, "staff considering the patient to be too ill to complete the HRQOL assessments" was the most commonly cited problem affecting the distribution of questionnaires, while patient refusal was the least cited problem. It is understandable that study personnel are reluctant to approach patients when they appear to be feeling particularly ill, but in order to minimize the bias from bracketing out these patients, all subjects should be given the option to complete the questionnaire. There may be ways of encouraging ill patients, specifically by providing conditions to make it as easy as possible for them to complete the questionnaire. When a patient refuses, that refusal must be respected.

Procedures for minimizing missing data are also critical to creating a high quality study. These procedures start with education of research personnel about the importance of the HRQOL data. Patient information sheets, which explain to the patient the rationale behind the HRQOL assessments, will minimize missing data. These sheets can contain messages about the importance of the patient's perspective, that there are no "correct" answers to the questions, the reasons it is important to respond to every question, and the importance of completing follow-up questionnaires. In addition to the persuasive information, the fact that patients can refuse without affecting their treatment or their relationship with their doctor should be included. Reminder systems will also minimize missing assessments. These reminder systems can be as grand as a calendar, which includes the scheduled follow-up assessments, to as small as reminder slips on the patient's chart. Linking the HRQOL assessments to other clinical assessments will provide a reminder to the research personnel to ask the patient to complete the HRQOL questionnaires. Clear instructions for follow-up procedures when a patient discontinues therapy are critical, especially when HRQOL assessments are to be continued and certain laboratory or other clinical assessments may be discontinued. Plans for follow-up by phone or mailing of questionnaires when a patient misses a visit will also minimize missing data. Finally, it is important to document the reasons for missing assessments. As part of this documentation, it is important to differentiate whether the reason is related or unrelated to their HRQOL. For example, if the patient felt too ill to complete the questionnaire, that is likely to be related to their HRQOL. Alternatively, if the visit was missed because of bad weather or staff forgetting to administer the questionnaire, is unlikely to be related to the patient's HRQOL.

Analysis

Most studies of health-related quality of life consider measurement from one of two perspectives. In the first, the endpoints are expressed in the metric of the HRQOL scales, whereas in the second, the outcome is expressed in the metric of time. The latter group includes outcomes such as QALYs (Feeny, 1998) and Q-TWiST (Gelber, 1998). In studies where the endpoints are expressed in the metric of the HRQOL scales, HRQOL assessment generally is incorporated into the study by administering questionnaires at multiple time points before, during, and sometimes after an intervention, with the goal of characterizing the patient's HRQOL in a longitudinal fashion. The number of planned assessments may be as few as three or as many as nine.

The choice of the appropriate analysis methods is influenced also by two other issues: missing data (Matthews, Altman, Campbell, & Royston, 1990) and multiple endpoints and comparisons (Korn & O'Fallon, 1990). Missing data is a concern because of the potential for biased estimates of HRQOL when the reasons for missing data are related to factors that affect the patient's HRQOL. The presence of multiple endpoints presents two potential problems: controlling type I errors for multiple comparisons and finding strategies for presenting HRQOL results in a way that is clinically meaningful and easily interpretable. These two issues are central to the discussion of alternative methods of analysis presented in this chapter.

Multiple Comparisons

One strategy for handling multiple testing is to specify a limited number of comparisons (no more than three) in the design of the trial (Gotay, Korn, McCabe, Moore, & Cheson, 1992). While this is a valid approach, in practice, investigators are reluctant to ignore the remaining data. There is also an ethical question about collection of data that are not intended for use in the analysis. One way to address this problem is to utilize a multiple comparisons procedure, such as the Bonferroni corrections or Hochberg sequential rejection procedure (Hochberg, 1988). The Bonferroni procedure is to accept as statistically significant only those tests with p-values that are less than α/K, where α is the overall type I error and K is the number of tests (or comparisons) performed. It is typical to have studies of two treatments with three to nine repeated measures and four to six measures of HRQOL, resulting in 12–54 potential multiple comparisons. If the type I error rate was set to be 5%, then comparisons would be statistically significant if the p-values were less than 0.001 for the study with 54 comparisons. The sequential rejection procedures, such as Hochberg sequential rejection procedure, are somewhat less conservative than the classical Bonferroni. The ordered p-values, $p_{[k]}$ are compared sequentially to $\alpha/(K - k + 1)$, $k = 1 \ldots K$, starting with the largest p-value. When $p_{[k]} < \alpha/(K - k + 1)$ for one of the comparisons, the null hypothesis is rejected for that comparison and all others with smaller p-values. While addressing the type I error problem, this approach significantly reduces the power to detect real differences in HRQOL.

Summary Measures
An alternative approach to either multiple univariate analyses or multivariate analyses is the use of summary measures (O'Brien, 1984; Pocock, Geller, & Tsiatis, 1987; Cox et al., 1992) or global statistics (Tandon, 1990). Examples of summary measures include post-treatment mean, mean change relative to baseline, last value minus baseline, average rate of change over time (or slope), maximum value, area under the curve, and time to reach

a peak or a prespecified value. There are several reasons for the use of summary measures in the analysis of a longitudinal study of HRQOL. The primary advantage of summary measures is that they are often easier to interpret than the multivariate methods described previously. Not only is the number of comparisons reduced, but measures such as the rate of change and the area under the curve are familiar concepts in clinical medicine. In addition, depending on which summary measure is selected, they often have greater ability to detect clinically relevant differences in HRQOL that persist over time.

Patterns of Change Across Time

The choice of summary measure selected for the endpoint in a clinical trial depends on the objective of the investigation, the research question, the expected pattern of change across time, and the patterns of missing data. Consider several possible patterns of change in HRQOL across time. One pattern might be a steady rate of change over time reflecting either a constant improvement in HRQOL over time or a constant decline over time. This pattern of change suggests that the rate of change or slope would be a good summary measure to select for this population. In contrast, other measures, such as the change from baseline to the last measure, might not be applicable if patients who fail earlier, and thus drop out from the study earlier, have smaller changes than those patients with longer follow-up.

An alternative profile might be a rapid change initially with a subsequent plateau after the maximum therapeutic benefit is realized. This profile illustrates the importance of identifying clinically relevant questions *a priori*. If the objective of the study is to identify the therapy that produces the most rapid improvement in HRQOL, the time to reach a peak or prespecified value would be a good measure to select. If, in contrast, it is more important to determine the ultimate level of benefit rather than the time to achieve the benefit, a measure such as the posttreatment mean or mean change relative to baseline might be more appropriate.

A third pattern of change might occur with a therapy that has transient benefits or toxicity. For example, individuals may experience transient benefits and then return to their baseline levels after the effect of the therapy has ceased. Alternatively, a toxic therapy for cancer may significantly reduce HRQOL during therapy but ultimately result in a better HRQOL following therapy than the patient was experiencing at the time of diagnosis. For these more complex patterns of change over time, a measure such as the area under the curve might be considered as a summary of both early and continued effects of the therapy.

Constructing Summary Measures

There are two approaches to constructing a summary measure. In the first approach, one summarizes the data within an individual subject by constructing a single value for each individual and then performing a univariate test. In the second approach, data are modeled within treatment groups across time and summary measures are constructed from these population estimates. For example, in the first approach, the rate of change experienced by each individual could be estimated using ordinary least squares (for individuals with at least two measurements), and a two-sample *t*-test could be used to compare the estimates in two treatment groups. In the second approach, the mean rate of change (i.e., slope) for each treatment group would be estimated using a mixed effects model and the differences in the slopes between the treatment groups are tested. If there are no missing data, then the two approaches are virtually identical. However, when there are missing data, missing assessments are handled on an individual basis in the first approach and on a population basis in the second approach.

On an individual basis, first consider the construction of summary measures that reduce the set of n (or n_{ik}) measurements (Y_{ijk}) on the ith individual in the kth group to a single value (S_{ik}) by computing a weighted sum of the measurements (Y_{ijk}) or a function of the measurements as follows:

$$(f(Y_{ijk})): \quad S_{ik} = \sum_{j=1}^{n_{ik}} w_j f(Y_{ijk}).$$

O'Brien (1984) proposed several methods for complete data. In the first, the measurements on all subjects are ranked at each time point and then the average of the ranks across the n time points is computed for each individual. If the reasons for missing data were known and one could make reasonable assumptions about the ranking of HRQOL assessments among patients at each time point, it is possible one could adapt this approach to a study with missing data. For example, it would be reasonable to assume that the HRQOL of patients who died or left the study due to excessive toxicity was worse than the HRQOL of those patients who remained on therapy. Individuals who died or experienced excessive toxicity would be assigned the lowest possible rank for measurements scheduled after death or during the time of excessive toxicity.

In the second approach proposed by O'Brien, the measurements at each time point are converted to z-scores by subtracting the overall mean ($\bar{Y}_j$) and dividing by the standard deviation of the pooled sample as follows: $z_{ijk} = (Y_{ijk} - \bar{Y}_j)/\text{s.d.}(Y_{ijk})$. The measurements are averaged by using either equal weights ($w_j = 1/n$) or weights derived by summing the columns of the inverse correlation (R^{-1}) of the repeated measures. This latter approach down-weights the more highly correlated measurements. Based on studies of the power and size of the test, O'Brien recommended the average of the ranks for general use and the second approach with the weights derived from the inverse correlation, for normally distributed data with moderate or large sample sizes.

Matthews and colleagues (1990) and Cox and colleagues (1992) suggest an approach that provides a measure of HRQOL over time. The summary statistic is the area under the curve (AUC) of the HRQOL scores (Y_{ijk}) plotted against time (t). The AUC for the ikth individual can be estimated using a trapezoidal approximation as follows:

$$S_{ik} = AUC_{ik} = \sum_{j=2}^{n} (t_j - t_{j-1})(Y_{ijk} + Y_{i(j-1)k})/2 \quad , \quad j = 1, \cdots n$$

When the data are complete, this computation is straightforward. However, with this approach, strategies for handling missing data need to be developed. For example, if intermediate observations are missing, one could interpolate between observations. If a patient dies during the study, the minimum HRQOL score could be assigned at that time point. For a patient who dropped out, the last measurement could be inferred either by carrying the last value forward or extrapolating from the last two observations. Each of these approaches makes assumptions that may or may not be reasonable in specific settings, and it would be advisable to examine the sensitivity of the conclusions to the various assumptions.

Initially, it would appear that one could present the AUC values calculated to the time of censoring of the HRQOL assessments as one would present survival data. This approach would appear to have the advantages of displaying more information about the distribution of the AUC values and accommodating administrative censoring. Unfortunately, administrative censoring is informative on the AUC scale (Gelber, Gelman, & Goldhirsch, 1989; Glasziou et al., 1990) and the usual Kaplan-Meier estimates are biased. Specifically, if the censoring mechanism is due to staggered entry and incomplete follow-up is identical for two groups, the group with poorer HRQOL will have lower values of the AUC and will be censored earlier on the AUC scale. An alternative strategy for handling censoring due to dropout or administrative censoring is proposed by Korn (1993). Korn describes a procedure to reduce the bias of the estimator by assuming that the probability of censoring in short intervals is independent of the HRQOL measures prior to that time. While this assumption is probably not true, if HRQOL is measured frequently and the relationship between HRQOL and censoring is weak, the violation may be small enough that the bias in the estimator will also be small.

Within an individual basis, the second approach to constructing summary measures is to obtain parameter estimates for each treatment group $g(\hat{\beta}_{jk})$ and then reduce the set of estimates to a single summary measure for each treatment group as follows: $\hat{S}_k = \sum_{j=1}^{n} g(\hat{\beta}_{jk})$. In general, $g(\hat{\beta}_{jk})$ are the estimates of the mean of the jth measurement of HRQOL in the kth treatment group adjusted for important covariates (Fairclough, 1997). Alternatively, $g(\hat{\beta}_{jk})$ may be a direct estimate of the summary measure, such as the slope. If the data are complete, one can use multivariate analysis of variance or growth curve models to estimate β_{kj}. When data are missing, one can use the appropriate methods discussed later in this chapter for obtaining unbiased estimates, depending on whether the data are missing at random or nonignorable. In practice, this second strategy may be preferable because it may be much easier to develop a model-based method for handling missing data than to examine every missing observation.

A simple example of this second class of summary measures is the average of the r post-baseline means. This approach of constructing summary measures can also be used to estimate AUC for the kth treatment group. The AUC can be estimated by using a weighted function of the means (trapezoidal approximation) as follows:

$$\hat{S}_k = \sum_{j=2}^{n} (t_j - t_{j-1})(\mu_{jk} + \mu_{(j-1)k})/2$$

Alternatively, if a polynomial model ($E[Y_{ijk}] = \sum_{l=0}^{L} \beta_{kl} t_{ij}^{l}$) is used to estimate the change over time then the AUC can be estimated by integration as follows:

$$\hat{S}_k = \int_0^{t_n} \sum_{l=0}^{L} \beta_{kl} t^l = \sum_{l=0}^{L-1} \beta_{lk} t^{l+1} / (l+1)$$

Pocock and colleagues (1987) suggest an extension of O'Brien's weighted average z-scores to the combination of any asymptotically normal test statistics, illustrating the concept with the log-rank statistics and a binary endpoint.

Analysis of Longitudinal Data

When the endpoints are expressed in the metric of the HRQOL scales, there are three basic approaches to the analysis of longitudinal studies. The first, a repeated measure design, is to conceptualize time as ordered categories, with assessments planned during particular phases of the patient's treatment and/or disease progression. An example is a study by the Eastern Cooperative Oncology Group of two adjuvant therapy regimens for patients with hormone receptor negative, node-positive breast cancer (Fetting et al., 1998). In this study, there were three planned assessments: one prior to therapy, another during therapy, and a final assessment 4 months following therapy, representing three phases of the patient's treatment. The second approach, a growth curve model, conceptualizes time as a continuous factor. This approach is appropriate in settings where duration of treatment may not be determined *a priori* but depends on disease status and continues as long as therapy appears to be effective, as often occurs in a patient with chronic or advanced disease. The third approach is to reduce the longitudinal information to a single summary measure (i.e., global statistic).

Repeated Measures

Multiple univariate analyses is the most commonly used method of analysis, which consists of univariate analyses at each time point using test procedures such as *t*-tests, Analysis of variance (ANOVA), or Wilcoxon rank sum test. While simple to implement, this approach has several disadvantages (de Klerk, 1986; Pocock, Hughes, & Lee, 1987; Matthews et al., 1990). As previously discussed, the large number of comparisons often fails to answer the clinical question, but rather presents a confusing picture, and the probability of concluding that there are significant differences in HRQOL when none exist (the type I error) increases as the number of comparisons increase. In some cases, these univariate methods can be difficult to implement if measurements are mistimed due to delays in therapy or other factors.

A second analytic approach for repeated measures is to perform multivariate analyses. These procedures include multivariate analysis of variance (MANOVA), which deletes all cases with missing assessments and likelihood-based multivariate methods, such as mixed effects or repeated measures models that utilize all available data (Dempster, Laird, &

Rubin, 1977; Jennrich & Schluchter, 1986). Multivariate tests such as Hotelling's T and Likelihood Ratio tests can be used to control the type I error of the multiple comparisons. These statistics, however, test a hypothesis of no treatment differences against a general alternative. They are not sensitive to persistent differences over time and ask the general question, "Are there differences in HRQOL at *any* point in time?" These tests may sometimes be hard to interpret when the results are counterintuitive (de Klerk, 1986). For example, the test may be "statistically" significant when HRQOL is better in one treatment arm at one time point and another treatment at another time point, and not measure as significant when one treatment appears to have consistently better HRQOL over time (Fairclough, 1997). As discussed previously, summary measures provide an alternative.

Growth Curve Models

Growth curve models are useful most often for clinical trials with missing and mistimed observations, time-varying covariates, and a large number of potential repeated measures. These models include polynomial, or piecewise, linear functions of the actual time of assessment relative to some reference point. While most studies employ the date of diagnosis, with treatment initiation or randomization as the reference point, alternatives such as the time prior to death may be appropriate when the research focus is the patterns of change in HRQOL over time prior to death (Hwang, Chang, Fairclough, Cogswell, & Kasimis, 2003).

Missing Data

Missing data are inevitable in any longitudinal study in which, over an extended period of time, patients potentially will experience morbidity or mortality due to disease or its treatment. Missing data may also result from administrative problems such as staff forgetting to give the forms to the patient during a very busy time. Other reasons are directly related to the patient's quality of life, such as the patient being unable to complete the questionnaire because of severe toxicity or death.

Three classes of missing data determine which methods of analysis are appropriate for longitudinal studies (Little & Rubin, 1987). Briefly, if the reasons for missing assessments are unrelated to the patient's HRQOL, then the data is considered to be missing completely at random (MCAR). Common sense and historical evidence suggest this assumption will not be true in most clinical trials. If the probability of a missing assessment only depends on the observed measures of HRQOL and other explanatory factors, but not on the HRQOL the patient was experiencing at the time of the planned assessment, we consider the data to be missing at random (MAR). Finally, missing data are considered to be not missing at random (NMAR), or nonignorable, if the probability that an observation is missing depends on the value of the missing observation. Formal definitions and further discussion of these three types of missing assessments are presented by Little (1995). There are various formal approaches to testing the assumption of MCAR (Little, 1988; Diggle, 1989; Ridout, 1991; Park & Davis, 1993).

Missing data present difficulties in the design and analysis of longitudinal HRQOL studies for several reasons. First, there is the loss of power to detect change over time or differences between groups as a result of a reduced number of observations. However, in many large (Phase III) trials, the sample size has been based on other clinical endpoints and the power to detect meaningful differences in HRQOL measures generally is adequate. If not, increasing the sample size of the trial may be feasible, depending on patient and economic resources.

The second problem with missing data is the potential for bias in the estimates as a result of nonrandomly missing data (Fairclough, Peterson, & Chang, 1998). For example, patients experiencing a negative impact of the disease or therapy on their quality of life may be less likely to complete the HRQOL assessments. In other settings, patients who have had an excellent response to therapy may feel that they no longer need to continue their participation in the treatment study. In either case, as will be illustrated in the following paragraphs, a clear understanding of the reasons for missing assessments is critical in the selection of the appropriate method of analysis for these longitudinal studies.

Analysis of Complete Cases (MCAR)

The most often used methods of analysis for longitudinal data are methods such as multivariate analysis of variance (MANOVA), or growth curve models, that include data from patients who have completed *all* of the scheduled assessments. This is sometimes referred to as complete case analysis. These methods are popular because they are taught in most intermediate statistical courses and are available in almost every statistical analysis package. If the proportion of subjects with any missing assessments is very small (<5% of the cases), these methods may be reasonable. However, in many studies with extended follow-up and patients who may be experiencing morbidity and/or mortality, these methods could easily exclude more than half of the subjects from the analysis. More critically, these approaches are based on the very strong assumption of MCAR; if that assumption is violated, then the estimates may be seriously biased. This assumption is that the probability an observation is missing does not depend on the HRQOL of the patient at the time of any of the planned assessments. An example of a study where this is not true is a longitudinal study conducted by the International Breast Study Group (IBCSG) of 1475 premenopausal breast cancer patients (Hurny et al., 1996). The relationship between the number of missing assessments and the available HRQOL scores from the Perceived Adaptation to Chronic Illness Scales (PACIS) (Hurny et al., 1992) was examined in patients who did not experience disease progression during the first 18 months of follow-up. After excluding patients with missing assessments due to disease progression, the individuals with fewer missing assessments reported better HRQOL when they were assessed than individuals with more missing assessments (Fairclough, Peterson, Cella, & Bonomi, 1998). Thus, the probability an observation was missing depended on the HRQOL that the patient was experiencing. The relationship is even stronger when all subjects (including those with disease progression) are included. Based on this evidence, the data cannot be considered MCAR. If the analysis had been limited to the complete cases (the 344 patients with all 7 assessments), the results would be biased and not representative of the entire group of patients.

Analysis of All Available Data (MAR)

The assumption that data are MCAR, required in the analysis of complete cases, can be relaxed to the assumption that data are missing at random (MAR) (Little, 1995) or ignorable (Laird, 1988). In either situation, the probability that an observation is missing may depend on observed data and covariates, but still must be independent of the value of the missing observation(s) after adjustment for the observed data and covariates. Likelihood based methods that use all the available data result in unbiased estimates when the data are MAR. These methods are also accessible in many of the major statistical software packages (The Mixed Procedure, 1992).

One approach to understanding the assumption of MAR is to consider a study where the assumption is incorrect. In this observational study (Fairclough, Peterson, Cella & Bonomi, 1998), 68 patients with metastatic or progressive disease completed an assessment of HRQOL every 3 to 6 weeks. When the data are analyzed using a model that assumes the data are MAR, there is only a small, statistically insignificant decrease in the estimates of HRQOL over time. However, when subjects were grouped by the duration of follow-up (or survival), patients who died earlier experienced a rapid rate of decline in HRQOL over time. However, because these subjects no longer were being observed, the estimates obtained from the MAR models describe the average HRQOL of the surviving patients rather than the decline in HRQOL of the entire group of terminal patients.

Strategies for Nonignorable Missing Data (NMAR)

Nonignorable missing data probably is the most likely type of missing data in HRQOL studies in clinical trials where there is dropout due to toxicity, disease progression, or therapeutic effectiveness. Studies with this type of missing data are also difficult to analyze. The primary reason is there are numerous potential models and it is impossible to verify statistically the correctness of any. A primary reason is because the data required to test the adequacy of the possible models are missing. A secondary reason is that software for these methods of analysis is not available in statistical analysis packages.

Little (1995) describes two general classes of models, selection, and pattern mixture. The choice between the two classes partially depends on whether the missing data mechanism is viewed to be solely a "nuisance" or not. In the class of selection models, a statistical model is specified for the missing data mechanism. In addition to adjusting the estimates for the missing data, these models allow the investigator to make inferences about the relationship of HRQOL and other explanatory factors causing missing observations. This would be particularly interesting, for example, if death or disease progression were the cause of dropout. In contrast to the selection models, pattern mixture models do not require specification of a particular model for the missing data mechanism. This advantage is balanced by the large number of potential patterns of missing data and the difficulties of estimating parameters in the under-identified models of dropout for some of the missing data patterns. The following two sections describe these two classes of models in more detail.

Selection models. Selection models for the analysis of studies with nonignorable missing data include models where the change in HRQOL over time is related functionally to the time of death, disease progression, or study dropout. Wu and Carroll (1988) proposed a probit model for the probability of dropout, which depends on the linear change in HRQOL over time. Wu and Bailey (1989) describe a conditional linear model where the rate of change in an individual is modeled as a polynomial function of the dropout time. Both methods are based on a growth curve model approach with the individual slope parameters related to censoring of later observations (right censoring) either through a linear random effects model with a probit model for the censoring process or a conditional linear model. Mori, Woodworth, and Woolson (1992) propose empirical Bayes estimates of the individual subject slopes that adjust for informative right censoring. When a patient is censored early, the time of censoring dominates the estimate of the change in HRQOL, whereas when censoring occurs later, the ordinary least squares estimate of the individual's slope dominates the estimate.

Shared parameter/joint models. One of the most popular recent strategies has been joint modeling of the longitudinal HRQOL assessments with survival or other events, such as discontinuation of therapy, disease progression, or dropout that are extensions of the random effects, or two-stage mixed effects, model. These approaches are applicable even when the change over time is not expected to be linear or the censoring times vary across patients. The time of censoring (or death) is incorporated into the model by allowing the time of censoring to be correlated with the random effects of the longitudinal model for HRQOL. For example, it is assumed the initial score and rate of change for an individual recorrelates with the time to dropout or death. Thus, patients who drop out early tend to have poorer HRQOL scores initially and decline more rapidly. Various models for the time to dropout include normal and log normal distributions (Schluchter, 1992; Schluchter, Konstan, & Davis, 2002; Schluchter, Greene, & Beck, 2001; DeGruttola & Tu, 1994) and piecewise exponential (Vonesh, Green, & Schluchter, 2006).

Pattern mixture models. The basic concept behind the pattern mixture models, described by Little (1995), is the distribution of the measures of HRQOL; Y_i, may differ across the K different missing data patterns, having different means, $\mu^{(k)}$ and variance, $\Sigma^{(k)}$. For example, patients who die earlier (with missing data due to death) may have lower HRQOL scores (different means) and also may have more or less variability in their scores (different variance) than patients who survive longer. The true distribution of the measures of HRQOL for the entire group of patients will be a mixture of the distributions of each of the K groups of patients. The general method of analysis is to stratify the patients by the missing data patterns. Then the mean and variance parameters ($\mu^{(k)}$, $\Sigma^{(k)}$) are estimated within each strata. Weights are determined by the proportion of subjects within each of the K missing data patterns ($w_k = n_k/N$). The population estimates are the weighted average of the estimates from the K missing data patterns ($\mu = \Sigma w_k \mu^{(k)}$). The advantage of these models is one doesn't have to define a model for the missing data mechanism. However, there are strong assumptions and restrictions associated with these models that may not be readily obvious, but are important nonetheless. One of the difficulties of this approach is the large number of missing data patterns that occur in actual studies where there may only be a few subjects with some patterns. More critically, for all but the one pattern where there are no missing observations, the model may be under-identified; there may not be enough data in certain patterns to estimate all the parameters of the model without making additional assumptions. The pattern where all the observations are missing is the most obvious example of an under-identified model. The assumptions required for the estimation of model parameters often are difficult to communicate and cannot be validated because they depend on the values of the missing data.

Imputation, estimating missing data. An alternative method of analysis uses the strategy of imputation to estimate the missing data (Crawford, Tennstedt, & McKinlay, 1995; Lavori, Dawson, & Shera, 1995; Rubin, 1987; Rubin & Schenker, 1991). The motivations for this approach are that complete data methods, such as MANOVA, can be used to analyze the imputed data sets, and information about the reasons for missing data can be incorporated into the imputation scheme. These methods include both single and multiple imputation using both model-based and sampling methods for imputation.

The choice of the method for imputation should consider the missing data mechanism. Most of the available methods, such as the Markov Chain Monte Carlo (MCMC) procedure for multivariate normal data, assume the data are MCAR or MAR. The danger is, if that assumption is not true, there is a false confidence about the results. Only if auxiliary information, such as surrogate measures and other strongly correlated measures, are included in the imputation model such that the data are missing at random, conditional on the observed data and auxiliary information, will estimates obtained from the imputed data be unbiased.

Single imputation methods include mean imputation and regression imputation. In mean imputation, the average value of the measure of HRQOL is substituted for the missing observations. In regression imputation, the predicted value of the measure of HRQOL is estimated using a regression model, and is substituted for the missing assessments. One implementation of this technique in SPSS is referred to as an expectation maximization (EM) imputation. The value imputed is the expected value of the missing observation. The criticism of all the single imputation methods is that the analysis treats imputed values just like observed values and underestimates uncertainty by ignoring the measurement error, among-subject variability, and the incomplete knowledge of the reason for nonresponse. Thus, single imputation strategies are ill-advised because they incorrectly underestimate the variance of the estimates and inflate test statistics (von Hippel, 2004). Multiple imputation retains many of the advantages of single imputation, but rectifies both problems. The basic strategy of multiple imputation is to impute three to ten sets of values for the missing data that incorporate both sampling variability and the uncertainty about the reasons for nonresponse. Methods of sampling can include explicit models such as the MCMC algorithm for multivariate normal data, or implicit models such as approximate Bayesian bootstrap. Each set of data is then analyzed using complete data methods and the analyses are combined in a way that reflects the extra variability due to missing data (Rubin, 1987; Rubin, 1996; Rubin & Schenker, 1991).

Lavori and colleagues (1995) propose a strategy for multiple imputation based on a propensity score of the probability of dropout. The idea is to find a univariate score that summarizes the multiple variables defining the history of each patient, stratify patients using the quintiles of the score, and then use an approximate Bayesian bootstrap (Rosenbaum & Rubin, 1984) to impute the missing values within each of the strata. A multistep process is used to compute the score for each of the planned observation times. One of the advantages of this approach is that a single set of propensity scores is computed, which can be used for multiple HRQOL outcomes. As the number of assessments increases with multiple causes for missing data, these strategies can quickly become very complex. The most critical assumption of this approach is that the data are MCAR within each of the strata. Specifically, this approach assumes that, within groups defined by a limited number of measured characteristics, the HRQOL of the subjects who completed an HRQOL assessment is no better or worse than the HRQOL of subjects who did not complete the assessment. For example, the strata might be defined by the value of the previous measure and demographic characteristics. We assume that scores for missing assessments have the same distribution as the observed assessments for subjects in each stratum.

A popular approach is to use the last observation (or value) carried forward (LOCF or LVCF), where the patient's last available assessment is substituted for each of the missing assessments. This approach has limited utility (Heyting, Tolboom, & Essers, 1992) and should be employed with great caution. For example, in a study where HRQOL is decreasing over time, a treatment with early dropout possibly could look better than a treatment where tolerance to the therapy was better.

Nonparametric Analysis Using Ranked Data

Gould (1980) describes a practical method for the analysis of clinical trials with withdrawal. If there is adequate documentation concerning the reasons for missing assessments, it may be possible to determine a reasonable ordering (or ranking) of HRQOL among the subjects. For example, it would be reasonable to assign patients who withdraw because of disease progression, excessive toxicity, or death a rank that is lower than that observed for patients remaining in the study. The advantage of this approach is we do not have to impute the specific value. However, Heyting and colleagues (1992) identified limitations, including multiple reasons for dropout that are not clearly ordered. Methods for nonparametric analysis of repeated measures are proposed by Wei and Johnson (1985).

Choice of Methods and Sensitivity Analyses

In practice, current application of methods (selection models and pattern mixture models) for nonignorable missing data is limited by several factors. The first is the large number of subjects required to distinguish between alternate models. The second is the restriction of some assumptions such as linear changes over time and the inability of any one technique to deal with both the monotone and nonmonotone patterns. In addition, the sophisticated programs required for these methods and the lack of generally available software are barriers to implementation. The most significant barrier, however, may be how to present these complicated models in a manner that is readily interpretable in clinical literature.

Given the numerous potential methods of analysis, how do we choose between different strategies? In some cases, we have information such as the reason for missing assessments or a clearly defined objective that will determine the so-called best approach. But although certain approaches may be eliminated from consideration, generally we will be left with several possibilities. A sensitivity analysis in which the effect of the different methods of analysis is examined may be informative (Fairclough, Peterson, Cella, & Bonomi, 1998). There are two likely outcomes of the sensitivity analysis. The first is that the conclusions are consistent regardless of the approach. The alternative outcome of a sensitivity analysis is that the conclusions are dependent on the method of analysis or the summary measure selected. When this occurs, the methods should be examined to ascertain the reason for the discrepancy.

Summary and Implications for Design and Conduct

With the incorporation of HRQOL into an increasing number of clinical trials, there is an urgent need to develop practical methods for the analysis of these longitudinal studies. Methods of analysis for trials where the data can safely be assumed to be MAR are well established with easily accessible software. However, in most trials some of the missing data associated with HRQOL assessment is likely to be nonignorable. The question is, when is it critical to use more sophisticated methods? For example, will it make a difference in the treatment comparisons if only 5% of the subjects have missing data? What about 10% or 20% missing data? Can we say, if the proportion of missing data is the same in two treatment arms, that treatment comparisons will be valid even if the estimates are biased? Clearly, there are many questions to be addressed in the context of actual clinical trials. The challenge will be to adapt theoretical methods to settings where there are multiple reasons for missing data.

The issues of missing data and multiple comparisons have strong implications for the design and conduct of these studies. The first step is to specify a well defined objective. Vague aims such as, "To compare the quality of life of patients on the two treatment arms" do not help investigators specify a limited number of endpoints or develop a strategy to minimize multiple comparisons. Clearly, strategies to minimize missing data will also be important (Fairclough, Peterson, Cella, & Bonomi, 1998). For example, linking the timing of the HRQOL assessments with another assessment may reduce the number of assessments that are omitted. Careful consideration of whether to continue HRQOL assessment when a patient discontinues treatment early will affect what hypotheses can be tested and the ability to generalize the results. Careful prospective documentation of the reasons for missing assessments will offer the analyst a basis for choosing a particular analysis strategy.

Interpretation and Reporting of Results

With the wealth of information coming from clinical trials, the most difficult question facing investigators is how to communicate the results in a way that is meaningful to patients, clinicians, third-party players, relatives, and society. How do we make HRQOL relevant to the development of new therapies and individual treatment? These challenges may be solved partially with future research if done carefully and with directed questions. We need, however, to pay as much attention to the way in which results of HRQOL assessment are presented and used as we have to the development of HRQOL measures and their incorporation into clinical trials.

One of the most critical issues is the interpretation of meaningful change in HRQOL scores. We must be able to communicate a sense of what it means to have a 1-point difference or a 10-point change over time in HRQOL scores, if that is observed in the study. Is that difference of sufficient clinical importance to consider the selection of one therapeutic approach over another? This determination will involve relating these scores to other measures that are meaningful to the audience. For clinicians, this might mean relating the scores to performance status or to an outcome measure. It may also involve assessing what patients perceive as a meaningful change (Osoba, Rodrigues, Myles, Zee, & Pater, 1998).

CONCLUSION

The inclusion of health-related quality-of-life assessments in clinical investigations promises to play an important role in our current healthcare system. Information from this research has the potential to promote communication between the patient and the healthcare provider; HRQOL assessment can provide quantitative information that can facilitate decisions on resource allocations. During the past three decades there has been considerable energy channeled into the development of HRQOL instruments and an increased incorporation of HRQOL assessment into clinical trials. As a result, there have been advances in our understanding of HRQOL.

We need to be looking to the future and considering how these investigations can best be designed, what questions truly are being addressed, and how resulting information is used to improve clinical practice. Before embarking on resource intensive studies, it is important to examine carefully the specific objectives for assessing HRQOL. Are the results likely to have an impact on clinical practice? If not, how will the results advance cancer investigation and ultimately benefit future patients? The issue of when to include HRQOL assessment in a clinical trial is not only about the conservation of resources, but more importantly, the protection of the patients who consent to participate in clinical trials.

REFERENCES

Brooks, M. M., Jenkins, L. S., Schron, E. B., Steinberg, J. S., Cross, J. A., & Paeth, D. S. (1998). Quality of life at baseline: Is assessment after randomization valid? The AVID (Antiarrhythmics Versus Implantable Defibrillators) Investigators. *Medical Care, 36*(10), 1515–1519.

Cella, D. F., Skeel, R. T., & Bonomi, A. E. (1993). *Policies and Procedures Manual.* (Available from the Eastern Cooperative Oncology Group: Quality of Life Subcommittee; Health Practices Committee).

Cella, D. F., Tulsky, D. S., Gray, G., Sarafian, B., Linn, E., Bonomi, A., et al. (1993). The Functional Assessment of Cancer Therapy scale: Development and validation of the general measure. *Journal of Clinical Oncology, 11*(3), 570–579.

Cohen, J. (1998). *Statistical power analysis for the behavioral sciences* (2nd ed.). Hillsdale, NJ: Lawrence Erlbaum Associates.

Cox, D. R., Fitzpatrick, R., Fletcher, A. E., Gore, S. M., Spiegelhalter, D. J., & Jones, D. R. (1992). Quality-of-life assessment: Can we keep it simple? *Journal of the Royal Statistical Society A, 155*(3), 353–393.

Crawford, S. L., Tennstedt, S. L., & McKinlay, J. B. (1995). A comparison of analytic methods for non-random missingness of outcome data. *Journal of Clinical Epidemiology, 48*(2), 209–219.

DeGruttola, V., & Tu, X. M. (1994). Modeling progression of CD4-lymphocyte count and its relationship to survival time. *Biometrics, 50*(4), 1003–1014.

de Klerk, N. H. (1986). Repeated warnings re-repeated measures. *Australian and New Zealand Journal of Medicine, 16*(5), 637–638.

Dempster, A. P., Laird, N. M., & Rubin, D. B. (1977). Maximum likelihood from incomplete data via the EM Algorithm. *Journal of the Royal Statistical Society (B), 39*(1), 1–38.

Diggle, P. J. (1989). Testing for random dropouts in repeated measurement data. *Biometrics, 45*(4), 1255–1258.

Fairclough, D. L. (1997). Summary measures and statistics for comparison of quality of life in a clinical trial of cancer therapy. *Statistics in Medicine, 16*(11), 1197–209.

Fairclough, D. L., & Cella, D. F. (1996). Eastern Cooperative Oncology Group (ECOG). *Journal of the National Cancer Institute Monographs, 20*, 73–75.

Fairclough, D. L., Peterson, H. F., Cella, D., & Bonomi, P. (1998). Comparison of several model-based methods for analysing incomplete quality of life data in cancer clinical trials. *Statistics in Medicine, 17*(5–7), 781–796.

Fairclough, D. L., Peterson, H. F., & Chang, V. (1998). Why are missing quality of life data a problem in clinical trials of cancer therapy? *Statistics in Medicine, 17*(5–7), 667–677.

Feeny, D. (1998). QALY: The application of decision theory to RCT. In M. Staquet, R. Hays, & P. Fayers (Eds.), *Quality of life assessment in clinical trials: Methods and practice.* Oxford, NY: Oxford University Press.

Feeny, D., Furlong, W., Barr, R. D., Torrance, G. W., Rosenbaum, P., & Weitzman, S. (1992). A comprehensive multiattribute system for classifying the health status of survivors of childhood cancer. *Journal of Clinical Oncology, 10*(6), 923–928.

Fetting, J. H., Gray, R., Fairclough, D. L., Smith, T. J., Margolin, K. A., Citron, M. L., et al. (1998). Sixteen-week multidrug regimen versus cyclophosphamide, doxorubicin, and fluorouracil as adjuvant therapy for node-positive, receptor-negative breast cancer: An Intergroup study. *Journal of Clinical Oncology, 16*(7), 2382–2391.

Gelber, R. (1998). TWiST and Q-TWiST. In M. Staquet, R. Hays, & P. Fayers (Eds.), *Quality of life assessment in clinical trials: Methods and practice.* Oxford; NY: Oxford University Press.

Gelber, R. D., Gelman, R. S., & Goldhirsch, A. (1989). A quality-of-life-oriented endpoint for comparing therapies. *Biometrics, 45*(3), 781–795.

Glasziou, P. P., Simes, R. J., & Gelber, R. D. (1990). Quality adjusted survival analysis. *Statistics in Medicine, 9*(11), 1259–1276.

Goldhirsch, A., Gelber, R. D., Simes, R. J., Glasziou, P., & Coates, A. S. (1989). Costs and benefits of adjuvant therapy in breast cancer: A quality- adjusted survival analysis. *Journal of Clinical Oncology, 7*(1), 36–44.

Gotay, C. C., Korn, E. L., McCabe, M. S., Moore, T. D., & Cheson, B. D. (1992). Building quality of life assessment into cancer treatment studies. *Oncology (Hunting), 6*(6), 25–28; discussion 30–32, 37.

Gould, A. L. (1980). A new approach to the analysis of clinical drug trials with withdrawals. *Biometrics, 36*(4), 721–727.

Groenvold, M., Klee, M. C., Sprangers, M. A., & Aaronson, N. K. (1997). Validation of the EORTC QLQ-C30 quality of life questionnaire through combined qualitative and quantitative assessment of patient-observer agreement. *Journal of Clinical Epidemiology, 50*(4), 441–450.

Heyting, A., Tolboom, J. T., & Essers, J. G. (1992). Statistical handling of drop-outs in longitudinal clinical trials. *Statistics in Medicine, 11*(16), 2043–2061.

Hicks, J. E., Lampert, M. H., Gerber, L. H., Glastein, E., & Danoff, J. F. (1985). Functional outcome update in patients with soft tissue sarcoma undergoing wide local excision and radiation. *Archives of Physical Medicine, 66,* 542–543.

Hochberg, Y. (1988). A sharper Bonferroni procedure for multiple tests of significance. *Biometrika, 75,* 800–802.

Hopwood, P., Harvey, A., Davies, J., Stephens, R. J., Girling, D. J., Gibson, D., et al. (1998). Survey of the Administration of quality of life (QOL) questionnaires in three multicentre randomised trials in cancer. From The Medical Research Council Lung Cancer Working Party the CHART Steering Committee. *European Journal of Cancer, 34*(1), 49–57.

Hurny, C., Bernhard, J., Coates, A. S., Castiglione-Gertsch, M., Peterson, H. F., Gelber, R. D., et al. (with the International Breast Cancer Study Group). (1996). Impact of adjuvant therapy on quality of life in women with node-positive operable breast cancer. *Lancet, 347*(9011), 1279–1284.

Hurny, C., Bernhard, J., Gelber, R. D., Coates, A., Castiglione, M., Isley, M., et al. (with the International Breast Cancer Study Group). (1992). Quality of life measures for patients receiving adjuvant therapy for breast cancer: An international trial. *European Journal of Cancer, 28*(1), 118–124.

Hwang, S. S., Chang, V. T., Fairclough, D. L., Cogswell, J., & Kasimis, B. (2003). Longitudinal quality of life in advanced cancer patients: Pilot study results from a VA medical center. *Journal of Pain and Symptom Management, 25*(3), 225–235.

Jennrich, R. I., & Schluchter, M. D. (1986). Unbalanced repeated-measures models with structured covariance matrices. *Biometrics, 42*(4), 805–820.

Korn, E. L. (1993). On estimating the distribution function for quality of life in cancer clinical trials. *Biometrika, 80*(3), 335–342.

Korn, E. L., & O'Fallon, J. (with the Statistics Working Group: Quality of life assessment in cancer clinical trials). (1990). *Statistical considerations: Report on the workshop on quality of life research in cancer clinical trials.* Division of Cancer Prevention and Control, National Cancer Institute.

Laird, N. M. (1988). Missing data in longitudinal studies. *Statistics in Medicine, 7,* 305–315.

Lavori, P. W., Dawson, R., & Shera, D. (1995). A multiple imputation strategy for clinical trials with truncation of patient data. *Statistics in Medicine, 14*(17), 1913–1925.

Little, R. J. A. (1988). A test of missing completely at random for multivariate data with missing values. *Journal of the American Statistical Association, 83*(404), 1198–1202.

Little, R. J. A. (1995). Modeling the drop-out mechanism in repeated-measures studies. *Journal of the American Statistical Association, 90*(431), 1112–1121.

Little, R. J. A., & Rubin, D. B. (1987). *Statistical analysis with missing data.* New York, NY: John Wiley & Sons.

Loprinzi, C. L., Laurie, J. A., Wieand, H. S., Krook, J. E., Novotny, P. J., Kugler, J. W., et al. (with North Central Cancer Treatment Group). (1994). Prospective evaluation of prognostic variables from patient-completed questionnaires. *Journal of Clinical Oncology, 12*(3), 601–607.

Matthews, J. N., Altman, D. G., Campbell, M. J., & Royston, P. (1990). Analysis of serial measurements in medical research. *British Medical Journal, 300*(6719), 230–235.

McNeil, B. J., Weichselbaum, R., & Pauker, S. G. (1981). Speech and survival: Tradeoffs between quality and quantity of life in laryngeal cancer. *New England Journal of Medicine, 305*(17), 982–987.

The Mixed Procedure. (1992). *SAS Technical Report T-229, SAS/STAT software, changes and enhancements* (pp. 289–366). Cary, NC: SAS Institute.

Mori, M., Woodworth, G. G., & Woolson, R. F. (1992). Application of empirical Bayes inference to estimation of rate of change in the presence of informative right censoring. *Statistics in Medicine*, *11*(5), 621–631.

O'Brien, P. C. (1984). Procedures for comparing samples with multiple endpoints. *Biometrics*, *40*(4), 1079–1087.

Osoba, D., Rodrigues, G., Myles, J., Zee, B., & Pater, J. (1998). Interpreting the significance of changes in health-related quality-of-life scores. *Journal of Clinical Oncology*, *16*(1), 139–144.

Park, T., & Davis, C. S. (1993). A test of the missing data mechanism for repeated categorical data. *Biometrics*, *49*(2), 631–638.

Pocock, S. J., Geller, N. L., & Tsiatis, A. A. (1987). The analysis of multiple endpoints in clinical trials. *Biometrics*, *43*(3), 487–498.

Pocock, S. J., Hughes, M. D., & Lee, R. J. (1987). Statistical problems in the reporting of clinical trials. A survey of three medical journals. *New England Journal of Medicine*, *317*(7), 426–432.

Ridout, M. S. (1991). Testing for random dropouts in repeated measurement data. *Biometrics*, *47*, 1617–1621.

Rosenbaum, P. R., & Rubin, D. B. (1984). Reducing bias in observational studies using subclassification on the propensity score. *Journal of the American Statistical Association*, *79*(387), 516–524.

Rubin, D. B. (1987). *Multiple imputation for nonresponse in surveys*. New York, NY: John Wiley and Sons.

Rubin, D. B. (1996). Multiple imputation after 18 + years. *J Am Stat Assoc*, *91*(434), 473–489.

Rubin, D. B., & Schenker, N. (1991). Multiple imputation in health-care databases: An overview and some applications. *Statistics in Medicine*, *10*(4), 585–598.

Schipper, H. (1990). Guidelines and caveats for quality of life measurement in clinical practice and research. *Oncology (Huntingt)*, *4*(5), 51–57; discussion 70.

Schluchter, M. D. (1992). Methods for the analysis of informatively censored longitudinal data. *Statistics in Medicine*, *11*(14–15), 1861–1870.

Schluchter, M. D., Greene, T., & Beck, G. J. (2001). Analysis of change in the presence of informative censoring: Application to a longitudinal clinical trial of progressive renal disease. *20*, 989–1007.

Schluchter, M. D., Konstan, M. W., & Davis, P. B. (2002). Jointly modeling the relationship between survival and pulmonary function in cystic fibrosis patients. *Statistics in Medicine*, *21*, 1271–1287.

Slevin, M. L., Stubbs, L., Plant, H. J., Wilson, P., Gregory, W. M., Armes, P. J., et al. (1990). Attitudes to chemotherapy: Comparing views of patients with cancer with those of doctors, nurses, and general public. *British Medical Journal*, *300*(6737), 1458–1460.

Slevin, M. L., Plant. H., Lynch, D., Drinkwater, J., & Gregory, W. M. (1988). Who should measure quality of life, the doctor or the patient? *British Journal of Cancer*, *57*, 109–112.

Sugarbaker, P. H., Barofsky, I., Rosenberg, S. A., & Gianola, F. J. (1982). Quality of life assessment of patients in extremity sarcoma clinical trials. *Surgery*, *91*(1), 17–23.

Tandon, P. K. (1990). Applications of global statistics in analysing quality of life data. *Statistics in Medicine*, *9*(7), 819–827.

Torrance, G. W., Thomas, W. H., & Sackett, D. L. (1971). A utility maximizing model for evaluation of health care programs. *Health Services Research*, *7*, 118–133.

Vonesh, E. F., Green, T., & Schluchter, M. D. (2006). Shared parameter models for the joint analysis of longitudinal data and event times. *Statistics in Medicine*, *25*(1), 143–163.

von Hippel, P. T. (2004). Biases in SPSS 12.0: Missing Value Analysis. *The American Statistician*, *58*, 160–164.

Weeks, J. (1992). Quality-of-life assessment: Performance status upstaged? *Journal of Clinical Oncology*, *10*(12), 1827–1829.

Wei, L. J., & Johnson, W. E. (1985). Combining dependent tests with incomplete repeated measurements. *Biometrika*, *72*(2), 359–364.

Wu, M. C., & Bailey, K. R. (1989). Estimation and comparison of changes in the presence of informative right censoring: Conditional linear model. *Biometrics, 45*(3), 939–955.

Wu, M. C., & Carroll, R. J. (1988). Estimation and comparison of changes in the presence of informative right censoring by modeling the censoring process. *Biometrics, 44*, 175–88.

Yabroff, K. R., Linas, B. P., & Schulman, K. (1996). Evaluation of quality of life for diverse patient populations. *Breast Cancer Research and Treatment, 40*(1), 87–104.

Zhang, J., Quan, H., Ng, J., & Stepanavage, M. E. (1997). Some statistical methods for multiple endpoints in clinical trials. *Controlled Clinical Trials, 18*(3), 204–221.

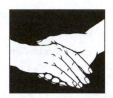

Chapter Twelve

Health-Related Quality-of-Life Studies Conducted Through the NCI Clinical Trials Networks

Ann M. O'Mara

Introduction

For over 50 years, the National Cancer Institute (NCI) has supported the Cooperative Group Program, which was established to develop and implement studies of chemotherapy for cancer. Since its inception, the program has expanded to include all types of treatment, not just chemotherapy, and currently includes twelve cooperative groups (Table 12-1), which place more than 22,000 new patients into cancer treatment clinical trials each year (National Cancer Institute, 2009). In 1983, recognizing that accrual to cancer treatment trials remained low, the NCI established the Community Clinical Oncology Program (CCOP) as a way to improve not only accrual numbers, but also to increase the racial, ethnic, and age distribution characteristics of eligible patients (National Cancer Institute, n.d.). This program also expanded the focus of clinical trials beyond treating the disease to preventing cancer and ameliorating and preventing the toxicities and side effects of the disease and its treatment. These two NCI-supported clinical trials networks have provided the infrastructure for assessing and evaluating health-related quality of life (HRQOL) of cancer patients participating in clinical trials.

Beginning in the late 1980s, results of the early disease treatment trials showed increased survival and improved tumor response came with a number of physical, psychosocial, and economic costs. A number of publications began to address these costs, namely HRQOL issues, as important outcomes in cancer clinical trials (Waalen, 1990; Lindley, 1990; Skeel, 1989). However, there was, and continues to be, a number of challenges to incorporating HRQOL assessments into multisite clinical trials. This chapter will do the following: (1) describe the outcomes of a 1985 NCI pilot project and several NCI meetings and workshops conducted between 1990 and 2005 on the challenges of incorporating HRQOL endpoints into NCI-approved clinical trials; (2) highlight findings from several major trials that included HRQOL endpoints; and (3) discuss the current status of incorporating HRQOL endpoints into disease treatment, symptom management, and cancer prevention clinical trials conducted through the NCI-supported clinical trials networks.

Table 12-1. **Current NCI-funded Cooperative Groups, 2007**

Cooperative Group	Acronym
1. American College of Surgeons Oncology Group	ACOSOG
2. American College of Radiology Imaging Network	ACRIN
3. Cancer and Leukemia Group B	CALGB
4. Children's Oncology Group	COG
5. Eastern Cooperative Oncology Group	ECOG
6. European Organization for Research and Treatment of Cancer	EORTC
7. Gynecologic Oncology Group	GOG
8. National Cancer Institute of Canada, Clinical Trials Group	NCIC
9. National Surgical and Adjuvant Breast and Bowel Project	NSABP
10. North Central Cancer Treatment Group	NCCTG
11. Radiation Therapy Oncology Group	RTOG
12. Southwest Oncology Group	SWOG

Status of HRQOL Studies in the 1980s

In addition to the methodological issues inherent in designing trials that include HRQOL endpoints, there are the logistics of implementing them. For the CCOP program in its early years, these issues were crucial. Most clinical trials were (and continue to be) conducted in busy outpatient settings, where patients are present for only a short period of time and the data are collected locally, but transmitted to and managed at remote sites. In 1985, NCI staff implemented a 4-month pilot project among six CCOP institutions in Illinois, Michigan, Ohio, Wisconsin, and Texas to determine the difficulties health personnel faced in collecting and transmitting HRQOL data in clinical trials (Yancik, Edwards, & Yates, 1987). Four areas of interest were feasibility of conducting the research in the various settings, patient burden, staff burdens, and obtaining useful data with the selected HRQOL measures. Findings from the study showed accrual was poor (156 out of 655 eligible patients were consented) and was due not only to lack of patient interest, but to staff forgetting to mention the study. When a patient was accrued, staff viewed the work as an additional burden, not an integral part of cancer care or clinical trials management. Patients were asked to complete four different measures, which took approximately 30 minutes to complete. Staff viewed this as burdensome to both patient and staff. Recommendations included ensuring that the HRQOL study was an integral part of a clinical trial and not a separate study, educating staff on the procedures for conducting the assessments, and using the briefest measures to gather the most information. The findings and recommendations from this small study were used to assist CCOP and research bases in the design and implementation of HRQOL studies, as well as to assist NCI staff in their review of the studies.

Progress During the 1990s

Disease Treatment Trials

In 1990, the National Cancer Institute and the Office of Medical Applications of Research convened a workshop of clinicians, social scientists, and statisticians from the Cooperative Groups, NCI-supported cancer centers, pharmaceutical companies, and the Food and Drug Administration (FDA) to (1) define elements of HRQOL relevant to clinical decision making and represent realistic endpoints in clinical trials; (2) evaluate currently available instruments for HRQOL assessment and strategies for implementation; (3) identify diseases in which HRQOL measures may be most useful; and (4) examine issues regarding the integration of findings from therapeutic evaluations and HRQOL measures (Nayfield, Ganz, Moninpour, Cella, & Hailey, 1992). For each of the objectives, workshop participants made several recommendations, which are summarized in Table 12-2. Although there was consensus on the recommendations, the exact role of HRQOL assessment in cancer clinical trials was not determined, nor was there agreement on the best measure. However, the working group did recommend a number of candidate measures that met the criteria of brevity, adequate coverage of key dimensions, and published evidence of psychometric evaluation. Since that meeting, HRQOL assessments have become common secondary endpoints on Phase III disease treatment and symptom management trials, and on very large prevention trials conducted through the NCI national clinical trials networks.

In a follow-up to the 1990 meeting, the NCI, in 1995, convened a similar group of clinicians, social scientists, and statisticians to assess the progress that had been made in NCI-sponsored HRQOL research during the past 5 years. The goals of the workshop were to (1) re-evaluate clinical research areas in which HRQOL questions were a priority, (2) address issues of implementation and collection of HRQOL data in NCI-sponsored clinical trials, and (3) focus on new methods of HRQOL research, such as outcome studies and methods of assessing HRQOL in culturally diverse populations (Varricchio, McCabe, Trimble, & Korn, 1996). One significant change in priority was the identification of clinical research areas. One of the recommendations from the earlier meeting was the identification of selected disease sites appropriate for HRQOL measurements. This recommendation was no longer considered the driving force for adding a HRQOL research question. Instead, recommendations focused on questions that would identify the full range of toxicities, compare treatments in a trial, and use HRQOL data as a predictor of response to future treatment, irrespective of the disease site (Cella & Tulsky, 1993). Cooperative group participants reported on their progress in studying HRQOL in both treatment and symptom management trials (Bradlyn & Pollock, 1996; Fairclough & Cella, 1996; Gallup & Cella, 1996; Kornblith, 1996; Loll, Moninpour, & Feigel, 1996; Loprinzi, 1996; MacLean, 1996; Wasserman, Bruner, & Scott, 1996) with most of the progress in the increased number of treatment trials having HRQOL endpoints (McCabe, 1996). Since 1990, the growth in adding HRQOL measures to disease treatment trials has been almost threefold, as seen in Table 12-3 (O'Mara et al., 2008). The groups also identified the most frequently used measures, which increased from ten in 1990 to over 20 in 1995. Measures

---

Table 12-2. **Summary Recommendations from 1990 NCI Workshop, "Quality of Life Assessment in Cancer Clinical Trials**

Objective	Recommendations
1. Define elements of quality of life (QOL) that are relevant to clinical decision-making and represent realistic endpoints in clinical trials	a. Patient best indicator of impact of cancer treatment, use proxies judiciously. c. QOL measures should include both generic and disease- or treatment-specific dimensions d. Age, race, gender, marital status should be obtained on all patients.
2. Evaluate currently available instruments for QOL assessment and strategies for implementation	a. Minimum of 2 assessment time points, baseline & one follow-up. Additional assessments driven by study objectives, course of disease & treatment b. Train personnel on gathering & managing QOL data prior to opening study
3. Identify diseases in which QOL measures may be most useful in comparing differential effect of toxicities between 2 arms.	a. Studies comparing organ sparing procedures; i.e., surgery vs. radiotherapy b. Adjuvant breast cancer studies c. Gynecologic malignancies d. Hematologic malignancies c. Bone marrow support for intensive therapy d. Pediatric tumors e. Symptom control
4. Examine issues regarding the integration of findings from therapeutic evaluations and QOL measures	a. Small number of primary QOL hypotheses with reduction in significance level for each hypothesis. b. Number of patients needed to answer secondary QOL questions may be less than for primary treatment questions. c. Minimize potential for missing data

---

such as the Mini-Mental State Exam and the Karnofsky Performance Scale were included as examples.

Early HRQOL findings from selected clinical trials, conducted through the cooperative groups, as well as through other international networks, revealed interesting and sometimes unexpected outcomes about how patients fared. In trials where survival was no different between two treatment modalities, HRQOL findings were particularly important. For example, in the breast cancer clinical trials where there was no survival advantage for mastectomy versus lumpectomy, the generally held assumption was women undergoing lumpectomies would fare better, both emotionally and physically. A review of 18 studies published in the 1980s found no differences on a number of psychological measures, with the exception of body image and sexual functioning, which favored the use of

Table 12-3. **Disease Specific Phase III Trials with QOL Endpoints, Active in 1990 and 2008**

Cancer Type	1990 Number of Trials	2008 Number of Trials
Pediatric Tumors	4	7
Breast	3	8
GYN	2	4
Lung	2	5
Hematologic	2	2
Bladder	1	0
Head & Neck	1	2
Prostate	1	9
Colorectal	0	4
Myeloma	0	3
Melanoma	0	1
Metastases	0	1
Trials with QOL components	**16**	**46**

breast-conserving treatment (Kiebert, de Haes, & van de Velde, 1991). Health-related quality-of-life findings of pediatric acute lymphoblastic leukemia survivors of the early 1990s revealed they were more likely than their sibling control subjects to enter a special education or learning disabilities program. The risk for special education increased with increasing dosages of cranial radiotherapy (Haupt Fears et al., 1994).

Cancer Prevention and Symptom Management Trials

Efforts in the early years of the clinical trials program were focused primarily on comparing HRQOL outcomes in disease treatment trials. With the initiation of the CCOP program in the 1980s and its emphasis on cancer prevention and symptom management, the role of measuring HRQOL expanded. In the breast cancer prevention arena, several important HRQOL findings have come to light.

The 1992 Breast Cancer Prevention Trial (BCPT), which enrolled over 13,000 women and was designed to test whether tamoxifen would lower a woman's risk for developing breast cancer in comparison to a placebo, had several important specific and overall HRQOL secondary findings. Among them were a lack of difference between the tamoxifen and placebo arms with regard to depression, overall physical or mental quality of life, and weight gain. Vasomotor (e.g., hot flashes) and gynecological (e.g., vaginal discharge) symptoms, as well as difficulties in certain domains of sexual functioning, were persistent problems for women on the tamoxifen arm (Day, 2001). In the 1994 follow-up study, Study of Tamoxifen and Raloxifene (STAR), which enrolled over 19,000 women, investigators were interested in identifying differences in vasomotor symptoms, selected physical symptoms, and sexual and cognitive function. The trial closed in 2004 and results from these assessments revealed no significant differences between the tamoxifen and raloxifene groups in physical health, mental health, and depression, although the tamoxifen group reported better sexual function. Women in the tamoxifen group reported more gynecological problems, vasomotor symptoms, leg cramps, and bladder control problems, whereas women in the raloxifene group reported more musculoskeletal problems, dyspareunia, and weight gain (Land et al., 2006).

The largest prostate prevention trial, the Selenium and Vitamin E Cancer Prevention Trial (SELECT), launched in 2001 and enrolled 35,000 men, was designed to determine whether one or both of these dietary supplements prevented prostate cancer. Unlike the breast cancer prevention trials where there were known toxicities for tamoxifen and raloxifene and potential effect on HRQOL, the agents used in SELECT had a very low toxicity profile, thus HRQOL would likely not be affected. However, investigators were interested in the potential of these agents to prevent or delay the onset of Alzheimer's disease. Participants who agreed to participate in this ancillary component of SELECT, called Prevention of Alzheimer's Disease by Vitamin E and Selenium (PREADVISE), underwent a 5-minute memory check every year during their yearly SELECT visits. If their memory checks suggested problems, they would be offered a slightly longer memory examination (PREADVISE, 2010). Results from the parent trial revealed selenium, or vitamin E, alone or in combination did not prevent prostate cancer in this population of relatively healthy men (Lippman et al., 2009). Results from PREADVISE have not been reported.

Because improving symptoms related to treatment or cancer has long been assumed to result in an improved HRQOL, measuring the effect of symptom relief on HRQOL has been of strong interest among CCOP investigators. However, recent publications in this area have not always been positive (Somerfield et al., 2003; Jatoi, Kumar, Sloan, & Nguyen, 2003). In 2005, Buchanan and colleagues (2005) published their review of all HRQOL research objectives, rationales, assessment instruments, symptoms treated, and types of interventions from the CCOP symptom management portfolio of clinical trials initiated since 1987. Their goal was to examine how HRQOL was prospectively conceptualized, defined, and measured in these clinical trials. They found that trials conducted in the early 1990s often used global HRQOL as the primary endpoint, but this became less frequent with increased use of symptom-specific measures. A total of 22 global HRQOL instruments were identified and two, the Functional Assessment of Cancer Treatment (FACT) (Cella et al., 1993) and the Uniscale, were used most frequently over this time period. Table 12-4 depicts the five most frequently used scales over the two decades. In addition, in trials where global HRQOL was an endpoint, investigators did not propose consistently either a definition of HRQOL or a conceptual framework. When a framework was presented, it was limited to univariate relationships between symptom relief and global improvements in HRQOL. Recommendations included more precise descriptions of conceptual frameworks that specify the hypothesized links between the specific

Table 12-4.   **Commonly Used HRQOL Scales in CCOP Symptom Management Trials, 1987–2004**

HRQOL Instrument Used	No. of Trials
Functional Assessment of Cancer Treatment (FACT)	36
Uniscale	19
Medical Outcomes Study Short Form – 36 (SF-36)	5
Spitzer Quality of Life Index (SQLI)	5
Functional Living Index (FLIC)	3
Rand General Well Being Scale (GWB)	3
European Organization for Research and Treatment of Cancer (EORTC)	3
Linear Analog Scale Assessment (LASA)	3
Subject Global Impression of Change (SGIC)	

symptom(s) being managed, interactions with other symptoms, different domains of HRQOL, and global HRQOL. One of the outcomes of this review was the convening of a group of symptom management and HRQOL investigators to recommend the future course of HRQOL endpoints in symptom management trials to NCI staff. The meeting was held in October, 2005 and the proceedings of the meeting have been published (O'Mara, 2007).

Current Status

Patient-Reported Outcomes

Over two decades of research has shown, to understand the patients' perceptions of their experiences with cancer and treatment-related toxicities, self-reports are the best method for obtaining the information. The Common Terminology Criteria for Adverse Events, volume 4, which is the standard method for assessing cancer treatment toxicities (US Department of Health and Human Services, 2010), is insufficient for conducting this evaluation as it requires a health professional to ask the patient. There are emerging data that reveal there is not consistent agreement when clinicians or other proxies report patient symptoms and patients complete a validated self-report of the same symptoms (Sneeuw, Sprangers, & Aaronson, 2002; Sneeuw et al., 1999; Basch et al., 2006). The release of the FDA's guidance on patient-reported outcomes in 2009 (US FDA, 2009) further supports the notion that symptoms and quality of life can be known only to and reported by the patient. Furthermore, most symptoms, such as feelings of depression, pain, and fatigue, cannot be verified by any laboratory test. Although these guidances are directed primarily to investigators seeking FDA drug approval, the information contained in this guidance is relevant also to investigators with a broader interest in assessing quality of life and confirms Buchanan and colleagues' (2005) recommendation of the importance of clearly describing the hypothesized relationship between improved symptoms and HRQOL or the effect of treatment-related toxicities on HRQOL. For example, in a Phase III cancer treatment trial where there are known toxicities, what research questions will give the most information about the current trial and inform future trials? Given the limited resources to conduct multiple assessments and the need to minimize patient burden, should investigators focus their questions on the patient's specific perceptions of several treatment-related symptoms, using a scale such as the MD Anderson Symptom Inventory (Cleeland et al., 2000), or should they question the effect of these known toxicities on global health-related quality of life? Bruner and colleagues' review of nonsmall cell lung cancer (NSCLC) treatment trials conducted through the Radiation Therapy Oncology Group (RTOG) (Bruner et al., 2004) provide insights to these questions. When they analyzed six Phase II and III NSCLC trials using the RTOG Outcomes Triad model, they found that esophagitis was the symptom affecting quality of life the greatest in elderly ($\geq$ 70 years) patients. This finding led to the development of a radioprotectant trial (RTOG 98-01) of amifostine to decrease the incidence and intensity of esophagitis.

Role of Nurses in HRQOL Research

Oncology nurses' unique understanding of symptom management practices, as well as clinical trial design and implementation, positions them to assume a prominent role in HRQOL research conducted through the NCI clinical trials networks. Trials that include patient-reported outcomes can potentially be labor intensive, and nurses have the most information on the feasibility of collecting these data. The multiple roles and responsibilities oncology nurses assume are pivotal in maintaining a balance between collecting essential patient data, implementing the particular treatment, and not burdening either the patient or staff. Each role of the nurse in the clinical trials arena brings a unique set of responsibilities (Klimaszewski et al., 2000), and these are displayed in Table 12-5.

The results of a survey of 61 CCOP administrators regarding the roles and responsibilities of nurses involved in symptom management clinical trials revealed the roles of the research and protocol nurses were similar to what has been described in the literature, meaning that developing marketing strategies and educating staff and patients about the availability of trials are crucial to successful accrual (O'Mara, Padberg, & Westendorp, 2004). There was wide variability in the use of nurses as clinical research associates and a limited role for advanced practice nurses (APNs) in symptom management trials. The limited role of APNs could be attributed to the fact that many CCOPs are small, located outside of large urban areas, and not part of academic medical centers. Finally, at the time of the survey three nurses were protocol chairs and since 2004, two protocols with nurses as protocol chairs have been added (Table 12-6).

Table 12-5. **Nurses' Roles & Knowledge in Symptom Management Trials**

Role	Unique Knowledge
Research/Protocol Nurse	Disease & Treatment-related symptoms
Data Managers	Symptom & QOL self-reported instruments (how to complete, report data)
Advanced Practice Nurse	Evidence-based symptom management practices
Nurse Researcher	Research methodology; instrument development

Table 12-6. **Nurses as Protocol Chairs of Symptom Management Trials**

Sponsoring Research Base Trial (Year Reported)	Nurse
Children's Oncology Group	
Difference in Parental Caregiving Demands in Childhood Acute Lymphoblastic Leukemia (ALL) by Length of Infusion Therapy (2004)	D. Keegan-Wells
Prevention of Mucositis in Children with AES-14 (IND #36978), a Glutamine Based Oral Care Regimen, for Patients Diagnosed with Solid Tumors: A Randomized Placebo-controlled Clinical Study (2007)	D. Betcher
Music Video and Adolescent/Young Adult Resilience During Transplant (2007)	J. Haase
North Central Cancer Treatment Group	
The Use of Testosterone to Enhance Libido in Female Cancer Survivors, A Phase III Randomized Placebo-Controlled, Double-Blind Crossover Study (2004)	D. Barton
The Use of Ginkgo Biloba for the Prevention of Chemotherapy related Cognitive Dysfunction (2004)	D. Barton
Radiation Therapy Oncology Group	
Treatment of Erectile Dysfunction in Patients Treated on RTOG 99-10 for Prostate Cancer: Impact of Patient and Partner Quality of Life (2004)	D. Watkins-Bruner

CONCLUSION

NCI clinical trials networks have been in existence for over 50 years and have provided the infrastructure for collecting and analyzing HRQOL data of patients enrolled in cancer treatment, prevention, and symptom management clinical trials. In the early 1980s, evidence began to emerge demonstrating cancer survival and tumor response can have an effect on a patient's HRQOL. A series of workshops and meetings sponsored by NCI were conducted between 1990 and 2005 to evaluate the evolving role of HRQOL in cancer treatment, prevention, and symptom management trials conducted through these networks. The overarching goal of assessing HRQOL has been, and continues to be, focused on evaluating the patient's experience with cancer and its related treatments. However, the measures used to assess HRQOL, development of conceptual frameworks to explain the associations between HRQOL and other variables, and the role of HRQOL data to inform future clinical trials remain an evolving field. Nurses play critical roles in the development and implementation of HRQOL studies and are increasingly playing more of a leadership role as protocol chairs.

REFERENCES

Basch, E., Iasonos, A., McDonough, T., Barz, A., Culkin, A., Kris, M. G., et al. (2006). Patient versus clinician symptom reporting using the National Cancer Institute Common Terminology Criteria for Adverse Events: Results of a questionnaire-based study. *The Lancet Oncology, 7*(11), 903–909.

Bradlyn, A. S., & Pollock, B. H. (1996). Pediatric oncology group (POG). *Journal of the National Cancer Institute Monographs,* (20), 89–90.

Bruner, D.W., Movsas, B., Konski A., Roach, M., Bondy, M., Scarintino, C., et al. (2004). Outcomes research in cancer clinical trial cooperative groups: The RTOG model. *Quality of Life Research, 13*(6), 1025–1041.

Buchanan, D. R., O'Mara, A. M., Kelaghan, J. W., & Minasian, L. M. (2005). Quality-of-life assessment in the symptom management trials of the National Cancer Institute-supported Community Clinical Oncology Program. *Journal of Clinical Oncology, 23*(3), 591–598.

Cella, D. F., Tulsky, D. S. (1993). Quality of life in cancer: Definition, purpose, and method of measurement. *Cancer Invest, 11*(3), 327–336.

Cella, D. F., & Tulsky, & D. S., Gray, G., Sarafian, B., Linn, E., Bonomi, A., et al. (1993). The Functional Assessment of Cancer Therapy (FACT) scale: Development and validation of the general measure. *Journal of Clinical Oncology, 11*(3), 570–579.

Cleeland, C. S., Mendoza, T. R., Wang, X. S., Chou, C., Harle, M. T., Morrissey, M., et al. (2000). Assessing symptom distress in cancer patients: The M.D. Anderson Symptom Inventory. *Cancer, 89*, 1634–1646.

Day, R. (2001). National Surgical Adjuvant Breast and Bowel Projet P-1 study (NSABP-1): Quality of life and tamoxifen in a breast cancer prevention trial: A summary of findings from the NSABP P-1 study. National surgical adjuvant breast and bowel project. *Annals of the New York Academy of Sciences, 949,* 143–150.

Fairclough, D. L., & Cella, D. F. (1996). Eastern Cooperative Oncology Group (ECOG). *Journal of the National Cancer Institute Monographs,* (20), 73–75.

Gallup, D. G., & Cella, D. F. (1996). Gynecologic Oncology Group (GOG). *Journal of the National Cancer Institute Monographs,* (20), 77–78.

Haupt, R., Fears, T. R., Robison, L. L., Mills, J. L., Nicholson, H. S., Zeltzer, et al. (1994). Educational attainment in long-term survivors of childhood autologous lymphoblastic leukemia. *Journal of the American Medical Association,* (272), 1427–1432.

Jatoi, A., Kumar, S., Sloan, J. A., & Nguyen, P. L. (2003). On appetite and its loss. *Journal of Clinical Oncology, 1*(21)(9 Suppl), 79s–81s.

Kiebert, G. M., de Haes, J. C., & van de Velde, C. J. (1991). The impact of breast-conserving treatment and mastectomy on the quality of life of early-stage breast cancer patients: A review. *Journal of Clinical Oncology,* 9(6), 1059–1070.

Klimaszewski, A. D., Aikin, J. L., Bacon, M. A., Distasio, S. A., Ehrenberger, H. E., & Ford, B. A. (Eds). (2000). *Manual for clinical trials nursing.* Pittsburgh, PA: Oncology Nursing Press.

Kornblith, A. B. (1996). Cancer and Leukemia Group B (CALGB). *Journal of the National Cancer Institute Monographs,* (20), 67–71.

Land, S. R., Wickerham, D. L., Costantino, J. P., Ritter, M. W., Vogel, V. G., Lee, M., et al. (2006). Patient-reported symptoms and quality of life during treatment with tamoxifen or raloxifene for breast cancer prevention: The NSABP Study of Tamoxifen and Raloxifene (STAR) P-2 trial. *Journal of the American Medical Association.* 295(23), 2742–2751.

Lindley, C. (1990). Outcome assessment: Functional status measures and quality of life as therapeutic endpoints in oncology. *Topics in Hospital Pharmacy Management,* 10(2), 54–63.

Lippman, S. M., Klein, E. A., Goodman, P. J. et al. (2009). Effect of selenium and vitamin E on risk of prostate cancer and other cancers: The Selenium and Vitamin E Cancer Prevention Trial (SELECT). *Journal of the American Medical Association.* 301(1), 39–51.

Loll, L. C., Moinpour, C. M., & Feigel, P. (1996). Southwest Oncology Group (SWOG). *Journal of the National Cancer Institute Monographs,* (20), 83–85.

Loprinzi, C. (1996). North Central Cancer Treatment Group (NCCTG). *Journal of the National Cancer Institute Monographs,* (20), 79–80.

MacLean, W. E. (1996). Children's Cancer Group (CCG), *Journal of the National Cancer Institute Monographs,* (20), 87–88.

McCabe, M. (1996). A cooperative group report on quality-of-life research: Lessons learned. *Journal of the National Cancer Institute Monographs,* (20), 63–65.

National Cancer Institute. (2009). NCI's clinical trials cooperative group program factsheet. Retrieved March 13, 2011, from http://www.cancer.gov/cancertopics/factsheet/NCI/clinical-trials-cooperative-group

National Cancer Institute. (n.d.). Community clinical oncology program (CCOP). Retrieved March 13, 2011, from http://prevention.cancer.gov/programs-resources/programs/ccop/about/history#2

Nayfield, S. G., Ganz, P. A., Moinpour, C. M., Cella, D. F., Hailey, & B. J. (1992). Report from a National Cancer Institute (USA) workshop on quality of life assessment in cancer clinical trials. *Quality of Life Research, 1*(3), 203–210.

O'Mara, A. (Ed.). (2007). Quality of life assessment in symptom management trials. *Journal of the National Cancer Institute, 37.*

O'Mara, A., Denicoff, A. M., Reeve, B. B., Schoenfeldt, M., Burns, R., & Trimble, E. L. (2008). An analysis of quality of life endpoints and measures in 2008 U.S. National Cancer Institute-sponsored Phase III cancer treatment trials. 15th Annual Conference. International Society for Quality of Life Research. Retrieved from http://www.isoqol.org/

O'Mara, A., Padberg, R. M., & Westendorp, J. (2004). Ensuring the success of symptom management trials in the community setting: The critical roles that oncology nurses play. *Oncology Nursing Forum, 31,* 448.

Prevention of Alzheimer's Disease by Vitamin E and Selenium (PREADVISE). Retrieved March 13, 2011, from http://clinicaltrials.gov/ct2/show/NCT00040378

Skeel, R. T. (1989). Quality of life assessment in cancer clinical trials—it's time to catch up. *Journal of the National Cancer Institute,* 81(7), 472–473.

Sneeuw, K. C., Aaronson, N. K., Sprangers, M. A., Detmar, S. B., Wever, L. D., & Schornagel, J. H. (1999). Evaluating the quality of life of cancer patients: Assessments by patients, significant others, physicians and nurses. *British Journal of Cancer, 1*(1), 87–94.

Sneeuw, K. C., Sprangers, M. A., & Aaronson, N. K. (2002). The role of health care providers and significant others in evaluating the quality of life of patients with chronic disease. *Journal of Clinical Epidemiology, 55*(11), 1130–1143.

Somerfield, M., Jatoi, A., Nguyen, P. L., Kumar, S., Sloan, J., & Loprinzi, C. L. (2003). Hazards of quality-of-life data for clinical decision making. *Journal of Clinical Oncology, 21*(9 Suppl), 82–83.

US Food and Drug Administration. (2009). Guidance for Industry. Patient Reported Outcome Measures: Use in Medical Product Development to Support Labeling Claims. Retrieved from http://www.fda.gov/

US Department of Health and Human Services. (2010). Common Terminology Criteria for Adverse Events, version 4.0. Retrieved March 13, 2011, from http://evs.nci.nih.gov/ftp1/CTCAE/CTCAE_4.03_2010-06-14_QuickReference_5x7.pdf

Varricchio, C. G., McCabe, M. S., Trimble, E., & Korn, E. L. (1996). Quality of life in clinical cancer trials. Introduction. *Journal of the National Cancer Institute Monographs,* (20), vii–viii.

Waalen, J. (1990). Experts debate quality of life as clinical trial endpoint. *Journal of the National Cancer Institute, 82*(17), 1381–1382.

Wasserman, T., Bruner, D., & Scott, C. (1996). Radiation Therapy Oncology Group (RTOG). *Journal of the National Cancer Institute Monographs,* (20), 81–85.

Yancik, R., Edwards, B. K., & Yates, J. W. (1987). Quality of life assessment: A pilot study report. National Cancer Institute, US Department of Health and Human Services.

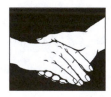

Practice

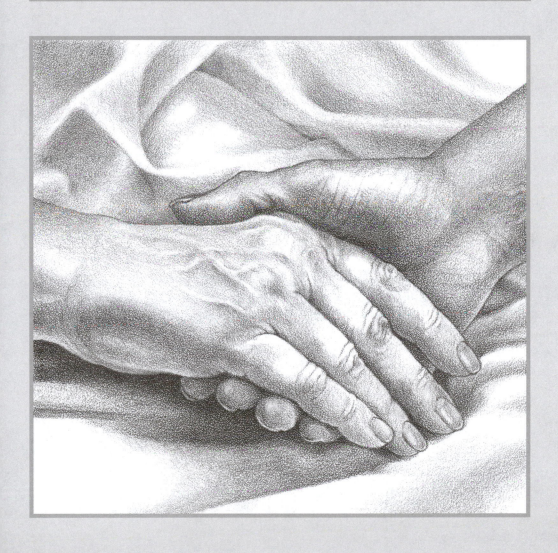

Quality-of-Life Issues in Breast and Prostate Cancer

LORRIE L. POWEL • KAREN M. MENESES

Introduction

Approximately 207,090 and 217,730 new cases of breast and prostate cancer, respectively, were diagnosed in the US in 2010 (American Cancer Society, 2010). Although breast and prostate cancers represent the most prevalent cancers among Americans, many questions are unanswered. The physical consequences of primary treatment frequently are life long, and often invoke difficult behavioral, emotional, and interpersonal changes that may diminish quality of life (QOL) in multiple ways (Fowler, McNaughton, Walker, Elliott, & Barry, 2002; Leventhal, Patrick-Miller, & Leventhal, 1998). Questions related to the impact of short- and long-term treatment outcomes on QOL beg our attention. Moreover, cancer survivors commonly suffer unexpected intrusive thoughts about the possibility that their cancer may recur. Cancer recurrence signifies that the best efforts for eradicating the disease have failed; it might be the most discouraging and difficult period patients face in their experience with cancer (Weisman & Worden, 1976). Significant gaps in our knowledge remain regarding the complicated treatment-related experiences breast and prostate cancer survivors face within the context of the fear of recurrence.

Of the 11.4 million Americans alive with a history of cancer in the United States today, breast and prostate cancer survivors comprise the largest group of male and female cancer survivors (American Cancer Society, 2010). As the baby boomers advance in age, the incidence and prevalence of breast and prostate cancers, and subsequently, the number of cancer survivors, is expected to further increase. Progress in the management of breast and prostate cancers requires continued QOL research to comprehensively and effectively addresses the concerns of the growing number of breast and prostate cancer survivors.

The purpose of this chapter is as follows:

- Identify research related to QOL in breast and prostate cancer.
- Describe the state of current knowledge in QOL interventions used in breast and prostate cancer research.
- Explore future QOL research directions and challenges in breast and prostate cancer survivorship research.

Research and Measurement in QOL and Breast Cancer

An impressive and cumulative body of research over the past two decades consistently has documented QOL outcomes in breast cancer. Some of the data examine specific aspects of QOL such as physical symptoms; psychological distress; social, family, and work relationships; and spiritual well-being, while other research focuses on multidimensional QOL outcomes 5-60.

Several QOL instruments were designed for use specifically in breast cancer research (Cella et al., 1993; Dow, Ferrel, Haberman, & Eaton, 1999; Fraser et al., 1993; Schag, Ganz, & Heinrich, 1991; Sprangers, Cull, Bjordal, Groenvold, & Aaronson, 1993). These measures contain varying domains of multidimensionality and have been used to evaluate treatment and disease side effects on physical, psychological, social, and spiritual well-being. The tools emphasize different aspects of QOL. For example, the Cancer Rehabilitation Evaluation System (CARES) includes a component of assessment for identifying high-risk individuals requiring psychosocial intervention (Schag, Guntz, & Heinrich, 1991). The QOL instrument developed by Dow and colleagues (1999) captures perceived changes in spiritual well-being such as transcendence, hopefulness, and uncertainty over the future. Sprangers and colleagues (1993) use a modular approach to QOL assessment in cancer clinical trials based on the European Organization for Research and Treatment of Cancer (EORTC) Study Group. The module incorporates a "core" instrument (QLQ-C30) covering a range of QOL issues along with a site-specific module for breast cancer used to assess aspects of QOL of particular importance to specific populations.

Interventions to Improve Quality of Life in Breast Cancer

The vast majority of QOL research in breast cancer has focused on women during active combined modality therapy. A variety of interventions to ameliorate individual symptoms and improve overall QOL, including selected aspects of QOL such as physical symptoms, psychological distress, social and family burden, and spiritual distress have generally produced successful outcomes (Institute of Medicine, 2004). Quality-of-life interventions constitute a wide range of methods that include individual psychoeducational support (Badger, Segrin, Meek, Lopez, & Bonham, 2004; Yates et al., 2005), cognitive-behavioral interventions (Braden, Mischel, & Longman, 1998), community-based group support (Golant, Altman, & Martin, 2003), relaxation and guided imagery (Hosaka et al., 2001), supportive expressive interventions (Sandgren & McCaul, 2006; Spiegel, Bloom, Kraemer, & Gottheil, 1989; Spiegel, Bloom, & Yalom, 1981), mind-body and spiritual interventions, and restorative support (Cimprich, 1993; Cimprich & Ronis, 2003).

Variations of QOL interventions have included a variety of approaches, including face-to-face or telephone (Marcus et al., 1998; Sandgren & McCaul, 2006), written (e.g., books, pamphlets, booklets, tip sheets), multimedia (e.g., audiotape, videotape) (Hoskins, 2001; Hoskins et al., 2001; Wilkins et al., 2006), CD, and online (Rawl et al., 2002; Shaw et al., 2006). Fewer intervention studies have been accomplished to date on improving our understanding of QOL among breast cancer survivors posttreatment, which is the period of time characterized by the Institute of Medicine (IOM, 2006) as the transition from cancer patient to cancer survivor. The following discussion is divided into two areas:

- QOL intervention studies initiated at the time of diagnosis or early into adjuvant treatment. Longitudinal evaluations continued into posttreatment survivorship.
- QOL intervention studies designed specifically for posttreatment survivorship.

QOL Intervention Studies Begun During Early Diagnosis or Treatment

Helgeson, Cohen, Schultz, and Yasko (2001), reported a 3-year follow-up study examining the effects of short 8-week support group interventions on QOL of women with newly diagnosed breast cancer. The researchers assigned women prior to or early entry into chemotherapy (n=312) to one of four treatment arms: control, education, peer discussion, and education. Their results showed the consistent positive benefits of education intervention, but little benefit of peer discussion. The follow-up study (Helgeson, Cohen, Schultz, & Yasko, 1999) supported the initial findings that education was effective in providing information, which enhanced women's control over the illness experience, increased self-esteem, and reduced intrusive thoughts. Education support statistically accounted for the greater improvement in QOL. However, peer discussion did not benefit women. This is likely due to the increase in negative downward comparison, more negative interactions with family and friends, and a short-term increase in psychosocial distress.

Hosaka and colleagues evaluated a psychiatric intervention comprised of five weekly structured group interventions and three follow-up group meetings among 34 Japanese women with breast cancer (Hosaka et al., 2001; Hosaka, Sugiyama, Hirai, & Sugawara, 2001; Hosaka et al., 2000). Weekly group intervention sessions consisted of psychoeducational support and supportive-expressive interventions (i.e., relaxation training and guided imagery). Subjects were referred by their surgeon to the study. Results showed the five weekly group interventions with follow-up were sufficient support for women with nonmetastatic breast cancer. However, women with nodal metastasis and/or adjustment disorders required additional psychiatric intervention (Pienta & Esper, 1993).

In another study of Japanese women with breast cancer, Okamura, Fukui, Nagasaka, and Koike (2003) conducted an exploratory study evaluating whether a 6-week psychoeducational intervention program was effective in reducing psychological distress among 41 patients with breast cancer. Six months post-intervention, investigators found significant increase in patient satisfaction with information about breast cancer ($p=.02$) and ways to cope with cancer ($p=.04$).

Hoskins (2001) reported her pilot results of phase-specific interventions related to diagnosis, surgical, adjuvant treatment, or recovery after breast cancer (Hoskins, 2001; Hoskins et al., 2001). Using a patient–partner approach, Hoskins and colleagues in both studies enrolled 128 women with breast cancer and 121 partners who were assigned to one of three intervention arms: standard education by videotape, telephone counseling, or a combination of the two interventions. Pilot results showed that phase-specific educational counseling and interventions were associated with a positive adjustment outcome.

Coleman and colleagues (2005), explored the effects of telephone social support and education on adaptation to breast cancer in the first year after diagnosis. The investigators used a two-group experimental design. Both experimental and control groups received a mailed educational resource kit, however, the experimental group also received 13 months of telephone social support and education. Results showed no significant differences between groups, with the mailed educational resource kit alone being as effective as telephone social support.

In a related study, Chamberlain-Wilmoth, Tulman, Coleman, Stewart, and Samarel (2006) randomized breast cancer patients to one of two treatment arms: education and social support, or education only. They also performed a content analysis of interviews to examine women's perceptions of emotional and interpersonal adaptation to breast cancer. Of the 106 women who participated in the clinical trial, 77 were interviewed at home. Results showed that 54% of women who received telephone support interventions and educational materials reported improvement compared with 43% who received only educational materials. Forty-six percent of women in the intervention group reported improved relationships with their spouses compared with 38% in the control group. Investigators concluded telephone social support helped improved survivor attitudes toward breast cancer and their relationship with spouses.

Yates and colleagues (2005) evaluated the efficacy of a psychoeducational intervention on cancer-related fatigue (CRF) among 109 women starting chemotherapy for breast cancer. Oncology nurses delivered the intervention in one face-to-face and two telephone interactions. The primary endpoint was CRF; secondary endpoints were QOL, and psychological well-being. Study results showed women in the control arm consistently experienced an increase in CRF by 50% more than women in the intervention arm. Women in the intervention group reported significantly greater mean increase in fatigue-management actions. Investigators concluded a brief psychoeducational intervention was effective in reducing CRF.

Sandgren and McCaul (2006) reported the outcomes of a trial that tested two telephone interventions on either health education or emotional expressions with standard control on QOL and distress. Women (n = 218) with stage I–III breast cancer were assigned randomly to one of the three arms. Oncology nurses delivered the interventions in six 30-minute individual telephone sessions. Subjects entered the study either after surgery or during adjuvant therapy. Standard QOL assessments were done pre- and post-intervention and 6 months after baseline. Results showed that health education was superior to either peer support or no intervention conditions. Furthermore, the results suggested time may have been a healing factor for the subjects.

In summary, the preceding QOL intervention studies were begun shortly after diagnosis and treatment and were completed by end of breast cancer therapy or posttherapy. A variety of interventions were used to ameliorate QOL problems and improve QOL.

QOL Interventions During Posttreatment Survivorship

Increasingly, QOL intervention studies are being conducted during the posttreatment phase of survivorship. Ganz and colleagues (2004) reported baseline QOL characteristics in 558 women with breast cancer in the Moving Beyond Cancer (MBC) project, a randomized trial of psychosocial, behavioral interventions. Subjects completed a mailed baseline survey of standard QOL measures and health outcomes. Baseline results showed the patients with mastectomy reported the poorest physical functioning ($p = .05$). Subjects on chemotherapy reported poorest sexual functioning. At the end of primary treatment, all groups reported good emotional functioning, as well as problems with physical functioning.

Stanton and colleagues (2005) reported on the follow-up to the MBC trial, using a three-arm intervention consisting of standard National Cancer Institute print materials; standard print material and peer-modeling videotape; or standard print material, videotape, and two sessions with a trained cancer educator, and informational workbook. The primary endpoints of interest were energy and fatigue and cancer-specific distress. Results showed a peer modeling videotape improves recovery of energy in the posttreatment survivorship phase.

Scheier and colleagues (2005) conducted a clinical trial evaluating whether an educational or nutritional intervention enhanced physical and psychological functioning among women younger than 50 years of age with breast cancer ($n = 252$). They randomly assigned women to one of three treatment arms: receiving standard medical care, educational intervention to provide information about the illness and ways to manage, or nutritional intervention promoting a healthy diet. Primary endpoints were physical and mental functioning, and depressive symptoms. Results showed participants assigned to one of the two treatment arms had less depressive symptoms and better physical functioning at the 13-month follow-up than those in the standard treatment arm. They concluded that tailored psychosocial interventions are effective in the adjustment of young women with breast cancer at the end of treatment.

Mishel and colleagues (2005) tested the efficacy of an uncertainty management intervention for older long-term breast cancer survivors. The sample consisted of 509 women with non-metastatic disease 5 to 9 years posttreatment. Subjects were assigned to one of two arms, usual care or intervention. Nurses delivered the intervention during four weekly telephone sessions. The nurses instructed survivors in using cognitive-behavioral strategies to manage uncertainty about recurrence and in using a self-help manual designed to help survivors understand the nature of long-term treatment side effects. Investigators found survivors in the treatment arm showed differences in outcomes in the areas of improved knowledge, cognitive reframing, problem solving, and social support compared with the control arm ($p = .01$).

Meneses, McNees, Loerzel, Su, Zhang, and Hassey (2007) examined the effectiveness of the Breast Cancer Education Intervention, also known as the BCEI. The BCEI was a psychoeducational support intervention delivered by oncology nurses face to face. Participants

(n = 256) were randomized to either the experimental or wait control group. The BCEI intervention consisted of three face-to-face QOL sessions and five monthly follow-up sessions. The wait control group received four monthly attention telephone calls and the BCEI intervention at the sixth month. Quality-of-life data were collected at baseline, 3, and 6 months post-study entry. Primary QOL endpoints were physical, psychological, social, spiritual, and overall QOL. No baseline differences were noted between the two groups. However, the intervention group reported a significantly improved QOL at 3 months while the wait control group reported a decline in QOL. Treatment effects continued between the two groups at 6 months post-study entry.

Research in QOL and Prostate Cancer

Current estimates indicate that nearly 200,000 men were diagnosed with prostate cancer in 2009, and 380,000 new cases per year are expected by 2025 (National Cancer Institute, 2007). As the most prevalent visceral cancer diagnosed in US males, prostate cancer will affect one in six men in the United States in their lifetime. It is estimated that 70% of men who survive to 80 years of age have evidence of histologic or latent prostate cancer (Pienta & Esper, 1993). Some researchers believe histologic prostate cancer eventually leads to clinically evident cancer (Meng & Carroll, 2001), while others suggest it has no impact on survival (Ahles et al., 2005; Ashing-Giwa, Padilla, Bohorquez, Tejero, & Garcia, 2006; Fogel, Albert, Schnabel, Ditkoff, & Neugut, 2002). Until recently, prostate-specific antigen (PSA) was used as a dichotomous biomarker of prostate cancer, with a value of widely adopted cut-off of 4 ng/ml being considered as *normal*. In 1997, Catalona, Beiser, and Smith (1997) suggested a lowered value of 2.5 ng/ml be adopted as a new cut-off value of *normal* to increase the sensitivity of the test. Depending on the institution and individual clinician, any value over the *normal* value of 4.0 ng/ml or 2.5 ng/ml prompted a prostate biopsy.

However, recent studies indicate prostate cancer may be present even when PSA levels are *normal* (Thompson et al., 2006). The Prostate Cancer Prevention Trial demonstrated that PSA is not a dichotomous biomarker but reflects a continuum of prostate cancer risk. To better assess prostate cancer risk, data were collected from the control group of the PCPT (n=5,519 ≥ 55 years). These men were followed for 7 years while receiving PSA and digital rectal exam (DRE) screening annually. Those in whom screening tests were abnormal underwent a prostate biopsy to further assess for the presence of prostate cancer. In addition, those who had not undergone a biopsy during the course of the study underwent prostate biopsy at the end of the study (Thompson et al., 2006). Findings from analysis of these data, as well as demographic data such as family history, race, age, and previous biopsy history, were used to develop the PCPT Prostate Cancer Risk Calculator (Thompson et al., 2006), a tool to aid clinicians in calculating an individual's risk of prostate cancer.

For example, for a 55-year-old African American man with a PSA of 3 ng/ml, a positive family history of prostate cancer, no history of previous biopsy, and a normal DRE, the risk of prostate cancer is 36% (95% CI = 32–39%), but the risk of high-grade prostate cancer is 10% (95% CI = 4.8–15.5%) (Parekh et al., 2006). Thus, by using the calculator to consider a number of risk-related variables, clinicians can convey risk more confidently and are also able to explain that risk to patients, rather than giving the patient raw data to interpret or interpreting it for him as normal or abnormal.

These data notwithstanding, the topic of PSA screening remains controversial among clinicians. Clinicians do not use such calculations always and, if used, the degree of risk is not discussed always with patients. More often than not, patients' perceptions of risk, and their understanding of next steps, (e.g., biopsy, potential treatment options) are not well informed. Some men report that being confronted with news of an elevated PSA necessitates immediate active treatment. These men, who are often frightened by the diagnosis, feel that taking no action to combat the disease is not a viable alternative. They later admit in retrospect their decision to undergo treatment was clouded by the fear of cancer. Moreover, not fully understanding treatment alternatives led them to make hasty treatment decisions and sacrifices regarding functional status they later regretted (Clark, Wray, & Ashton, 2001; Powel, 2002, 2003, 2006).

This knee-jerk response is particularly problematic when trying to help men interpret the implications of a PSA value as it relates to the next course of action. Using the calculator to counsel patients with an elevated PSA can help them understand what an elevated PSA really means for them and help them make a decision whether treatment is necessary, and if it is, what treatment option makes the most sense.

Despite this breakthrough in our understanding of risk, little is known about patient and/or physician characteristics that can influence a patient's decision to undergo treatment (Powel et al., 2009). Men diagnosed with early stage prostate cancer choose between a growing number of primary treatment alternatives, including radical prostatectomy, laparoscopic prostatectomy, external beam radiotherapy, brachytherapy, cryosurgery, and observation (such as watchful waiting or active surveillance). Patients treated with active treatment are at risk for the often problematic aftereffects of urinary, bowel, and sexual dysfunction. Thus, the overwhelming majority of studies examining prostate cancer-related QOL outcomes have focused on the influence of these aftereffects on QOL (Bhatnagar, Stewart, Huynh, Jorgensen, & Kaplan, 2006; Bishoff et al., 1998; Lepore, Helgeson, Eton, & Schulz, 2003; McNaughton-Collins, Walker-Corkery, & Barry, 2004; Powel, 2002; Powel & Clark, 2005; Talcott et al. 1998). In 2002, the US Preventative Care Task Force (USPCTF) stated in *Screening for Prostate Cancer: Recommendation and Rationale* (2002), routine prostate cancer screening did not affect overall survival, yet both providers and patients have been reluctant to forego screening. Moreover, an elevated PSA value most often results in active treatment. Further research examining QOL outcomes prior to treatment, such as those related to diagnosis and treatment decision making, is warranted.

Although aftereffects often occur as a result of active treatment, virtually all men treated for early prostate cancer survive 5 or more years. Nonetheless biochemical recurrence is increasingly common, occurring as early as 3 years after primary treatment (D'Amico et al., 1998; Meng & Carroll, 2001). Research examining QOL outcomes in men with metastatic disease is less common. Thus, while the risk of treatment side effects has been well characterized, we only are beginning to fully appreciate the experiences prostate cancer survivors may encounter in their journey from diagnosis through posttreatment cancer survivorship, which includes the possibility of recurrence (Powel et al., 2007).

An area only recently investigated is the influence of socioeconomic status (SES) on prostate cancer, diagnosis, treatment, and prognosis. That is, although studies have been done of various ethnic groups, mostly related to comparisons of African American and Caucasian men, the influence of specific variables is masked by the moderating role of SES (Powel, Pugh, & Elnitsky, 2002). For example, Kudadjie-Gyamfi, Consedine, and Magai (2006) found typical groups of White, Black, and Latino often used to code aggregate data obscured their ability to examine coping and other psychological variables in prostate cancer survivors. However, Gore and colleagues (Gore, Krupski, Kwan, Fink, & Litwin, 2005) found, even when controlling for income, Latino ethnicity was negatively associated with mental health of prostate cancer survivors. In a study of mono- and bilingual Latino men of Mexican heritage, Powel, Hopkins, Kozlovsky, and Parekh, (2009) found principles such as machismo, allocentrism, power distance and simpatia (e.g., those principles that typify Latino morals) influence the manner in which Latino men approach prostate cancer screening, assess treatment decisions, and react to treatment-related aftereffects. Indeed their socialization as Latino men, as well as language congruence with healthcare providers, put them at increased risk for distress following prostate cancer treatment (Powel et al., 2009; Gonzalez, Powel, Kozlovsky, Parekh, & Ford, 2009). This socialization difference also influenced their ability to reclaim wellness as a cancer survivor (Powel, Hopkins, Kozlovsky, & Parekh, 2009; Powel et al., 2009; Gonzalez, Powel, Kozlovsky, Parekh, & Ford, 2009). Issues relevant to specific ethnic groups must be examined in order to provide care that is culturally and linguistically appropriate, as seen in *Mi Decisiçon—PCa: A Prostate Cancer Decision Aid for Latino Men* (2009).

QOL Tools Used in Prostate Cancer Research

The influence of prostate cancer treatment on health-related QOL outcomes typically includes instruments that assess generic or global QOL, cancer-specific QOL, prostate cancer-specific QOL, or a combination thereof. The most frequently used instrument in assessing global QOL in prostate cancer is the Mental Health Subscale of the Medical Outcomes Study Short-form Health Survey (SF-36) (Ware, Jr. & Sherbourne, 1992). The SF-36 is designed to measure health status in the Medical Outcomes Study (MOS) and focuses on distinct dimensions of current health status including general health perceptions, physical functioning, role performance, emotional limitations, bodily pain and pain-related limitations, general mental health, vitality, and social functioning. Cancer-specific QOL in prostate cancer is assessed most commonly using the European Organization for Research and Treatment of Cancer QLQ-C30 (EORTC-QLQ-C30) (Ware, Jr. & Sherbourne, 1992); it uses a modular approach that includes a composite inventory coupled with disease-specific modules designed to assess HRQOL in patients with cancer. This tool has been and is used widely in numerous studies around the world. EORTC-QLQ-C30 incorporates nine multi-item scales: five functional scales (physical, role, cognitive, emotional, and social);

three symptom scales (fatigue, pain, and nausea and vomiting); and a global health and quality-of-life scale. The most commonly used instrument to assess disease-specific QOL is the University of California, Los Angeles, Prostate Cancer Index (UCLA-PCI) (Litwin et al., 1998). It includes 20 items related to urinary, sexual, and bowel (dys) function, as well as bother (i.e., how much the patient is troubled by the dysfunction). Participants are instructed to select one of the following response choices that best fits their experience: (1) no problem, (2) very small problem, (3) moderate problem, (4) big problem. The UCLA-PCI has been used to measure prostate-specific QOL in men with early or late stage prostate cancer (Litwin & Penson, 1998). In addition to these instruments, other instruments are used in studies of QOL in prostate cancer. They include the Functional Assessment of Cancer Therapy–Prostate (FACT-P) (Esper et al., 1997), a 12-item subscale to the FACT measurement system, which assesses attributes of weight loss, appetite changes, and urinary and sexual problems; the Prostate Cancer Specific Quality of Life Instrument (PROSQOLI) (Stockler, Osoba, Corey, Goodwin, & Tannock, 1999), which is a 20-item instrument focusing on domains specific to men with advanced hormone-resistant metastatic disease (very different from the domains common to men with localized prostate cancer); the PCTO-Q (Cheryl, Janice, Carol, & Charles, 1997), a 41-item instrument that assesses patients' perceptions of changes in the severity of urinary, sexual, and bowel functioning after prostate cancer therapy; and the Expanded Prostate Cancer Index Composite (EPIC) (Wei, Dunn, Litwin, Sandler, & Sanda, 2000), which includes 50 items related to the three domains important in the measurement of QOL in men with prostate cancer (i.e., urinary, sexual, bowel). The EPIC also includes items related to irritative urinary symptoms and hormonal changes, which are symptoms more likely to be seen as a consequence of radiotherapy and/or hormone ablation therapy.

Within the last few years other instruments focusing on assessing QOL with greater sensitivity have been developed. The EORTC QLQ-PR25 (van Andel et al., 2008) is a more recent version of the EORTC-C30 and is designed to measure HRQOL in prostate cancer patients. The EORTC QLQ-PR25 assesses urinary, bowel, and sexual symptoms and functioning, as well as the side effects of hormonal treatment. Forty-five healthcare professionals and 56 patients in 9 countries were interviewed in order to identify the most prevalent symptoms and functional problems. The initial instrument underwent two additional phases of testing prior to resulting in the 25-item questionnaire assessing urinary and bowel symptoms, sexual activity and functioning, and side effects of treatment. To evaluate psychometric properties of the EORTC QLQ-PR25, it was tested in 509 patients from 13 countries. Multi-trait scaling analysis confirmed the hypothesized scale structure of the instrument. Internal consistency ranged between α coefficient of 0.70–0.86, indicating good internal consistency for the urinary symptoms and sexual function scales, but an α coefficient of < 0.70 for the bowel and side-effect scales. The module was able to discriminate between clinically distinct patient subgroups and was responsive to changes in health status over time. Although some caution should be used when interpreting the bowel and side effects of hormonal scales, the instrument demonstrates acceptable psychometric properties and clinical validity.

Interventions to Improve Quality of Life in Prostate Cancer

Interventions to improve QOL in prostate cancer have focused on interventions specific to QOL in patients who receive a type of treatment, exhibit certain treatment or disease-specific symptoms, or are at a particular disease stage, such as early stage or metastatic disease. Few studies have examined prostate cancer survivorship specifically. Therefore, the following discussion focuses on those QOL intervention studies seen predominately in the current literature.

Prostate Cancer QOL Intervention Studies

Lepore and colleagues (Lepore, Helgeson, Eton, & Schulz, 2003) reported on their efforts to improve prostate cancer knowledge, health behaviors, and general QOL outcomes in 250 men recruited one month following treatment for localized prostate cancer. Subjects were randomized to control, group education (GE), or group education plus facilitator-led group discussion (GED). The group-education intervention was comprised of six weekly 1-hour lectures on the biology and epidemiology of prostate cancer, control of physical symptoms, nutrition and cancer, stress and coping, relationships and sexuality, and follow-up care concerns. Ninety-three subjects were included in each condition, with assessments at 2 (baseline), 4, 10, and 16 months following primary treatment. Outcome measures were prostate cancer knowledge, positive healthcare behaviors, and overall QOL. The investigators hypothesized that less educated subjects (non-college grads) would gain more from the intervention arms than more educated subjects (college grads) because they would have access to information previously not available or understood. Both the GE and the GED intervention increased prostate cancer knowledge. Men in the GED group were less likely to be bothered by sexual dysfunction than those in the control group, and GED participants were more likely than either the control or the GE groups to remain steadily employed. The findings indicated that non-college grads in the GE and GED groups were more likely to increase physical functioning than the control group and those in the GED group demonstrated more positive health behaviors than the GE or control groups. College graduates, in all groups, improved physical functioning and demonstrated more positive health behaviors compared with baseline.

One of the often identified dilemmas of reports of QOL in men treated for prostate cancer is that, after brief declines in global QOL following treatment, QOL returns to baseline within 12 months of treatment despite reports from men regarding distress and bother resulting from treatment-related consequences. Indeed, patients treated for prostate cancer often are reluctant to report postoperative symptoms (Powell, 2003; Powell et al., 2009) for these four reasons: they are reluctant to challenge their care, and by extension, their care provider (Powell & Clark, 2005); they think their problem is not severe enough to warrant seeking medical attention (Bhatnagar, Stewart, Huynh, Jorgensen, & Kaplan, 2006); they may be uncomfortable disclosing issues related to private experiences such as urinary incontinence and erectile dysfunction (McNaughton-Collins, Walker-Corkery, & Barry, 2004); or they are grateful to have been *cured* of their cancer and thus accept the symptoms as a tradeoff (Lepore et al., 2003; McNaughton-Collins et al., 2004).

Thus, Penedo and colleagues (2004) designed a stress management skills training intervention to address the cognitive, emotional, and behavioral strategies that may contribute to the distress men experience as a result of posttreatment urinary incontinence and erectile dysfunction. The goal of this training intervention was to improve QOL by helping participants identify and effectively manage stressful experiences associated with treatment-related consequences. Investigators randomly assigned 92 men, who had completed either radical prostatectomy or external beam therapy for prostate cancer within the previous 18 months, to either a 10-week cognitive-behavioral stress management (CBSM) intervention or a half-day seminar on improving QOL (Penedo et al., 2004).

The CBSM intervention consisted of one 2-hour per week session of 90 minutes of didactic instruction, 30 minutes of relaxation, and homework. The half-day seminar (control) group received one 4-hour seminar on stress management skills and had an opportunity to practice relaxation. Assessments were made at two time points (pre- and post-intervention) using the Functional Assessment of Cancer Therapy—General Module (FACT-G) and the Measure of Current Status Instrument (MOCS), a measure of perceived stress management skill.

A hierarchical regression model was used to predict post-intervention QOL. Predictors and covariates (income, baseline QOL, ethnicity, and group condition) explained 62.1% of the variance, and group assignment was a significant predictor of QOL even when controlling for covariates. The MOCS change score accounted for 14% of the variance in QOL after the intervention, indicating that subjects in the CSBM group made significant improvements in stress management skills, whereas their counter parts in the control group did not.

In a prospective, multi-site study, Giesler and colleagues (2005) compared a nurse-driven QOL intervention to usual care in 99 men treated for prostate cancer 6 weeks previously. The QOL intervention was tailored individually to problems identified by subjects using a computer-assisted program. Using evidence-based strategies, nurses provided education and support regarding the identified need and monitored responses to the strategies each month for 6 months (twice in person and four times by telephone). The outcome variables included disease-specific QOL (urinary, sexual, and bowel symptoms, and cancer worry), depression, dyadic adjustment, and global QOL. Assessments were made at baseline, 4, 7, and 12 months following treatment. Patients in the intervention arm experienced long-term improvements related to sexual function and cancer worry when compared to subjects in the control arm. Patients with depression improved over time without regard to treatment condition.

Daubenmier and colleagues (2006) examined the influence of lifestyle on HRQOL in men managed with active surveillance for early stage prostate cancer. Ninety-three men were randomized to the lifestyle intervention ($n=44$) or control ($n=49$). The lifestyle intervention consisted of a low-fat vegan diet, 3 hours of moderate exercise weekly, 1 hour per day of stress management practice, and weekly support groups. Subjects in the intervention group participated in a 1-week residential retreat to learn the intervention program. Measures assessed included HRQOL, perceived stress, sexual function, and lifestyle behavior. Assessments were completed at baseline and 12 months. Data were analyzed using repeated measures analysis of variance and multiple logistic regression. Intervention participants significantly improved their lifestyle by 12 months and those with healthy lifestyles reported improved mental and physical QOL and sexual function. Those who improved their lifestyles over time reported improved physical QOL and decreased perceived stress (Daubenmier et al., 2006).

Canada and colleagues (2005) reported on the findings of their pilot intervention study to enhance sexual rehabilitation in men treated locally with radical prostatectomy or external beam therapy 3 months to 5 years previously, as well as their female partners. Four educational and counseling sessions focused on prostate cancer, sexual function, options to treat erectile dysfunction (ED), sexual communication, and stimulation skills. Couples were assigned randomly to one of two conditions: the man attending the sessions alone, or the couple attending the sessions together. Partners in both groups completed behavioral homework. The outcome variables were sexual function, marital adjustment, psychological distress, and utilization of medical treatment for erectile dysfunction. Of the 84 dyads originally recruited, 51 completed the intervention, with 26 couples assigned to the man-alone group and 25 couples assigned to the couples group. Improvement in male overall distress, male global sexual function, and female global satisfaction were apparent at 3 months; however improvement waned by 6 months following the intervention, with the exception of the use of ED treatments, which improved from 31% at baseline to 49% at 6 months. Partner attendance did not affect the outcomes (Canada et al., 2005).

Carmack-Taylor et al, (2004) described the design and baseline characteristics of a randomized controlled clinical trial aimed at improving QOL by increasing physical activity. Investigators randomized 134 men treated with androgen ablation therapy for 1 year or more to a 6-month lifestyle intervention, a 6-month educational support intervention, and standard care. The lifestyle intervention included 16 weekly sessions and four bimonthly sessions comprised of a 60-minute active physical activity skills training followed by 30 minutes of discussion. The educational intervention was structured identically, except the didactic portion of the intervention related to education about prostate cancer. Measures assessed global QOL, including physical and emotional health status, depression, pain, and anxiety, in addition to variables that could potentially mediate the effects of QOL or physical activity. Assessments were completed at baseline, following the intensive intervention (6 months), and at a 6-month follow-up (12 months). Results from this study promise to inform both providers and patients about physical exercise in men with prostate cancer (Carmack-Taylor et al., 2004).

In a randomized controlled study of patients 65 years and older with advanced cancer, Kornblith and colleagues compared the effectiveness of an intervention providing educational materials (EM) alone to an intervention of educational materials combined with telephone follow-up (EM + TM) focusing on reducing distress in 192 patients with breast, colon, or prostate cancer. The EM intervention included written materials regarding cancer-related psychosocial issues and available resources, whereas the EM + TM group also included a monthly telephone call for 6 months. Of those subjects with prostate cancer, 32% and 35%, respectively of the total sample, were included in the EM alone and EM + TM groups. Measures assessed QOL, anxiety and depression, and social support at baseline and

6 months. At 6 months, subjects in the EM + TM group reported significantly less anxiety, depression, and overall distress than those in the EM-alone group (Kornblith et al. 2006).

Similar to the previously reported Canada study, Harden and her colleagues (2009) examined 69 men with prostate cancer and their spouses in a descriptive, comparative design guided by a theoretical framework that linked an adult developmental and family stress framework. Participants were in one of three groups: middle age (50–64 years), young-old (65–74 years), and old-old (over 75 years) (Harden et al., 2009). Study end-points were QOL, psychosocial factors including work and family obligations, self-efficacy, appraisal of illness, and appraisal of caregiving. Study variables were assessed using instruments previously tested for reliability and validity in patients with prostate cancer, with the exception of the Lewis Cancer Self-Efficacy Scale (CASE), which reported acceptable psychometric and clinical validity in patients with breast cancer. The following instruments were used: SF-36, EPIC, Appraisal of Illness Scale (AIS), Appraisal of Caregiving Scale (ACS), CASE, and the Omega Screening Questionnaire (OSQ). Analysis of covariance (ANCOVA) and multivariate analysis of covariance (MANCOVA) were used to determine differences among age groups. Participants in the young-old group had better QOL and self-efficacy than those in the middle-age group, and less negative appraisal of their illness compared to those in the middle-age and old-old groups. Middle-age spouses had greater distress regarding their partner's sexual dysfunction; spouses in the youngest and oldest groups reported greater bother related to hormonal changes than their counterparts in the young-old group.

In a longitudinal analysis of predictors of QOL in patients and spouses, Kershaw and colleagues (2008) examined whether baseline antecedent coping and stress variables predicted coping and QOL. One hundred twenty-one patient–spouse dyads were assessed at three time points for self-efficacy, current concerns, communication, symptoms, negative appraisal, hopelessness, and uncertainty. Socioeconomic status, age, and phase of illness were also assessed at baseline. Analyses included a single integrated path model using structural equation modeling. The stress-coping model accounted for a significant portion of the variance in mental and physical activity. Appraisal mediated the effects of antecedent variables on QOL (Kershaw et al., 2008).

Issues for Future QOL Research in Breast and Prostate Cancer

Based on the review and the authors' combined research experience in breast and prostate cancer research and QOL, several significant areas for future QOL research are presented. First, the importance of QOL in posttreatment survivorship cannot be overemphasized. Given the Institute of Medicine report on cancer survivors being lost in transition, the development of targeted interventions in posttreatment survivorship is critical to decrease the chance of being lost in transition. Such interventions can aim at improving health after cancer treatment, improving cancer surveillance, and managing living with cancer recurrence (Institute of Medicine, 2005).

Second, the most efficacious QOL interventions deserve further consideration. What different types of targeted interventions are most effective and for which type of cancer survivor? Future QOL interventions also need to target to health disparities between breast and prostate cancer survivors. For example, can interventions delivered by low-tech methods, such as telephone, decrease the potential for being lost in transition in at-risk breast and prostate cancer survivors?

Third, age-related differences, as they influence QOL across breast and prostate cancer survivors, deserve consideration. The bulk of studies relating to breast cancer are conducted with middle-age to older women, while the majority of studies in prostate cancer focus on younger men.

The measurement of QOL in breast cancer has remained largely constant over the past 10 years. The EORTC-breast cancer version and physical functioning tools such as the SF-36 are, more often than not, seen in QOL breast cancer studies. There is movement toward more symptom-specific problem scales such as sleep disturbance, menopausal symptoms, and pain that complement the general QOL and physical functioning scales. Similarly, instruments assessing QOL in patients with prostate cancer have focused on increasing sensitivity, relying on patient interviews, and attending to changes in health status over time. The measurement of QOL in prostate cancer has improved over the last two decades as research has moved from the ultimate goal of survival to include a focus on patient-centered assessment of QOL. However, a number of issues impede interpretation of published reports of QOL. Among them are conflicting stances on such basic issues as the definition of incontinence and erectile dysfunction and the heterogeneous nature of prostate cancer. Thus, by definition, a variety of perspectives are commonly studied. For example, studies may focus on type of treatment (e.g., open radical protatectomy, laparoscopic prostatectomy, external beam therapy, brachytherapy, observation), techniques (e.g., nerve sparing, non-nerve sparing surgery), symptoms (e.g., urinary incontinence, bowel or erectile dysfunction), or disease trajectory (e.g., early stage versus metastatic disease). This diverse orientation presupposes that different attributes of QOL are studied and different instruments are used to measure them, making the synthesis of overall QOL in men with prostate cancer complex.

To assess the dimensions or attributes of health that capture the illness or treatment experience adequately, measurement of QOL ideally should include indices of global, disease-specific, and domain- or dimension-specific QOL. Most studies of QOL in prostate cancer include instruments that assess domains of general (i.e., global) and disease-specific QOL; however, items sensitive to specific symptoms are not always well articulated in these instruments (Aaronson, 1988; Ware, 1984).

CONCLUSION

Research examining QOL in breast and prostate cancer survivors has been fruitful. In breast cancer, the vast majority of QOL intervention studies have been conducted during active treatment. Far fewer studies have been identified in posttreatment survivorship. Although a variety of methods have been used to deliver QOL interventions, the most efficacious are not yet well described, particularly for underserved and at-risk survivors. Given that breast and prostate cancer survivors represent a significant proportion of all cancer survivors, QOL research must continue.

REFERENCES

Aaronson, N. K. (1988). Quality of life: What is it? How should it be measured? *Oncology (Williston Park)*, 2(5), 69–76, 64.

American Cancer Society. (2010). *ACS Facts & Figures 2010*. Retrieved March 13, 2011, from www.cancer.org/research/cancerfactsfigures/cancerfactsfigures/cancer-facts-and-figures-2010

Ahles, T. A., Saykin, A. J., Furstenberg, C. T., Cole, B., Mott, L.A., Titus-Ernstoff, L. et al. (2005). Quality of life of long-term survivors of breast cancer and lymphoma treated with standard-dose chemotherapy or local therapy. *Journal of Clinical Oncology, 23*(19), 4399–4405.

Ashing-Giwa, K. T., Padilla, G. V., Bohorquez, D. E., Tejero, J. S., & Garcia, M. (2006). Understanding the breast cancer experience of Latina women. *Journal of Psychosocial Oncology, 24*(3), 19–52.

Badger, T., Segrin, C., Meek, P., Lopez, A. M., & Bonham, E. (2004). A case study of telephone interpersonal counseling for women with breast cancer and their partners. *Oncology Nursing Forum, 31*(5), 997–1003.

Bhatnagar, V., Stewart, S. T., Huynh, V., Jorgensen, G., & Kaplan, R. M. (2006). Estimating the risk of long-term erectile, urinary and bowel symptoms resulting from prostate cancer treatment. *Prostate Cancer Prostatic Diseases, 9*(2), 136–146.

Bishoff, J. T., Motley, G., Optenberg, S. A., Stein, C. R., Moon, K. A., Browning, S. M. et al. (1998). Incidence of fecal and urinary incontinence following radical perineal and retropubic prostatectomy in a national population. *The Journal of Urology, 160*(2), 454–458.

Braden, C. J., Mishel, M. H., & Longman, A. J. (1998). Self-Help Intervention Project: Women receiving breast cancer treatment. *Cancer Practice, 6*(2), 87–98.

Canada, A. L., Neese, L. E., Sui, D., & Schover, L. R. (2005). Pilot intervention to enhance sexual rehabilitation for couples after treatment for localized prostate carcinoma. *Cancer, 104*(12), 2689–2700.

Carmack-Taylor, C. L., Smith, M. A., de Moor, C., Dunn, A.L., Pettaway, C., Sellin, R. et al. (2004). Quality of life intervention for prostate cancer patients: Design and baseline characteristics of the active for life after cancer trial. *Controlled Clinical Trials, 25*(3), 265–285.

Catalona, W. J., Beiser, J. A., & Smith, D. S. (1997). Serum free prostate specific antigen and prostate specific antigen density measurements for predicting cancer in men with prior negative prostatic biopsies. *The Journal of Urology, 158*(6), 2162.

Cella, D. F., Tulsky, D. S., Gray, G., Sarafian, B., Linn, E., Bonomi, A. et al. (1993). The Functional Assessment of Cancer Therapy scale: Development and validation of the general measure. *Journal of Clinical Oncology, 11*(3), 570–579.

Chamberlain-Wilmoth, M., Tulman, L., Coleman, E. A., Stewart, C. B., & Samarel, N. (2006). Women's perceptions of the effectiveness of telephone support and education on their adjustment to breast cancer. *Oncology Nursing Forum, 33*(1), 138–144.

Cheryl, L. S. B., Janice, L. K., Carol, P. M., & Charles, L. M. (1997). Quality of life and treatment outcomes. *Cancer, 79*(10), 1977–1986.

Cimprich, B. (1993). Development of an intervention to restore attention in cancer patients. *Cancer Nursing, 16*(2), 83–92.

Cimprich, B., & Ronis, D. L. (2003). An environmental intervention to restore attention in women with newly diagnosed breast cancer. *Cancer Nursing, 26*(4), 284–292; quiz 293–284.

Clark, J. A., Wray, N. P., & Ashton, C. M. (2001). Living with treatment decisions: Regrets and quality of life among men treated for metastatic prostate cancer. *Journal of Clinical Oncology, 19*(1), 72–80.

Coleman, E. A., Tulman, L., Samarel, N., Wilmoth, M.C., Rickel, L., Rickel, M. et al. (2005). The effect of telephone social support and education on adaptation to breast cancer during the year following diagnosis. *Oncology Nursing Forum, 32*(4), 822–829.

D'Amico, A. V., Whittington, R., Malkowicz, S. B., Schultz, D., Blank, K., Broderick, G.A. et al. (1998). Biochemical outcome after radical prostatectomy, external beam radiation therapy, or interstitial radiation therapy for clinically localized prostate cancer. *Journal of the American Medical Association, 280*(11), 969–974.

Daubenmier, J. J., Weidner, G., Marlin, R., Crutchfield, L., Dunn-Emke, S., Chi, C. et al. (2006). Lifestyle and health-related quality of life of men with prostate cancer managed with active surveillance. *Urology, 67*(1), 125–130.

Dow, K. H., Ferrell, B. R., Haberman, M. R., & Eaton, L. (1999). The meaning of quality of life in cancer survivorship. *Oncology Nursing Forum, 26*(3), 519–528.

Esper, P., Mo, F., Chodak, G., Sinner, M., Cella, D., & Pienta. K. J. (1997). Measuring quality of life in men with prostate cancer using the functional assessment of cancer therapy-prostate instrument. *Urology, 50*(6), 920–928.

Fogel, J., Albert, S. M., Schnabel, F., Ditkoff, B. A., & Neugut, A. I. (2002). Internet use and social support in women with breast cancer. *Health Psychology, 21*(4), 398–404.

Fowler, F. J., Jr., McNaughton Collins, M., Walker Corkery, E., Elliott, D. B., & Barry, M. J. (2002). The impact of androgen deprivation on quality of life after radical prostatectomy for prostate carcinoma. *Cancer, 95*(2), 287–295.

Fraser, S. C., Ramirez, A. J., Ebbs, S. R., Fallowfield, L.J., Dobbs, H.J., Richards, M.A. et al. (1993). A daily diary for quality of life measurement in advanced breast cancer trials. *British Journal of Cancer, 67*(2), 341–346.

Ganz, P. A., Kwan, L., Stanton, A. L., et al. (2004). Quality of life at the end of primary treatment of breast cancer: First results from the moving beyond cancer randomized trial. *Journal of the National Cancer Institute, 96*(5), 376–387.

Giesler, R. B., Given, B., Given, C. W., Rawl, S., Monahan, P., Burns, D., et al. (2005). Improving the quality of life of patients with prostate carcinoma: A randomized trial testing the efficacy of a nurse-driven intervention. *Cancer, 104*(4), 752–762.

Golant, M., Altman, T., & Martin, C. (2003). Managing cancer side effects to improve quality of life: A cancer psychoeducation program. *Cancer Nursing, 26*(1), 37–44; quiz 45–36.

Gonzalez, C. E., Powel, L., Kozlovsky, K., Parekh, D., & Ford, C. (2009). Specific concerns of Latino men following robotic-assisted laparoscopic prostatectomy: An examination of field notes. *Proceedings of the Annual Meeting of the National Association of Hispanic Nurses.* San Antonio, TX.

Gore, J. L., Krupski, T., Kwan, L., Fink, A., & Litwin, M. S. (2005). Mental health of low income uninsured men with prostate cancer. *The Journal of Urology, 173*(4), 1323.

Harden, J., Falahee, M., Bickes, J., Schafenacker, A., Walker, J., Mood, D. et al. (2009). Factors associated with prostate cancer patients' and their spouses' satisfaction with a family-based intervention. *Cancer, 32*(6), 482–492.

Helgeson, V. S., Cohen, S., Schulz, R., & Yasko, J. (2001). Long-term effects of educational and peer discussion group interventions on adjustment to breast cancer. *Health Psychology 20*(5), 387–392.

Helgeson, V. S., Cohen, S., Schulz, R., & Yasko, J. (1999). Education and peer discussion group interventions and adjustment to breast cancer. *Archives of General Psychiatry, 56*(4), 340–347.

Hosaka, T., Sugiyama, Y., Hirai, K., & Sugawara, Y. (2001). Factors associated with the effects of a structured psychiatric intervention on breast cancer patients. *Tokai Journal of Experimental and Clinical Medicine, 26*(2), 33–38.

Hosaka, T., Sugiyama, Y., Tokuda, Y., Okuyama, T., Sugawara, Y., & Nakamura, Y. (2000). Persistence of the benefits of a structured psychiatric intervention for breast cancer patients with lymph node metastases. *Tokai Journal of Experimental and Clinical Medicine, 25*(2), 45–49.

Hosaka, T., Sugiyama, Y., Hirai, K., Okuyama, T., Sugawara, Y., & Nakamura, Y. (2001). Effects of a modified group intervention with early-stage breast cancer patients. *General Hospital Psychiatry, 23*(3), 145–151.

Hoskins, C. N. (2001). Promoting adjustment among women with breast cancer and their partners: A program of research. *Journal of the New York State Nurses Association, 32*(2), 19–23.

Hoskins, C. N., Haber, J., Budin, W. C., Cartwright-Alcarese, F., Kowalski, M. O., Panke, J. et al., (2001). Breast cancer: Education, counseling, and adjustment-a pilot study. *Psychological Reports, 89*(3), 677–704.

Institute of Medicine, National Research Council (2004). *Meeting psychosocial needs of women with breast cancer.* Washington, DC: National Academies Press.

Institute of Medicine (2005). IOM report recommends 'survivorship care plan' to guide growing number of Americans living with cancer . *Hospitals & Health Networks, 79*(12), 64.

Institute of Medicine, National Research Council (2006). *From cancer patient to cancer survivor: Lost in transition.* Washington, DC: The National Academies Press.

Kershaw, T. S., Mood, D.W., Newth, G., Ronis, D. L., Sanda, M. G., Vaishampayan, U., et al. (2008). Longitudinal analysis of a model to predict quality of life in prostate cancer patients and their spouses. *Annals of Behavioral Medicine: A Publication of the Society of Behavioral Medicine, 36*(2), 117.

Kornblith, A. B., Dowell, J. M., Herndon, J. E., 2nd, Engelman, B. J., Bauer-Wu, S., Small, E. J. et al. (2006). Telephone monitoring of distress in patients aged 65 years or older with advanced stage cancer: A cancer and leukemia group B study. *Cancer, 107*(11), 2706–2714.

Kudadjie-Gyamfi, E., Consedine, N. S., & Magai, C. (2006). On the importance of being ethnic: Coping with the threat of prostate cancer in relation to prostate cancer screening. *Cultural Diversity and Ethnic Minority Psychology, 12*(3), 509.

Lepore, S. J., Helgeson, V. S., Eton, D. T., & Schulz, R. (2003). Improving quality of life in men with prostate cancer: A randomized controlled trial of group education interventions. *Health Psychology, 22*(5), 443–452.

Leventhal, H., Patrick-Miller, L., & Leventhal, E. A. (1998). It's long-term stressors that take a toll: Comment on Cohen et al. *Health Psychology, 17*(3), 211–213.

Lewis, J. A., Manne, S. L., DuHamel, K. N., Vickburg, S. M., Bovbjerg, D. H., Currie, V., et al. (2001). Social support, intrusive thoughts, and quality of life in breast cancer survivors. *Journal of Behavioral Medicine, 24*(3), 231–245.

Litwin, M. S., Hays, R. D., Fink, A., Ganz, P. A., Leake, B., & Brook, R. H. (1998). The UCLA Prostate Cancer Index: Development, reliability, and validity of a health-related quality of life measure. *Medical Care, 36*(7), 1002–1012.

Litwin, M. S., & Penson, D. F. (1998). Health-related quality of life in men with prostate cancer. *Prostate Cancer and Prostatic Diseases, 1*(5), 228–235.

Marcus, A. C., Garrett, K. M., Cella, D., Wenzel, L. B., Brady, M. J., Crane, L. A., et al. (1998). Telephone counseling of breast cancer patients after treatment: A description of a randomized clinical trial. *Psychooncology, 7*(6), 470–482.

McNaughton-Collins, M., Walker-Corkery, E., & Barry, M. J. (2004). Health-related quality of life, satisfaction, and economic outcome measures in studies of prostate cancer screening and treatment, 1990–2000. *Journal of the National Cancer Institute Monographs, 33*, 78–101.

Meng, M. V., & Carroll, P. R. (2001). Local therapy for prostate-specific antigen recurrence after definitive treatment. *Prostate Cancer and Prostatic Diseases, 4*(1), 20–27.

Meneses, K., McNees, P., Loerzel, V., Su, X., Zhang, Y., & Hassey, L. (2007). Transition from treatment to survivorship: Effects of a psychoeducational intervention on quality of life in breast cancer survivors. *Oncology Nursing Forum, 34*, 1007–1116.

Mishel, M. H., Germino, B. B., Gil, K. M., Belyea, M., Laney, I. C., Stewart, J., et al. (2005). Benefits from an uncertainty management intervention for African-American and Caucasian older long-term breast cancer survivors. *Psychooncology, 14*(11), 962–978.

National Cancer Institute. (2007). *Surveilllance, Epidemiology, & End Results: Cancer of the Prostate.* Bethesda, MD: Author.

Okamura, H., Fukui, S., Nagasaka, Y., Koike, M., & Uchitomi, Y. (2003). Psychoeducational intervention for patients with primary breast cancer and patient satisfaction with information: An exploratory analysis. *Breast Cancer Research and Treatment, 80*(3), 331–338.

Parekh, D. J., Pauler Ankerst, D., Higgins, B. A., Hernandez, J., Canby-Hagino, E., Brand, T., et al. (2006). External validation of the prostate cancer prevention trial risk calculator in a screened population. *Urology, 68*(6), 1152.

Penedo, F. J., Dahn, J. R., Molton, I., Gonzalez, J. S., Kinsinger, D., Roos, B. A., et al. (2004). Cognitive-behavioral stress management improves stress-management skills and quality of life in men recovering from treatment of prostate carcinoma. *Cancer, 100*(1), 192–200.

Pienta, K. J., & Esper, P. S. (1993). Risk factors for prostate cancer. *Annals of Internal Medicine, 118*(10), 793–803.

Powel, L. (2002). Incontinence Morbidity Following Radical Prostatectomy: Measuring the Effect on Psychosocial Adjustment to Illness. *Proceedings of the 9th Annual International Society for Quality of Life Research Meeting.* Orlando, FL.

Powel L. L. (2002). *Incontinence morbidity, psychosocial adjustment to illness, and quality of life after prostatectomy.* Unpublished doctoral dissertation, University of Maryland, Baltimore.

Powel, L. (2003). It's not just black and white: Examining perceptions of urinary incontinence postprostatectomy in men of diverse ethnic backgrounds. *Proceedings of the Gerontological Society of America Annual Meeting.* San Diego, CA.

Powel, L. (2003). Men's Characterizations of the Psychosocial Effects of Radical Prostatectomy. *Proceedings of the 7th Biennial Oncology Nursing Research Conference.* San Diego, CA.

Powel, L. (2004). Cognitive representations and emotional responses to postprostatectomy urinary incontinence in men of diverse ethnic backgrounds. *Proceedings of the Society of Behavioral Medicine's 25th Annual Meeting & Scientific Sessions.* Baltimore, MD.

Powel, L. (2006). Characterizations of the Impact of Laparoscopic Prostatectomy on Adaptation to Prostate Cancer. *Proceedings of the American Psychosocial Oncology Society 3rd Annual Meeting.* Amelia Island, FL.

Powel, L. L., & Clark, J. A. (2005). The value of the marginalia as an adjunct to structured questionnaires: Experiences of men after prostate cancer surgery. *Quality of Life Research, 14*(3), 827–835.

Powel, L., Harper, M., Decker, J., Edmonson, K., Moore, D., Velez, G., et al. (2007). Adaptation to Prostate Cancer. *Proceedings of the US Department of Defense Prostate Cancer Research Program Meeting: Innovative Minds in Prostate Cancer Today (IMPaCT).* Atlanta, GA.

Powel, L., Gonzalez, C. E., Kozlovsky, K., Marquise, O., Chen, J., Ford, C., et al. (2009). Mi decisi_on-PCa: A prostate cancer decision aid for Latino men. *Proceedings of the Annual Meeting of the National Association of Hispanic Nurses.* San Antonio, TX.

Powel, L. L., Hopkins, M., Kozlovsky, K., & Parekh, D. (2009). Experiences of bilingual and monolingual Latino men following robotic laparoscopic prostatectomy: Examination of field notes. *Proceedings of the Annual Meeting of the National Hispanic Nurses Association.* San Antonio, TX.

Powel, L. Kozlovsky, K., Reed, A., Thompson, I. M., Berndt, A., Marcus, J., et al. (2009). Factors that influence patients with elevated PSA to chose or decline prostate biopsy. *Proceedings of the 2nd European Congress on the Aging Male.* Budapest, Hungary.

Powel, L., Pugh, M. J. V., & Elnitsky, C. (2002). Diverse methods of evaluating disparities: Thinking outside of the box. *Proceedings of the Primary Care Research Methods & Statistics Conference, The University of Texas Health Sciences Center.* San Antonio, TX.

Rawl, S. M., Given, B. A., Given, C. W., Champion, V. L., Kozachik, S.L., Barton, D., et al. (2002). Intervention to improve psychological functioning for newly diagnosed patients with cancer. *Oncology Nursing Forum, 29*(6), 967–975.

Sandgren, A. K., & McCaul, K. D. (2006). Long-term telephone therapy outcomes for breast cancer patients. *Psychooncology, 16*(1), 38–47.

Schag, C. A., Ganz, P. A., & Heinrich, R. L. (1991). Cancer Rehabilitation Evaluation System-short form (CARES-SF). A cancer specific rehabilitation and quality of life instrument. *Cancer, 68*(6), 1406–1413.

Scheier, M. F., Helgeson, V. S., Schulz, R., Colvin, S., Berga, S., Bridges, M.W., et al. (2005). Interventions to enhance physical and psychological functioning among younger women who are ending nonhormonal adjuvant treatment for early-stage breast cancer. *Journal of Clinical Oncology, 23*(19), 4298–4311.

Screening for prostate cancer: Recommendation and rationale. (2002). *Annals of Internal Medicine, 137*(11), 915–916.

Shaw, B. R., Hawkins, R., Arora, N., McTavish, F., Pingree, S., & Gustafson, D. H. (2006). An exploratory study of predictors of participation in a computer support group for women with breast cancer. *Computers Informatics Nursing, 24*(1), 18–27.

Spiegel, D., Bloom, J. R., Kraemer, H. C., & Gottheil, E. (1989). Effect of psychosocial treatment on survival of patients with metastatic breast cancer. *Lancet, 2*(8668), 888–891.

Spiegel, D., Bloom, J. R., & Yalom, I. (1981). Group support for patients with metastatic cancer: A randomized outcome study. *Archives of General Psychiatry, 38*(5), 527–533.

Sprangers, M. A., Cull, A., Bjordal, K., Groenvold, M., & Aaronson, N. K. (1993). The European Organization for Research and Treatment of Cancer Approach to quality of life assessment: Guidelines for developing questionnaire modules. EORTC Study Group on Quality of Life. *Quality of Life Research, 2*(4), 287–295.

Stanton, A. L., Ganz, P. A., Kwan, L., Meyerowitz, B. E., Bower, J. E., Krupnick, J. L., et al. (2005). Outcomes from the Moving Beyond Cancer psychoeducational, randomized, controlled trial with breast cancer patients. *Journal of Clinical Oncology, 23*(25), 6009–6018.

Stockler, M. R., Osoba, D., Corey, P., Goodwin, P. J., & Tannock, I. F. (1999). Convergent, discriminitive, and predictive validity of the Prostate Cancer Specific Quality of Life Instrument (PROSQOLI) assessment and comparison with analogous scales from the EORTC QLQ-C30 and a trial-specific module. European Organisation for Research and Treatment of Cancer. Core Quality of Life Questionnaire. *Journal of Clinical Epidemiology, 52*(7), 653–666.

Talcott, J. A., Rieker, P., Clark, J. A., Propert, K. J., Weeks, J. C., Beard, C. J., et al. (1998). Patient-reported symptoms after primary therapy for early prostate cancer: Results of a prospective cohort study. *Journal of Clinical Oncology, 16*(1), 275–283.

Thompson, I. M., Ankerst, D. P., Chi, C., Goodman, P. J., Tangen, C. M., Lucia, M. S., et al. (2006). Assessing prostate cancer risk: Results from the prostate cancer prevention trial. *Journal of the National Cancer Institute, 98*(8), 529–534.

van Andel, G., Bottomley, A., Fosså, S. D., Efficace, F., Coens, C., Guerif, S., et al. (2008). An international field study of the EORTC QLQ-PR25: A questionnaire for assessing the health-related quality of life of patients with prostate cancer. *European Journal of Cancer, 44*(16), 2418.

Ware, J. E., Jr. (1984). Methodology in behavioral and psychosocial cancer research: Conceptualizing disease impact and treatment outcomes. *Cancer, 53*(10, Suppl.), 2316–2326.

Ware, J. E., Jr., & Sherbourne, C. D. (1992). The MOS 36-item short-form health survey (SF-36). I. Conceptual framework and item selection. *Medical Care, 30*(6), 473–483.

Wei, J. T., Dunn, R. L., Litwin, M. S., Sandler, H. M., & Sanda, M. G. (2000). Development and validation of the expanded prostate cancer index composite (EPIC) for comprehensive assessment of health-related quality of life in men with prostate cancer. *Urology, 56*(6), 899–905.

Weisman, A. D., & Worden, J. W. (1976). The existential plight in cancer: Significance of the first 100 days. *International Journal of Psychiatry in Medicine, 7*(1), 1–15.

Wilkins, E. G., Lowery, J. C., Copeland, L. A., Goldfarb, S. L., Wren, P. A., & Janz, N. K. (2006). Impact of an educational video on patient decision making in early breast cancer treatment. *Medical Decision Making, 26*(6), 589–598.

Yates, P., Aranda, S., Hargraves, M., Mirolo, B., Clavarino, A., McLachlan, S., et al. (2005). Randomized controlled trial of an educational intervention for managing fatigue in women receiving adjuvant chemotherapy for early-stage breast cancer. *Journal of Clinical Oncology, 23*(25), 6027–6036.

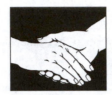

Chapter Fourteen

Clinical Implications of Quality of Life

CYNTHIA R. KING • ANNETTE BAKER HINES

Introduction

Quality of life (QOL) for oncology patients and QOL research are relevant to oncology nursing clinical practice. One of the primary goals of any type of nursing care is to assess human response to illness. Nurses understand that human responses to illness, specifically to cancer, are influenced not only by the disease, but also by psychological influences, social influences (e.g., interpersonal, family, cultural), and spiritual issues. These four areas of influence are similar to the four domains of QOL displayed in the City of Hope Medical Center Conceptual Model of Quality of Life (Figure 14-1). Thus, there is a tie between the concept of QOL and oncology nursing goals across the illness trajectory. But how in clinical

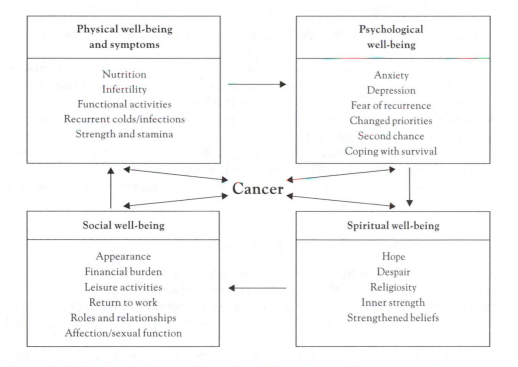

Figure 14-1. **Quality-of-life model for cancer survivors.**
Source: Adapted with permission from Ferrell, Grant et al., at City of Hope Medical Center.

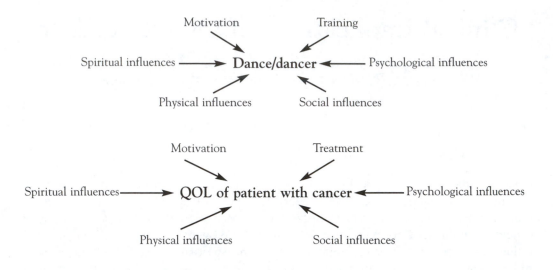

Figure 14-2. **Similarity of dance and quality of life.**
Permission granted from ONS. King, C. R. *Dance of Life* (2001).

practice do oncology nurses directly tie the concept of QOL to, and apply QOL research in, clinical practice?

First, imagine that a newly diagnosed cancer patient is like a novice dancer and an experienced nurse is the dance instructor. As the patient develops a relationship with the nurse, they begin dancing. The dance may be a duet (a nurse and a patient together), a performance by a company of dancers (nurse and patient along with family, caregivers, or other healthcare professionals), or a solo (patient dances and the nurse, family, and others support from the sidelines). The cancer dance is not only about movement, but also about attitude, motivation, and physical, psychological, social, and spiritual influences (Figure 14-2). For the cancer patient, this dance is analogous to living with a positive attitude and not concentrating on dying (King, 2001).

Nurses' Perceptions of Quality of Life

Nurses play an integral role in the care of all oncology patients. Unfortunately, nurses in clinical practice cannot assume they know how patients and families feel about their quality of life while living with cancer or undergoing treatment. Several studies have been conducted to assess nurses' perceptions of quality of life. In one study, King, Ferrell, Grant, and Sakurai (1995) explored nurses' perceptions of the impact of bone marrow transplantation (BMT) on the QOL of survivors. The study was conducted using the City of Hope Medical Center Conceptual Model of QOL (Figure 14-3). The nurses' responses to a QOL questionnaire were compared with the responses of the BMT survivors. Significant differences were revealed between the nurses' and patients' perceptions of the effect of BMT on quality of

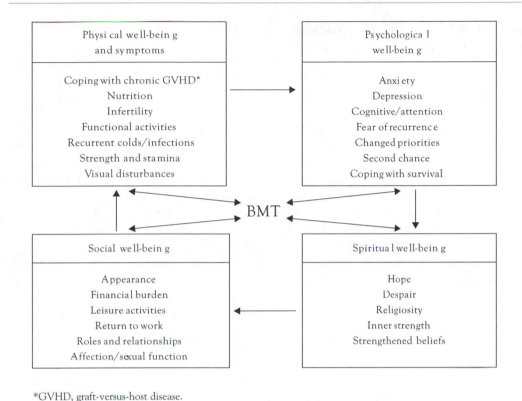

Figure 14-3. Quality-of-life model for bone marrow transplant survivors.
Source: Adapted with permission from Ferrell, Grant et al., at City of Hope Medical Center.

life. Although nurses could describe both positive and negative consequences of BMT, they perceived patients to have a poorer QOL than that actually reported by patients.

Other nursing studies have reported similar discrepancies in perceptions of the patient's QOL between the patient, nurse, and physician (Aaronson, 1986; Carr & Higginson, 2001; Cochran & Ganong, 1989; Dow, Ferrell, Haberman, & Eaton, 1999; Farrell, 1991; Ferrell & Dow, 1996; Johnston, 1982; Larson, 1984; Larson, 1986; Mayer, 1987; Mellon, 2002; Schipper & Levitt, 1985; von Essen & Sjoden, 1991; Wilson, Dowling, Abdollel, & Tannock, 2000; Zhao, Kanda, Liu, & Mao, 2003). Nurses had a 46% agreement rate and a 15% large discrepancy rate in comparison with QOL ratings with patients in a 1999 study (Sneeuw et al., 1999). Additionally, 86% of healthcare practitioners equate treatment efficacy with extension of survival, whereas 45% of patients view treatment efficacy as preserving QOL, 29% view it as extension of expected life, and 13% perceive it as delaying disease progression (Crawford et al., 1997; Weinfurt, 2007). Unfortunately, these misperceptions can result in lack of appropriate, comprehensive care for patients, provision of care not required by patients, or lack of attention to issues other than physical ones.

Barriers to Providing Nursing Care Focused on Quality-of-Life Issues

Although nurses in clinical practice are in an ideal position to support the importance of QOL as an outcome measure of cancer treatment, numerous obstacles prevent nurses from assessing QOL and providing support to this important concept. Lindley and Hirsch (1994) conducted a study to assess oncology nurses' attitudes, perceptions, and knowledge of QOL in patients with cancer. An exploratory survey was conducted at the 1990 Oncology Nursing Society Congress. Six hundred twenty-one nurses completed two questionnaires regarding the effect of treatment on QOL, the importance of QOL assessment, barriers to measuring QOL, and knowledge about QOL measurement issues. Lindley and Hirsch concluded that nurses value QOL as an outcome measure, but lack knowledge regarding its measurability, especially related to reliable tools and sufficient time to assess QOL in clinical practice. Specifically, 68% of the respondents indicated that a lack of time was a barrier to measuring QOL in clinical practice, while 63% responded that a lack of valid tools for measuring patient QOL was a barrier. Other obstacles cited were lack of physician and patient time, patient unwillingness to complete questionnaires, healthcare professionals' unwillingness to administer questionnaires, nurses not liking research, and healthcare professionals believing it is an invasion of patient's privacy to measure QOL.

It appears, from this study, that nurses have difficulty overcoming barriers to the use of QOL as an outcome or measure. Despite the fact that QOL can best be assessed by the patient, and that many reliable and valid self-administered questionnaires for patients exist, nurses perceive the amount of time healthcare professionals would need to administer QOL tools as a major obstacle.

In 1995, the Oncology Nursing Society held a state-of-the-knowledge conference concerning QOL issues for patients with cancer, their families, and healthcare providers. A recommendation from this conference was to evaluate the applicability of available information about QOL to nurses in clinical practice (King et al., 1997). This recommendation, combined with the knowledge that there are barriers to assessing and measuring QOL, led to research by King, Hinds, Dow, Schum, and Lee (2002). This qualitative research by King and associates explored patients' QOL as defined by nurses and examined the knowledge needed to apply QOL outcomes in clinical practice. Focus group discussions were held with adult and pediatric oncology nurses in three states in the United States. Participants were asked to read the article "Quality of life and the cancer experience: The state-of-the-knowledge" (King et al., 1997) prior to the discussion. Forty-seven unique themes were reported in response to three key questions used to facilitate discussions. The three questions were as follows: (1) Could you say what the term QOL means to you in terms of your practice?; (2) what helps you to use QOL information in your own nursing practice on any day?; and (3) was there any particular content in the article that you found helpful about QOL? The six most frequently reported themes were as follows: using the patient's standard; nursing strategies; differences (e.g. cultural, economic) decrease QOL care; maintenance of social interest; insightful relations with patient; and nurse–patient communication.

The theme "using the patient's standard" represents nurses' beliefs that the best measure of QOL is what the patient believes it to be, which can vary by situation. Using the patients' standard of measure was the most frequently reported code in response to question one. "Nursing strategies" is about recognizing that nurses can implement certain tactics and procedures to increase a patient's QOL. This was the second most common theme in response to question one, but also was a common theme in response to questions two and three. The theme "differences decrease QOL care" recognizes that cultural, economic, and behavioral differences may create barriers for nurses attempting to assess or improve QOL for patients. "Maintenance of social interest," "insightful relations with patient," and "nurse–patient communication" were common themes in response to question three. In the theme of "maintenance of social interest" nurses recognized the importance of patients remaining involved in life events as part of QOL. The themes of "insightful relations with patient" and "nurse–patient communication" both acknowledge the importance of the nurse–patient relationship in improving QOL. From this research and key themes, it is apparent that clinically based oncology nurses did not find research-based information relevant to their clinical practice for assessment of QOL or interventions to positively affect QOL (King et al., 2002). In the current climate of evidence-based practice, programs are needed to facilitate the translation of research into practice (Cooke et al., 2004; King, 2006).

Using this research, King and colleagues (2002) developed a conceptual model of the nurses' relationship-based perception of patients' QOL (Figure 14-4 and Table 14-1). This model demonstrates that an oncology nurse's QOL assessment is based mostly on a strong nurse–patient relationship.

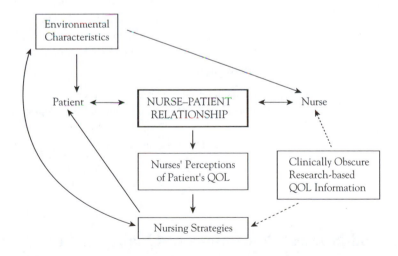

Figure 14-4. **Nurses' relationship-based perception of patient's quality of life.**
> *Legend:* A solid line means a strong influence for clinical nurses, while a dashed line means the researched-based QOL information is not helpful for clinical purposes so it is infrequently used. Adapted from King, Hinds, Dow, Schum, & Lee (2002). Used with permission from ONS Press.

Table 14-1. **Model Concepts and Their Definitions**

Concept	Definition
Nurse–Patient Relationship	Nurses rely on establishing strong rapport with patients and their family members, being physically present, being technically competent to complete quality-of-life assessments, and to adjust their own behavior, mood, and pace of providing treatment-related information.
Nurses' Perceptions of Patients' Quality of Life	Nurses' recognize that their most valid measure of an individual's quality of life is what that individual believes it to be, and that this belief could differ from what others (including healthcare professionals and family members) believe it to be, and that this belief could vary by situation.
Nursing Strategies	Actions initiated by nurses and directed toward improving the patient's physical condition, functional abilities, and social interests, and implemented in consideration of the patient's values, preferences, definition of normalcy, and need for hope.
Clinically Obscure Research-based QOL Information	Nurses' belief that the lack of (a) a single or clear definition of quality of life, (b) clinical guidelines to assess a patient's quality of life, and (c) population-specific strategies to influence quality of life all contribute to their conclusion that the findings from studies on quality of life are not useful to them and contribute to the low likelihood of their using the findings in their practice.
Environmental Characteristics	Nurses describe how rules and procedures and the general atmosphere of a healthcare setting as well as coworkers' views can affect a patient's quality of life and the nurses' abilities to influence patient's quality of life.

Adapted from King, Hinds, Dow, Schum, & Lee (2002). Used with permission from ONS Press.

Patients' and Nurses' Perceptions of Quality of Life

Despite the research demonstrating that nurses cannot assume they understand how patients view their QOL and illustrating potential barriers to providing nursing care focused on QOL, nurses have learned recently that information gained from patients regarding QOL issues throughout the cancer trajectory may be useful in clinical practice.

For instance, information gained from cancer patients regarding QOL issues at diagnosis may be used by nurses to provide newly diagnosed patients with realistic expectations of the impact of cancer and therapies on QOL. From this knowledge, nurses and patients can work together to train other patients and provide support and encouragement through the cancer journey (King, 2001).

One way to obtain this knowledge is through patients' stories. Nurses can gather stories from patients individually or in groups to help them understand patients' perspectives of QOL. King and Hinds (1998) and others (Howell, Fitch, & Caldwell, 2002; King, 2001) have identified several key characteristics throughout numerous patients' stories regarding QOL. These include (a) a profound sense of vulnerability; (b) inability to avoid frightening aspects of cancer and treatment; (c) changes in priorities in life; (d) a desire to make life better for others; (e) a need to be respected by other individuals; (f) a need for loving connections with other individuals; (g) learning to deal with alienation from the norms of society; (h) greater appreciation of daily life and activities; and (i) a need to be taken seriously. Listening to patients' stories and finding common experiences such as vulnerability and changes in priorities can be helpful for nurses to share with patients as they start and continue their "dance of life" with cancer.

Patients' Perceptions of What Nurses Can Do to Improve Quality of Life

Although nurses perceive numerous barriers to assessing and supporting the concept of QOL, patients have reported specific interventions nurses and physicians can employ to improve QOL for patients. In 1992, Ferrell and colleagues surveyed bone marrow transplant (BMT) survivors concerning the meaning of QOL. One of the questions asked was, "What could physicians or nurses do to improve QOL?" Six themes were identified from 119 responses. The first theme was for healthcare providers to be accessible. Specifically, survivors wanted physicians and nurses to be available to respond to questions and problems. The second theme focused on survival and was identified as discovering a cure. The third theme, providing support groups to benefit patients and their families, is a recurrent theme for BMT survivors, as well as all cancer survivors. The fourth theme involved a need to reinforce current education. Survivors and families continue to need both support and information or education posttreatment. Specifically, survivors want information concerning long-term effects and symptoms. Providing additional coping strategies was the fifth theme. Survivors and families suggested support groups, as well as individual counseling, to enhance coping. Lastly, respondents suggested that providers increase patient participation in decision making. Survivors wanted to continue to make informed decisions. Having cancer, undergoing treatment, and surviving cancer are considered out-of-control situations. Survivors felt that having information to make informed decisions helped them to maintain control in an out-of-control situation. This study validated the need for nurses to be involved throughout the many stages of cancer and to be concerned about QOL issues for patients and families (Table 14-2). It is important for nurses to understand QOL changes over time in relationship to individual patients and how they respond to cancer.

Table 14-2. **Tips for Positively Affecting QOL for Patients with Cancer**

Increase knowledge and skills related to QOL:
  Attend presentations, seminars, workshops.
  Read articles, books.
  Use the Internet.
  Network with colleagues.
  Start a journal club.
Assess QOL, specifically, how patients perceive their illness, treatment, and recovery.
Understand that QOL is evaluated subjectively by the patient.
Help patients and families identify what makes their QOL better or worse.
Be accessible to patients and families.
Be sensitive to individual situations.
Provide support groups for patients and families.
Provide information/education for patients/families.
  Concentrate on concrete objective information.
  Provide information on symptoms and symptom management.
Be aware of potential long-term effects of treatment and the impact on QOL.
Encourage patients to participate in activities that improve QOL.
Address the negative effects of cancer treatments on QOL.
Help patients learn new coping techniques:
  Guided imagery
  Progressive muscle relaxation
  Meditation

How Clinical Nurses Can Affect Quality of Life for Patients with Cancer

Knowing that controversies regarding the definition and measurement of QOL prevail, how can clinical nurses positively affect QOL for patients with cancer? The first step is for clinical nurses to increase their knowledge and skills regarding QOL issues (Table 14-2). Few, if any, QOL courses for nurses exist, however nurses can attend presentations, seminars, or workshops on QOL. Books, articles, and the Internet are useful resources for clinical nurses. Networking with colleagues in nursing organizations such as the National Oncology Nursing Society can offer valuable insight into how other clinical nurses have assessed QOL and developed interventions to positively affect QOL. Because nurses are present throughout the cancer journey, they develop a relationship or partnership with the patient and family and seek to help them cope with living with cancer. King and colleagues (2002) found that nurses rely on these relationships with patients to assess the patient's QOL, rather than using available clinical tools. As nurses continue to help cancer patients with problems such as fatigue, pain, nausea and vomiting, organ toxicities, sexual dysfunction, and suffering, they are ultimately working to improve each patient's QOL (Howell et al., 2002; King, 2001).

As Grant and Dean point out in Chapter 1, some factors of QOL may not be amenable to nursing intervention (e.g., diagnosis, family illness history, predisposing characteristics, medical treatment). Yet, other factors are amenable to nursing interventions (e.g., the environment, information provided to patients and families, symptom management). Additional recommendations for clinical practice are presented in Table 14-2.

Nurses in clinical practice can use what has been learned from QOL research, patient stories, and their relationship with patients to do the following:

- Use established tools to assess the QOL of patients throughout the cancer experience
- Understand that QOL is evaluated subjectively
- Evaluate symptoms within a framework of QOL and developing interventions for symptom management
- Help patients and families determine what makes QOL better or worse
- Provide education and support groups to patients and families
- Address the negative impact of cancer treatments on QOL (Cooke et al., 2004; King et al., 1997; King, 2006).

In Chapter 17, "Fatigue and Sleep Disturbances: Symptoms that Cluster and Adversely Affect Quality of Life," Barton-Burke and colleagues describe fatigue as a clinical symptom requiring intervention. In discussing fatigue as a symptom that significantly affects QOL, Burke offers practical interventions to reduce fatigue and improve QOL. She also provides examples of teaching tools to conserve energy. Eilers and King stress the importance of providing appropriate symptom management and appropriate information and education to transplant patients and their families in their chapter "Quality-of-Life Issues Related to Marrow Transplantation" (Chapter 15). In Chapter 9, "Quality of Life and Symptoms," Borneman and Economou describe how clinically managing symptoms is an important QOL concern across settings of cancer care (e.g., acute, home care, outpatient). In Chapter 13, Powel and Meneses highlight the importance of patient education, exercise interventions, coping skills in behavioral and cognitive management, and support groups in improving QOL in patients with breast cancer.

CONCLUSION

Even though nurses and other healthcare professionals cannot know exactly what any specific patient experiences on the cancer journey, the nurses are still instructors or leaders along the journey. Nurses play an important role with cancer patients and their families because they have direct, and prolonged, contact with them. This places nurses in an optimal position to assess and affect the quality of life of oncology patients in a positive way. Nurses need to learn from each patient what physical, psychological, social, and spiritual aspects increase or decrease QOL. As advocates, educators, and leaders of the dance, nurses can use their relationship-based perceptions of patients' QOL to help patients understand strengths, needs, and important physical, psychological, social, and spiritual aspects of QOL during the cancer journey. It is essential also that clinicians develop knowledge and skills in order to be a significant force in affecting the QOL of patients with cancer. Currently, nursing curricula stress the physical and social skills (e.g., communication, counseling). Little, if any, content is offered regarding QOL issues for patients and families. The knowledge and skills of oncology nurses, and nurses in general, are critical to advancing QOL as an accepted treatment outcome.

REFERENCES

Aaronson, N. K. (1986). Methodological issues in psychosocial oncology with special reference to clinical trials. In V. Ventafridda, F. S. A. M. van Dam, R. Yancik, & M. Tamburini (Eds.), *Assessment of quality of life and cancer treatment* (pp. 29–41). Amsterdam: Excerpta Medica.

Carr, A. J., & Higginson, I. J. (2001). Are quality of life measures patient centered? *British Medical Journal, 322*, 1357–1360.

Cochran, J., & Ganong, L. H. (1989). A comparison of nurses' and patients' perceptions of intensive care unit stressors. *Journal of Advances in Nursing, 14*, 1038–1043.

Cooke, L., Smith-Idell, C., Dean, G., Gememill, R., Steingass, S., Sun, V., et al. (2004). Research to practice: A practical program to enhance the use of evidence-based practice at the unit level. *Oncology Nursing Forum, 31*, 825–832.

Crawford, E. D., Benneti, C. L., Stone, N. N., Knight, S. J., De Anton, E., Sharp, L., et al. (1997). Comparison of perspectives on prostate cancer: Analysis of survey data. *Urology, 50*, 366–372.

Dow, K. H., Ferrell, B. R., Haberman, M. R., & Eaton, L. (1999). The meaning of quality of life in cancer survivorship. *Oncology Nursing Forum, 26*, 519–528.

Farrell, G. A. (1991). How accurately do nurses perceive patients' needs? A comparison of general and psychiatric settings. *Journal of Advances in Nursing, 16*, 1062–1070.

Ferrell, B. R., & Dow, K. H. (1996). Portraits of cancer survivorship: A glimpse through the lens of survivors' eyes. *Cancer Practice, 4*, 76–80.

Grant, M., Ferrell, B., Schmidt, G. M., Fonbuena, P., Niland, J. C., & Forman, S. J. (1992). Measurement of quality of life in bone marrow transplantation survivors. *Quality of Life Research, 1*(6), 375–384.

Howell, D., Fitch, M., & Caldwell, B. (2002). The impact of interlink community cancer nurses on the experience of living with cancer. *Oncology Nursing Forum, 29*, 715–723.

Johnston, M. (1982). Recognition of patients' worries by nurses and other patients. *British Journal of Clinical Psychology, 21*, 255–261.

King, C. R. (2001). The dance of life. *Clinical Journal of Oncology Nursing, 5*(1).

King, C. R. (2006). Advances in how clinical nurses can evaluate and improve quality of life for individuals with cancer. *Oncology Nursing Forum, 33*(1, Suppl.), 5–12.

King, C. R., Ferrell, B. R., Grant, M., & Sakurai, C. (1995). Nurses' perceptions of the meaning of quality of life for bone marrow transplant survivors. *Cancer Nursing, 18*, 118–129.

King, C. R., Haberman, M., Berry, D. L., Bush, N., Butler, L., Dow, K. H., et al. (1997). Quality of life and the cancer experience: The state-of-the-knowledge. *Oncology Nursing Forum, 24*(1), 27–41.

King, C. R., & Hinds, P. (1998). Quality of life from nursing and patient perspectives (3rd. ed.). Sudbury, MA: Jones and Bartlett.

King, C. R., Hinds, P. Dow, K. H., Schum, L., & Lee, C. (2002a). The nurse's relationship-based perceptions of patient quality of life. *Oncology Nursing Forum, 29*, E118–E126.

Larson, P. J. (1984). Important nurse caring behaviors perceived by patients with cancer. *Oncology Nursing Forum, 11*, 46–50.

Larson, P. J. (1986). Cancer nurses' perceptions of caring. *Cancer Nursing, 9*, 86–91.

Lindley, C. M., & Hirsch, J. D. (1994). Oncology nurses' attitudes, perceptions, and knowledge of quality-of-life assessment in patients with cancer. *Oncology Nursing Forum, 21*(1), 103–110.

Mayer, D. K. (1987). Oncology nurses' versus cancer patients' perceptions of nurse caring behaviors: A replication study. *Oncology Nursing Forum, 14*, 48–52.

Mellon, S. (2002). Comparisons between cancer survivors and family members on meaning of the illness and family quality of life. *Oncology Nursing Forum, 29*, 1117–1125.

Schipper, H., & Levitt, M. (1985). Measuring quality of life: Risks and benefits. *Cancer Treatment, 69*, 1115–1123.

Sneeuw, K. C., Aaronson, N. K., Detmar, S. B., Wever, L. D., & Schornagel, J. H. (1999). Evaluating the quality of life of cancer patients: Assessments by patients, significant others, physicians, and nurses. *British Journal of Cancer, 81*(1), 87–94.

von Essen, L., & Sjoden, P. O. (1991). Patient and staff perceptions of caring. *Journal of Advances in Nursing, 16*, 1363–1374.

Weinfurt, K. P. (2007). Value of high-cost cancer care: A behavioral science perspective. *Journal of Clincial Oncology, 25*(2), 223–227.

Wilson, K. A., Dowling, A. J., Abdolell, M., & Tannock, I. F. (2000). Perception of quality of life by patients, partners, and treating physicians. *Quality of Life Research, 9*, 1041–1052.

Zhao, H. Kanda, K., Liu, S., & Mao, X. (2003). Evaluation of quality of life in Chinese patients with gynecological cancer: Assessments by patients and nurses. *International Journal of Nursing Practice, 9*, 40–49.

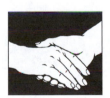

Chapter Fifteen

Quality-of-Life Issues Related to Marrow Transplantation

June G. Eilers • Cynthia R. King

Introduction

Although bone marrow transplantation (BMT) was attempted as early as 1891 and again in the late 1950s and early 1960s, limited information is available regarding the health-related quality of life (HRQOL) of the early BMT recipients. Bone marrow transplantation in the 1950s and 1960s encountered numerous difficulties, resulting in limited success with few long-term survivors. This degree of difficulty was due, in part, to inadequate tissue typing, lack of adequate supportive care during aplasia, and side effects associated with the high doses of cytotoxic therapy (Wingard, Curbow, Baker, & Piantadosi, 1991). As knowledge expanded and support therapies, such as blood products and antibiotics, became available, results improved. Great advances occurred in the 1980s and 1990s with increased understanding regarding marrow typing, improved approaches for aplasia management, and the utilization of critical care support therapies. As technology and knowledge continue to advance, new information has been integrated into the transplant field, leading to improved results with larger numbers of transplants in the 2000s. The new decade heralded by 2010 holds continued promise for the integration of expanded knowledge into evidence-based practice that will benefit even greater numbers of individuals.

As a result of the potential for multiple problems associated with BMT, much of the initial effort primarily focused on survival during the acute phases of transplant, and on extension of the length of survival. Thus, limited data exist regarding HRQOL for early transplant recipients. As the survival rates from the acute phase improved and posttransplantation cure rates increased, practitioners broadened their concern beyond merely length of survival to HRQOL. In fact, there has been an increased acknowledgment of the importance of including HRQOL measures as clinical study outcomes (Bevans et al., 2006). Response to the ever upward spiraling cost of health care also fuels examination of quality-of-life outcomes in light of procedure cost. This chapter will address HRQOL in BMT and issues related to the examination of HRQOL in this arena.

Transplantation as a Treatment

Bone marrow transplantation (BMT) is the term that had been used traditionally to describe the treatment modality used to replace malfunctioning marrow in a person whose marrow is diseased or deficient due to conditions such as leukemia, aplastic anemia, and immune deficiencies. This form of treatment is used also to replace or "rescue" the marrow destroyed by high doses of cytotoxic treatment in individuals with cancers such as lymphoma, multiple myeloma, and germ cell tumors that have not responded adequately to traditional doses of therapy. In these situations, the goal of the high-dose cytotoxic treatment is to destroy all cancer cells. Due to their high mitotic index, the cells in the marrow (i.e., white blood cells, red blood cells, and platelets) are also destroyed. Thus, the marrow must be recovered, or "rescued," to overcome the otherwise potentially lethal state of the cytotoxic-induced aplasia.

Traditionally, bone marrow itself was the primary source of the cells used for the replacement or rescue of the marrow through a collection process similar to a bone marrow biopsy. These cells, called pluripotent stem cells, have the potential to produce the early forms of red blood cells, white blood cells, and platelets. With additional laboratory study in the 1980s, hematopoietic stem cells capable of reconstituting the marrow were also identified in the peripheral circulation (Juttner et al., 1988; Kessinger, Armitage, Landmark, Smith, & Weisenburger, 1988; Reiffers et al., 1986) and umbilical cord blood (Gluckman et al., 1989). As these sources of stem cells became more widely used, different terminology for marrow transplantation evolved. *Hematopoietic stem cell transplant* (HSCT) is now the term used to encompass the marrow, peripheral circulation, and umbilical cord blood as sources of the stem cells used in transplantation. This term became more prevalent in the 1990s (Pavletic & Armitage, 1996) and remains applicable. The transplant itself merely involves the infusion of the pluripotent stem cells in a process very similar to a blood transfusion.

Transplantation brought together many of the medically related advances developed over the years into a treatment modality that offered hope to individuals with otherwise life-threatening conditions (Thomas, 1994). Discovery of the role of stem cells in the production of the cells in the marrow laid the groundwork for the rescue of the marrow. Human leukocyte antigen (HLA) typing allowed for the identification of potential donors for individuals whose marrow was malfunctioning (Beatty et al., 1985). Advances regarding dose-response curves for chemotherapy agents led to the administration of higher drug doses for optimal cell kill in HSCT. The ability to administer pluripotent stem cells intravenously for marrow engraftment and repopulation of the marrow decreased the concern regarding marrow aplasia seen with the high doses of chemotherapy. New and more effective antimicrobial agents and better management of aplasia-related infections have been crucial to increased survival during transplant, which was seen in the 1980s (Wingard et al., 1991). Transplantation has both utilized and fostered continued advances in the treatment of disease and in the management of treatment-related side effects in the 2000s.

Although not all transplant recipients require dialysis and mechanical ventilation, an understanding of these approaches, which provide major organ support, has been essential to supporting patients with preexisting comorbidities and transplant-related acute toxicities through transplantation. The administration of pharmaceuticals, including diuretics, volume expanders, and vasopressors, has contributed to the success of supportive care during the crises that can occur with HSCT. In addition to the use of blood products, growth factors have been used to enhance peripheral stem cell collection and hematopoietic recovery, thus shortening the duration of aplasia and, consequently, reducing the risk of infection. Nutritional support to facilitate normal cell recovery from the cytotoxic treatments and recovery of the immune system continues to improve the overall success in the 2000s. Careful orchestration of each of these components of the whole process is critical to the success of HSCT today and into the future.

Fortunately, transplantation often can be performed without major complications, especially in the autologous arena, in which clients with limited disease receive their own cells. This process contributed greatly to the increased interest in HSCT, leading to the skyrocketing increase in the number of transplants performed and an increased number of transplant programs in place by the mid-1990s (Horowitz, 1995). Multiple programs now perform small numbers of transplants using a variety of protocols; the numbers of transplants continue to rise. According to the Center for International Blood and Marrow Transplant Research and the American Society of Blood and Marrow Transplantation (Rizzo et al., 2006), over 40,000 HSCTs are performed worldwide each year, leading to improved access for individuals requiring transplant. The increase in procedures has also influenced the ability to track the success of this treatment modality and to follow the HSCT recipients.

Due to the significant improvements discussed previously, more HSCT recipients are surviving free of their original disease; it is estimated that tens of thousands of HSCT survivors are alive today (Rizzo et al., 2006) as a result. Consequently, the individuals who are living longer now must deal with the potential of long-term late effects of treatment. The survivorship movement has helped to prompt an increased focus in this area (For more information, go to http://www.iom.edu/CMS/28312/4931.aspx, http://www.canceradvocacy.org, and http://www.ed.gov/cancer/survivorship/). What then is the best way to measure success in transplantation, and what place does HRQOL have in that measurement?

As discussed in other chapters, HRQOL has evolved as a significant theme in the healthcare literature over the last several decades. This increased interest in HRQOL also has been experienced in the transplant setting. Several factors combine to provide the basis for the perceived importance of HRQOL research in HSCT.

Transplantation as a Unique Experience

Awareness of the unique aspects of transplantation facilitates an enhanced understanding of HRQOL for this population. Generally, candidates for HSCT are most of the individuals diagnosed with life-threatening conditions. They have been informed they will most likely die prematurely, secondary to the disease process unless a more aggressive treatment strategy is used. Therefore, these potential HSCT recipients, and their loved ones, must come to terms with the issue of possible premature death. The immediacy of the life-threatening phase of the disease varies for each individual and depends on such factors as age, diagnosis, and the extent of disease. Hematopoietic stem cell transplant is a more aggressive treatment strategy that offers these individuals an alternative. It is not, however, without significant risk. Candidates are informed of the potential complications of the procedure. These include the risk of premature death secondary to complications seen with the toxicity of the high-dose cytotoxic therapy. Hematopoietic stem cell transplant patients and their families then must face the paradox that the treatment offering them hope, against fairly certain death, actually may result in premature death. They must be willing to acknowledge and accept the significance of the risk of death from the disease in order to be willing to face the risk of life-threatening complications from the treatment. It is this hope of a new lease on life, coupled with awareness that, with the excellent support therapies available some recipients have few major problems and actually do very well, that enables them to face this risk (Eilers, 1991). The impact of this paradox on HRQOL will be addressed in more detail later in the chapter.

Potential HSCT recipients have a wide variety of diseases and are in different stages of the disease process. Additionally, they have had varying amounts and types of treatments and experience with symptoms and complications prior to HSCT. Therefore, no two recipients enter the world of HSCT at the same point in terms of disease trajectory; symptom, complication, and treatment history; comorbidities; and risk for complications.

Different types of transplants are used, depending on the underlying disease process and patient age. The type of transplants used are identified based on the donor of the pluripotent stem cells for the rescue of the marrow (Table 15-1). Allogeneic transplants utilize stem cells from an HLA-matched donor. Initially used primarily for individuals with leukemia, these transplants were the mainstay of the modality of transplant through the 1970s and into the 1980s. Over time, the principle of marrow rescue with hematopoietic stem cells was applied in autologous transplants for other malignancies. These transplants use the individual's own stem cells for collection, storage, and later reinfusion post-preparatory treatment. Syngeneic transplants, which are much fewer in number, involve the use of stem cells from an identical twin. Because the donor and recipient are HLA identical, syngeneic transplants are similar to autologous transplants.

Although the different types of transplants use the same principle of marrow rescue, allogeneic transplants differ significantly from autologous and syngeneic transplants. The major difference is related to the potential complication of graft-versus-host disease (GVHD) in allogeneic transplantation. Allogeneic transplantation can result in the graft, or new hematopoietic system, actually rejecting its host (the recipient). Due to this risk,

Table 15-1. **Types of Hematopoietic Stem Cell Transplants**

Type of Transplant	Source of Cells
Autologous	Patient
Syngeneic	Identical twin
Allogeneic	Donor
Related	Dnor is HLA-matched relative
Unrelated	Donor is HLA-matched nonrelative
Mismatched	Donor is not complete HLA match

allogeneic recipients require additional immune suppression, increasing the risk for infections throughout the period of suppression. In addition to the difference between allogeneic transplants and autologous and syngeneic transplants, there is a potential difference within the grouping of allogeneic transplants based on donor match. Unrelated and mismatched transplants, used when an HLA-matched sibling is not available, have an increased risk of complications related to GVHD.

Not only do the types of transplants differ, the cytotoxic protocols used have varied toxicities and therefore have potentially different effects on the HSCT recipients and their families. Some patients have relatively simple, uncomplicated courses with minimal side effects; others experience multiple life-threatening complications and latent effects.

Potentially, HSCT is a very costly procedure requiring a well organized system of support services for optimum outcomes (Franco & Ford, 2007). The need for multiple support therapies and the necessary high level of critical care support both contribute to the costs involved in transplantation. Although practitioners have attempted to provide transplant at a lower cost with a movement to the outpatient setting (Rizzo et al., 1999), costs remain a significant factor in HSCT. In fact, a 2009 Agency for Healthcare Research and Quality (AHRQ) report identified bone marrow transplant as the procedure with the fastest growing costs between 2004 and 2007 (Stranges, Russo, & Friedman, 2009). Pharmaceuticals alone comprise a significant portion of the costs. Bed availability also presents a challenge in some transplant centers as does the availability of family member caregivers for outpatient transplant (Frey et al., 2002; Jagannath et al., 1997; Meisenberg et al., 1998; Ritchie, 2005).

Due to the cost involved and the potential level of toxicity, both in the acute and long-term phases, as well as the limited availability of resources, HRQOL is especially important to consider in HSCT. Mast (1995) identified that, historically, a major goal of HRQOL research has been to justify the expensive and often toxic treatment regimens in terms of patients' psychosocial, functional, and pathophysiologic responses to treatment. Awareness of HRQOL posttransplant is vital for pretransplant counseling, informed consent, and evaluation of outcomes after different types of conditioning therapy. Moreover, this awareness can help care providers limit problems by providing appropriate rehabilitative support and counseling regarding long-term expectations. Knowing that HSCT is a costly, life-threatening procedure with a potentially lasting impact on HRQOL, healthcare providers are frequently challenged with the question: Is HSCT worth the risk and cost? This chapter addresses issues related to determining the HRQOL outcomes of HSCT.

Information regarding the HRQOL of HSCT recipients is essential in answering the question posed previously. As the results in transplantation improve and increasing numbers of HSCT recipients survive, there is an expanding pool of potential subjects for HRQOL studies (Rizzo et al., 2006). Because the recipients live longer after HSCT, not only is there an expanded time period for potential study of HRQOL, but also more knowledge is gained regarding longer-term complications and late effects that may not have had time to develop in the short-term survivors of the past. This is especially timely in light of increased acknowledgment by healthcare providers of survivorship issues related to cancer and cancer treatment. Reports regarding these survivorship issues can be found at http://www.iom.edu/CMS/28312/4931.aspx and http://www.canceradvocacy.org.

The changes over time in HSCT that led to improved results and wider application of the treatment modality also affect the generalizability of HRQOL findings from survivors of the early transplants. As discussed previously, because supportive therapies have advanced and treatment results have improved, HSCT has been utilized in a broader spectrum of diagnoses. With the advances in technology and knowledge, transplant teams have learned how to respond to clinical situations when they occur to decrease the morbidity and mortality related to treatment during the acute phase of HSCT. Components of transplant that may have contributed to the impact on the recipient in the past may no longer be state of the art, and it becomes challenging to track specific HSCT treatment programs and their outcomes. Late effects that can impact HRQOL for transplant survivors include ophthalmologic, pulmonary, cardiac, endocrine, renal, gastrointestinal, musculoskeletal, immune reconstitution, secondary malignancy, and neurocognitive late effects. This is an ever changing field; HRQOL is an important area for us to address, and patients who have survived with or without recurrent disease deserve our ongoing support and research.

Measuring HRQOL in HSCT recipients requires an awareness of the heterogeneity of the population being studied and an understanding of the differences in the procedures being used currently as compared to those of the past. Not only is there heterogeneity in the types of transplant (e.g., autologous versus allogeneic, related versus unrelated, and matched versus mismatched), there are also differences in terms of the level of wellness of the individual at the time of transplant, the level of aggressiveness of the underlying disease, and the age of the HSCT recipient. Furthermore, the various treatment protocols have different toxicities. Thus, it becomes difficult to compare outcomes across the entire spectrum of HSCT.

Theoretical Approach to HRQOL

The volume of literature in the area of transplantation has increased dramatically since the 1980s. Evidence of this increase is found in the emergence of journals that focus on bone marrow transplantation, such as *Bone Marrow Transplantation, Pediatric Transplantation, Progress in Transplantation, Transplant Immunology,* and *Transplant Infectious Disease.* However, as was apparent at the time of the earlier version of this chapter (Eilers & King, 2003), investigators made limited progress during the 1980s and 1990s in terms of systematic, theory-driven analysis of HRQOL related to HSCT. Numerous early articles on HSCT addressed physical complications sometimes seen with transplantation and included topics related to marrow engraftment (Buchsel & Kelleher, 1989; Corcoran-Buchsel, 1986; Eilers, Berger, & Petersen, 1988; Ersek, 1992; Ezzone et al., 1993; Ford & Ballard, 1988; Ford & Eisenberg, 1990; Franco & Gould, 1994; Haberman, 1988; Hutchison & King, 1983; Klemm, 1985; McConn, 1987; McGuire et al., 1993; Nims & Strom, 1988; Parker & Cohen, 1983; Shaffer & Wilson, 1993; Wujcik, Ballard, & Camp-Sorrell, 1994). Psychological and emotional factors during and after treatment were addressed in a number of early studies (Andrykowski, Henslee, & Barnett, 1989; Hengeveld, Houtman, & Zwaan, 1988; Wolcott, Wellisch, Fawzy, & Landsverk, 1986a, 1986b). However, these earlier articles focused primarily on the allogeneic transplant recipient and donor. Furthermore, the use of a theoretical approach to studies in this area has been limited. Prior to the late 1990s, only a limited number of the studies of HRQOL in transplant identified the conceptual or theoretical framework for the study (Andrykowski, Greiner et al., 1995; Baker et al., 1994; Belec, 1992; Bush, Haberman, Donaldson, & Sullivan, 1995; Ferrell et al., 1992a, 1992b; Grant et al., 1992; Haberman, Bush, Young, & Sullivan, 1993; Molassiotis, Boughton, Burgoyne, & van den Akker, 1995; Nespoli et al., 1995; Schmidt et al., 1993). Unfortunately, this neglect of conceptual or theoretical framework is also consistent for much of the research reported since 2000, as will be discussed later. Researchers are more consistently referring to the multidimensional nature of HRQOL. Interestingly, it is nursing research that is more likely to address the theoretical approach used in HRQOL research.

Although not realistic in young children, there does appear to be agreement that HRQOL is dependent on the client's perception. Nevertheless, due to ambiguity regarding its meaning (Ferrans, 1990b), consensus has not been reached regarding conceptual or operational definitions for HRQOL (Cella & Tulsky, 1990; Hacker, 2003; King et al., 1997; Mast, 1995). In fact, prior to the late 1990s, some studies did not even offer a definition of HRQOL before attempting to measure it (Andrykowksi, Greiner et al., 1995; Belec, 1992; Bush et al., 1995; Gaston-Johansson & Foxall, 1996; Grant et al., 1992; Haberman et al., 1993; Nespoli et al., 1995; Schmidt et al., 1993). One definition that was used by several researchers presents HRQOL as the degree of satisfaction with present life circumstances, as perceived by the individual (Belec, 1992; Gaston-Johansson & Foxall, 1996). Hacker (2003) conducted a critical evaluation of quantitative quality-of-life (QOL) measurement in adults receiving transplants published between January 1990 and January 2000 and summarized the variety of definitions used for quality of life.

Just as there has been a lack of consistent definition for HRQOL, there has been a lack of agreement regarding the dimensions, or domains, of HRQOL on which to focus (Hacker, 2003; King et al., 1997). Some researchers examined only physical aspects of transplantation, while others included social, economic, and spiritual components. In earlier studies, the spiritual component was most likely to be present in studies including narrative questioning or building on the City of Hope model for QOL (Ferrell et al., 1992a.) A study by Andrykowski and colleagues (2005) examined spiritual well-being, and a study by Vickberg and colleagues (2001) explored global meaning as areas of change in HSCT recipients. The varied and atheoretical approaches to the study of HRQOL have limited the ability to build theory, to establish sound tools for measuring HRQOL, and to develop and test interventions to improve outcomes in the HSCT population.

Early in HRQOL research, Ferrell and colleagues developed a model to examine the impact of BMT on HRQOL (Ferrell et al., 1992a). This model was based on previous research and surveys of long-term BMT survivors. The conceptual model includes the four domains of physical well-being and symptoms, psychological well-being, social well-being, and spiritual well-being (Figure 15-1). Health-related quality of life is depicted as a series of interrelationships between the domains. Ferrell and colleagues (1992b) used this model in a sequential article to discuss the results of a survey of long-term survivors. Subsequently, the model has been used by other investigators; Byar and colleagues (1999), Saleh and Brockopp (2001), and Whedon and associates (1995) used the model in a HRQOL study

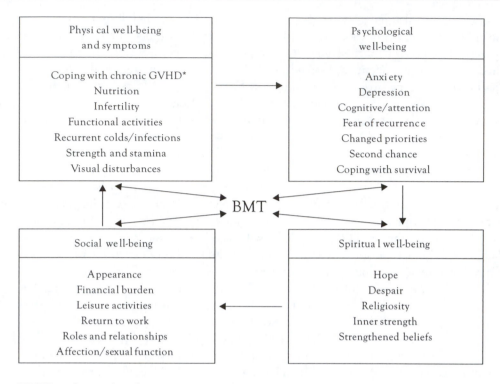

*GVHD, graft-versus-host disease.

Figure 15-1. **Quality-of-life model for bone marrow transplant survivors.**
Source: Adapted with permission from Ferrell, Grant et al., at City of Hope Medical Center.

of long-term survivors of autologous transplant; Dow and Ferrell (1994) used this model to compare the meanings of changes in HRQOL for HSCT, breast cancer, and thyroid cancer patients; and King, Ferrell, Grant, and Sakurai (1995) used the model in a study of nurses' perceptions of HRQOL in transplant. This model has seen only limited use in transplant since 2000, and further research is needed to determine the applicability of the model to groups beyond those included in the studies to date.

Ferrans and Powers have also worked on the development of a model to measure life satisfaction (Ferrans, 1990a; Ferrans & Powers, 1985, 1992). Their tool, the Quality-of-Life Index (QLI), has been used in patients with cancer and who are undergoing transplantation (Belec, 1992; Ferrans 1990a; Hacker & Ferrans, 2003; Hacker et al., 2006). The QLI produces an overall QOL score and subscale scores for four specific domains: health and functioning, social and economic, psychological or spiritual, and family. This instrument also requires further evaluation to determine its applicability for quality of life in transplantation.

Early Research

Most early HRQOL-related studies of transplant patients examined psychological aspects from a case study or anecdotal approach (Brown & Kelly, 1976; Gardner, August, & Githens, 1977; Patenaude, Szymanski, & Rappeport, 1979; Pfefferbaurn, Lindamood, & Wiley, 1978; Popkin, Moldow, Hall, Branda, & Yarchoan, 1977; Wolcott, Fawzy, & Wellisch, 1987; Wolcott, Wellisch, Fawzy, & Landsverk, 1986a, 1986b). As the number of HSCT recipients increased and survival rates improved, interest in HRQOL for these individuals increased. Advances in research, knowledge, and the availability of larger samples facilitated research in the area.

A number of earlier reviews of studies regarding HRQOL in HSCT have been presented in the literature, with some overlap across the reviews. In 1994, Whedon and Ferrell reviewed reports of post-HSCT studies to examine the findings regarding HRQOL beyond the first year posttransplant. Their review included the numbers of subjects, their ages, the types of transplant, the time post-HSCT, the measures used in the studies, and the major findings. King (1995) presented a review of the physical, psychological, social, and spiritual residual effects of transplantation remaining after 1 year, with particular emphasis on the incidence of the physical effects. Decker's (1995) review of a select group of transplant studies highlighted specific psychosocial concerns of transplant recipients before, during, and after HSCT, including perceived HRQOL after transplant, and the impact of family, friends, and caregivers on the hospitalization and recovery phases of HSCT. The most extensive early review of studies and abstracts assessing HRQOL and psychosocial issues in adults with cancer who had been treated with HSCT was completed by Hjermstad and Kaasa (1995). Their review of 48 HRQOL studies included type of transplant and number of subjects, use of a comparison group, study design, times of measurement, methods of assessment (i.e., tools), inclusion of performance status, and conclusions. In terms of overall results, generally the participating subjects in each of the reviews reported fairly good HRQOL (although specific symptoms and problems have emerged from the findings of the studies reviewed). A later review by Neitzert and colleagues (1998) focused on residual difficulties in transplant survivors, including fatigue and general functioning/psychological distress, sexual functioning, and endocrine functioning. Once again the reviewers noted that although there are residual difficulties, survivorship is often associated with high global QOL.

As an overview of this early work, with the exception of one chart review study for endocrine function, sample size in the studies reviewed ranged from 6 to 238, with allogeneic as the most common type of transplant. The majority of the subjects were adults. Most of the studies were cross-sectional or retrospective, with the time post-HSCT ranging from 3 months to more than 12 years. Only a limited number of studies included data from the time of admission or pretransplant. Few of the longitudinal studies followed subjects for longer than 1 year posttransplant. The studies used chart data, mailed questionnaires, phone interviews, and personal interviews to collect QOL data. Comparison groups were used infrequently and the instruments used varied greatly. Although progress was made in the study of HRQOL in HSCT, significant gaps and weaknesses remained.

A number of studies of HRQOL in HSCT, which were not included in the reviews and were published between 1995 and 2000, added to the knowledge base by addressing some areas of weakness. Longitudinal designs were used by Andrykowski, Bruehl, Brady, and Henslee-Downey (1995), McQuellon and colleagues (1996), Meyers and associates (1994), McQuellon and colleagues (1998), and Molassiotis, van den Akker, Milligan, and Goldman (1997). Rodique and colleagues (1999) used a pre- versus posttransplant design to examine the contribution of psychological variable to posttransplant outcomes. The study by Broers and colleagues, reported in two articles (Broers et al., 1998; Broers, Kaptein, LeCessie, Fibbe, & Hengeveld, 2000) included data from pretransplant to 3 years post-transplant in an attempt to identify changes over time. The longitudinal study by Andrykowski and associates (1997) involved survivors at least 12 months (mean of 43.5 months) posttransplant and again 18 months later. More such studies are needed to establish the trajectory of recovery.

Cross-sectional studies have examined subjects at a variety of time points posttransplant. Kopp and colleagues (1998, 2000) grouped their data to compare subjects less than 1 year posttransplant with those more than 1 year out. Five studies included individuals from as early as 1 month posttransplant with those many years posttransplant, with clustering for the expected differences in HRQOL during the initial year posttransplant as compared to beyond the first year (Hann et al., 1997; Heinonen et al. 2001; Molassiotis et al., 1996a; McQuellon et al., 1998; Sutherland et al., 1997). Parsons, Barlow, Levy, Supran, and Kaplan (1999) conducted follow-up on children less than 6 months and greater than 12 months posttransplant. Another by Andrykowski and colleagues (1999) studied recipients within a range of 3–62 (mean of 17) months posttransplant to identify psychosocial concerns present over time posttransplant, finding some concerns are common across the trajectory of time (such as recurrent disease, energy level, and returning to "normal"), whereas others are more of a concern early (such as quality of medical care received or others being overprotective), and some are more of a concern with the passage of time (such as feeling tense or anxious, sexual life, poor sleep, and relationship with spouse/partner). This pattern of both consistent and changing concerns reinforces the need for more longitudinal studies over time rather than across time.

Several HRQOL studies focused on the time after the first year posttransplant. This is when subjects could be expected to be more stable (Zittoun et al., 1997; Fromm, Andrykowski, & Hunt, 1996). During this period, the recipients are still recovering from the acute effects of the treatment and attempting to "return to normal."

Data collection continued to involve numerous self-report instruments (Table 15-2). The use of narrative/interview data to enhance findings is seen in a number of studies reported during this time (Fromm, Andrykowski, & Hunt, 1996; Molassiotis & Morris, 1998; McQuellon et al., 1998).

As autologous transplants became more prevalent, autologous subjects also became more common in HRQOL research studies. Most HRQOL studies included both autologous and allogeneic subjects. In some studies, the number of autologous and allogeneic subjects were similar (Andrykowski et al., 1997; Baker, Marcellus, Zabora, Polland, & Jodrey, 1997; Broers et al., 1998; Broers et al., 2000; Fromm, Andrykowski, & Hunt, 1996; Meyers

Table 15-2. Instruments Used in Quality-of-Life Studies of Hematopoietic Stem Cell Transplant Recipients

Instrument	Studies Using Instrument
A Brief Measure of Social Support (SSQ6)	Heinonen, Volin, Uutela, Zevon, Barrick, & Ruutu, 2001
Achenbach Behavior Check List (ABCL)	Lesko, Ostroff, Mumma, Mashberg, & Holland, 1992; Phipps, Brenner, Heslop, Krance, Jayawardene, & Mulhern, 1995
Affect Balance Scale (ABS)	Schimmer, Elliott, Abbey, Raiz, Keating, Beanlands, et al., 2001
Atkinson Life Happiness Rating	Schimmer, Elliott, Abbey, Raiz, Keating, Beanlands, et al., 2001
Beck Depression Inventory (BDI)	Ahles, Tope, Furstenberg, Hann, & Mills, 1996; Gaston-Johansson & Foxall, 1996; Gaston-Johansson, Franco, & Zimmerman, 1992; Hengeveld, Houtman, & Zwaan, 1988; Rodrigue, Boggs, Weiner, & Behen, 1993; Schimmer, Elliott, Abbey, Raiz, Keating, Beanlands, et al., 2001; Syrjala, Chapko, Vitaliano, Cummings, & Sullivan, 1993
Beery Development Test of Visual Motor Integration (VMI)	Phipps, Brenner, Heslop, Krance, Jayawardene, & Mulher, 1995
Bradburn Positive and Negative Affect Scale (BPNAS)	Andrykowski, Bruehl, Brady, & Henslee-Downey, 1995; Baker, Curbow, & Wingard, 1991; Bush, Haberman, Donaldson, & Sullivan, 1995
Brief Symptom Inventory (BSI)	Lesko, Ostroff, Mumma, Mashberg, & Holland, 1992; Mumma, Mashberg, & Lesko, 1992; Syrjala, Chapko, Vitaliano, Cummings, & Sullivan, 1993
Busnelli Anxiety Scale	Nespoli, Verri, Locatelli, Bertuggia, Taibi, & Burgio, 1995
Cantril Self-Anchoring Ladder of Life Scale (CSAL)	Baker, Curbow, & Wingard, 1991; Bush, Haberman, Donaldson, & Sullivan, 1995; Curbow, Somerfield, Baker, Wingard, & Legro, 1993; Wingard, Curbow, Baker, Zabora, & Piantadosi, 1992; Saleh & Brockopp, 2001

continues

Table 15-2. **Instruments Used in Quality-of-Life Studies of Hematopoietic Stem Cell Transplant Recipients (continued)**

Instrument	Studies Using Instrument
Center for Epidemiologic Studies—Depression Scale (CES-D)	Baker, Marcellus, Zabora, Polland, & Jordrey, 1997; McQuellon, Craven, Russell, Hoffman, Cruz, Perry, et al., 1996; McQuellon, Russell, Rambo, Craven, Radford, Perry, et al., 1998; Schimmer, Elliott, Abbey, Raiz, Keating, Beanlands, et al., 2001
Children's Depression Scale	Nespoli, Verri, Locatelli, Bertuggia, Taibi, & Burgio, 1995
City of Hope Quality of Life-BMT QOL-BMT-Survivors Tool	Grant, Ferrell, Schmidt, Fonbuena, Niland, & Forman, 1992; Saleh & Brockopp, 2001; Whedon, Stearns, & Mills, 1995
Composite International Diagnostic Interview	Jenkins, Liningtton, & Whittaker, 1991; Jenkins, Lester, Alexander, & Whittaker, 1994; Murphy, Jenkins, & Whittaker, 1996
Coping Strategy Questionnaire (CSQ)	Gaston-Johansson, Franco, & Zimmerman, 1992
Death Anxiety Questionnaire (DAQ)	Mumma, Mashberg, & Lesko, 1992
Demands of BMT Recovery Inventory	Bush, Haberman, Donaldson, & Sullivan, 1995
Dementia Rating Scale (DRS)	Meyers, Weitzner, Byrne, Valentine, Champlin, & Przepiorka, 1994
Derogatix Sexual Functioning Scale (DSF)	Lesko, Ostroff, Mumma, Mashberg, & Holland, 1992; Mumma, Mashberg, & Lesko, 1992
DSM III	Lesko, Ostroff, Mumma, Mashberg, & Holland, 1992
ECOG Performance Status Rating Scale (PSR)	Hann, Jacobsen, Martin, Kronish, Azzarello, & Fields, 1997; McQuellon, Russell, Rambo, Craven, Radford, Perry, et al., 1998

Table 15-2. continued

Instrument	Studies Using Instrument
European Organization for Treatment and Research of Cancer QOL Questionnaire (EORTC QLQ0Q30)	Bush, Haberman, Donaldson, & Sullivan, 1995; Kopp, Schweigkofler, Holzner, Nachbaur, Niedwewieser, Fleischhacker, et al., 1998; Kopp, Schweigkofler, Holzner, Nachbaur, Niedwewieser, Fleischhacker, et al., 2000; Zittoun, Suciu, Watson, Solbu, Muus, Mandelli, et al., 1997
Eysenck Personality Questionnaire (EPQ)	Jenkins, Liningtton, & Whittaker, 1991
FACES Life Satisfaction	Wingard, Curbow, Baker, Zabora, & Piantadosi, 1992
Family APGAR	Baker, Wingard, Curbow, Zabora, Jodrey, Fogarty, et al., 1994; Baker, Marcellus, Zabora, Polland, & Jordrey, 1997
Functional Assessment of Cancer Therapy—Bone Marrow Transplant (FACT-BMT)	Heinonen, Volin, Uutela, Zevon, Barrick, & Ruutu, 2001; Kopp, Schweigkofler, Holzner, Nachbaur, Niedwewieser, Fleischhacker, et al., 1998; Kopp, Schweigkofler, Holzner, Nachbaur, Niedwewieser, Fleischhacker, et al., 2000; McQuellon, Craven, Russell, Hoffman, Cruz, Perry, et al., 1996; McQuellon, Russell, Rambo, Craven, Radford, Perry, et al., 1998; Saleh & Brockopp, 2001
Functional Limitations Battery (FLB)	Broers, Hengeveld, Kaptein, LeCessie, van de Loo, & de Vries, 1998; Broers, Kaptein, LeCessie, Fibbe, & Hengeveld, 2000
Functional Living Index Cancer (FLIC)	Andrykowski, Altmaier, Barnett, Otis, Gingrich, & Henslee-Downey, 1990; Andrykowski, Bruehl, Brady, & Henslee-Downey, 1995; Andrykowski, Henslee, & Barnett, 1989; Andrykowski, Henslee, & Farrall, 1989; Andrykowski, Carpenter, Greiner, Altmaier, Burish, Antin, et al., 1997; Broers, Hengeveld, Kaptein, LeCessie, van de Loo, & de Vries, 1998

continues

Table 15-2. **Instruments Used in Quality-of-Life Studies of Hematopoietic Stem Cell Transplant Recipients (continued)**

Instrument	Study Using Instrument
General Health Questionnaire (GHQ)	Broers, Hengeveld, Kaptein, LeCessie, van de Loo, & de Vries, 1998; Fromm, Andrykowski, & Hunt, 1996; Prieto, Saez, Carreras, Atala, Sierra, Rovira, et al., 1996
Health Locus of Control	Broers, Hengeveld, Kaptein, LeCessie, van de Loo, & de Vries, 1998
Health Perceptions Questionnaire	Bush, Haberman, Donaldson, & Sullivan, 1995
Hospital Anxiety and Depression Scale (HADS)	Bush, Haberman, Donaldson, & Sullivan, 1995; Jenkins, Liningtton, & Whittaker, 1991; Jenkins, Lester, Alexander, & Whittaker, 1994; Leigh, Wilson, Burns, & Clark, 1995; Molassiotis, Boughton, Burgoyne, & van den Akker, 1995; Molassiotis, van den Akker, Milligan, Goldman, Boughton, Holmes, et al., 1996
Illness Intrusiveness Rating Scale	Schimmer, Elliott, Abbey, Raiz, Keating, Beanlands, et al., 2001
Impact of Event Scale (IES)	Lesko, Ostroff, Mumma, Mashberg, & Holland, 1992; Mumma, Mashberg, & Lesko, 1992
Internal–External Locus of Control Scale	Kopp, Schweigkofler, Holzner, Nachbaur, Niedwewieser, Fleischhacker, et al., 1998
Jalowiec Coping Scale	Molassiotis, van den Akker, Milligan, & Goldman, 1997
Leukemia-BMT module	Zittoun, Suciu, Watson, Solbu, Muus, Mandelli, et al., 1997
Life Questionnaire Test	Baker, Marcellus, Zabora, Polland, & Jordrey, 1997; Curbow, Somerfield, Baker, Wingard, & Legro, 1993

Table 15-2. **continued**

Instrument	Study Using Instrument
Mastery Scale	Baker, Marcellus, Zabora, Polland, & Jordrey, 1997
Medical Coping Modes Questionnaire (MCMQ)	Litwins, Rodrigue, & Weiner, 1994; Rodrigue, Boggs, Weiner, & Behen, 1993
Medical Outcomes Study—Short Form-36 (MOS SF-36)	Hann, Jacobsen, Martin, Kronish, Azzarello, & Fields, 1997; Heinonen, Volin, Uutela, Zevon, Barrick, & Ruutu, 2001; McQuellon, Craven, Russell, Hoffman, Cruz, Perry, et al., 1996; McQuellon, Russell, Rambo, Craven, Radford, Perry, et al., 1998; Sutherland, Fyles, Adams, Hao, Lipton, Minden, et al., 1997
Memorial Symptom Assessment Scale (MSAS)	Hann, Jacobsen, Martin, Kronish, Azzarello, & Fields, 1997
Mental Attitude to Cancer Scale	Jenkins, Lester, Alexander, & Whittaker, 1994; Murphy, Jenkins, & Whittaker, 1996
Mental Health Inventory (MHI)	Lesko, Ostroff, Mumma, Mashberg, & Holland, 1992
Multidimensional Health Locus of Control (MHLC)	Gaston-Johansson, Franco, & Zimmerman, 1992
Minnesota Multiphasic Personality Inventory (MMPI)	Rodrigue, Boggs, Weiner, & Behen, 1993
Neuropsychologic Battery [Trail Making Test B, Visual Retention Tests (VRT), Controlled Oral Work Association (COWA), Temporal Oral Orientation all from the Benton Iowa Screening Battery for Mental Decline]	Ahles, Tope, Furstenberg, Hann, & Mills, 1996
Norbeck Social Support Questionnaire	Kopp, Schweigkofler, Holzner, Nachbaur, Niedwewieser, Fleischhacker, et al., 1998; Molassiotis, van den Akker, Milligan, Goldman, Boughton, Holmes, et al., 1996
Nottingham Health Profile	Prieto, Saez, Carreras, Atala, Sierra, Rovira, et al., 1996

continues

Table 15-2. **Instruments Used in Quality-of-Life Studies of Hematopoietic Stem Cell Transplant Recipients (continued)**

Instrument	Study Using Instrument
Offer Self-Image Questionnaire	Nespoli, Verri, Locatelli, Bertuggia, Taibi, & Burgio, 1995
Pain-o-Meter (PoM)	Gaston-Johansson, Franco, & Zimmerman, 1992
Perceived Health Questionnaire (PHQ)	Andrykowski, Altmaier, Barnett, Otis, Gingrich, & Henslee-Downey, 1990; Andrykowski, Greiner, Altmaier, Burish, Antin, Gingrich, et al., 1995
Perceived Quality of Life Questionnaire (PQOL)	Andrykowski, Greiner, Altmaier, Burish, Antin, Gingrich, et al., 1995
Personality Research Form	Neuser, 1988
Piers-Harris Self Concept, Play Performance Scale for Children	Phipps, Brenner, Heslop, Krance, Jayawardene, & Mulhern, 1995
Pittsburgh Sleep Quality Index	Andrykowski, Carpenter, Greiner, Altmaier, Burish, Antin, et al., 1997
Play Performance Scale for Children	Phipps, Brenner, Heslop, Krance, Jayawardene, & Mulhern, 1995
Positive and Negative Affect Scale (PNAS)	Andrykowski, Brady, Greiner, Altmaier, Burish, Antin, et al., 1995; Fromm, Andrykowski, & Hunt, 1996
Present State Examination (PSE)	Leigh, Wilson, Burns, & Clark, 1995
Princess Margaret Hospital—Symptom Experience Report	Schimmer, Elliott, Abbey, Raiz, Keating, Beanlands, et al., 2001

Table 15-2. **continued**

Instrument	Study Using Instrument
Profile of Mood State (POMS)	Andrykowski, Altmaier, Barnett, Burish, Gingrich, & Henslee-Downey, 1990; Andrykowski, Altmaier, Barnett, Otis, Gingrich, & Henslee-Downey, 1990; Andrykowski, Brady, Greiner, Altmaier, Burish, Antin, et al., 1995; Andrykowski, Bruehl, Brady, & Henslee-Downey, 1995; Andrykowski, Carpenter, Greiner, Altmaier, Burish, Antin, et al., 1997; Andrykowski, Greiner, Altmaier, Burish, Antin, Gingrich, et al., 1995; Andrykowski, Henslee, & Barnett, 1989; Andrykowski, Henslee, & Farrall, 1989; Baker, Curbow, & Wingard, 1991; Baker, Wingard, Curbow, Zabora, Jodrey, Fogarty et al., 1994; Baker, Marcellus, Zabora, Polland, & Jordrey, 1997; Bush, Haberman, Donaldson, & Sullivan, 1995; Curbow, Somerfield, Baker, Wingard, & Legro, 1993; Fromm, Andrykowski, & Hunt, 1996; Heinonen, Volin, Uutela, Zevon, Barrick, & Ruutu, 2001; Jenkins, Lester, Alexander, & Whittaker, 1994; Molassiotis, van den Akker, Milligan, Goldman, Boughton, Holmes, et al., 1996, Molassiotis, van den Akker, Milligan, Goldman, & Boughton, 1996; Molassiotis, van den Akker, Milligan, & Goldman, 1997; McQuellon, Craven, Russell, Hoffman, Cruz, Perry, et al., 1996; McQuellon, Russell, Rambo, Craven, Radford, Perry, et al., 1998; Saleh & Brockopp, 2001
Psychiatric Diagnostic Interview (PDI)	Ahles, Tope, Furstenberg, Hann, & Mills, 1996
Psychosexual Functioning Questionnaire	Molassiotis, van den Akker, Milligan, Goldman, Boughton, Holmes, et al., 1996
Psychosocial Adjustment to Illness Scale (PAIS)	Andrykowski, Altmaier, Barnett, Burish, Gingrich, & Henslee-Downey, 1990; Andrykowski, Altmaier, Barnett, Otis, Gingrich, & Henslee-Downey, 1990; Andrykowski, Brady, Greiner, Altmaier, Burish, Antin, et al., 1995; Andrykowski, Bruehl, Brady, & Henslee-Downey, 1995; Fromm, Andrykowski, & Hunt 1996; Jenkins, Liningtton, & Whittaker, 1991; Molassiotis, Boughton, Burgoyne, & van den Akker, 1995; Molassiotis, van den Akker, Milligan, Goldman, Boughton, Holmes, et al., 1996; Mumma, Mashberg, & Lesko, 1992; Saleh & Brockopp, 2001

continues

Table 15-2. Instruments Used in Quality-of-Life Studies of Hematopoietic Stem Cell Transplant Recipients (continued)

Instrument	Study Using Instrument
Pryer Personality Assessment Scale	Leigh, Wilson, Burns, & Clark, 1995
Quality of Life Index (QLI)	Gaston-Johansson & Foxall, 1996
Recovery of Function Scale (ROF)	Andrykowski, Brady, Greiner, Altmaier, Burish, Antin, et al., 1995
Relational Support Scale	Baker, Wingard, Curbow, Zabora, Jodrey, Fogarty, & Legro, 1994; Baker, Marcellus, Zabora, Polland, & Jordrey, 1997
Rey Auditory–Verbal Learning Task	Phipps, Brenner, Heslop, Krance, Jayawardene, & Mulhern, 1995
Rosenberg Self-Esteem Scale (RSE)	Andrykowski, Brady, Greiner, Altmaier, Burish, Antin, et al., 1995; Baker, Wingard, Curbow, Zabora, Jodrey, Fogarty, et al., 1994; Broers, Hengeveld, Kaptein, LeCessie, van de Loo, & de Vries, 1998; Fromm, Andrykowski, & Hunt, 1996; Molassiotis, van den Akker, Milligan, Goldman, Boughton, Holmes, et al., 1996
Rotterdam Symptom Checklist	Molassiotis, van den Akker, Milligan, Goldman, Boughton, Holmes, et al., 1996
Satisfaction with Life Domains Scale	Baker, Curbow, & Wingard, 1991; Baker, Wingard, Curbow, Zabora, Jodrey, Fogarty, et al., 1994; Schimmer, Elliott, Abbey, Raiz, Keating, Beanlands, et al., 2001; Wingard, Curbow, Baker, Zabora, & Piantadosi, 1992
Self Report Karnofsky Performance Scale	Baker, Marcellus, Zabora, Polland, & Jordrey, 1997

Table 15-2. **continued**

Instrument	Study Using Instrument
Sickness Impact Profile (SIP)	Andrykowski, Altmaier, Barnett, Burish, Gingrich, & Henslee-Downey, 1990; Andrykowski, Altmaier, Barnett, Otis, Gingrich, & Henslee-Downey, 1990; Andrykowski, Bruehl, Brady, & Henslee-Downey, 1995; Andrykowski, Henslee, & Barnett, 1989; Fromm, Andrykowski, & Hunt, 1996; Litwins, Rodrigue, & Weiner, 1994; Syrjala, Chapko, Vitaliano, Cummings, & Sullivan, 1993
Simmons Scale	Wolcott, Wellisch, Fawzy, & Landsverk, 1986b
Sleep, Energy, and Appetite Scale (SEAS)	Andrykowski, Altmaier, Barnett, Otis, Gingrich, & Henslee-Downey, 1990; Andrykowski, Bruehl, Brady, & Henslee-Downey, 1995
Sleep Experience Report (SER)	Andrykowski, Carpenter, Greiner, Altmaier, Burish, Antin, et al., 1997
Social Adjustment Scale (SAS)	Leigh, Wilson, Burns, & Clark, 1995; Lesko, Ostroff, Mumma, Mashberg, & Holland, 1992; Wolcott, Willisch, Fawzy, & Landsverk, 1986b
Spielberger State-Trait Anxiety Inventory	Ahles, Tope, Furstenberg, Hann, & Mills, 1996; Gaston-Johansson, Franco, & Zimmerman, 1992; Gaston-Johansson & Foxall, 1996; Rodrigue, Boggs, Weiner, & Behen, 1993; Kopp, Schweigkofler, Holzner, Nachbaur, Niedwewieser, Fleischhacker, et al., 1998
Symbol Digits Modality Test (SDMT)	Phipps, Brenner, Heslop, Krance, Jayawardene, & Mulhern, 1995
Symptom Check-List 90-R (SCL-90-R)	Broers, Hengeveld, Kaptein, LeCessie, van de Loo, & de Vries, 1998
Symptom Distress Scale (SDS)	Molassiotis, van den Akker, Milligan, Goldman, Boughton, Holmes, et al., 1996; Molassiotis, van den Akker, Milligan, & Goldman, 1997
Symptom Experience Report (SER)	Andrykowski, Altmaier, Barnett, Otis, Gingrich, & Henslee-Downey, 1990; Andrykowski, Bruehl, Brady, & Henslee-Downey, 1995; Andrykowski, Brady, Greiner, Altmaier, Burish, Antin, et al., 1995

continues

Table 15-2. **Instruments Used in Quality-of-Life Studies of Hematopoietic Stem Cell Transplant Recipients (continued)**

Instrument	Study Using Instrument
State-Trait Anger Expression Inventory (STAXI)	Rodrigue, Boggs, Weiner, & Behen, 1993
Weschler Intelligence	Phipps, Brenner, Heslop, Krance, Jayawardene, & Mulhern, 1995
Wide Range Achievement Test (WRAT-R)	Phipps, Brenner, Heslop, Krance, Jayawardene, & Mulhern, 1995
Zung Depression Inventory	Kopp, Schweigkofler, Holzner, Nachbaur, Niedwewieser, Fleischhacker, et al., 1998

et al., 1994; Zittoun et al., 1997). Allogeneic subjects were more common in the following studies: Kopp and associates (1998), with 16 autologous and 40 allogeneic subjects; Kopp and colleagues (2000), with the same group as their 1998 study; Molassiotis, van den Akker, Milligan, and Goldman (1997), with 10 autologous and 21 allogeneic subjects; and Prieto and colleagues (1996), with 43 autologous and 70 allogeneic subjects. In contrast, autologous subjects outnumbered allogeneic subjects in studies by Andrykowski and colleagues (1999), with 96 autologous and 14 allogeneic; Molassiotis and colleagues (1996), with 53 autologous and 38 allogeneic subjects; and McQuellon and associates (1998), with 70 autologous and 16 allogeneic subjects. Subjects were restricted to autologous transplant recipients in the studies conducted by Gaston-Johansson and Foxall (1996); Whedon, Stearns, and Mills (1995), Ahles, Tope, Furstenberg, Hann, and Mills (1996); McQuellon and colleagues (1996). In contrast, the study reported by Sutherland and colleagues (1997) evaluated 231 allogeneic (5% syngeneic) subjects and the study performed by Molassiotis and Morris (1998) reported results from 28 unrelated allogeneic transplant recipients. With mixed populations in a study, it is difficult to determine whether concerns are specific to the type of transplant or more related to recovery from the underlying disease and the acute effects of the treatment. Allogeneic recipients generally are regarded to have more long-term effects due to the prolonged immunosuppression and graft-versus-host disease.

With the exception of the study by McQuellon and associates (1996) that focused on breast cancer transplant subjects, the diagnosis of the subjects within the studies varied greatly. The most common diagnoses included lymphoma (Hodgkin's and non-Hodgkin's), leukemia, breast cancer, multiple myeloma, aplastic anemia, and myelodysplastic syndrome. Although recognized in research as important, the use of a comparison group was reported only in four studies: Prieto and colleagues (1996), Hann and associates (1997), Molassiotis and associates (1996), and Zittoun and colleagues (1997). As oncology/hematology teams acknowledged and reported neuro/cognitive changes with high doses of antineoplastic therapy, awareness of and concern for the neuro/cognitive changes with transplantation began to surface in HRQOL studies (Ahles et al., 1996; Meyers et al., 1994).

Pediatric HRQOL studies were few in number. Studies by Kanabar and colleagues (1995), Nespoli and colleagues (1995), Phipps and colleagues (1995), and Arvidson and colleagues (1999) focused on HRQOL in pediatric recipients of transplants. Felder-Puig and associates (1999) focused on pediatric allogeneic transplant survivors 15–27 years old who were from 2 to 13 years (mean of 7 years) posttransplant. Three research groups included teenagers in their studies with adult subjects. These studies were reported by Prieto and colleagues (1996), including individuals 15–54 years old; Jenkins, Lester, Alexander, and Whittaker (1994), including individuals 15–56 years old; and Sutherland and associates (1997), including 16–56 individuals years old. Parsons, Barlow, Levy, Supran, and Kaplan (1999) compared children's scores with parents and also with physician disease severity ratings. In general, the respondents (and their parents) reported limited problems. Difficulties included neuropsychological disturbances; declines in social competence, self-esteem, and general emotional well-being; and anxiety regarding recurrence.

In summary, the research regarding HRQOL for HSCT prior to 2000 was improving over time, but continued to demonstrate consistent weaknesses. The early research, although not ideal, did set the stage for the research that was to follow. Findings generally indicated that transplant recipients in general were satisfied with their quality of life, and even in the presence of persistent physical and psychosocial concerns, they were grateful to be alive.

Research Reported Since 2000

HRQOL research in HSCT has continued to advance, as evidenced in several ways discussed in this section. Although some studies continue to have smaller sample size, as in Conner-Spady and colleagues (2005) with 52 subjects, Kiss and colleagues (2002) with 26 subjects, Schulz-Kindermann and colleagues (2007) with 39 subjects, and Wong and colleagues (2003) with 29 subjects, more studies are involving a larger sample size, as shown below:

- Andrykowski and colleagues (2005) with 662 survivors recruited through International Bone Marrow Transplant Registry (IBMTR) and Autologous Blood and Marrow Transplant Registry (ABMTR) from 40 centers
- Beanlands and colleagues (2003) with 90 subjects
- Chiodi and colleagues (2000) with 244 subjects
- Foster and colleagues (2004) with 131 subjects
- Grant, Cooke, Bhatia, and Forman (2005) with 100 subjects
- Gruber, Fegg, Buchmann, Kolb, and Hiddemann (2003) with 163 subjects
- Heinonen and colleagues (2001) with 109 adults
- Kettmann and Altmaier (2008) with 86 subjects multisite
- Lee and colleagues (2006) with 96 patients

- Loberiza and colleagues (2002) with 193 subjects
- Syrjala and colleagues (2004) with 94 subjects
- Vickberg and colleagues (2001) with 85 subjects

A major challenge to larger sample sizes is the ability to maintain an adequate number of subjects in a longitudinal study due to treatment-related morbidity and mortality, and ability to reach subjects further out from a transplant who have most likely moved, as demonstrated in the following studies:

- Altmaier and colleagues (2006) with 314 randomized in main trial, 309 at baseline, 179 at 100 days, 137 at 6 months, 103 at 1 year, and 81 at 3 years
- Broberger, Sprangers, and Tishelman (2006) with 126 main project, 115 at 3 months, and 89 at 6 months
- Byar, Eilers, and Nuss (2005) with 197 eligible, 166 available, 93 responded to invitation, and data available on 92
- Chang and colleagues (2005) with 114 eligible, 84 initial and 6 months, and 75 at 12 months
- Humphreys and colleagues (2007) with 242 baseline, 79 at 1 year, and 59 at 3 years
- Worel and colleagues (2002) with 307 patients treated, 155 disease-free for 2 years or more, 127 patients alive at time of survey, and 106 patients responded to survey.

These decreasing numbers over time essentially are unavoidable in this population and, often, initial sample size is limited by numbers of transplants performed at the center(s).

A number of pediatric studies were added to the transplant QOL literature during this time period. Barrera and associates (2000) studied 26 children and adolescents and their mothers. The results indicated improvement of QOL for 6 month survivors' family cohesion, children's adaptive functioning associated with QOL, and adjustment of survivors. Dobkin and colleagues (2000) conducted a study over 6.5 years to accrue 68 pediatric subjects. These findings showed initial prognosis estimated by the treating physician was the only significant predictor of survival. Felder-Puig and colleagues (2006) reported the results of a 5-year, longitudinal prospective study of 68 allogeneic patients. These findings indicated HRQOL was the worst shortly after transplant and then improved, although not always in a linear fashion. Forinder, Löf, and Winiarski (2005) assessed 52 children, aged 9 and over, who were at least 3 years beyond allogeneic transplant for leukemia or nonmalignant diseases. Most of the subjects were subjectively and objectively in good health. Helder and colleagues (2004) studied youth who were at least 5 years old at time of transplant and at least 16 years old at time of the study. Sixty-one subjects were invited to participate and 22 actually participated. The comparison with healthy reference individuals indicated the scores of the transplant recipients on generic measures of QOL were not significantly different from those of the healthy individuals. Kupst and colleagues (2002) examined cognitive and psychosocial functioning of HSCT patients, with 2 years of data, on 74 of the original 153 children. The results indicated stability of IQ scores over time, with the strongest predictor being pre-HSCT cognitive function. Nuss and Wilson (2007) studied youth under the age of 19. Thirty-one recipients participated, as well as 35 mothers and 28 fathers. Overall, transplant recipients and their parents reported moderately high

HRQOL. Phipps, Dunavant, Lensing, and Rai (2002) reported differences based on age and type of transplant in the medical and demographic determinants of 153 children undergoing HSCT. Simms and colleagues (2002) reported the cognitive, behavioral, and social outcome for 47 childhood survivors as not detrimentally affected 2 years after transplant. In summary, pediatric transplant survivors reported satisfactory HRQOL. Several findings of added interest include noting differences in scoring by patients versus parents and/or teachers, with patients scores typically being higher (Forinder, Lof & Winiarski, 2006). This is similar to the 1999 report by Arvidson, Larsson, and Lönnerholm. An editorial by Dreyer (2009) reiterated the importance of following up on pediatric transplant patients into adulthood. Retention of subjects will be a challenge in this endeavor.

A number of reviews since 2000 have been identified. Clarke, Eiser, and Skinner (2008) reviewed 15 studies of 12 separate cohorts, concluding HRQOL was comparable to or better than population norms 6 months to 8 years posttransplant; Hacker (2003) critically reviewed quantitative HRQOL measurement in adults; Hoodin and Weber (2003) conducted a systematic review of 15 studies (3 pediatric and 12 adult); Ortega and colleagues (2005) conducted a review of secondary malignancies and quality of life after transplant; and Redaelli and colleagues (2004) reviewed 21 HRQOL studies of individuals treated for acute myeloid leukemia (AML). Watson and colleagues (2004) also examined AML patients in a review of clinical trial data comparing transplant and chemotherapy only. A review of HRQOL following HSCT in children included ten research studies (Tsimicalis, Stinson, & Stevens, 2005).

Although most of the research continues to be cross-sectional and retrospective in nature, a number of research teams have used a prospective design (Chang et al., 2005; Conner-Spady et al., 2005; Dobkin et al., 2000; Frick, Rieg-Appleson, Tyroller, and Bumeder, 2005; Hacker et al., 2006; Humphreys et al., 2007; Kettmann, 2008; Lee et al., 2006; Prieto et al., 2005; Schulmeister, Quiett, & Mayer, 2005). Additionally, Hayes and colleagues (2004) conducted an intervention study to determine the effect of a mixed-type moderate intensity exercise program on HRQOL.

Another change in HRQOL research during this time has been the incorporation of a more focused approach by some researchers. Andrykowski and colleagues (2005) focused on spiritual well-being in adult survivors; Beanlands and colleagues (2003) focused on self-concept as a BMT patient, illness intrusiveness, and engulfment; Edman, Larsen, Hägglund, and Gardulf (2001) focused on sense of coherence in adult allogeneic survivors; Epstein and colleagues (2002) focused on oral function, taste, and smell; Hacker and colleagues (2006) focused on patterns of fatigue, physical activity, health status, and HRQOL; Harder and colleagues (2002, 2006) focused on cognitive function; Humphreys and colleagues (2007) conducted a longitudinal study of sexual function; Loberiza and colleagues (2002) focused on depressive syndrome and survival; Molassiotis (2003) focused on anorexia and weight loss; and Sherman and colleagues (2004) focused on pretransplant identification of deficits among myeloma patients during initial evaluation prior to treatment.

Family members have also been the focus of some research studies. Barrera and colleagues (2000) concentrated on pediatric patients and their mothers; Boyle and colleagues (2000) concentrated on HSCT survivors and caregivers; Eldredge and colleagues (2006) concentrated on caregiver role strain after transplant; Gaston-Johansson and colleagues (2004) concentrated on psychological distress and burdens in primary caregivers of transplant recipients for breast cancer; and Morris, Grant, and Lynch (2007) concentrated on the review of data from five cross-sectional surveys regarding family. Transplant is, indeed, a stressful experience for family members as originally stated by Patenaude and colleagues (1979). However, families are able to cope and the long-term effects of that stress has not been as prevelant in the research findings as might be indicated by the original statement. Family members involved and/or present during the transplant experience require support, guidance, and education to help them accomplish the tasks they are expected to do.

Use of comparison groups continues to be rather limited. Although the importance of a comparison group is accepted, it is difficult to identify which group actually would be the best "control" group. Goetzmann and colleagues (2006) compared lung, liver, and marrow transplant recipients. Pretransplant psychosocial variables were lower than community norms, as would be expected due to the intensity of the procedures and life-threatening nature of the illness. Quality of life for all of the recipients improved posttransplant, although perceived social support decreased. A 24-month follow-up of heart, lung, liver, kidney and allogeneic bone marrow patients by Goetzman and colleagues (2008) identified two clusters, or subgroups: one with good-to-optimal psychosocial profile before and after transplant, and the second, slightly smaller group, with lower mental health pretransplant that did not improve in 6 months and declined in the following 18 months. Kopp and colleagues(2005), comparing 34 HSCT patients having a mean of 9.6 years posttransplant with a data baseline of healthy controls, found that, although HRQOL is in some ways comparable, transplant recipients do have specific long-term sequelae that encompass physical and social functioning and financial difficulties. The element that cannot be factored in to these studies is what the HRQOL of the transplant recipient would have been without the transplant process—many would have died of their disease.

The HRQOL findings in the majority of the research studies since 2000 are similar to earlier reports. For the most part, subjects report a fairly good quality of life and satisfaction with their current HRQOL. It remains important to note, however, the majority of the studies still restrict accrual to individuals free of recurrent disease, thus the research is focusing primarily on the "success stories," the applicability of which may or may not hold true for those with recurrent disease. Because transplant recipients fear recurrence (Andrykowski et al., 1999), shouldn't our research expand to include those who do recur so the "what then?" questions can be answered?

Measurement of HRQOL in HSCT

As the estimated number of transplants has risen annually to over 40,000 (Rizzo et al., 2006) and there are increased numbers of survivors, HRQOL research has been increasingly recognized as critical. However, there remains a need for increased rigor in the research conducted, starting with measurement. In spite of the growing interest in HRQOL and the awareness of its importance, ambiguity prevails regarding the measurement of the concept (Ferrans, 1990b; Hacker 2003; King et al., 1997). Various tools and global life satisfaction questions have been used to assess HRQOL in HSCT. Table 15-2 provides a listing of tools that have been used. In addition, studies frequently include specific, researcher-developed questions and instruments. At times, studies have included questions pertaining only to specific physical aspects of HRQOL, such as pain, and have made global reference to HRQOL. In such instances, it is important to acknowledge only one domain of the multidimensional concept has been addressed, and then only partially. Although this dimension is a component of HRQOL, one must be cautious regarding generalization to global HRQOL. Although it is important to include quality-of-life measures as endpoints for clinical trials, another area of concern as expressed by both Gralla in 2002 and Klepin in 2006, is the need to be certain we ask the right questions and to carefully consider a fit between the reason for evaluating quality of life in the clinical trial and components of available instruments. As will be noted by examination of Table 15-2, many of the tools used in reported research do not focus on the multidimensional aspects of HRQOL. In fact, some of those listed are not truly HRQOL measures and are regarded as insufficient measures of HRQOL (Osoba, 1994).

Measurement of global HRQOL offers another area needing attention. The ability of single items to measure this multidimensional concept is worth questioning. If the level of function in the different domains is not similar, subjects may have difficulty identifying an overall rating. When the level of function varies across domains, the question about the ability of single items measuring this concept may be answered, based on the influence of a particular domain in subjects' lives. Is overall HRQOL intended to be a numeric average of other scores? How should it be determined?

The combination of disease-specific scales and global aspects of HRQOL, such as life satisfaction, is seen as an effort to address specific health situation concerns and the global aspects perceived as important by many of the individuals being evaluated (Mast, 1995). Several studies (Byar et al., 2005; King, Dobson, & Harnett, 1996) are noteworthy for their comparison of HRQOL instruments. Although it is important for HRQOL tools to address disease- and treatment-specific areas of concern, the development and use of unique tools impacts the ability to compare results with other populations. In contrast, some of the tools currently available do not specifically address areas pertaining to HSCT survivors in terms of long-term effects of the transplant. Examination of cognitive changes is one example of an area of concern (Ahles et al., 1996; Harder et al., 2002; Meyers et al., 1994).

Another area of concern is the development of tools by a specific discipline. If HRQOL truly is dependent on the perception or interpretation of the individual whose quality of life is being assessed, is there a need for discipline-specific tools? We must then ask, should interventions to improve HRQOL be discipline or subject specific?

The best instrument for measurement of HRQOL in pediatric subjects also is an area of concern (Parsons et al., 1999). Instruments used in most HRQOL studies to date have been developed and tested on adults. One exception is the Pediatric Quality of Life Inventory by Varni and colleagues (Varni, Burwinkle, Katz, Meeske, & Dickinson, 2002; Varni, Seid, & Kurtin, 2001; Varni, Seid, & Rode, 1999). Numerous questions regarding the best approach to measure HRQOL in children need to be addressed, as the numbers of long-term survivors of pediatric HSCT are increasing (Ljungman et al., 2006). In addition to the heterogeneity issues related to type of transplant, disease process, and treatment because of the normal developmental changes that occur in the pediatric patient, age at the time of transplant, and at the time of study, must also be taken into account. Pediatric research has focused primarily on physiologic and psychologic effects of HSCT, rather than attempting to address the concept of HRQOL from the perspective of the recipient in this population.

Mast (1995) encouraged researchers to address the appropriateness of the match of the HRQOL instruments and definitions of HRQOL in proposed studies. Hacker (2003) reviewed a series of six different definitions of HRQOL in HSCT to emphasize the wide range of definitions used. The list of questions Mast identified to be addressed in the process of instrument selection includes those shown in Table 15-3.

Qualitative studies, such as those by Haberman and colleagues (1993), Molassiotis and Morris (1998), and Sherman and colleagues (2005), have been helpful in tapping into HSCT recipients' dynamic, highly individual, and often very positive, HRQOL experiences. The use of narrative questions, such as those in the City of Hope Quality of Life in Bone Marrow Transplant Survivors has also produced rich data (Byar et al., 1999; Saleh & Brockopp, 2001). Open-ended questions allow subjects to tell their story. Qualitative data can also be collected during face-to-face or telephone interviews. Due to the current state of HRQOL instrument development and the ever changing status of HSCT treatment protocols, the triangulation of quantitative data and descriptive qualitative data should be given strong consideration in order to describe and measure this multidimensional concept adequately (Eilers, Byar, & Nuss, 2000).

Future Research

The majority of current HRQOL research in HSCT has consisted of retrospective, cross-sectional studies of relatively small numbers of adults who have had transplants. There is a need for baseline pretransplant data to determine if the QOL changes noted are secondary

---

Table 15-3. **Questions Used to Select an Instrument**

---

1. Which measures reflect your conceptual definition of QOL?

2. What degree of detail in QOL measurement is useful and practical, yet consistent with your conceptual definition?

3. Which of the operational definitions of QOL can you justify theoretically to suit the purpose and aims of measurement?

4. Are indicators of QOL in the instruments derived from actual patient responses rather than professional opinion?

5. Do the measures address areas of specific and overall QOL concern for your patients that are influenced by your nursing interventions?

6. Is a cancer-specific, disease-specific, or general-illness-specific QOL measure most useful?

Source: Adapted from Mast, 1995, p. 963. Used with permission.

to the HSCT conditioning regimen, or perhaps are the effects of the disease, treatments received prior to transplant, or other unknown factors. Longitudinal studies that follow subjects over time will contribute to the knowledge base regarding the normal recovery pattern and provide information regarding the point at which the effects noted become long-term effects as compared to being merely a delay in recovery, as anticipated to be the case in long-term allogeneic HSCT subjects in the study by Chiodi and colleagues (2000).

A particular challenge in HRQOL research in HSCT is the significant decrease in the numbers of subjects that remain available over time and their response rates to studies. Such a decrease in numbers must be taken into account when planning longitudinal studies. In some instances, it may be necessary to conduct multisite studies in order to accrue adequate subject numbers and enhance generalizablity of findings. However, the use of multiple sites raises a concern regarding differences in care delivery that might influence HRQOL outcomes.

Careful documentation of interventions is essential if the intent is to not merely describe HRQOL changes noted, but to begin to show relationships between dependent and independent variables. Rehabilitation efforts must also be addressed. For instance, did transplant survivors with less physical, psychological, social, and spiritual problems receive more rehabilitation or have fewer side effects or did they have better coping skills?

The majority of studies have examined QOL in adults, which is certainly important because adults comprise the majority of marrow transplants. Yet, in terms of long-term effects, the potential impact of HSCT on the surviving child should not be overlooked, especially with the increasing numbers of long-term pediatric survivors (Ljungman et al., 2006; Tsimicalis et al., 2005). Assessment of the real impact of HSCT on long-term physical and psychosocial functioning has been hampered by the paucity of prospective research that begins with pre-HSCT data and follows subjects of all ages for an extended period posttransplant.

The longitudinal, prospective studies of the future that follow larger numbers of subjects over a longer period of time must be theory driven, using consistent, valid, and reliable instruments. Studies should be carefully conceptualized in order to ensure selected measures will provide the data essential to answering the proposed questions. Due to the heterogeneity of HSCT recipients, large samples are essential to allow for broader generalization of findings. Careful study design would also help overcome problems seen when individuals from a few months to many years posttransplant are studied as one group. Although the group of choice may be difficult to identify, use of comparison groups would add strength to the findings of well designed, theory-driven studies.

There is a need for additional research studies to look at the impact of transplant on the families involved in HSCT, both when the recipient is an adult or a child. Two interesting areas of concern include when the recipient is an adult child of older parents and when the recipient is a parent of an otherwise independent adult child. As early as 1979, Patenaude identified transplant as one of the most difficult things for a family to experience, yet research on family members remains limited. This is true for those who are involved in caregiving, as there has been a transitioning of care to alternative settings, and it is true for those who are less involved in direct caregiving.

Family members can provide information regarding the assessment of the HSCT recipient's experience and the effect of the transplant on the QOL of the recipient's family. The family member's assessment of QOL may involve dimensions less focused on the physical health of the individual and more focused on psychosocial, financial, and spiritual aspects. This is especially important to consider when HSCT recipients must travel great distances to tertiary treatment centers and when treatment for graft-versus-host disease (GVHD) necessitates extended stays near the transplant center. As with other types of family research, one must address which family member to ask to provide the data and how to handle the family data obtained (e.g., as one unit with the HSCT recipient or as individuals). Responses will depend on multiple factors, including the family member's relationship with the recipient, their direct involvement with care, their physical proximity to the transplant center, their added family and work responsibilities, the nature of the transplant course, and the outcome of the transplant. In earlier research by Eilers (1991, 1992), family members interviewed at the time of the recipient's admission for transplant frequently discussed the sense of "preparing for the worst and hoping for the best." This paradox keeps family members in a consistent state of uncertainty. It is not known whether this state of uncertainty remains typical for family members planning for HSCT. Another factor to be considered is the residual effect on family survivors when the HSCT recipient dies early in the transplant process or due to factors related to the effectiveness of the transplant.

Clinicians and researchers must collaborate to address questions regarding research methods and study design in a joint effort to expand our body of knowledge regarding the impact of HSCT on HRQOL and to determine clinically meaningful effect sizes (Cella et al., 2002). Although consensus exists regarding the need for baseline data, the best time for obtaining the data is less clear. Due to the heterogeneity of potential HSCT candidates, baseline data may demonstrate a large variation in HRQOL, pre-HSCT, regarding baseline neurocognitive function. The intent of the baseline measures should be to determine not only the impact of the disease and previous treatment on HRQOL, but also recent changes in HRQOL secondary to the disease or treatment. For example, has the individual been in a fairly stable, declining, or improving state?

Perhaps, rather than HRQOL measures during the acute phase of HSCT, it would be more important to have consistent and accurate assessment of the morbidity associated with transplant, similar to symptom inventory assessment by Anderson and colleagues (2007). This assessment could then be taken into account as researchers attempt to determine changes in HRQOL from pre- to post-HSCT. The experience of severe side effects may seem less significant to the recipients who recover fully from their disease than those that have long-term, late effects that are unrelated to the acute effects experienced. Bush and colleagues (2005) provide an example of a Web-based system for monitoring symptom self-assessment posttransplant.

The exclusion of individuals with active recurrent disease from research continues to have significant implications that must be addressed. While it is important to protect vulnerable subjects, exclusion of these individuals from the samples studied only tells us the HRQOL of the individuals for whom HSCT successfully eradicated their disease. What about those who continue to struggle with disease, are living with recurrent disease, or have a new treatment-related diagnoses? Andrykowski and colleagues (1999) identified fear of recurrence as a prevalent psychosocial concern over the recovery trajectory for survivors. More information is needed to adequately support individuals facing this concern. Does HSCT affect the end-stage disease experience for these individuals? While some of this information could be obtained from the medical records, investigators must identify approaches for sensitively obtaining additional information in this area. The difficulty that persists is determining the alteration, if any, in the expected disease trajectory that has been caused by the transplant. For example, how would the person have died if HSCT had not been attempted? Such information is essential to assist individuals considered at high risk for death from their initial disease to make an informed decision regarding consenting to transplant or considering another treatment option. How do HSCT recipients whose disease has relapsed feel about their transplant-related QOL? How about individuals who were expecting only to "buy" time, not be cured? Does transplant alter symptomatology as the recipients die? What about the transplant recipients who die some time after or during transplant; can we do a better job of palliative care for these individuals?

When to study HRQOL is also an issue to consider. Studies frequently have set 1-year post-HSCT as the criterion for inclusion in research samples for recovery from transplant. Although the rationale for this approach can be justified based on waiting for stabilization and avoiding unnecessary subject burden during recovery, it has resulted in a gap in our knowledge base. We do not have a clear picture of HRQOL during the posttransplant recovery phase, and, thus, do not know the time trajectory of the recovery process.

The time period from 100 days to 1 year posttransplant is marked by many physical effects and frequent checkups. Perhaps this time period is more accurately viewed as a continuation of acute posttreatment recovery. During this time, the patient's status may be very labile in all HRQOL domains. Rehabilitation and support needs during this time period also require further articulation. Beyond the first year, many latent physical effects resolve. Yet, some continue as chronic health problems. Existence during the first year is characterized as a tightrope walk, or roller coaster, because the individual is moving cautiously forward through each month of survival beyond the state of having chronic cancer and very slowly reaching toward a desired identity of cure. Shouldn't healthcare providers be concerned regarding the impact these first-year challenges have on HRQOL? Focused assessment and monitoring is important, especially because this is also the time when HSCT recipients may die with recurrent disease and/or experience significant treatment effects such as decreased thyroid function and osteoporosis that ultimately impact their well-being.

Studies to date have focused on the time beyond 1 year and as far out as 20-plus years posttransplant without breakdowns for different lengths of time. Is it appropriate to combine recipients from such a large range of time into one group? What about the many changes in treatment protocols over that time? If longitudinal studies were used more extensively, the question of when to study might shift to the intervals at which survivors should be followed.

Researchers must look not only at when the transplant was performed, but also at the type of transplant and type of preparatory regimen to determine if generalization can be made to other types of HSCT. Perhaps some of the findings apply only to autologous, related allogeneic, or unrelated allogeneic transplants. At times the findings may apply only to certain preparatory regimens, especially with the rapidity of changes in HSCT.

Although involved individuals can provide supplemental information, the primary source of the data should be the subject of the study. The exception to this is a young child who is unable to supply the information in a reliable manner. Family members can contribute in terms of how they see their loved one functioning and relationships, but they cannot determine the transplant recipient's HRQOL. Using other sources for supplemental information could increase our understanding of HRQOL in a broader context, but the intent of approaching each source must be clearly understood in order to facilitate appropriate utilization of the information collected. Professionals can provide information regarding performance status for Karnofsky, and similar scales, based on observation and input from the patients, but they cannot determine the HRQOL for that individual. Nurses who work closely with patients and form well established relationships with patients and family members can assess and positively affect HRQOL for those individuals (King, 2006).

Concerns and Challenges Related to Assessing HRQOL in HSCT

A number of underlying concerns must be considered when assessing HRQOL in HSCT recipients. In earlier research, survivors were seen as reporting an unexpectedly high HRQOL (Whedon & Ferrell, 1994). Gradually, as findings were similar across multiple studies, it was no longer an "unexpected" finding. It may be that survivors do not want to appear ungrateful to care providers, or they may be so consumed with "being alive" they de-emphasize physical changes related to their disease and treatment. What is the best approach to explore this issue? According to Andrykowski and colleagues (1999) perhaps simply being "grateful to be alive" translates into minimization of HRQOL concerns; this may be reinforced by healthcare professionals who indicate survivors should "count their blessings" and not worry about things that are not life-threatening.

Does the experience of a life-threatening condition such as cancer alter an individual's outlook on life, and thus, influence assessment of issues related to QOL? Just as paraplegics after critical accidents have adjusted to disability and identify their HRQOL higher than may be expected by others, do individuals with cancer experience a similar change in their assessment of priorities? Does dealing with a life-threatening illness alter one's concept of HRQOL? Are survivors just happy to be alive and not as concerned regarding alterations from *normal*? Of interest is a conversation the first author (JE) had with an individual sharing airport sitting space while waiting for a delayed flight and at risk of missing a connecting flight. The woman, not previously known by the author, was a 15-year survivor of a transplant for ovarian cancer. Although her cancer had recurred twice in that time period, she initiated the conversation and indicated she focused on how well she was doing, had a purpose in life, and knew there was hope in her future. Can research support this anecdotal narrative, thereby offering researchers and healthcare providers additional insight into HRQOL?

At the same time, if HRQOL assessment is to be provided by HSCT recipients as is widely accepted, how can we question whether their views have been altered by the experience of having a life-threatening condition? Perhaps we need to take into account that, just as HSCT recipients tend to evaluate satisfaction with care higher due to a sense of indebtedness (Ferrell et al., 1992b), they may tend to be more accepting of residual effects of HSCT seen as less desirable by others. What role does response shift as discussed by Tierney, Facione, Padilla, and Dodd (2007) play in satisfaction with HRQOL? What is the best approach to use to assess this shift (Schwartz & Sprangers, 1999)?

A statement provided by a subject in a HRQOL study demonstrates what is seen as a response shift:

> You have asked no questions regarding the absolutely most important aspects of living, of surviving, of gratitude for just being here. (*Subjects had been given three well established QOL tools to complete.*) I bet that I enjoy sitting on my deck, feeling the sun on my face, the blue sky above, and the birds singing much more than many or most people enjoy all their "doingness." "Quality" of life is actually not about what we do, but rather how we are. These questionnaires are typical of our culture which is so focused on produce! produce! and leaves no place for actually enjoying time. Living life fully means just that—being fully present...Experiencing life fully means actually experiencing it—not just rushing from activity to activity as a diversion from life. Many if not all of the cancer patients I know speak of the gifts which come from not taking anything for granted. This is a dimension which often leads them to slowing down, choosing what is of real importance to them and finding a new or renewed connection with their own sense of the Divine—whether that be God, nature, love, art..."

How can we capture this sense of quality of life in our studies? This "gift," if captured and shared with others on their transplant journey, could facilitate a high sense of well-being.

One challenge is to evaluate the adjustment to limitations experienced by HSCT recipients. Studies using instruments that allow subjects to not only identify changes experienced, but also assess the significance of the alteration for their overall HRQOL, would add to our understanding of the true impact for the individual. Such an effort would not merely be in an attempt to alter the adjustment, but rather to provide rehabilitation to decrease limitations and facilitate coping in individuals with residual effects of transplant. As the survivorship movement gains momentum, more information regarding long-term effects of treatment will be available (Curtiss, Haylock, & Hawkins, 2006; Houldin, Curtiss, & Haylock, 2006; Syrjala et al., 2005, 2007).

How do the following influence the quantitative measurement of the philosophically abstract and contextually dependent concept of HRQOL: the paradox of risking death to live; the meaning of the experience; and the second opportunity for life? Additionally, are the symptoms and problems experienced by HSCT recipients in adaptation mediated by the individual's perspective on his or her situation, as was proposed by Altmaier, Gingrich, and Fyfe (1991)? If such is the case, the most commonly used data analysis approaches in HRQOL research may be inadequate.

Another factor that is difficult to assess is the impact of what was expected by the individuals prior to HSCT. If the current level of function or outcome is much less than expected, does that influence assessment of the current situation and HRQOL? Likewise, if the expectation of HSCT was to merely buy time, are those individuals more accepting of residual effects? Also, how do expectations influence or alter the recipient's and family's reception and understanding during the informed consent process, and thus their evaluation of posttransplant HRQOL?

In their 1995 work, Whedon and colleagues questioned whether some aspects of HRQOL are trait-like and prone to more stability, while others are state-like and predisposed to instability. Although the numbers are not known, not all individuals who are encouraged to consider transplant select it as an option. Because potential candidates are well informed regarding the significant risks associated with HSCT, one might assume, as was suggested by Eilers (1991, 1992), that the individuals who decide to have a transplant are perhaps more optimistic. These individuals were able to express awareness of the dangers involved with transplant; they saw it as their only hope. Are these aspects that are trait-like similar across transplant recipients and family members, or are these aspects trait-like for some and state-like for others? When examining changes in QOL over time after transplant, how do we interpret improvements in some domains and declines in others?

Because transplant treatment protocols are ever changing, there will be a potentially ever changing spectrum of residual effects. Frequently, the long-term, late effects are not really known before protocols are altered to improve short-term results. Thus, researchers must address the unique challenge of attempting to account for differences in treatment protocols and morbidity during the acute phase of transplant.

There has been a gradual evolution toward improved quality in research that addresses the concept of HRQOL in HSCT. But, as healthcare providers have improved the quality of research, changes in protocols and improved supportive treatment may actually have altered the potential impact of the complications previously identified. New medications may potentially increase or decrease the effect on HRQOL. We need to continue to strive to improve our research studies by making them current to treatment protocol trends.

It may not always be easy to identify relationships between alterations from disease and HSCT as causative factors. When HSCT recipients are dealing with progressive disease and/or nonresponse to the transplant therapy, how can we ascertain if the impact on HRQOL is secondary to the underlying disease process or secondary to the treatment administered as part of the transplant? The importance of some changes or residual effects, such as alterations in fertility, probably will be different for the 22-year-old HSCT recipient, as compared to the 56-year-old. Other residual effects, such as fatigue and pain, may function as confounding variables that actually affect assessment of HRQOL. Are these symptoms or effects that should be managed more appropriately, or irreversible residual effects? If the latter, how can professionals provide the necessary counseling to patients and families? In addition, some effects may actually be related to underlying disease or treatment prior to HSCT, such as sterility caused by disease or previous treatment.

Although it would be helpful to compare HSCT survivors with another group, identification of the appropriate comparison group remains unclear, especially when attempting to identify one that is equivalent. Chemotherapy patients have been used in comparison studies (Altmaier et al., 1991; Hjermstad, Evensen, Kvaløy, Fayers, & Kaasa, 1999; Litwins, Rodrigue, & Weiner, 1994; Molassiotis et al., 1996; Watson et al., 2004; Zittoun et al., 1997).

Felder-Puig and associates (1999) compared three groups: pediatric transplant survivors, individuals with bone cancer, and normal individuals. Goetzmann and colleagues (2006) compared lung, liver, and marrow transplant recipients. Andrykowski and colleagues (1990) used renal transplant recipients as a comparison group and proposed that the solid organ transplant recipients, patients treated for other life-threatening conditions, and even the general population could serve as comparisons for HSCT recipients. Wolcott and associates (1986b) compared HSCT recipients with donors in a study of psychological adjustment. When generic instruments are included, subjects actually are compared to population norms (Hann et al., 1997; Kopp et al., 2005). While each of the comparison groups used to date helps to expand our awareness, additional work is needed to identify appropriate comparison groups.

Implications for Practice

Nursing implications will be discussed in terms of application for nurses working with potential transplant candidates, nurses directly involved in transplant, and nurses caring for individuals posttransplant. The implications will be addressed for the same three time periods in terms of transplantation—pretransplant, during the acute phase, and posttransplant, with discussion of both immediate and long-term posttransplant. Accurate information regarding HRQOL posttransplant is essential for nurses providing care to recipients and family members in this arena. As discussed in the study by King and colleagues (1995), nurses' knowledge regarding QOL has the potential to affect the care delivered. This knowledge, or lack of it, can influence both the information shared with potential recipients and families, as well as the direct care delivered. Obtaining this information and remaining current regarding the implications for practice is not always an easy task for the nurse. As indicated in focus groups of nurses conducted in multiple sites, nurses most often base their assessment of HRQOL on established relationships with their patients (King et al., 2002).

Because HSCT encompasses a broad spectrum of recipients, both in terms of diagnoses and treatment protocols, HRQOL outcomes for one segment of individuals may or may not be applicable to others. Thus, it is important for nurses to know the outcomes related to similar scenarios. Due to the time required for adequate identification and verification of treatment-related, long-term effects, and the rapidity with which transplant protocols change, frequently this information is not readily available. Therefore, it is often the role of staff working with potential transplant recipients and family members to facilitate information gathering and interpretation of the applicability of the findings for a particular scenario. This is especially important in light of the fact that, because potential recipients often are dealing with a life-threatening diagnosis, they may have an intense need to "hear" only stories with positive outcomes. In other situations, they may have difficulty sorting through information shared by former recipients and family members. At times, such information may not be applicable to a given situation and may require some interpretation by knowledgeable professionals who can assist patients and family members. This is only possible, however, when the professionals are adequately knowledgeable. Thus it is important for the relevant information to be made available to widespread audiences of professionals, not just those working directly in HSCT.

The process of adequately informing potential recipients and family members regarding transplantation is a transdisciplinary responsibility that occurs in both formal and informal settings. Nurses caring for individuals receiving traditional treatment for high-risk diseases may find themselves being approached with statements such as, "The doctor mentioned that we might have to consider other options in the future, such as transplant. What do you think?" or "Have you ever taken care of anyone who has had a transplant? Is it really as bad as it sounds?" Verbal and nonverbal responses in such situations have the potential to influence the individual's decisions regarding treatment choices. It is important that all nurses caring for potential HSCT recipients have adequate knowledge to be able to respond appropriately and understand how to refer individuals for additional information. All of the information shared with potential HSCT recipients and family members prior to the consent signing must be accurate and up to date to allow them to make the most appropriate decision regarding treatment for their unique situation. Nurses not directly involved in transplant and, therefore, not in possession of current knowledge, need to be aware of available resources to which they can refer the potential recipient and family for the information they are seeking. Lack of sufficient data regarding the HRQOL of HSCT recipients over time interferes with this process.

Nurses caring for individuals scheduled for HSCT preparatory regimens must ensure that the individuals have an understanding of transplant and have had the opportunity to get questions answered clearly. The nurse attempting this affirmation process must proceed with astute caution and be aware of indications that the recipient may have been informed of probable death secondary to disease if more aggressive treatment is not used. The positive attitude often displayed by the recipient may be a manifestation of "hoping for the best" in light of having been "prepared for the worst" (Eilers, 1991, 1992). Once the transplant process has been initiated, recipients and family members must be supported in their decision. Nurses must exercise caution to avoid a sense of concern regarding the appropriateness of the decision for transplant once the preparatory treatment has begun.

Although there are limited outcomes data in HSCT to link specific nursing interventions with decreased posttransplant morbidity, astute nursing care is regarded as important. During HSCT, adequate symptom management, especially in terms of nausea, vomiting, and pain control, can decrease the discomfort associated with the acute phase of the treatment. Prevention of infections and other complications will decrease the likelihood of long-term effects related to major organ failure. Family members require support during this phase to decrease the negative impact of HSCT on them. Often family members can benefit from additional educational sessions regarding the process, side effects, and care expectations. Sharing what to expect, offering an explanation of changes, and having a discussion of the cause of certain signs and symptoms can both provide information and decrease the stress for many families.

Support groups can decrease the sense of isolation and aloneness that family members may experience. Maintaining a whole-person focus decreases the psychosocial and spiritual distress often experienced by recipients and family members. Professionals teaching and providing support groups during the acute phase of HSCT must be aware of expected outcomes, so information can be accurately shared as questions arise. This awareness includes not generalizing from one aspect of one domain identified in a given study to the impact on the multidimensional concept of QOL in general related to transplant.

After the acute phase of transplant, recipients and family members require reinforcement of earlier education regarding what to expect as they anxiously seek a return to what they see as normal. Therefore, staff must have adequate information regarding usual patterns of recovery. Awareness of these patterns also can guide decisions to initiate appropriate rehabilitative measures to expedite optimal recovery.

For some individuals there may be a need to facilitate the process. Mishel and Murdaugh (1987) referred in their early research with cardiac transplant as "redesigning the dream." HSCT recipients and family members may have approached transplant in anticipation of full recovery and now find themselves dealing with a new array of unanticipated recovery problems, especially in the case of allogeneic recipients experiencing persistent difficulties with GVHD. These individuals may require support as the concept of an evolving, or new, "normal" becomes reality for them. Nursing can have a key role in providing support and making referrals for supportive counseling.

HSCT recipients participating in early research in this area identified "finding a cure" as an important thing for staff to do as related to HRQOL (Ferrell et al., 1992a, 1992b). Professionals must work together to facilitate study in this area and collect the essential data regarding HRQOL post-HSCT. Participating in clinical trials and multidisciplinary studies will increase the awareness of activities in various disciplines. Multidisciplinary, collaborative approaches can also help to identify the preferred approach for working together in the most cost-effective manner to achieve the desired outcome in terms of survival and optimum HRQOL. Ultimately, with continued improvement in treatment protocols, and thus results, we can progress toward the goal of identifying a cure for the diseases currently requiring HSCT as a treatment.

Long-term follow-up care and support has become increasingly relevant as survival numbers improve. It is estimated that there are now tens of thousands of transplant survivors alive today (Rizzo et al., 2006). The Institute of Medicine report on cancer survivorship (http://www.iom.edu/CMS/28312/4931.aspx) emphasizes the importance of cancer survivors having a long-term plan for ongoing care that is diagnosis and treatment relevant. This need carries over to long-term transplant survivors who will require follow-up related to the treatments they received. Antin (2002) discusses the importance of transplant recipients having healthcare professionals who are knowledgeable regarding risks and residual effects directing their long-term care.

CONCLUSION

Many advances have been made in the field of HSCT since the first transplant in 1891. These include technology, care delivery, and supportive services, as well as increased research-focused study. As overall survival rates have improved and we have moved beyond a "be happy you are alive" mentality, there has been increased concern with HRQOL issues for transplant survivors. QOL measures are seen as important outcomes for clinical trials.

HSCT is a costly, potentially life-threatening procedure with a potential for significant long-term effects on HRQOL. Although interest in HRQOL has increased significantly, there have been limited systematic, theory-driven analyses of HRQOL related to HSCT. The critiques of research to date remain consistent. Few studies identify the conceptual or theoretical framework used, and some studies have failed to define HRQOL before measuring this concept. Furthermore, studies have frequently measured only one domain of HRQOL, and few of the tools used to measure HRQOL in transplant survivors have specifically addressed issues related to transplant. There is an even more critical need now for theory-driven, longitudinal prospective studies from patients' perspectives using reliable and valid tools. Clinicians must have information regarding HRQOL in order to provide accurate information and education to potential patients and families during and after transplant and to improve the care delivered across the trajectory. Nurses caring for patients scheduled for HSCT are responsible for ensuring patients and families understand the transplant process and HRQOL issues, yet often lack adequate information themselves.

Additionally, information gathered through research about symptoms experienced and psychological, social, and spiritual problems will help nurses improve symptom management and provide support for patients and families. As more information regarding long-term HRQOL is available, clinicians will be able to increase their focus on rehabilitative measures to decrease the problems identified. Transplant continues to offer hope and promise for the future.

References

Ahles, T. A., Tope, D. M., Furstenberg, C., Hann, D., & Mills, L. (1996). Psychologic and neuropsychologic impact of autologous bone marrow transplantation. *Journal of Clinical Oncology, 14*(5), 1457–1462.

Altmaier, E. M., Ewell, M., McQuellon, R., Geller, N., Carter, S. L., Henslee-Downey, J., et al. (2006). The effect of unrelated donor marrow transplantation on health-related quality of life: A report of the unrelated donor marrow transplantation trial (T-cell depletion trial). *Biology of Blood and Marrow Transplantation, 12*(6), 648–655.

Altmaier, E. M., Gingrich, R. D., & Fyfe, M. A. (1991). Two-year adjustment of bone marrow transplant survivors. *Bone Marrow Transplantation, 7*(4), 311–316.

Anderson, K. O., Giralt, S. A., Mendoza, T. R., Brown, J. O., Neumann, J. L., Mobley, G. M., et al. (2007). Symptom burden in patients undergoing autologous stem-cell transplantation. *Bone Marrow Transplantation, 39*(12), 759–766.

Andrykowski, M. A., Altmaier, E. M., Barnett, R. L., Otis, M. L., Gingrich, R., & Henslee-Downey, P. (1990). The quality of life in adult survivors of allogeneic bone marrow transplantation: Correlates and comparison with matched renal transplant recipients. *Transplantation, 50*(3), 399–406.

Andrykowski, M. A., Bishop, M. M., Hahn, E. A., Cella, D. F., Beaumont, J. L., Brady, M. J., et al. (2005). Long-term health-related quality of life, growth, and spiritual well-being after hematopoietic stem-cell transplantation. *Journal of Clinical Oncology, 23*(3), 599–608.

Andrykowski, M. A., Brady, M. J., Greiner, C. B., Altmaier, E. M., Burish, T. G., Antin, J. H., Gingrich, R., McGarigle, C., & Henslee-Downey, P. J. (1995). Returning to normal' following bone marrow transplantation: outcomes, expectations and informed consent. *Bone Marrow Transplantation, 15*(4), 573–581.

Andrykowski, M. A., Bruehl, S., Brady, M. J., & Henslee-Downey, P. (1995). Physical and psychosocial status of adults one-year after bone marrow transplantation: A prospective study. *Bone Marrow Transplantation, 15*(6), 837–844.

Andrykowski, M. A., Carpenter, J. S., Greiner, C. B., Altmaier, E. M., Burish, T. G., Antin, J. H., et al. (1997). Energy level and sleep quality following bone marrow transplantation. *Bone Marrow Transplantation, 20*(8), 669–679.

Andrykowski, M. A., Cordova, M. J., Hann, D. M., Jacobsen, P. B., Fields, K. K., & Phillips, G. (1999). Patients' psychosocial concerns following stem cell transplantation. *Bone Marrow Transplantation, 24*(10), 1121–1129.

Andrykowski, M. A., Greiner, C. B., Altmaier, E. M., Burish, T. G., Antin, J. H., Gingrich, R., et al. (1995). Quality of life following bone marrow transplantation: Findings from a multicentre study. *British Journal of Cancer, 71*(6), 1322–1329.

Andrykowski, M. A., Henslee, P. J., & Barnett, R. L. (1989). Longitudinal assessment of psychosocial functioning of adult survivors of allogeneic bone marrow transplantation. *Bone Marrow Transplantation, 4*(5), 505–509.

Antin, J. H. (2002). Clinical practice: Long-term care after hematopoietic-cell transplantation in adults. *New England Journal of Medicine, 347*(1), 36–42.

Arvidson, J., Larsson, B., & Lönnerholm, G. (1999). A long-term follow-up study of psychosocial functioning after autologous bone marrow transplantation in childhood. *Psycho-Oncology, 8*(2), 123–134.

Baker, F., Curbow, B., & Wingard, J. R. (1991). Role retention and quality of life of bone marrow transplant survivors. *Social Science Medicine, 32*(6), 697–704.

Baker, F., Marcellus, D., Zabora, J., Polland, A., & Jodrey, D. (1997). Psychological distress among adult patients being evaluated for bone marrow transplantation. *Psychosomatics, 38*(1), 10–19.

Baker, F., Wingard, J. R., Curbow, B., Zabora, J., Jodrey, D., Fogarty, L., et al. (1994). Quality of life of bone marrow transplant long-term survivors. *Bone Marrow Transplantation, 13*(5), 589–596.

Barrera, M., Boyd-Pringle, L., Sumbler, K., & Saunders, F. (2000). Quality of life and behavioral adjustment after pediatric bone marrow transplantation. *Bone Marrow Transplantation, 26*(4), 427–435.

Beanlands, H. J., Lipton, J. H., McCay, E. A., Schimmer, A. D., Elliott, M. E., Messner, H. A., et al. (2003). Self-concept as a "BMT patient," illness intrusiveness, and engulfment in allogeneic bone marrow transplant recipients. *Journal of Psychosomatic Research, 55*(5), 419–425.

Beatty, P. G., Clift, R. A., Mickelson, E. M., Nisperos, B. B., Flournoy, N., Martin, P. J., et al. (1985). Marrow transplantation from related donors other than HLA-identical siblings. *New England Journal of Medicine, 313*(13), 765–771.

Belec, R. H. (1992). Quality of life: Perceptions of long-term survivors of bone marrow transplantation. *Oncology Nursing Forum, 19*(1), 31–37.

Bevans, M. F., Marden, S., Leidy, N. K., Soeken, K., Cusack, G., Rivera, P., et al. (2006). Health-related quality of life in patients receiving reduced-intensity conditioning allogeneic hematopoietic stem cell transplantation. *Bone Marrow Transplantation, 38*(2), 101–109.

Boyle, D., Blodgett, L., Gnesdiloff, S., White, J., Bamford, A. M., Sheridan, M., et al. (2000). Caregiver quality of life after autologous bone marrow transplantation. *Cancer Nursing, 23*(3), 193–203.

Broberger, E., Sprangers, M., & Tishelman, C. (2006). Do internal standards of quality of life change in lung cancer patients? *Nursing Research, 55*(4), 274–282.

Broers, S., Hengeveld, M. W., Kaptein, A. A., LeCessie, S., van de Loo, F., & de Vries, T. (1998). Are pretransplant psychological variables related to survival after bone marrow transplantation? A prospective study of 123 consecutive patients. *Journal of Psychosomatic Research, 45*(4), 341–351.

Broers, S., Kaptein, A. A., LeCessie, S., Fibbe, W., & Hengeveld, M. W. (2000). Psychological functioning and quality of life following bone marrow transplantation: A 3-year follow-up study. *Journal of Psychosomatic Research, 48*(1), 11–21.

Brown, H. N., & Kelly, M. J. (1976). Stages of bone marrow transplantation: A psychiatric perspective. *Psychosomatic Medicine, 38*(6), 439–446.

Buchsel, P. C., & Kelleher, J. (1989). Bone marrow transplantation. *The Nursing Clinics of North America, 24*(4), 907–938.

Bush, N., Donaldson, G., Moinpour, C., Haberman, M., Milliken, D., Markle, V., et al. (2005). Development, feasibility and compliance of a web-based system for very frequent QOL and symptom home self-assessment after hematopoietic stem cell transplantation. *Quality of Life Research, 14*(1), 77–93.

Bush, N. E., Haberman, M., Donaldson, G., & Sullivan, K. M. (1995). Quality of life of 125 adults surviving 6–18 years after bone marrow transplantation. *Social Science & Medicine, 40*(4), 479–490.

Byar, K., Eilers, J. E., & Vose, J. (1999). Quality of life of individuals at least five years or more past autologous blood and marrow stem cell transplant [Abstract #132A]. *Oncology Nursing Forum, 26*(2), 387,

Byar, K. L., Eilers, J. E., & Nuss, S. L. (2005). Quality of life 5 or more years post-autologous hematopoietic stem cell transplant. *Cancer Nursing, 28*(2), 148–157.

Cella, D., Eton, D. T., Fairclough, D. L., Bonomi, P., Heyes, A. E., Silberman, C., et al. (2002). What is a clinically meaningful change on the functional assessment of cancer therapy-lung (FACT-L) questionnaire? Results from eastern cooperative oncology group (ECOG) study 5592. *Journal of Clinical Epidemiology, 55*(3), 285–295.

Cella, D. F., & Tulsky, D. S. (1990). Measuring quality of life today: Methodological aspects. *Oncology, 4*(5), 29–38.

Chang, G., Orav, E. J., McNamara, T. K., Tong, M., & Antin, J. H. (2005). Psychosocial function after hematopoietic stem cell transplantation. *Psychosomatics, 46*(1), 34–40.

Chiodi, S., Spinelli, S., Ravera, G., Petti, A. R., van Lint, M. T., Lamparelli, T., et al. (2000). Quality of life in 244 recipients of allogeneic bone marrow transplantation. *British Journal of Haematology, 110*(3), 614–619.

Clarke, S., Eiser, C., & Skinner, R. (2008). Health-related quality of life in survivors of BMT for paediatric malignancy: A systematic review of the literature. *Bone Marrow Transplantation, 42*(2), 73–82.

Conner-Spady, B. L., Cumming, C., Nabholtz, J.-M., Jacobs, P., & Stewart, D. (2005). A longitudinal prospective study of health-related quality of life in breast cancer patients following high-dose chemotherapy with autologous blood stem cell transplantation. *Bone Marrow Transplantation, 36*(3), 251–259.

Corcoran-Buchsel, P. (1986). Long-term complications of allogeneic bone marrow transplantation: Nursing implications. *Oncology Nursing Forum, 13*(6), 61–70.

Curbow, B., Somerfield, M. R., Baker, F., Wingard, J. R., & Legro, M. W. (1993). Personal changes, dispositional optimism, and psychological adjustment to bone marrow transplantation. *Journal Behavioral Medicine, 16*(5), 423–443.

Curtiss, C. P., Haylock, P. J., & Hawkins, R. (2006). Improving the of care cancer survivors. Anticipating, assessing for, and managing the effects of cancer and its treatment. *The American Journal of Nursing, 106*(3), 48–52.

Decker, W. A. (1995). Psychosocial considerations for bone marrow transplant recipients. *Critical Care Nursing Quarterly, 17*(4), 67–73.

Dobkin, P. L., Poirier, R. M., Robaey, P., Bonny, Y., Champagne, M., & Joseph, L. (2000). Predictors of physical outcomes in pediatric bone marrow transplantation. *Bone Marrow Transplantation, 26*(5), 553–558.

Dow, K. H., & Ferrell, B. R. (1994). Long-term cancer survival: A quality of life model. *Quality of Life— Nursing Challenge, 3*(4), 81–86.

Dreyer, Z. E. (2009). Follow-up into adulthood is critically important for survivors of pediatric transplant. *Bone Marrow Transplantation, 43*(6), 433.

Edman, L., Larsen, J., Hägglund, H., & Gardulf, A. (2001). Health-related quality of life, symptom distress and sense of coherence in adult survivors of allogeneic stem-cell transplantation. *European Journal of Cancer Care, 10*(2), 124–130.

Eilers, J. (1991). *Family member perception of bone marrow transplant: A qualitative pilot study.* Unpublished manuscript.

Eilers, J. (1992). *Uncertainty in family members of bone marrow transplant patients.* Unpublished manuscript.

Eilers, J., Berger, A. M., & Petersen, M. C. (1988). Development, testing, and application of the oral assessment guide. *Oncology Nursing Forum, 15*(3), 325–330.

Eilers, J., Byar, K., & Nuss, S. (2000). The lived experience of autologous blood and marrow stem cell transplant survivors [Abstract #202]. *Oncology Nursing Forum, 27*(2), 352,

Eilers, J., & King, C. (2003). Quality of life issues related to marrow tranplantation. In C. R. Kink, & P. S. Hinds (Eds.), *Quality of life from nursing and patient perspectives* (2nd ed., pp. 273–313). Sudbury, MA: Jones & Bartlett.

Eldredge, D. H., Nail, L. M., Maziarz, R. T., Hansen, L. K., Ewing, D., & Archbold, P. G. (2006). Explaining family caregiver role strain following autologous blood and marrow transplantation. *Journal of Psychosocial Oncology, 24*(3), 53–74.

Epstein, J. B., Phillips, N., Parry, J., Epstein, M. S., Nevill, T., & Stevenson-Moore, P. (2002). Quality of life, taste, olfactory and oral function following high-dose chemotherapy and allogeneic hematopoietic cell transplantation. *Bone Marrow Transplantation, 30*(11), 785–792.

Ersek, M. (1992). The process of maintaining hope in adults undergoing bone marrow transplantation for leukemia. *Oncology Nursing Forum, 19*(6), 883–889.

Ezzone, S., Jolly, D., Replogle, K., Kapoor, N., & Tutschka, P. J. (1993). Survey of oral hygiene regimens among bone marrow transplant centers. *Oncology Nursing Forum, 20*(9), 1375–1381.

Felder-Puig, R., di Gallo, A., Waldenmair, M., Norden, P., Winter, A., Gadner, H., et al. (2006). Health-related quality of life of pediatric patients receiving allogeneic stem cell or bone marrow transplantation: Results of a longitudinal, multi-center study. *Bone Marrow Transplantation, 38*(2), 119–126.

Felder-Puig, R., Peters, C., Matthes-Martin, S., Lamche, M., Felsberger, C., Gadner, H., et al. (1999). Psychosocial adjustment of pediatric patients after allogeneic stem cell transplantation. *Bone Marrow Transplantation, 24*(1), 75–80.

Ferrans, C. E. (1990a). Development of a quality of life index for patients with cancer. *Oncology Nursing Forum, 17*(3), 15–19.

Ferrans, C. E. (1990b). Quality of life: Conceptual issues. *Seminars in Oncology Nursing, 6*(4), 248–254.

Ferrans, C. E., & Powers, M. J. (1985). Quality of life index: Development and psychometric properties. *Advances in Nursing Science, 8*(1), 15–24.

Ferrans, C. E., & Powers, M. J. (1992). Psychometric assessment of the quality of life index. *Research in Nursing & Health, 15*(1), 29–38.

Ferrell, B., Grant, M., Schmidt, G. M., Rhiner, M., Whitehead, C., Fonbuena, P., et al. (1992a). The meaning of quality of life for bone marrow transplant survivors, part 1: The impact of bone marrow transplant on quality of life. *Cancer Nursing, 15*(3), 153–160.

Ferrell, B., Grant, M., Schmidt, G. M., Rhiner, M., Whitehead, C., Fonbuena, P., et al. (1992b). The meaning of quality of life for bone marrow transplant survivors, part 2: Improving quality of life for bone marrow transplant survivors. *Cancer Nursing, 15*(4), 247–253.

Ford, R., & Ballard, B. (1988). Acute complications after bone marrow transplantation. *Seminars in Oncology Nursing, 4*(1), 15–24.

Ford, R., & Eisenberg, S. (1990). Bone marrow transplant. Recent advances and nursing implications. *The Nursing Clinics of North America, 25*(2), 405–422.

Forinder, U., Löf, C., & Winiarski, J. (2005). Quality of life and health in children following allogeneic SCT. *Bone Marrow Transplantation, 36*(2), 171–176.

Forinder, U., Löf, C., & Winiarski, J. (2006). Quality of life following allogeneic stem cell transplantation, comparing parents' and children's perspective. *Pediatric Transplantation, 10*(4), 491–496.

Foster, L. W., McLellan, L. J., Rybicki, L. A., Sassano, D. A., Hsu, A., & Bowell, B. J. (2004). Survival of patients who have undergone allogeneic bone marrow transplantation: The relative importance of in-hospital lay care-partner support. *Journal of Psychosocial Oncology, 22*(2), 1–20.

Franco, T., & Ford, R. C. (2007). Models of care delivery for hematopoietic stem cell transplant patients. In Ezzone & Schmit-Pokorny (Ed.), *Blood and marrow stem cell transplantation* (pp. 423–439). Sudbury, MA: Jones & Bartlett.

Franco, T., & Gould, D. A. (1994). Allogeneic bone marrow transplantation. *Seminars in Oncology Nursing, 10*(1), 3–11.

Frey, P., Stinson, T., Siston, A., Knight, S. J., Ferdman, E., Traynor, A., et al. (2002). Lack of caregivers limits use of outpatient hematopoietic stem cell transplant program. *Bone Marrow Transplantation, 30*(11), 741–748.

Frick, E., Rieg-Appleson, C., Tyroller, M., & Bumeder, I. (2005). Social support, affectivity, and the quality of life of patients and their support-givers prior to stem cell transplantation. *Journal of Psychosocial Oncology, 23*(4), 15–34.

Fromm, K., Andrykowski, M. A., & Hunt, J. (1996). Positive and negative psychosocial sequelae of bone marrow transplantation: Implications for quality of life assessment. *Journal of Behavioral Medicine, 19*(3), 221–240.

Gardner, G. G., August, C. S., & Githens, J. (1977). Psychological issues in bone marrow transplantation. *Pediatrics, 60*(4), 625–631.

Gaston-Johansson, F., & Foxall, M. (1996). Psychological correlates of quality of life across the autologous bone marrow transplant experience. *Cancer Nursing, 19*(3), 170–176.

Gaston-Johansson, F., Franco, T., & Zimmerman, L. (1992). Pain and psychological distress in patients undergoing autologous bone marrow transplantation. *Oncology Nursing Forum, 19*(1), 41–48.

Gaston-Johansson, F., Lachica, E. M., Fall-Dickson, J., & Kennedy, M. J. (2004). Psychological distress, fatigue, burden of care, and quality of life in primary caregivers of patients with breast cancer undergoing autologous bone marrow transplantation. *Oncology Nursing Forum, 31*(6), 1161–1169.

Gluckman, E., Broxmeyer, H. A., Auerbach, A. D., Friedman, H. S., Douglas, G. W., Devergie, A., et al. (1989). Hematopoietic reconstitution in a patient with fanconi's anemia by means of umbilical-cord blood from an HLA-identical sibling. *New England Journal of Medicine, 321*(17), 1174–1178.

Goetzmann, L., Klaghofer, R., Wagner-Huber, R., Halter, J., Boehler, A., Muellhaupt, B., et al. (2006). Quality of life and psychosocial situation before and after a lung, liver or an allogeneic bone marrow transplant. *Swiss Medical Weekly, 136*(17-18), 281–290.

Goetzmann, L., Ruegg, L., Stamm, M., Ambühl, P., Boehler, A., Halter, J., et al. (2008). Psychosocial profiles after transplantation: A 24-month follow-up of heart, lung, liver, kidney and allogeneic bone-marrow patients. *Transplantation, 86*(5), 662–668.

Gralla, R. J. (2002). Problems and progress for quality of life as a clinical trial endpoint. MASCC/ISSO *14th International Symposium Supportive Care in Cancer,* 25–26.

Grant, M., Cooke, L., Bhatia, S., & Forman, S. (2005). Discharge and unscheduled readmissions of adult patients undergoing hematopoietic stem cell transplantation: Implications for developing nursing interventions. *Oncology Nursing Forum, 32*(1), E1–E8.

Grant, M., Ferrell, B., Schmidt, G. M., Fonbuena, P., Niland, J. C., & Forman, S. J. (1992). Measurement of quality of life in bone marrow transplantation survivors. *Quality of Life Research, 1*(6), 375–384.

Gruber, U., Fegg, M., Buchmann, M., Kolb, H., & Hiddemann, W. (2003). The long-term psychosocial effects of haematopoetic stem cell transplantation. *European Journal of Cancer Care, 12*(3), 249–256.

Haberman, M. R. (1988). Psychosocial aspects of bone marrow transplantation. *Seminars in Oncology Nursing*, 4(1), 55–59.

Haberman, M., Bush, N., Young, K., & Sullivan, K. M. (1993). Quality of life of adult long-term survivors of bone marrow transplantation: A qualitative analysis of narrative data. *Oncology Nursing Forum*, 20(10), 1545–1553.

Hacker, E. D. (2003). Quantitative measurement of quality of life in adult patients undergoing bone marrow transplant or peripheral blood stem cell transplant: A decade in review. *Oncology Nursing Forum*, 30(4), 613–629.

Hacker, E. D., & Ferrans, C. E. (2003). Quality of life immediately after peripheral blood stem cell transplantation. *Cancer Nursing*, 26(4), 312–322.

Hacker, E. D., Ferrans, C., Verlen, E., Ravandi, F., van Besien, K., Gelms, J., et al. (2006). Fatigue and physical activity in patients undergoing hematopoietic stem cell transplant. *Oncology Nursing Forum*, 33(3), 614–624.

Hann, D. M., Jacobsen, P. B., Martin, S. C., Kronish, L. E., Azzarello, L. M., & Fields, K. K. (1997). Quality of life following bone marrow transplantation for breast cancer: A comparative study. *Bone Marrow Transplantation*, 19(3), 257–264.

Harder, H., Cornelissen, J. J., van Gool, A. R., Duivenvoorden, H. J., Eijkenboom, W. M. H., & van den Bent, M. J. (2002). Cognitive functioning and quality of life in long-term adult survivors of bone marrow transplantation. *Cancer*, 95(1), 183–192.

Harder, H., Duivenvoorden, H. J., van Gool, A. R., Cornelissen, J. J., & van den Bent, M. J. (2006). Neurocognitive functions and quality of life in haematological patients receiving haematopoietic stem cell grafts: A one-year follow-up pilot study. *Journal of Clinical and Experimental Neuropsychology*, 28(3), 283–293.

Hayes, S., Davies, P. S. W., Parker, T., Bashford, J., & Newman, B. (2004). Quality of life changes following peripheral blood stem cell transplantation and participation in a mixed-type, moderate-intensity, exercise program. *Bone Marrow Transplantation*, 33(5), 553–558.

Heinonen, H., Volin, L., Uutela, A., Zevon, M., Barrick, C., & Ruutu, T. (2001). Quality of life and factors related to perceived satisfaction with quality of life after allogeneic bone marrow transplantation. *Annals of Hematology*, 80(3), 137–143.

Helder, D. I., Bakker, B., de Heer, P., van der Veen, F., Vossen, J. M. J. J., Wit, J. M., et al. (2004). Quality of life in adults following bone marrow transplantation during childhood. *Bone Marrow Transplantation*, 33(3), 329–336.

Hengeveld, M. W., Houtman, R. B., & Zwaan, F. E. (1988). Psychological aspects of bone marrow transplantation: A retrospective study of 17 long-term survivors. *Bone Marrow Transplantation*, 3(1), 69–75.

Hjermstad, M. J., Evensen, S. A., Kvaløy, S. O., Fayers, P. M., & Kaasa, S. (1999). Health-related quality of life 1 year after allogeneic or autologous stem-cell transplantation: A prospective study. *Journal of Clinical Oncology*, 17(2), 706–718.

Hjermstad, M. J., & Kaasa, S. (1995). Quality of life in adult cancer patients treated with bone marrow transplantation: A review of the literature. *European Journal of Cancer*, 31A(2), 163–173.

Hoodin, F., & Weber, S. (2003). A systematic review of psychosocial factors affecting survival after bone marrow transplantation. *Psychosomatics*, 44(3), 181–195.

Horowitz, M. M. (1995). New IBMTR/ABMTR slides summarize current use and outcome of allogeneic and autologous transplants. *IBMTR Newsletter*, 2, 1–8.

Houldin, A., Curtiss, C. P., & Haylock, P. J. (2006). Executive summary: The state of the science on nursing approaches to managing late and long-term sequelae of cancer and cancer treatment. *The American Journal of Nursing*, 106(3), 54–59.

Humphreys, C. T., Tallman, B., Altmaier, E. M., & Barnette, V. (2007). Sexual functioning in patients undergoing bone marrow transplantation: A longitudinal study. *Bone Marrow Transplantation, 39*(8), 491–496.

Hutchison, M. M., & King, A. H. (1983). A nursing perspective on bone marrow transplantation. *The Nursing Clinics of North America, 18*(3), 511–522.

Jagannath, S., Vesole, D. H., Zhang, M., Desikan, K. R., Copeland, N., Jagannath, M., et al. (1997). Feasibility and cost-effectiveness of outpatient autotransplants in multiple myeloma. *Bone Marrow Transplantation, 20*(6), 445–450.

Jenkins, P. L., Lester, H., Alexander, J., & Whittaker, J. (1994). A prospective study of psychosocial morbidity in adult bone marrow transplant recipients. *Psychosomatics, 35*(4), 361–367.

Jenkins, P. L., Linington, A., & Whittaker, J. A. (1991). A retrospective study of psychosocial morbidity in bone marrow transplant recipients. *Psychosomatics, 32*(1), 65–71.

Juttner, C. A., To, L. B., Ho, J. Q., Bardy, P. G., Dyson, P. G., Haylock, D. N., et al. (1988). Early lympho-hemopoietic recovery after autografting using peripheral blood stem cells in acute non-lymphoblastic leukemia. *Transplantation Proceedings, 20*(1), 40–42.

Kanabar, D. J., Attard-Montalto, S., Saha, V., Kingston, J. E., Malpas, J. E., & Eden, O. B. (1995). Quality of life in survivors of childhood cancer after megatherapy with autologous bone marrow rescue. *Pediatric Hematology and Oncology, 12*(1), 29–36.

Kessinger, A., Armitage, J. O., Landmark, J. D., Smith, D. M., & Weisenburger, D. D. (1988). Autologous peripheral hematopoietic stem cell transplantation restores hematopoietic function following marrow ablative therapy. *Blood, 71*(3), 723–727.

Kettmann, J. D., & Altmaier, E. M. (2008). Social support and depression among bone marrow transplant patients. *Journal of Health Psychology, 13*(1), 39–46.

King, C. R. (1995). Latent effects and quality of life one year after marrow and stem cell transplantation. *Quality of Life—Nursing Challenge, 4*(2), 40–45.

King, C. R. (2006). Advances in how clinical nurses can evaluate and improve quality of life for individuals with cancer. *Oncology Nursing Forum, 33*(1), 5–12.

King, C. R., Ferrell, B. R., Grant, M., & Sakurai, C. (1995). Nurses' perceptions of the meaning of quality of life for bone marrow transplant survivors. *Cancer Nursing, 18*(2), 118–129.

King, C. R., Haberman, M., Berry, D. L., Bush, N., Butler, L., Dow, K. H., et al. (1997). Quality of life and the cancer experience: The state-of-the-knowledge. *Oncology Nursing Forum, 24*(1), 27–41.

King, C. R., Hinds, P., Dow, K. H., Schum, L., & Lee, C. (2002). The nurse's relationship-based perceptions of patient quality of life. *Oncology Nursing Forum, 29*(10), E118–E126.

King, M. T., Dobson, A. J., & Harnett, P. R. (1996). A comparison of two quality-of-life questionnaires for cancer clinical trials: The functional living index-cancer (FLIC) and the quality of life questionnaire core module (QLQ-C30). *Journal of Clinical Epidemiology, 49*(1), 21–29.

Kiss, T. L., Abdolell, M., Jamal, N., Minden, M. D., Lipton, J. H., & Messner, H. A. (2002). Long-term medical outcomes and quality-of-life assessment of patients with chronic myeloid leukemia followed at least 10 years after allogeneic bone marrow transplantation. *Journal of Clinical Oncology, 20*(9), 2334–2343.

Klemm, P. (1985). Cyclosporin A: Use in preventing graft versus host disease. *Oncology Nursing Forum, 12*(5), 25–32.

Klepin, H. D., & Hurd, D. D. (2006). Autologous transplantation in elderly patients with multiple myeloma: Are we asking the right questions? *Bone Marrow Transplantation, 38*(9), 585–592.

Kopp, M., Holzner, B., Meraner, V., Sperner-Unterweger, B., Kemmler, G., Nguyen-Van-Tam, D. P., et al. (2005). Quality of life in adult hematopoietic cell transplant patients at least 5 yr after treatment: A comparison with healthy controls. *European Journal of Haematology, 74*(4), 304–308.

Kopp, M., Schweigkofler, H., Holzner, B., Nachbaur, D., Niederwieser, D., Fleischhacker, W. W., et al. (1998). Time after bone marrow transplantation as an important variable for quality of life: Results of a cross-sectional investigation using two different instruments for quality-of-life assessment. *Annals of Hematology, 77*(1-2), 27–32.

Kopp, M., Schweigkofler, H., Holzner, B., Nachbaur, D., Niederwieser, D., Fleischhacker, W. W., et al. (2000). EORTC QLQ-C30 and FACT-BMT for the measurement of quality of life in bone marrow transplant recipients: A comparison. *European Journal of Haematology, 65*(2), 97–103.

Kupst, M. J., Penati, B., Debban, B., Camitta, B., Pietryga, D., Margolis, D., et al. (2002). Cognitive and psychosocial functioning of pediatric hematopoietic stem cell transplant patients: A prospective longitudinal study. *Bone Marrow Transplantation, 30*(9), 609–617.

Lee, S. J., Kim, H. T., Ho, V. T., Cutler, C., Alyea, E. P., Soiffer, R. J., et al. (2006). Quality of life associated with acute and chronic graft-versus-host disease. *Bone Marrow Transplantation, 38*(4), 305–310.

Leigh, S., Wilson, K. C., Burns, R., Clark, R. E. (1995). Psychosocial morbidity in bone marrow transplant recipients: A prospective study. *Bone Marrow Transplantation, 16*(5), 635–640.

Lesko, L. M., Ostroff, J. S., Mumma, G. H., Mashberg, D. E., & Holland, J. C. (1992). Long-term psychological adjustment of acute leukemia survivors: impact of bone marrow transplantation versus conventional chemotherapy. *Psychosomotic Medicine, 54*(1), 30–47.

Litwins, N. M., Rodrigue, J. R., & Weiner, R. S. (1994). Quality of life in adult recipients of bone marrow transplantation. *Psychological Reports, 75*(1), 323–328.

Ljungman, P., Urbano-Ispizua, A., Cavazzana-Calvo, M., Demirer, T., Dini, G., Einsele, H., et al. (2006). Allogeneic and autologous transplantation for haematological diseases, solid tumours and immune disorders: Definitions and current practice in europe. *Bone Marrow Transplantation, 37*(5), 439–449.

Loberiza, F. R., Jr., Rizzo, J. D., Bredeson, C. N., Antin, J. H., Horowitz, M. M., Weeks, J. C., et al. (2002). Association of depressive syndrome and early deaths among patients after stem-cell transplantation for malignant diseases. *Journal of Clinical Oncology, 20*(8), 2118–2126.

Mast, M. E. (1995). Definition and measurement of quality of life in oncology nursing research: Review and theoretical implications. *Oncology Nursing Forum, 22*(6), 957–964.

McConn, R. (1987). Skin changes following bone marrow transplantation. *Cancer Nursing, 10*(2), 82–84.

McGuire, D. B., Altomonte, V., Peterson, D. E., Wingard, J. R., Jones, R. J., & Grochow, L. B. (1993). Patterns of mucositis and pain in patients receiving preparative chemotherapy and bone marrow transplantation. *Oncology Nursing Forum, 20*(10), 1493–1502.

McQuellon, R. P., Craven, B., Russell, G. B., Hoffman, S., Cruz, J. M., Perry, J. J., et al. (1996). Quality of life in breast cancer patients before and after autologous bone marrow transplantation. *Bone Marrow Transplantation, 18*(3), 579–584.

McQuellon, R. P., Russell, G. B., Rambo, T. D., Craven, B. L., Radford, J., Perry, J. J., et al. (1998). Quality of life and psychological distress of bone marrow transplant recipients: The 'time trajectory' to recovery over the first year. *Bone Marrow Transplantation, 21*(5), 477–486.

Meisenberg, B. R., Ferran, K., Hollenbach, K., Brehm, T., Jollon, J., & Piro, L. D. (1998). Reduced charges and costs associated with outpatient autologous stem cell transplantation. *Bone Marrow Transplantation, 21*(9), 927–932.

Meyers, C. A., Weitzner, M., Byrne, K., Valentine, A., Champlin, R. E., & Przepiorka, D. (1994). Evaluation of the neurobehavioral functioning of patients before, during, and after bone marrow transplantation. *Journal of Clinical Oncology, 12*(4), 820–826.

Mishel, M. H., & Murdaugh, C. L. (1987). Family adjustment to heart transplantation: Redesigning the dream. *Nursing Research, 36*(6), 332–338.

Molassiotis, A. (2003). Anorexia and weight loss in long-term survivors of haematological malignancies. *Journal of Clinical Nursing, 12*(6), 925–927.

Molassiotis, A., Boughton, B. J., Burgoyne, T., & van den Akker, O. B. (1995). Comparison of the overall quality of life in 50 long-term survivors of autologous and allogeneic bone marrow transplantation. *Journal of Advanced Nursing, 22*(3), 509–516.

Molassiotis, A., & Morris, P. J. (1998). The meaning of quality of life and the effects of unrelated donor bone marrow transplants for chronic myeloid leukemia in adult long-term survivors. *Cancer Nursing, 21*(3), 205–211.

Molassiotis, A., van den Akker, O. B., Milligan, D. W., & Goldman, J. M. (1997). Symptom distress, coping style, and biological variables as predictors of survival after bone marrow transplantation. *Journal of Psychosomatic Research, 42*(3), 275–285.

Molassiotis, A., van den Akker, O. B., Milligan, D. W., Goldman, J. M., & Boughton, B. J. (1996a). Psychological adaptation and symptom distress in bone marrow transplant recipients. *Psycho-Oncology, 5,* 9–22.

Molassiotis, A., van den Akker, O. B., Milligan, D. W., Goldman, J. M., Boughton, B. J., Holmes, J. A., et al. (1996b). Quality of life in long-term survivors of marrow transplantation: Comparison with a matched group receiving maintenance chemotherapy. *Bone Marrow Transplantation, 17*(2), 249–258.

Morris, M. E., Grant, M., & Lynch, J. C. (2007). Patient-reported family distress among long-term cancer survivors. *Cancer Nursing, 30*(1), 1–8.

Mumma, G. H., Mashberg, D., & Lesko, L. M. (1992). Long-term psychosexual adjustment of acute leukemia survivors: impact of marrow transplantation versus conventional chemotherapy. *General Hospital Psychiatry, 14*(1), 43–55.

Murphy, K. C., Jenkins, P. L., Whittaker, J. A. (1996). Psychosocial morbidity and survival in adult bone marrow transplant recipients--a follow-up study. *Bone Marrow Transplantation, 18*(1), 199–201.

Neitzert, C. S., Ritvo, P., Dancey, J., Weiser, K., Murray, C., & Avery, J. (1998). The psychosocial impact of bone marrow transplantation: A review of the literature. *Bone Marrow Transplantation, 22*(5), 409–422.

Nespoli, L., Verri, A. P., Locatelli, F., Bertuggia, L., Taibi, R. M., & Burgio, G. R. (1995). The impact of paediatric bone marrow transplantation on quality of life. *Quality of Life Research, 4*(3), 233–240.

Neuser J. (1988). Personality and survival time after bone marrow transplantation. Journal *Psychosomatic Research, 32*(4-5), 451–455.

Nims, J. W., & Strom, S. (1988). Late complications of bone marrow transplant recipients: Nursing care issues. *Seminars in Oncology Nursing, 4*(1), 47–54.

Nuss, S. L., & Wilson, M. E. (2007). Health-related quality of life following hematopoietic stem cell transplant during childhood. *Journal of Pediatric Oncology Nursing, 24*(2), 106–115.

Ortega, J. J., Olivé, T., de Heredia, C. D., & Llort, A. (2005). Secondary malignancies and quality of life after stem cell transplantation. *Bone Marrow Transplantation, 35,* S83–S87.

Osoba, D. (1994). Lessons learned from measuring health-related quality of life in oncology. *Journal of Clinical Oncology, 12*(3), 608–616.

Parker, N., & Cohen, T. (1983). Acute graft-versus-host disease in allogeneic marrow transplantation. *The Nursing Clinics of North America, 18*(3), 569–577.

Parsons, S. K., Barlow, S. E., Levy, S. L., Supran, S. E., & Kaplan, S. H. (1999). Health-related quality of life in pediatric bone marrow transplant survivors: According to whom? *International Journal of Cancer Supplement, 12,* 46–51.

Patenaude, A. F., Szymanski, L., & Rappeport, J. (1979). Psychological costs of bone marrow transplantation in children. *The American Journal of Orthopsychiatry, 49*(3), 409–422.

Pavletic, Z. S., & Armitage, J. O. (1996). Bone marrow transplantation for cancer: An update. *The Oncologist, 1,* 159–168.

Pfefferbaum, B., Lindamood, M., & Wiley, F. M. (1978). Stages in pediatric bone marrow transplantation. *Pediatrics, 61*(4), 625–628.

Phipps, S., Brenner, M., Heslop, H., Krance, R., Jayawardene, D., & Mulhern, R. (1995). Psychological effects of bone marrow transplantation on children and adolescents: Preliminary report of a longitudinal study. *Bone Marrow Transplantation, 15*(6), 829–835.

Phipps, S., Dunavant, M., Lensing, S., & Rai, S. N. (2002). Acute health-related quality of life in children undergoing stem cell transplant, part II: Medical and demographic determinants. *Bone Marrow Transplantation, 29*(5), 435–442.

Popkin, M. K., Moldow, C. F., Hall, R. C., Branda, R. F., & Yarchoan, R. (1977). Psychiatric aspects of allogeneic bone marrow transplantation for aplastic anemia. *Diseases of the Nervous System, 38*(11), 925–927.

Prieto, J. M., Atala, J., Blanch, J., Carreras, E., Rovira, M., Cirera, E., et al. (2005). Patient-rated emotional and physical functioning among hematologic cancer patients during hospitalization for stem-cell transplantation. *Bone Marrow Transplantation, 35*(3), 307–314.

Prieto, J. M., Saez, R., Carreras, E., Atala, J., Sierra, J., Rovira, M., et al. (1996). Physical and psychosocial functioning of 117 survivors of bone marrow transplantation. *Bone Marrow Transplantation, 17*(6), 1133–1142.

Redaelli, A., Stephens, J. M., Brandt, S., Botteman, M. F., & Pashos, C. L. (2004). Short- and long-term effects of acute myeloid leukemia on patient health-related quality of life. *Cancer Treatment Reviews, 30*(1), 103–117.

Reiffers, J., Bernard, P., David, B., Vezon, G., Sarrat, A., Marit, G., et al. (1986). Successful autologous transplantation with peripheral blood hemopoietic cells in a patient with acute leukemia. *Experimental Hematology, 14*(4), 312–315.

Ritchie, L. (2005). Outpatient stem cell transplant: Effectiveness and implications. *British Journal of Community Nursing, 10*(1), 14–20.

Rizzo, J. D., Vogelsang, G. B., Krumm, S., Frink, B., Mock, V., & Bass, E. B. (1999). Outpatient-based bone marrow transplantation for hematologic malignancies: Cost saving or cost shifting? *Journal of Clinical Oncology, 17*(9), 2811–2818.

Rizzo, J. D., Wingard, J. R., Tichelli, A., Lee, S. J., Van Lint, M. T., Burns, L. J., et al. (2006). Recommended screening and preventive practices for long-term survivors after hematopoietic cell transplantation: Joint recommendations of the European Group for Blood and Marrow Transplantation, the Center for International Blood and Marrow Transplant Research, and the American Society of Blood and Marrow Transplantation. *Biology of Blood and Marrow Transplantation, 12*(2), 138–151.

Rodrigue, J. R., Boggs, S. R., Weiner, R. S., & Behen, J. M. (1993). Mood, coping style, and personality functioning among adult bone marrow transplant candidates. *Psychosomatics, 34*(2), 159–165.

Rodrigue, J. R., Pearman, T. P., & Moreb, J. (1999). Morbidity and mortality following bone marrow transplantation: Predictive utility of pre-BMT affective functioning, compliance, and social support stability. *International Journal of Behavioral Medicine, 6*(3), 241–254.

Saleh, U. S., & Brockopp, D. Y. (2001). Quality of life one year following bone marrow transplantation: Psychometric evaluation of the quality of life in bone marrow transplant survivors tool. *Oncology Nursing Forum, 28*(9), 1457–1464.

Schimmer, A. D., Elliott, M. E., Abbey, S. E., Raiz, L., Keating, A., Beanlands, H. J., McCay, E., Messner, H. A., Lipton, J. H., & Devins, G. M. (2001). Illness intrusiveness among survivors of autologous blood and marrow transplantation. *Cancer, 15, 92*(12), 3147–3154.

Schmidt, G. M., Niland, J. C., Forman, S. J., Fonbuena, P. P., Dagis, A. C., Grant, M. M., et al. (1993). Extended follow-up in 212 long-term allogeneic bone marrow transplant survivors. Issues of quality of life. *Transplantation, 55*(3), 551–557.

Schulmeister, L., Quiett, K., & Mayer, K. (2005). Quality of life, quality of care, and patient satisfaction: Perceptions of patients undergoing outpatient autologous stem cell transplantation. *Oncology Nursing Forum, 32*(1), 57–67.

Schulz-Kindermann, F., Mehnert, A., Scherwath, A., Schirmer, L., Schleimer, B., Zander, A. R., et al. (2007). Cognitive function in the acute course of allogeneic hematopoietic stem cell transplantation for hematological malignancies. *Bone Marrow Transplantation, 39*(12), 789–799.

Schwartz, C. E., & Sprangers, M. A. (1999). Methodological approaches for assessing response shift in longitudinal health-related quality-of-life research. *Social Science & Medicine, 48*(11), 1531–1548.

Shaffer, S., & Wilson, J. N. (1993). Bone marrow transplantation: Critical care implications. *Critical Care Nursing Clinics of North America, 5*(3), 531–550.

Sherman, A. C., Simonton, S., Latif, U., Spohn, R., & Tricot, G. (2004). Psychosocial adjustment and quality of life among multiple myeloma patients undergoing evaluation for autologous stem cell transplantation. *Bone Marrow Transplantation, 33*(9), 955–962.

Sherman, R. S., Cooke, E., & Grant, M. (2005). Dialogue among survivors of hematopoietic cell transplantation support-group themes. *Journal of Psychosocial Oncology, 23*(1), 1–24.

Simms, S., Kazak, A. E., Golomb, V., Goldwein, J., & Bunin, N. (2002). Cognitive, behavioral, and social outcome in survivors of childhood stem cell transplantation. *Journal of Pediatric Hematology/Oncology, 24*(2), 115–119.

Stranges, E., Russo, C. A., & Friedman, B. (2009). Procedures with the most rapidly increasing hospital costs, 2004–2007. Agency for Healthcare Research and Quality Statistical Brief # 82. Retrieved from http://www.hcup-us.ahrq.gov/reports/statbriefs/sb82.jsp

Sutherland, H. J., Fyles, G. M., Adams, G., Hao, Y., Lipton, J. H., Minden, M. D., et al. (1997). Quality of life following bone marrow transplantation: A comparison of patient reports with population norms. *Bone Marrow Transplantation, 19*(11), 1129–1136.

Syrjala, K. L., Chapko, M. K., Vitaliano, P. P., Cummings, C., & Sullivan, K. M. (1993). Recovery after allogeneic marrow transplantation: prospective study of predictors of long-term physical and psychosocial functioning. *Bone Marrow Transplant, 11*(4), 319–327.

Syrjala, K. L., Langer, S. L., Abrams, J. R., Storer, B. E., & Martin, P. J. (2005). Late effects of hematopoietic cell transplantation among 10-year adult survivors compared with case-matched controls. *Journal of Clinical Oncology, 23*(27), 6596–6606.

Syrjala, K. L., Langer, S. L., Abrams, J. R., Storer, B., Sanders, J. E., Flowers, M. E. D., et al. (2004). Recovery and long-term function after hematopoietic cell transplantation for leukemia or lymphoma. *JAMA, 291*(19), 2335–2343.

Syrjala, K. L., Martin, P., Deeg, J., & Boeckh, M. (2007). Medical and psychosocial issues in transplant survivors. In Gantz (Ed.), *Cancer survivorship* (pp. 188–214). New York, NY: Springer.

Thomas, E. D. (1994). The nobel lectures in immunology. The nobel prize for physiology or medicine, 1990. Bone marrow transplantation: Past, present and future. *Scandinavian Journal of Immunology, 39*(4), 339–345.

Tierney, D. K., Facione, N., Padilla, G., & Dodd, M. (2007). Response shift: A theoretical exploration of quality of life following hematopoietic cell transplantation. *Cancer Nursing, 30*(2), 125–138.

Tsimicalis, A., Stinson, J., & Stevens, B. (2005). Quality of life of children following bone marrow transplantation: Critical review of the research literature. *European Journal of Oncology Nursing, 9*(3), 218–238.

Varni, J. W., Burwinkle, T. M., Katz, E. R., Meeske, K., & Dickinson, P. (2002). The PedsQL in pediatric cancer: Reliability and validity of the pediatric quality of life inventory generic core scales, multidimensional fatigue scale, and cancer module. *Cancer, 94*(7), 2090–2106.

Varni, J. W., Seid, M., & Kurtin, P. S. (2001). PedsQL 4.0: Reliability and validity of the pediatric quality of life inventory version 4.0 generic core scales in healthy and patient populations. *Medical Care, 39*(8), 800–812.

Varni, J. W., Seid, M., & Rode, C. A. (1999). The PedsQL: Measurement model for the pediatric quality of life inventory. *Medical Care, 37*(2), 126–139.

Vickberg, S. M., Duhamel, K. N., Smith, M. Y., Manne, S. L., Winkel, G., Papadopoulos, E. B., et al. (2001). Global meaning and psychological adjustment among survivors of bone marrow transplant. *Psycho-Oncology, 10*(1), 29–39.

Watson, M., Buck, G., Wheatley, K., Homewood, J. R., Goldstone, A. H., Rees, J. K. H., et al. (2004). Adverse impact of bone marrow transplantation on quality of life in acute myeloid leukaemia patients: Analysis of the UK medical research council AML 10 trial. *European Journal of Cancer, 40*(7), 971–978.

Whedon, M., & Ferrell, B. R. (1994). Quality of life in adult bone marrow transplant patients: Beyond the first year. *Seminars in Oncology Nursing, 10*(1), 42–57.

Whedon, M., Stearns, D., & Mills, L. E. (1995). Quality of life of long-term adult survivors of autologous bone marrow transplantation. *Oncology Nursing Forum, 22*(10), 1527–1535.

Wingard, J. R., Curbow, B., Baker, F., & Piantadosi, S. (1991). Health, functional status, and employment of adult survivors of bone marrow transplantation. *Annals of Internal Medicine, 114*(2), 113–118.

Wingard, J. R., Curbow, B., Baker, F., Zabora, J., & Piantadosi, S. (1992). Sexual satisfaction in survivors of bone marrow transplantation. *Bone Marrow Transplantation, 9*(3), 185–190.

Wolcott, D. L., Fawzy, F. I., & Wellisch, D. K. (1987). Psychiatric aspects of bone marrow transplantation: A review and current issues. *Psychiatric Medicine, 4*(3), 299–317.

Wolcott, D. L., Wellisch, D. K., Fawzy, F. I., & Landsverk, J. (1986a). Adaptation of adult bone marrow transplant recipient long-term survivors. *Transplantation, 41*(4), 478–484.

Wolcott, D. L., Wellisch, D. K., Fawzy, F. I., & Landsverk, J. (1986b). Psychological adjustment of adult bone marrow transplant donors whose recipient survives. *Transplantation, 41*(4), 484–488.

Wong, R., Giralt, S. A., Martin, T., Couriel, D. R., Anagnostopoulos, A., Hosing, C., et al. (2003). Reduced-intensity conditioning for unrelated donor hematopoietic stem cell transplantation as treatment for myeloid malignancies in patients older than 55 years. *Blood, 102*(8), 3052–3059.

Worel, N., Biener, D., Kalhs, P., Mitterbauer, M., Keil, F., Schulenburg, A., et al. (2002). Long-term outcome and quality of life of patients who are alive and in complete remission more than two years after allogeneic and syngeneic stem cell transplantation. *Bone Marrow Transplantation, 30*(9), 619–626.

Wujcik, D., Ballard, B., & Camp-Sorrell, D. (1994). Selected complications of allogeneic bone marrow transplantation. *Seminars in Oncology Nursing, 10*(1), 28–41.

Zittoun, R., Suciu, S., Watson, M., Solbu, G., Muus, P., Mandelli, F., et al. (1997). Quality of life in patients with acute myelogenous leukemia in prolonged first complete remission after bone marrow transplantation (allogeneic or autologous) or chemotherapy: A cross-sectional study of the EORTC-GIMEMA AML 8A trial. *Bone Marrow Transplantation, 20*(4), 307–315.

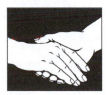

Chapter Sixteen

A European Perspective on Quality of Life of Stem Cell Transplantation Patients

Monica C. Fliedner

Introduction

Nursing aspects related to the quality of life (QOL) of patients who underwent a bone marrow transplantation (BMT) or peripheral blood cell transplantation (PBCT) have been assessed for many years. Several organizations investigate aspects of QOL. The most important oncology organization in Europe, the European Group for Blood and Marrow Transplantation (EBMT), primarily examines all medical and nursing aspects of the stem cell transplanted (SCT) patient. In 1975, a group of ten physicians from Switzerland, France, and the Netherlands started discussing medical and scientific aspects of BMT annually. Two years later, scientists from Germany, Italy, and Great Britain joined this growing organization. All other European countries followed in time. In 1985, the first EBMT nurses' conference was organized to improve networking around bone marrow (and later blood cell) transplantations. Since then the conference has been organized on an annual basis, and the number of attendees has grown from 20 to more than 400 per conference. This conference is offered at the same time as the EBMT conference for physicians, scientists, and data managers. Since the beginning, the physicians and nurses have worked closely together, resulting in joint sessions since 1995. The medical side of the EBMT is comprised of many different working parties or committees, such as acute leukemia, solid tumors, aplastic anemia, and infection. The late effect, pediatric, and infection working parties may be of special interest to nurses and allied healthcare professionals.

The purpose of this chapter is to provide an overview of the many studies and clinical experiences related to the QOL of the SCT patient presented at the EBMT nurses conferences between 1985 and 2009. This overview will facilitate international communication among nurses working on units where blood or marrow transplantations are performed. Geographical differences between participating countries who perform SCT (Goldman 1993; Gratwohl, Hermans, Goldman, & Gahrton, 1993) will be considered in the overview.

It is important for the patient to understand the impact that transplantation may have on his or her later life. Therefore, nurses need to define at-risk patients and areas where special attention is required to promote, enhance, and support the quality of the patients' lives. Some of the goals of nursing, therefore, must focus on promoting the strength of the patients to optimize their abilities and to improve their QOL. Consideration of QOL should play an important role each time the nursing and medical staff, together with the patient and his or her family, discuss the continuity of treatment (Fliedner, 1992). However, how can nurses improve the QOL of patients after a transplantation if the concept is unclear and if the goal is ambiguous? The caring medical staff should realize that nurses, doctors, and the patient perceive the quality of the patient's life differently. To measure and evaluate the QOL of the patient, there should be an agreed upon definition of QOL. Other chapters of this book discuss definitions of QOL; therefore, it is not the purpose of this chapter to define QOL, but to provide an overview of different aspects of QOL on which nurses, working with the transplant patients, may choose to focus.

The meaning of life is altered immediately once a patient is diagnosed with cancer. When a person is evaluated for SCT, everything that promotes life satisfaction, in a sense, is taken away. The independence of the person is restricted *significantly*. The individual is limited in his or her freedom do whatever pleases him or her when or where it pleases him or her. Typically, the person must remain close to the unit or hospital, and during the aplastic phase or the isolation period, he or she is even more restricted. The person's intimacy with loved ones can be interrupted as it takes energy for the individual to stay in contact physically and mentally. One's sense of well-being, vitality, and health becomes distorted by the treatment; it takes quite a long time for the patient to feel healthy again. The struggle to survive the disease and its treatment can overshadow concern for QOL for each patient. What makes the patient's life worth living and what contributes to his or her QOL are different for each patient and, if asked, each patient would give a different answer. It seems obvious that QOL is unique for every individual and QOL can also change over time, even during a given day. Cultural, spiritual, ethical, and religious values, and other life experiences influence perceptions of meaning and consequences of QOL (Zhan, 1993). Since the phrase QOL was first coined, soon after World War II, the concept has become a significant consideration for society in general and, specifically, with regard to health and health care. It was not until 1977 that the term QOL first received a separate heading in the *Index Medicus* (Frank-Stromborg, 1992).

An overall definition of QOL cannot be found in the literature. There seems as many definitions as there are people who use it. Nearly all authors emphasize the subjective and individualized nature of QOL. Often, satisfaction of needs in the physical, psychological, social, activity, material, and structural domains of life are evaluated (Meeberg, 1993). Other authors look at QOL dimensions in terms of fulfillment of life plans or emotional well-being. It is important to accept that QOL is what the person thinks and says it is, relevant to that particular moment, because it can change quickly. It is not always possible to reduce QOL to a simple measurement because it is a multifaceted phenomenon (Yang, 1990). An inability to define QOL makes it hard to understand in a society that is more and more materialistic and in which things are only considered real when they can be measured and made visible (Yang, 1990). Happiness and a feeling of well-being will result from attending to issues that improve QOL. When individuals rate their life quality as high, they are experiencing a positive sense of self-esteem, self-concept, and pride.

Most clinical trials also include examining how QOL is affected by medical treatment. Specific questions should be included when investigating the SCT population. However, it is important that outcomes of the research not be analyzed only, but also considered when developing a new protocol. Five major dimensions should be included in any assessment of QOL (Aaronson, 1988; Ferrell et al., 1992a, 1992b; Haberman, Bush, Young, & Sullivan, 1993; Spilker, 1990):

1. *Physical status* and functional abilities, such as activity level and/or physical symptoms, including infertility
2. *Psychological status*, such as life satisfaction, achievement of life goals, affect, perceived stress, self-esteem, psychological defense mechanisms, and coping
3. *Social interactions*, such as friendship, social support, family, and marriage, including sexual satisfaction
4. *Economic status*, such as occupation, education, and financial status
5. *Spiritual aspects*, such as religiosity, inner strength, hope, and despair.

A stem cell transplantation has a serious impact on divergent dimensions of life. Stem cell transplantation influences physical well-being, contributes to problems of infertility, creates a need to cope with chronic graft-versus-host disease (GVHD), impairs nutrition and cataracts, and creates ongoing fatigue. Psychological well-being is influenced by anxiety, depression, and the need to cope with survival. SCT affects social well-being by causing changes in roles and relationships, and by burdening caregivers. Spiritual well-being also is affected through altered beliefs, changes in values, and changes in religiosity (Ferrell et al., 1992a, 1992b). Economic well-being might be affected by financial impacts brought on by changes in work environment, as well as increased out-of-pocket costs for the patient and family.

Prior to conducting research involving patients and/or families or partners, one should consider that participating in tests might contribute another stress factor. However, most patients and family members welcome being asked how they feel and might appreciate the attention given to them. It must be realized that participation in a research project evaluating the psychosocial burden of a transplantation usually does not involve any other therapeutic actions or interventions. Thus, it is important to follow up after completion of the study, or develop specific interventions for this vulnerable group of patients as needed.

EBMT Nurses Group Research

In the past 15 years, European nurses have contributed valuable projects and studies to research on the concept of QOL. Quality of life prior to, during, and after transplantation has been a topic since the beginning of the EBMT conferences. Work by nurses has developed over the years from describing personal experiences to empirical research studies. More and more, systematic approaches are being used to look more closely at how QOL is affected by treatment and how nurses play a role in promoting QOL. These approaches have been published in the proceedings of the EBMT nurses conference from 1985 to 1991. Since 1992, many presentations have been published in the *EBMT Nurses Group Newsletter*, which changed its name in 1993 to *EBMT Nurses Group Journal*. In 2002, the *EBMT Nurses Group Journal* stopped publication. Since then specific, practice-related articles are published in the *EBMT Nurses Group Newsletter*, however scientific articles can be published in any peer-reviewed journal at the discretion of the authors.

Aspects of Adult Psychosocial Care Prior to the Transplantation

Patients diagnosed with a life-threatening disease, such as leukemia, are confronted with important decisions that will change their lives. It is crucial these patients are closely involved in the informed consent procedure, and that they understand their disease, prognosis, and any problems or challenges that might arise prior to, during, and after transplantation (Dillon, 1985). Usually these patients are still in the prime of their life; they might be finishing school, starting their career, recently married, or starting a family. All these factors should be considered in the communication and support the patients receive throughout the entire transplantation process. Patients can show extreme anxiety prior to their SCT (Keogh, O'Riordan, McCann, & McNamara, 1995). This anxiety usually diminishes after the first steps for the transplantation are taken, when patients reach a "point of no return" and must continue with the transplantation procedure.

By providing adequate information beforehand (Larsen, Stenstrup, Lerche, & Olesen, 1989) caregivers can anticipate and mitigate difficulties during admission for transplantation or after discharge. Although there is always discussion regarding the extent to which patients and families should be informed about the risk factors (Morgan, 1991), it is certain that patients and families must be told what they can expect in easily understandable terms. In many countries, it is required by law to inform patients undergoing an intensive treatment about the risk factors and short- and long-term side effects. Such disclosure facilitates two-way communication between the patient and the healthcare providers. In addition to verbal information, folders, videos, illustrated booklets, and even interactive computerized teaching programs have been developed to provide additional information and help the patient visualize the procedure (Boyd, 1994; Defendini, Midon, & Perrot, 1994; Haupt & Keller, 1989; Kersteman & van de Loo, 1991; Keskimäki & Tammisto, 1994; Larsen et al. 1989; Saudubray, Tellaa, Feral, Moarau, & André, 1989). Authors agree that this written or audiovisual information should not be a substitute for the conversation between the physician and nurse on one hand and the patient and family on the other hand. Information sharing should be planned carefully so as to not over inform patients inappropriately or make them more frightened than necessary. Many patients will share the written information with their families (Boyd, 1994) and feel they can share the burden of transplantation with others.

Patients who undergo peripheral stem cell transplantation need special attention during the phase of stem cell harvesting. In addition, healthcare professionals should also pay specific attention to the donors who are mobilizing stem cells for harvest. The psychological pressure of the mobilization and harvesting for the patient or donor should not be underestimated. Feelings of fear, anxiety, and worry could be experienced by patients or donors (Charley, 1996). Initially, the written information about the procedure itself prepares the patient for the procedure (such as eating breakfast beforehand and drinking milk during the harvest). Privacy is important to patients, as is having a close friend or relative accompany them. Given the fact the harvest procedure takes time, nurses can be creative by suggesting the patient listen to music or watch movies during the procedure. In using the nursing process, when a thorough assessment of risk factors and coping strategies is obtained, important information for the transplant patient can be provided to the team responsible for the patient's care.

Aspects of Adult Care During the Transplantation

The care of the patient during the admission phase of the transplantation is both intensive and challenging for healthcare professionals. All aspects of QOL must receive attention in order to support the patient fully. Assessing the needs of the SCT patient is important as a basis for nursing care planning. One model used that offers a framework for the nursing process is the Mead Model, adapted from the intensive care unit of a hospital in London (Kretzer, Morgan, & Swan, 1994). The Mead Model uses a dependence or independence continuum to assess the needs of the patient. The goals are established within a short-term time frame, which are achievable within 24 hours. The patient is scored for every criterion. There are five stages, ranging from total independence via intervention and prevention to total dependence. The scores indicate the independence or dependence of the patient. Based on this information, interventions can be planned and executed.

Physical Status

It is important to consider the experience of the patient in previous treatment phases and the patient's reaction to possible physical side effects of chemotherapy or irradiation. Physical symptoms such as nausea and vomiting, mucositis, diarrhea, and pain can affect the QOL during transplantation to a high degree. Nutritional status is influenced by these symptoms, and the bacterial limitations of the type of food patients are allowed to eat can limit the energy level. Lienhart (2001) suggests several complementary therapy methods to prevent or relieve side effects of high-dose treatment, such as nausea and vomiting. Among the possibilities described are acupuncture, acupressure, aromatherapy, and several relaxation techniques. Lienhart suggests these treatments should only be applied in addition to, and not a substitute for, conventional drugs. Foot massage is another possibility to improve coping with side effects (Chabot & Legaré, 1997).

One strategy to overcome physical limitations and to keep in shape is any kind of physiotherapy and specifically active and passive kinesiology and isometric exercises (Planzer & Baumann, 1987), although space can be very limited in isolation rooms. Active kinesiology can be used to maintain physical fitness of the patient. It is important for the patient to maintain mobility by special movement and stretching exercises. If the condition of the patient no longer allows active exercises, passive kinesiology should be applied to stimulate circulation and prevent thrombosis and other side effects of immobility (Planzer & Baumann, 1987). To prevent pneumonia and stimulate proper and deep breathing, active or passive respiration therapy can be applied (Planzer & Baumann 1987). The positioning of the patient during respiration therapy is essential for a maximum effect.

Increasingly, research is being undertaken to look at specific symptoms during the transplantation, such as mucositis, pain, and optimal care for the central venous access device of the patient. These studies might require a meta-analysis in the near future to suggest consensus on the state-of-the-art care of handling these often distressing symptoms.

Additional research on several symptoms, as well as an easy-to-use and reliable measurement tool for clinical practice is still required.

Psychological Status

Many patients have difficulties with the lifestyle changes required during the transplantation procedure. Signs of anxiety and depression have been evaluated during the different stages of treatment (Gloriod et al., 1992). Studies show a correlation between the physical condition and signs of depression. In some cases, psychiatric interventions are necessary to support the patient in coping with the situation. Many patients have a feeling of deprivation because, when they enter the isolation period, they have to leave behind small things that characterize their personality, such as their wallet, special clothes, jewelry, and other personal things from home (Dillon, 1985). They experience helplessness and try to escape by engaging in unusual behavior, such as retreat, regression, or aggression (Baumgartner, 1990). Therefore, it is important patients remain responsible for themselves. It is important to break through the vicious cycle and encourage the patient to use appropriate and constructive defense mechanisms.

For many patients, the completion of the conditioning regimen brings feelings of relief and optimism because they have passed what they see to be the point of no return (Dillon, 1985). Many patients experience the feeling of being able to make a new start and often celebrate their transplantation day as their second birthday. Although many allogeneic transplanted patients do not worry initially about infection or GVHD (Dillon, 1985), they realize that a period of waiting for the blood counts to return can be emotional and that potential complications are yet to come. The first contact with the donor is crucial for patients (Baumgartner, 1990) because patients often worry about the well-being of the donor after the donation.

Physical exercise is necessary, not only for the prevention of side effects of the treatment due to immobility, but to support the motivation of the patient (Planzer & Baumann, 1987) by providing a feeling of self-confidence, resulting from the ability to do something rather than having things done for him or her. Other recreational outlets, such as playing games, watching television or movies, writing letters or a diary, and listening to music can be important in offering patients an opportunity to occupy themselves (Amrane & Legree, 1991; Baumgartner, 1990). Some patients look for mental support using complementary therapies such as meditation and relaxation, visualization, guided imagery, and special diets (Naylor, 1987). These techniques help patients survive the isolation period, view the transplantation as a positive experience, and maintain control of the situation as much as possible. Patients also can discover something about the reality and mystery of the quality of their own lives (Yang, 1990). To give structure to the isolation period, patients are advised to have a daily routine and to keep busy, making the time pass more quickly (Naylor, 1987). Many centers emphasize the importance of creating a personal atmosphere for each patient. This can include not only a personal caring approach, but also accepting personal belongings of the patient within the limitations of the protective care policy. Patients might want to bring pictures or photographs of their friends, fill the room with artificial flowers, or bring their own computers or stereos. Isolation restrictions allow for many possibilities, and the team should consider carefully the wishes of the patient.

Survivors who at one time were in the same position as the patient (e.g., similar age, similar background) but have successfully gone through therapy for a malignancy may serve as volunteers and can offer mental and emotional support for patients and families during the transplant procedures (Ilves, Salovaara, Vepsäläinen, & Tuomarila, 1990). However, these volunteers should not answer medical and nursing questions, and the importance of confidentiality also needs to be emphasized. Volunteers are valuable in sharing their experience; encouraging patients and families; offering realistic, practical advice for daily life; and sharing information on services for cancer patients. It is important patients also share with volunteers experiences and feelings, which might be too difficult to share with family members.

Social Interaction

Patients are admitted to the hospital as part of a family unit in which each member has a personal role (Hucklesby, 1992). The patient must understand that social interaction during the transplant period is limited considerably from their lives before the transplant. Patients may have to deal with lack of privacy as well. Although patients show admirable flexibility and adaptation, studies also indicate having decreased contact with friends might lead to depression, demotivation, decrease of mobility, sleeping disorders, boredom, apathy, and introversion (Van Nierop, 1992; Neyens, 1987). In this circumstance, it is important for nurses to listen—not only to what is said, but also to what is not said or is said between the lines. Silence can be indicative of a patient worrying. Transplantation places the patient in a complex situation requiring special care. Thus, nurses should pay extra attention to signs of social isolation. It is also very important for SCT patients to receive mail or phone calls from family and friends on a regular basis (Naylor, 1987). This provides the feeling of still being in contact with the outside world. Patients should be able to stay in contact through frequent visitors (on a planned and regular basis), the daily newspaper or television, or school courses (Baumgartner, 1990).

Relatives, partners, and children play an important role, not only in supporting and encouraging the patient throughout the transplant procedure (Andersson, 1991; Entonen & Wirén, 1992; Hucklesby, 1992; Keskimäki, Tammisto, & Uotinen, 1997; Wendel, van Benthem, & Fliedner, 1991), but also in helping with physical needs. Often the presence of a relative is required to actively assist in the care of the patient (Goldberg, Segal, Armeli, Sharon, & Akerling, 1992). The patient should decide whether or not to have a family caregiver involved in all aspects of care and who that family caregiver should be. Many relatives find the intensive time with the patient valuable. However, economic, social, and psychological burden for the patient's family members, relatives, or support persons who are assisting in caregiving should not be underestimated when considering their specific need for contact, information, and advice. Feelings of fear, anxiety, loneliness, and psychological distress among close friends or partners of the patient have been identified (Toy, 1989). Often family members or partners feel neglected by their friends because much love and attention is given to the patient. Family or close friends should be included in patient care and may require help and special support. However, managing the situation without help from professionals can be a part of family caregiver coping strategy (Hucklesby, 1992).

Wilke, Rudolph, Grande, Siegert, and Sowade (1989) gave specific attention to the interaction between family members and the nursing team. Wilke and colleagues proposed regular, multidisciplinary conferences on the unit to exchange experiences with patients and family members and to gain a certain professional distance from the patient. Family caregivers have to be prepared in advance for their role and responsibilities and to be taught required caregiving tasks. Family caregivers should be supported by professional caregivers throughout the transplantation period (Goldberg et al., 1992).

A support group for relatives of patients with hematological malignancies was initiated in Sweden (Valdman & Lundqvist, 1995) because of the importance in counseling relatives in their support of the patient. While family members are expected to show strength and support, they also have to cope with the fear of losing a loved one. The goal of support groups, such as this one, is to not only support the family members, but to provide facts and enhance knowledge about the process patients experience. Family members learn coping and other strategies, such as relaxation exercises, which they can use at home. Changed roles within the family are discussed and methods for handling associated difficulties are shared in group sessions. These sessions are not only focused on the hospital stay, but also on the period when the patient returns home. Members can be counseled about the changes to expect in all of their lives and ways to handle these changes.

Economic Status

In addition to increasing the patient's comfort with the social aspect of their lives, it is important for patients to go into the transplantation period with the knowledge that everything in their professional life has been taken care of. The transplantation period is difficult not only for patients who have their own company, business, or farm, but also for people who are not self-employed. Losing work or status at work can be difficult to accept (Entonen & Wirén, 1992). Finding an alternative to work, such as going back to school or learning a new skill, can become important to increasing the patient's self esteem or in providing a distraction from thinking too much about illness and its sequelae.

Spiritual Aspects

The spiritual aspect of QOL increasingly is becoming recognized around the world as an important domain of QOL and is further described in Chapter 5. Many patients experience support from their personal view of spirituality. Each individual has different beliefs and values; it is important to continue to live life despite the restricted environment of the treatment procedure. Support can be found, not only in religion, but also in free or abstract spiritual ideas such as positive thinking, appreciating life as it is, and making the best of the situation. Several centers offer consultation with professionals such as psychologists or spiritual advisors (Baumgartner, 1990). These professionals can help structure the confused thoughts of patients and support them as they discover where these thoughts will take them.

Aspects of Care After Discharge of the Adult Transplant Patient

The first year after transplantation is the most crucial year in terms of psychosocial and physical adaptation. It is important for the patient and his or her family to know that how they define QOL will be different—though not necessarily worse—after SCT (Fliedner, 1992). The majority of patients and their families experience this period as more difficult than they expected. This can be due to the fact that the majority expect life after SCT to be exactly as before SCT (Wendel et al., 1991). The associated disappointment can result in both disillusionment and decreased morale. Many QOL studies are designed to examine the period after transplantation and explore ways to understand this phenomenon and to help the patient and family cope with any impairment or change in their lives. Patients are influenced in their development not only by their self-concept, but also by their environment.

The transition from the protective environment of the transplant unit to home is difficult for many patients. Being dependent on family, friends, and the hospital makes it difficult for patients to rebuild their lives again after surviving a life-threatening illness. Ongoing community support should be available during this time. A nurse coordinator responsible for continuity of care should work to maintain close contact with professionals in the community to meet the needs of the patient and his or her family members (Toy, 1989). Lines of communication should be established with agencies in the community, such as social services or home health agencies to provide additional care, identify potential problems, and prevent family breakdown.

Physical Status

After transplantation, while some patients indicate initially they feel physically stronger (Baier, Schmid, Werner-Dreissler, & Schuster, 1987) or they are in good physical condition (Fradique, Heitor, & Costa, 1994), more patients feel less physically able to perform normal daily activities, such as housekeeping or shopping. Chronic symptoms of fatigue or lack of energy are experienced in patients after both autologous and allogeneic transplantation. Changes in body image due to factors such as GVHD or changes in weight play an important role in the daily life of the patient.

It can be important as well to demonstrate how healthcare workers are influenced by the appearance of patients when determining how well they are doing (Haupt & Fliedner, 1992). On one hand, a healthcare provider might meet a patient a long time after he or she has been discharged and determine he or she looks very good. A conversation with that person, however, may reveal feelings of loss of self-esteem and QOL that stems from the patient's perceived change in appearance. On the other hand, some patients with severe chronic GVHD who may be assumed to be impaired in daily life may be, in actuality, well adapted.

The physical changes patients must deal with include baldness, "moon-face" due to the use of corticosteroids, changes of the oral mucosa resulting in dry saliva, and changes in the taste buds. Unexpected and prolonged alopecia or poor hair growth of patients who received busulfan/cyclophosphamide as a conditioning regimen prior to allogeneic SCT have also been reported (Inder, 1990). Another problem for patients can be weight and muscle loss (Hirsch, Claisse, Tabani, & Gluckman, 1994). These changes of body image can lead to embarrassment, insecurity, and emotional vulnerability (Toy, 1989). Evans, Barrett, and Horsler (1988) concluded in their study on the QOL of patients 4 to 9 years after SCT that, despite important physical and developmental changes, these patients show considerable adaptation to their problems and are able to develop new approaches to life. One way to overcome difficulties in resuming a normal lifestyle quickly is to follow a physical and mental rehabilitation program organized by nurses and physicians, together with other practitioners such as physical therapists and social workers (Harris & Hyde, 1993; Molassiotis, Boughton, Burgoyne, & van den Akker, 1994). By following a comprehensive exercise program, the patient is able to readjust, and regain strength, confidence, and motivation at home and work. Other physical impairments, such as cataracts, can be a problem in recovering from the treatment and returning to an active life after transplantation. Patients should know about these possible complications in order to be prepared to either address them or learn to live with them.

In order to gain independence from the hospital, patients and their families should be taught as soon as possible about food precautions and the prevention of potential infections, as well as interventions to be used if infections develop. Technical aspects, such as taking care of the Hickman catheter, must be taught as well (Dannie, 1988).

The sexuality of men and women can be affected by the transplantation treatment and its sequelae (Atlan, Kalayoglu-Besisik, & Sargin, 1999; Fliedner, 1993; Muir, 2000). Both men and women experience changes in their sex lives due to physical impairments such as symptoms of GVHD and vaginal dryness. The degree of these changes depends, among other factors, on the age at transplantation, the conditioning regimen, the kind of transplantation, and the severity of GVHD. Men might be impaired by a lack of interest, erectile failure, "dry ejaculation," or premature or retarded ejaculation (Baruch et al., 1991). Women can experience symptoms of early menopause due to failure of the reproductive organs to produce hormones, with consequences such as bone demineralization (Inder, 1990; Toy, 1989). Women who experience ovarian failure might need estrogen replacement therapies. Often, estrogen creams are prescribed to overcome vaginal dryness, although reported side effects (e.g., carcinogenic effects) should not be underestimated (Inder, 1990).

Healthcare professionals may feel uncomfortable or embarrassed addressing the issue of sexuality. They may feel a certain lack of knowledge (Kelly, 1997), have limited education and experience, or have personal reservations about discussing sexual issues. Studies show that nurses feel more confident than other healthcare professionals in discussing fertility issues or changes in body image (Kelly, 1997). A patient's partner must be included in the discussion. Nurses can suggest alternative methods, such as olive oil, for overcoming the impediment of resultant vaginal dryness during intercourse. Additionally, some patients and their partners might be in need of sexual counseling (Muir, 2002; Toy, 1989) to cope with long-term effects of treatment, such as infertility. It is important male patients receive accurate information about sperm banking and female patients learn about the possibility of storing embryos (Braat, 2001). Knowing about such opportunities can mitigate tension, communication problems, and anger between couples (Pugh & Toy, 1989).

Medical staff must realize the importance of fertility and sexuality for patients with life-threatening disease, although the priority for many patients at diagnosis might simply be survival. This does not take away the desire to have a family after surviving the treatment. It is wrong to assume patients do not need information about fertility options because they already have children. Medical staff should be educated on treatment impact to fertilization and associated risk factors in order to provide accurate information to the patient and his or her partner. One option is to refer patients to a specialty unit for counseling and treatment of fertility problems (Slater, Bass, Boraks, Price, & Marcus, 1995).

Psychological Status

Psychological problems can occur for some time after SCT (Baier et al., 1987), because the patient anticipates being cured and expects life to return to as it was before treatment. Potential difficulties or risk factors should be assessed as early after SCT as possible. In this phase, it is important to know about the behaviors patients demonstrate with regard to self-image, such as denial, compensation, or projection (van de Loo & Mentink 1987). The ability to solve problems may determine an individual's QOL, because every person has his or her own limit of accepting health impairments. By undergoing transplantation, the patient has to extend those limits with each step of the treatment (Fliedner, 1992). Feelings of insecurity and inadequacy can limit patients in their daily lives (Haupt & Fliedner, 1992). Feelings of anxiety due to the risk of an unsuccessful treatment or fearing unforeseen complications can play an important role in the psychological state of patients (Holtkamp et al., 1996). Problems related to social isolation, loss of motivation, and depression are signals of psychological changes (Harris & Hyde, 1993). In addition, many patients might experience physical and mental fatigue and fear of relapse, or additional complications such as infections, GVHD, or late graft failure after transplantation. These feelings and side effects are normal and generally go away with time and good results, but can affect patients psychologically (Baier et al., 1987; Dannie, 1988; van de Loo & Mentink, 1987). Fatigue often remains a common, long-lasting symptom in cancer patients and is often underestimated or unrecognized (Lenssen, 2000). Van den Brand (2001) describes vividly her own feeling of fatigue even a decade after her transplantation and offers professionals suggestions on how to help affected patients. First of all, a subjective assessment of the symptoms is mandatory in order to judge the severity of the problem and to oversee possible areas of improvement (Lenssen, 2000). One major asset is the caregiver's ability to recognize the problem. A thorough preparation of the patient, including the surroundings, would be supportive according to van den Brand (2001). In addition to the medical staff intervention, management of fatigue requires a comprehensive collaboration of different professionals such as dieticians, psychologists, and physiotherapists. After all, it remains a very personal symptom requiring a customized strategy (Lenssen, 2000). Physical changes, such as alopecia—or lesions or scars from central venous catheters or other invasive procedures—might affect the psychological status of the patient due to a changed body image and require attention.

Specific symptomatic differences in psychological dysfunction have been found between autologous and allogeneic transplant patients (Molassiotis et al., 1994). After autologous transplantation, patients tend to develop more symptoms of anxiety and depression. Nevertheless, most of the time they overcome the debilitating effects and are able to lead an active and meaningful life (Dannie, 1988, 1991). Keogh and associates' study (1995) of anxiety and depression in the posttransplant phase revealed that patients tend to experience more depression from isolation or dependency during the first 3 months after transplantation. At 6 months posttransplantation, the patient might show symptoms of anxiety. These feelings are largely resolved by 1 year posttransplantation. Although patients may think it is hard to go on with the changed conditions of their lives (Fradique & Costa, 1994) or feel discouraged (Hirsch et al., 1994), it is important that they maintain their hope for the future and attempt to live each day as fully as possible. Positive thinking and complementary therapies such as aromatherapy or relaxation techniques, music, and art can support patients' coping mechanisms (Boyd, 1994). Again a thorough assessment of the risk factors and resources is recommended. Careful counseling and good teaching to prevent additional stress factors must follow this assessment.

Neuropsychologic aspects such as loss of memory, behavior changes, and lack of concentration may develop in patients who undergo multiple courses of high-dose chemotherapy followed by autologous PBCT (Holtkamp et al., 1996).

Quality of life can improve drastically in the moment someone shows an active interest in a patient (Yang, 1990). Patients can feel good when someone they trust asks at the end of the day how they really feel and understands that something may be bothering them. Nurses often identify patients' need for attention and should have experience when asking patients or their loved ones about how things are going—they will get the whole story of past difficulties and joys, present concerns, and future expectations. Patients often expect nurses to listen to their concerns and appreciate when they do.

Social Interactions

Some patients have difficulties in their relationships due to anger and aggressive behavior after transplantation (Baier et al., 1987; Haupt & Fliedner, 1992). The relationship between partners is put under considerable pressure. The patient is expected to be the same as before transplantation, but this is usually not the case due to physical impairment or psychological stressors. It is important to resume the old pattern of life as much as possible, although many patients indicate various difficulties in their social interactions and the lack of acceptance and understanding by their families for years after their transplantation. These difficulties are the consequence not only of physical impairment (e.g., continuing fatigue, lack of concentration, infertility), but also of personality changes.

Friends and family are very important to patients after transplantation. Patients want to be accepted in society again. The circle of friends may change after SCT, because the transplantation period spreads over a long period of time in which life for other people moves forward and often in a different direction than the patient. Patients report that some friends become much closer and others move away (Baier et al., 1987). It is very important that patients and families or significant others take the time to socialize again and plan social and cultural activities. Resuming professional or school life often helps patients to feel that they have returned to a normal lifestyle (Hirsch et al., 1994).

The expectation of both partners that sexual life will be resumed shortly after discharge might lead to disappointment. Keogh and colleagues (1995) have shown that problems regarding sexual interest and activity may be present prior to the transplantation and during the first 3 months after transplantation. Frequently by 1 year post SCT, sexual interest and activity are restored. Talking about sexuality is not easy for many patients and their partners. Both patients and partners must find a way to express their feelings and satisfy their needs for love and understanding. Partners often say that they have to get to know each other again, as if it is their first time. Delayed recovery of satisfying sexual relations may be experienced (Hirsch et al., 1994). The patient may be influenced by a fear for infection due to low white blood cell counts, a fear of bleeding due to low platelets, or painful intercourse due to vaginal dryness. The partner might be influenced by the need to spare and protect the patient. Body image and other physical impairments play an important role in the resumption of sexual activity (van de Loo & Mentink, 1987). Emotional factors such as changes in self-image, mental fatigue, and fear of relapse or complications can cause feelings of unattractiveness and social isolation. Physical and emotional impairments might lead to feelings of guilt, shame, and frustration. An extended role for nurses when caring for patients with psychosexual problems after SCT may be to provide information and guidance to help them overcome minor problems. In any rehabilitation program, both the patient and his or her partner should be included in order to restore interpersonal intimacy and sexual satisfaction to optimum levels. Every person has the potential for sexual rehabilitation with the help of suitable support and counseling (Goren, 1990).

Patients' relationships with family members, especially the donor, might modify. Often the donor becomes the most important person to the allogeneic transplantation recipient for a certain period of time, and this importance may increase the bond between them. Patients may feel guilty because they feel they are obligated to the donor for the rest of his or her life (van de Loo & Mentink, 1987).

Changes in the social roles of the patient are very important to consider. The housewife may have to change her duties and go to work or the father, who always earned a living for the family, may have to stay at home and take care of the kids. Many problems may arise, and it is important to assess the social situation carefully and look for potential difficulties and resources, as well as prepare the family for possible changes and support the family in the process of change (Keogh et al., 1995). Often partners want to stop working during the transplant procedure and recovery period to be with the patient as much as possible, or they may find that their work is affected by the burden of the situation. Social life and leisure activities of the family members are affected by the transplantation because much time is spent in and around the hospital area. Having convenient access to support from the informal network (i.e., family and friends) is therefore crucial.

Dependency is often also a problem for patients as well as their family. Individuals who never depended on others now need assistance from others to master activities of daily living, while other individuals who were always in the position of the dependent person might become even more dependent and passive, possibly resulting in depression (van de Loo & Mentink, 1987).

A multidisciplinary approach to problems that might arise after SCT has to start before the transplantation procedure to prevent as many problems as soon as possible or to treat them in an early stage.

In several countries, support groups for patients undergoing an SCT have been established. In the Netherlands the ex-SCT contact group meets on a regular basis to talk about problems, exchange experiences, and support each other in establishing a normal life (De Bruyn et al., 2001; Fliedner, 1992). In Finland (Ilves, Tuomarila, & Jussila, 1988), patients who survived a successful SCT were asked to function as supportive individuals for recently diagnosed patients who would soon undergo a transplantation. They received specific training to help other patients in their preparation for the SCT. It is often helpful for patients to share experiences with someone who has survived a transplantation. Informal support group meetings have been established and supported by nurses (Bilbrough, 1997; Jones, Burley, & Heron, 1995) who coordinate and organize the group. Other organizations developed formal courses that last from 1 to 2 weeks, in which patients share information, work on a specific subject within small groups, exercise, and rest (Salovaara, Riitta, Ilves, & Kauppila, 1999). The goals of these groups are to promote the coping process and adjust to a new situation.

Economic Status

Many patients experience financial difficulties as a result of disruption in employment (Molassiotis et al., 1994; Toy, 1989). Many lose their job or cannot resume the same work after their transplantation. Countries differ in their social security systems and how much sickness benefit may be collected. It is obvious, however, that many patients lose a portion of their usual salary. Financial aid is not always sufficient (Fradique et al., 1994). Patients, therefore, need mental and organizational support to feel comfortable when getting back to work after a long period of treatment and convalescence. It is important that work colleagues accept the patient when returning to work even if there are still impairments such as ongoing fatigue the patient has to deal with.

Spiritual Aspects

SCT patients are in a very vulnerable situation and may look for support in spirituality. Baier and associates (1987) found that some patients become more religious or spiritual during this time. Some patients experience a change in values and are grateful to have encountered and conquered a life-threatening illness (Entonen & Wirén, 1992). Some patients state that they appreciate life more than they did prior to SCT and pay more attention to the small joys of life (Baier et al., 1987). One patient described the experience by stating that previously everything had been black and white and after the transplantation there was color in his life (Bach, Hijort, & Mathiesen, 1995). Faith in one's spiritual leader or God can support patients in their daily struggle (Boyd, 1994). Despite difficult, temporary or lasting impairment, a patient has the potential to adjust in the hope of a new and prolonged life (Haupt & Fliedner, 1992).

Psychosocial Aspects of the Care for Children Prior to Transplantation

Depending on the age of the child undergoing the transplantation, he or she will need to be included in the decision-making process (Karaiskou et al., 1997). In this process, contact with another family who already underwent the procedure might be helpful. To get an impression of the environment of the unit in which the transplantation will take place, the unit should be visited by the family, including the parents, the patient, the potential donor, and any other siblings. Open and honest answers to the children's concerns are mandatory. Children may want to know the length of admission. Seasonal events and holidays may help to get a feeling of the time and will help to pass time. A play therapist might be an asset to the multidisciplinary team.

Pot-Mees and Zeitlin (1985) interviewed parents of young patients within the first week of admission prior to transplantation. A second interview was conducted in order to look at the behaviors of the child, the siblings, and the parents' own mental states and marital relationships. The team evaluated the psychological state of the child prior to transplantation, focusing on the intellectual and self-perception of the child. During the treatment period, they evaluated the adjustment of the child and its parents on a weekly basis. They found effects on the entire family from the moment a SCT was proposed. Most of the children appeared to be less influenced by the treatment option than their parents were. Anxiety, depression, periodic lack of cooperation, and developmental regression in the children, as well as social and financial difficulties within the families, were found. An increase in psychosocial support was found to be necessary.

Nilsson (1987) suggested that most parents are not influenced by the information given to them prior to the transplantation, but that they follow the recommendation of the doctor to offer the child the best treatment available. Parents do not feel as if they have a choice for their child. According to Pot-Mees and Zeitlin (1985), the patients lead a relatively normal life during the months prior to the transplantation with normal participation in school and family life. Only one child showed major behavioral problems. On the other hand, parents reported signs of persistent distress and depression during this phase. The parents realized that they would be putting the child through a very stressful treatment that was the only option for cure. Feelings of doubt were evident despite their decision to proceed with the treatment.

To reduce feelings of isolation and frustration, communication with the referring physician and the treatment center are of great importance. Although many parents are not able to pay attention to their child's fear of dying, it is important that the child is able to express his or her fear of death to prevent distortion of an honest communication (Vecchi & Coppola, 1991).

The donor siblings can show considerable signs of distress and ambivalent feelings, and it is very important to communicate with them about their feelings, especially if the family is more occupied with the child who will undergo the transplantation. Siblings who are neither the donor nor the sick child also show mixed feelings about the situation. They may feel relieved about not having to go to the hospital, while also experiencing feelings of rejection and being shoved aside, because they feel that they can't do anything to help their brother or sister.

Psychosocial Aspects of the Care for Children During and After the Transplantation

The admission of a child to the hospital changes the whole lifestyle and rhythm of the family. In many countries, one of the parents is admitted simultaneously with the patient to give the child the opportunity to stay together with a significant person he or she can trust during the treatment (Pot-Mees & Zeitlin, 1985). This might reduce anxiety, although the feeling of fear is normal for both the patient and his or her parents (Nilsson, 1987). Parents also need assistance in maintaining as normal a life as possible for the other children at home (Dennis, 1989).

During the period of transplantation, a child is restricted in many activities of daily life. Many children have to stay in a cubicle or sterile tent for a long time during the aplastic phase. This limits their space to play. Food is also restricted at this phase, with only certain foods allowed in a sterile tent or isolation. However, the isolation procedures have been minimized over the years and many centers allow children to do things in an as normal way as possible, such as wearing their own clothes. For children, it is very important to have close eye or skin contact with friends, a significant caregiver, or other patients. All centers have developed one or more ways for young patients to have contact with friends (Hansson & Kerstin, 1990).

A way to communicate with children and to understand some of their inner feelings, joys, and fears is to have children draw, paint, or use other materials (Monteiro de Barros & Pot-Mees, 1994). Spontaneous drawings can provide new insights into the care of children because they show not only the reality, but also unconscious feelings such as anxieties due to the unknown, anger, and isolation, particularly at the beginning of the treatment and before discharge. Children can express feelings of insecurity and vulnerability in drawings. In addition, it is important to observe changes a child goes through, adapting to the situation, and experiencing a process of surviving treatment for a life-threatening disease. Another theme that can be seen in drawings is the relationship between the children and persons close to them. For caregivers it is important to consider the personality of the child and his or her cultural background to correctly interpret and understand the drawings of the child's inner world.

Another interesting way to stimulate children to express their experiences during the transplant phase is with humor by clowns (Simonds, Serge Beaussier, & Vissuzaine, 1994). Clowns should be a part of the team around the child. It is important to be sensitive to the changing mood on the unit and to be able to take into consideration the stage the child is in. Although children need their rest, clowns can be very helpful in initiating spontaneous laughter, singing, or even giving space for more serious emotions. Through their ability to create a magical environment, children can live in their own fantasies and dreams. Dissolving some of the stresses and tensions not only in children but also in their parents and staff is an important contribution to care.

Children younger than 5 years old tend to lose their self-help and self-management skills. Some children stop eating and drinking on their own, and some might become incontinent again. Signs of loss of speech and mobility are often observed. Children between 5 and 16 show signs of boredom, frustration, depression, overdependency on their parents, and sometimes an increasing lack of compliance. The feeling of losing control over the situation can cause children to try to control the situation by refusing to eat or take medication.

Body image plays an important role not only for adults but also for children (Harbin & Richardson, 1991) after transplantation. Children develop a sense of differences in appearance in simple terms (i.e., beautiful and ugly) at the age of 3 or 4 when they start to socialize with other children in playgroups or kindergarten. An alternative view on the typical body image should be carefully attended to.

After transplantation, physical and mental development can be impaired (Vickers, 1994). Although most children have initially delayed growth patterns, girls or boys might need further growth hormone therapy. Food tolerance can be influenced by GVHD. Food intolerance is seldom a permanent impairment, but usually children stay on a hypoallergenic diet for some time, depending on the recovery of their immune system. Taking into consideration the wide variation of physical and mental development in all children, children after transplantation may show delays in development such as in crawling, walking, and talking (e.g., speech and language development) (Vickers, 1994). Parents have to be prepared for these impairments and be able to anticipate their children's needs and support them in any further development.

Returning to school after such an intensive treatment might be a problem, depending on the age and stage of development of the child. Peykerli and colleagues (2002) evaluated 55 children (mean age 14.2 ± 3.1 years) and looked at reasons why children might not be able to return to school within a reasonable time. Reasons for not returning or returning to school after a long period of absence were chronic GVHD and severe immunosuppression, fear of being unsuccessful in school, and disrupted body image.

Siblings of Children Undergoing SCT

So far not much has been published about the effects the transplantation has on the siblings of the patient. Pot-Mees and Zeitlin (1985) examined the adaptation difficulties of siblings of transplanted children. In their study, 6 out of 19 siblings showed signs of behavioral problems including enuresis, eating and sleep disturbances, disobedience, and difficulties in school. The researchers concluded that not only the patient but also the rest of the family need special attention during the transplantation procedure.

Care for Parents of Children Undergoing SCT

The treatment period places tremendous pressure on the relationship of the parents, not only socially and emotionally, but also financially as they face extra out-of-pocket living and traveling costs (Hostrup, 1996; Vickers, 1994). Because the parents are usually separated over a longer period of time, they may keep in touch through many expensive phone calls or new communication tools. Sometimes a closer relationship between the partners can be seen (Hostrup, 1996). It is important to realize that the parent who takes care of the situation at home may have the feeling of being left out, because immediate input regarding the care of the transplant child may not be possible. Many parents show a high rate of anxiety and distress. Parents have also complained of claustrophobic feelings because the space in the hospital is limited. In addition, they may suffer from sleep disturbance and increased mental and physical fatigue or exhaustion (Nilsson, 1987). To protect the role of the parents as someone giving love and comfort, the parents should actively participate in the care for the child. They should not be involved in any painful or distressing care (Hansson &

Kerstin, 1990), though they should be present when the child has to undergo a specific treatment. Support of a psychologist, partner, or sexual counselor may be necessary for the parents to live through the SCT experience and keep their relationship together.

Asian parents of children undergoing transplantation can show difficulties with role changes (Pot-Mees & Zeitlin, 1985). In Asian families, the father is usually the decision maker, but if the mother stays at the hospital with the child, she may be the one who is involved in important or daily decisions for the child. This puts an extra pressure on the relationships of the partners and the whole family.

In addition to regular contact with doctors and nurses to clarify questions and understand the procedure, strategies to support the child, siblings, and parents may include having the child visit with a psychologist for talking, drawing, painting, and play therapy (Hansson & Kerstin, 1990). Parents, on the other hand, may need contact with a social worker, spiritual counselor, or psychologist who can help them work through their feelings and provide mental, emotional, or spiritual support. Next to a thorough preparation before discharge, Peykerli and colleagues (2002) suggest a need for continuing psychological support for school-age children, their siblings, and their parents.

Nurses Impact on QOL

Patients often ask nurses to assist them in obtaining the best possible quality of their lives. One of the goals of nursing, therefore, is to promote the strengths of patients and their surroundings and to optimize their abilities and improve their QOL (Fliedner, 1994). It is important to look at difficulties from the patients' perspective, to recognize their beliefs, feelings, judgments, and decisions, and not to assume we know what is best for them. Next to a firm knowledge base regarding transplantation, skills such as effective communication, confidence, and determination to pass the knowledge on to others are mandatory (Boyd, 1994). Nurses working with oncology patients and patients who undergo a SCT can affect the QOL of patients and families by being concerned with QOL as part of the treatment. To prepare patients for changes in their lives after SCT, nurses should support them in reevaluating their value system and reassure them of the value of life itself (Fliedner, 1992). Nursing care based on knowledge and skills as well as sympathy and empathy can have a significant impact on the experience of the SCT patient and his or her surrounding.

Barbieri and colleagues (1998) describe the nurse's role and point out that the trusting relationship between patient and nurse must be based on the unconditional acceptance of the other, self-awareness and understanding of one's own actions and responses, and recognition of the difference between thoughts, words, and actions. The strong relationship between good clinical practice and technical skills, including homogenous actions, is just as important as the awareness of what the patient says in words and body language.

Patients expect nurses to possess excellent professional skills, as well as be able to consider the individuality of a patient, and offer mental or other forms of support (Keskimäki et al., 1997). Some patients critique the care they receive while undergoing SCT. Keskimäki and associates (1997) found that patients were not sufficiently informed about nutritional aspects, consequences of SCT, hygiene, and other required activities. Patients' also felt that the socioeconomic consequences of the treatment were underestimated and not sufficiently described.

Nurses, working together with a multidisciplinary team, are the primary caregivers for patients and often share the most intimate, emotional aspects of their lives. A multidisciplinary approach to problems that might arise after SCT has to start prior to the transplantation procedure to prevent as many problems as possible or to treat them at an early stage. The multidisciplinary team must address all dimensions of QOL (Fradique et al., 1994) and look at the patient from a holistic point of view (Haupt & Fliedner, 1992).

Nurses often serve as advocates for patients and families who are too devastated to be their own advocates. Mental support of patients during and after SCT must be available. Nurses are frequently seen as the second most important supporter of the patient, next to the spouse and the family (Wirén, Hämäläinen, & Entonen, 1993). The essence of SCT nursing should be seen as relieving the suffering of patients and their loved ones. "Being there" for the patient in the most private moments of distress or joy is our responsibility, and it can be seen as a contribution to the patient's QOL. Patients need to discuss the potential changes caused by the illness and its treatment and talk about social relationships and everyday matters. Wendel and associates (1991) found it important to give structured and clear information at the right time and in the right manner, based on the individual patient's needs (Rafi et al., 1999). Nurses, therefore, play a pivotal role in the multidisciplinary team by educating the patient in a structured way (Desouza, Glogoski, Norcott, & Rennell, 2000). Evaluations of nursing care can guide quality changes by aiming at improving care and starting with the pretransplant information, including improving the support and care of patients after SCT in the outpatient setting.

Asking patients what really concerns them, what their coping strategies are, and how they have dealt with side effects in prior treatment phases or other stressful times of life may help them remember these strategies at a later time, and they may use them again. Defining the concept of QOL for each individual patient will direct attention to appropriate interventions for enhancing QOL following transplantation (Fliedner, 1992). Some patients, such as those with chronic leukemia, have never had any experience with aggressive treatment regimens. Nurses may want to ask these patients prior to SCT how they have dealt with any signs of being sick so far, evaluate the resources of the patient, and help identify suitable coping strategies.

Based on regular assessments of sexuality and intimacy, nurses can support patients and their partners who are experiencing sexual difficulties to find a new self-concept and redefine their sexual relationships. Nurses can assist by providing sexual health education, accurate information, and specific suggestions for problems. Continued periodic assessment can be helpful to adjust nursing care plans aimed at enhancing the quality of intimacy after transplantation (Fliedner, 1993).

The mind–body relationship should be taken seriously, as medical care should not be limited to "mechanical engineering" (Yang, 1990). Nurses can help prevent harm by providing accurate and timely information about the known long-term complications of SCT (Haberman et al., 1993). Nurses can assist the patient in taking the first steps into the experience of life after SCT (Fliedner, 1994). Dannie (1988) emphasized the fact that watchful outpatient care is as essential as inpatient care, especially within the first 3 months after discharge. It is also essential that nurses on the SCT unit provide nursing care in a consistent manner so that patients and families do not worry or become insecure (Hansson & Kerstin, 1990). Evidence-based standard care protocols should be developed for any technical and physical procedure to provide consistent care for patients.

To promote continuity of care after discharge, a care coordinator should be appointed, either by the hospital (Verhoeven & Smiet, 1995) or funded by a project from the community (Jones et al., 1995). The coordinator or liaison nurse is an important link between the different caregivers and quality of care provided. A thorough assessment of the needs of patients and their close surroundings is crucial to establishing a care plan, monitoring the implementation of the planned interventions, and evaluating the care together with patients. Careful planning of the logistical conditions, such as using a rotating patient chart and communicating with community workers on a regular basis, is the most important factor contributing to the success and continuity of care. Other tasks of the liaison nurse include psychological support, education, management, and communication. The nurse can function as a resource for information and support, not only for patients, but also for relatives and staff members inside and outside the hospital (Jones et al., 1995). The liaison nurse can offer to teach healthcare workers not familiar with the treatment to better serve patients and their families. After discharge from the hospital nurses can serve as consultants by answering the many questions the patients' might have via the phone or Internet. A close collaboration, including guidelines, about when to contact the physician needs to be developed and given to the patient upon discharge from the hospital. Documentation of the information and instructions provided is mandatory to ensure continuity of care.

Despite recent advances that allow outpatient autologous and allogeneic treatments (Bracha et al., 1999; Leather, Herrmann, Cannell, Buffery, & Seward, 1998; Svahn, 1999) or transplantation without isolation procedures (Stotts & Bouchard, 1997), it is essential that nurses realize that the nursing care remains the same. Outpatients need the same support and care as SCT inpatients. Some patients "shop around" to undergo SCT in an environment that fits their personal needs and expectations. Yet, all SCT patients need the same thorough education and care facilities prior to, during, and after this intensive treatment. The informal caregiver, usually a family member, should not be forgotten during this phase. He or she requires the same education, training, and care. In addition, nurses now need to organize a 24-hour a day, 7-day a week service to ensure continuity of care throughout the process (Leather et al., 1998).

CONCLUSION

Nurses must be aware that patients have to go through a normal process of adaptation and coping, which includes periods of joy and happiness on one hand and depression and anxiety on the other. But if patients cannot resolve these problems within a reasonable time, or the problems become too severe, interventions should be planned and incorporated into the care for patients after SCT. The multidisciplinary team should compare the patient's condition after transplantation with the situation prior to the transplantation when deciding on the most appropriate intervention. Additional prospective nursing research and qualitative studies on issues such as the effects of the treatment on patients and their social networks, and appropriate nursing interventions, are necessary in the near future.

References

Aaronson, N. K. (1988). Quality of life: What is it? How should it be measured? *Oncology*, *12*(5), 69–74.

Amrane, F., & Legree, N. (1991). The leisures in L.A.F. room. *Proceedings of the 7th Meeting of the EBMT Nurses Group* (p. 83). Cortina d'Ampezzo, Italy.

Andersson, C. (1991). An active role of the relatives during the bone marrow transplant procedure. *Proceedings of the 7th Meeting of the EBMT Nurses Group* (pp. 17–18). Cortina d'Ampezzo, Italy.

Atlan, N., Kalayoglu-Besisik, S., & Sargin, D. (1999). The sexual relationship in hematopoietic stem cell transplantation survivors. *EBMT Nurses Group Journal*, *2*, 5–7.

Bach, K., Hijort, K., & Mathiesen, A. M. (1995). A method to improve nursing care and its effect on the rehabilitation of patients undergoing autologous bone marrow transplantation. *EBMT Nurses Group Journal*, *1*, 36–38.

Baier, E., Schmid, A., Werner-Dreissler, M., & Schuster, V. (1987). Life after BMT: Psychological aspects after discharge. *Proceedings of the 3rd Meeting of the EBMT Nurses Group* (pp. 63–69). Interlaken, Switzerland.

Barbieri, S., Ventura, O., Prati, R., Canepa, M., Nobili, A., Agresta, M., et al. (1998). Experience: Nurses in the mirror. *EBMT Nurses Group Journal*, *2*, 6–8.

Baruch, J., Benjamin, S., Treleaven, J., Wilcox, A. H., Barron, J. L., & Powles, R. (1991). Male sexual function following bone marrow transplantation for hematological cancer. *Bone Marrow Transplantation*, *7*(2), 52.

Baumgartner, M. (1990). The problems and support of BMT patients in the laminar airflow unit: Observations of a nursing care team. *Proceedings of the 6th Meeting of the EBMT Nurses Group* (pp. 89–95). The Hague, Netherlands.

Bilbrough, C. (1997). Pioneering a haematology support network. *EBMT Nurses Group Journal*, *1*, 16–21.

Boyd, C. (1994). Quality of life: Patient education for bone marrow transplant patients, is it more effective if your patient is a healthcare professional? *EBMT Nurses Group Journal*, *1*, 16–20.

Braat, D. D. M. (2001). Fertility following bone marrow transplantation. *EBMT Nurses Group Journal*, *2*, 24–26.

Bracha, D., Raz, H., Sarelli, R., Grinberger, A., Rizel, S., Hardan, I., et al. (1999). Outpatient transplant: Safe, feasible, and well accepted by the patients. *EBMT Nurses Group Journal*, *2*, 10–12.

Chabot, L. F., & Legaré, C. (1997). The implementation of a programme of foot massage to enhance patients and family coping during bone marrow transplant. *EBMT Nurses Group Journal*, *2*, 18–21.

Charley, C. (1996). The patient's response to the peripheral blood stem cells programme. *EBMT Nurses Group Journal*, *1*, 13–22.

Dannie, E. (1988). Outpatient care of BMT patients. *Proceedings of the 4th Meeting of the EBMT Nurses Group* (pp. 35–41). Chamonix, France.

Dannie, E. (1991). Quality of life after bone marrow transplantation. *Proceedings of the 7th Meeting of the EBMT Nurses Group* (pp. 29–30). Cortina d'Ampezzo, Italy.

De Bruyn, I., Pol, M., Koppejan, M., Brand, I., Baeten, F., ter Beek, J., et al. (2001). Ten years of psychosocial support for patient and family—Contact group bone marrow transplantation, the Netherlands. *EBMT Nurses Group Journal*, *2*, 20–21.

Defendini, C., Midon, N., & Perrot, R. (1994). Preparing the patient for entering the air flow room: The support of a booklet. *EBMT Nurses Group Newsletter, 2,* 28–30.

Dennis, J. (1989). Preparation and support for the patient and family during displacement bone marrow transplantation. *Proceedings of the 5th Meeting of the EBMT Nurses Group* (pp. 9–15). Badgastein, Austria.

Desouza, S., Glogoski, G., Norcott, J., & Rennell, D. (2000). Is a multi-disciplinary pre-transplant assessment clinic useful in blood cell transplant? *EBMT Nurses Group Journal, 2,* 25–32.

Dillon, I. (1985). Psychological and emotional problems of patients undergoing bone marrow transplantation. *Proceedings of the 1st Meeting of the EBMT Nurses Group* (pp. 64–69). Bad Hofgastein (Salzburg), Austria.

Entonen, A., & Wirén, R. (1992). Adaptation to severe intestinal GVHD after BMT. *EBMT Nurses Group Newsletter, 2,* 15–17.

Evans, M. G. C., Barrett, A. J., & Horsler, H. (1988). Quality of life and late effects in 31 patients more than 4 years after BMT for leukemia. *Proceedings of the 4th Meeting of the EBMT Nurses Group* (p. 43). Chamonix, France.

Ferrell, B. R., Grant, M., Schmidt, G. M., Rhiner, M., Whitehead, C., Fonbuena, P., et al. (1992a). The meaning of quality of life for bone marrow transplant survivors, part 1: The impact of bone marrow transplant on quality of life. *Cancer Nursing, 15*(3), 153–160.

Ferrell, B. R., Grant, M., Schmidt, G. M., Rhiner, M., Whitehead, C., Fonbuena, P., et al. (1992b). The meaning of quality of life for bone marrow transplant survivors, part 2: Improving quality of life for bone marrow transplant survivors. *Cancer Nursing, 15*(4), 247–253.

Fliedner, M. (1992). Contribution to the panel discussion on quality of life. *EBMT Nurses Group Newsletter, 1,* 26–29.

Fliedner, M. (1993). Sexual satisfaction and functioning after BMT—A review of the literature. *EBMT Nurses Group Newsletter, 1,* 41–44.

Fliedner, M. (1994). Quality of life after BMT—A review of the literature. *EBMT Nurses Group Journal, 2,* 50–57.

Fradique, E., Heitor, M. J., & Costa, E. F. (1994). Quality of life after bone marrow transplantation. *EBMT Nurses Group Journal, 1,* 7–15.

Frank-Stromborg, M. (1992). *Instruments for clinical nursing research.* Sudbury, MA: Jones and Bartlett.

Gloriod, A., Morel, N., Devillers, A., Guillaume, S., Tiberghien, P., Flesh, M., et al. (1992). Evaluation of anxiety and/or depression in patients undergoing allogeneic BMT for hematological malignancies. *EBMT Nurses Group Newsletter, 1,* 4–8.

Goldberg, L., Segal, J., Armeli, N., Sharon, R., & Akerling, S. (1992). The attitude of family members of patients toward the work demanded of them as care givers in the hospital. *EBMT Nurses Group Newsletter, 1,* 12–16.

Goldman, J. M. (1993). Bone marrow transplantation in Europe—Can the geographical differences be explained? *Journal of Internal Medicine, 233,* 311–313.

Goren, E. (1990). BMT and sexuality: In search of an extended nursing role. *Proceedings of the 6th Meeting of the EBMT Nurses Group* (pp. 123–129). The Hague, the Netherlands.

Gratwohl, A., Hermans, J., Goldman, J. M., & Gahrton, G. (1993). Bone marrow transplantation in Europe: Major geographical differences. *Journal of Internal Medicine, 233,* 333–341.

Haberman, M., Bush, N., Young, K., & Sullivan, K. M. (1993). Quality of life of adult long-term survivors of bone marrow transplantation: A qualitative analysis of narrative data. *Oncology Nursing Forum, 20*(10), 1545–1553.

Hansson, G., & Kerstin, A. (1990). The psychological care of children undergoing bone marrow transplantation. *Proceedings of the 6th Meeting of the EBMT Nurses Group* (pp. 61–67). The Hague, the Netherlands.

Harbin, P., & Richardson, V. (1991). Body image—A pediatric BMT unit perspective. *Proceedings of the 7th Meeting of the EBMT Nurses Group* (pp. 43–46). Cortina d'Ampezzo, Italy.

Harris, J. L., & Hyde, H. L. (1993). A study to show the benefit of a rehabilitation programme following bone marrow transplantation. *EBMT Nurses Group Newsletter, 1,* 12–14.

Haupt, K., & Fliedner, M. (1992). Quality of life after bone marrow transplantation. *EBMT Nurses Group Newsletter, 2,* 31–33.

Haupt, K., & Keller, K. (1989). The written information for patient and donor. *Proceedings of the 5th Meeting of the EBMT Nurses Group* (p. 175). Badgastein, Austria.

Hirsch, I., Claisse, J. P., Tabani, K., & Gluckmann, E. (1994). Bone marrow transplantation with a matched unrelated donor: Quality of life a year after. *EBMT Nurses Group Journal, 1,* 52–53.

Holtkamp, M. J., Roodbergen, R., van der Wall, E., van Dam, F. S. A. M., Gualtherie van Weezel, L. M., Muller, M., et al. (1996). Nursing implications associated with changes in concentration and memory following multiple courses of high-dose chemotherapy with autologous peripheral blood stem cell transplantation. *EBMT Nurses Group Journal, 2,* 27–31.

Hostrup, H. (1996). Investigating the families' experience of the nursing care of children undergoing ABMT. *EBMT Nurses Group Journal, 2,* 19–23.

Hucklesby, E. (1992). Role of the relatives. *EBMT Nurses Group Newsletter, 2,* 22–25.

Ilves, L., Tuomarila, T., & Jussila, L. (1988). Patients after successful bone marrow transplantation (BMT) as volunteer supporting persons. *Proceedings of the 4th Meeting of the EBMT Nurses Group* (p. 81). Chamonix, France.

Ilves, L., Salovaara, H., Vepsäläinen, P., & Tuomarila, T. (1990). Experiences of help by voluntary supporting persons (SP) in the treatment of bone marrow transplant patients. *Proceedings of the 6th Meeting of the EBMT Nurses Group* (pp. 33–35). The Hague, the Netherlands.

Inder, A. (1990). Long-term effects of bone marrow transplantation at Christchurch Hospital. *Proceedings of the 6th Meeting of the EBMT Nurses Group* (pp. 81–86). The Hague, the Netherlands.

Jones, S. G., Burley, R. C., & Heron, D. (1995). The role of the community liaison nurse for the leukemia and transplant unit at the Christie Hospital. *EBMT Nurses Group Journal, 1,* 45–48.

Karaiskou, A., Malama, S., Sphigou, T., Alexopoulou, A., Loumidi, D., & Koutseli, V. (1997). Health care in a paediatric BMT unit: Illustrating two years experience of psychosocial support by the nursing staff. *EBMT Nurses Group Journal, 1,* 60–64.

Kelly, M. (1997). Sexuality: Do nurses address sexual issues in the bone marrow transplant patient? *EBMT Nurses Group Journal, 2,* 4–13.

Keogh, F., O'Riordan, J. M., McCann, S. R., & McNamara, C. (1995). Bone marrow transplantation: Assessing the need for psychological intervention. *EBMT Nurses Group Journal, 1,* 29–35.

Kersteman, J., & van de Loo, F. (1991). Using the video film for patient introduction. *Proceedings of the 7th Meeting of the EBMT Nurses Group* (p. 79). Cortina d'Ampezzo, Italy.

Keskimäki, R., & Tammisto, M. (1994). Instructions after bone marrow transplantation for adults. *EBMT Nurses Group Journal, 1,* 49–51.

Keskimäki, R., Tammisto, M., & Uotinen, H. (1997). Quality of life after allogeneic or autologous bone marrow or peripheral blood stem cell transplantation. *EBMT Nurses Group Journal, 1,* 48–59.

Kretzer, D. A., Morgan, T., & Swan, N. (1994). Adaptation of the Mead Model for nursing for use in a bone marrow transplant (BMT) unit. *EBMT Nurses Group Journal, 2,* 31–34.

Larsen, J., Stenstrup, K., & Lerche Olesen, S. (1989). The development of a means of communication information to prospective bone marrow transplant patients. *Proceedings of the 5th Meeting of the EBMT Nurses Group* (pp. 63–69). Badgastein, Austria.

Leather, M. J., Herrmann, R. P., Cannell, P. K., Buffery, S., & Seward, C. (1998). Nursing Challenges: Autologous transplantation patient treated at home. *EBMT Nurses Group Journal, 1,* 11–14.

Lenssen, P. (2000). Cancer-related fatigue. *EBMT Nurses Group Journal, 2,* 17–19.

Lienhart, V. (2001). Complementary therapies for nausea and vomiting. *EBMT Nurses Group Journal, 1,* 13–16.

Meeberg, G. A. (1993). Quality of life: A concept analysis. *Journal of Advanced Nursing, 18,* 32–38.

Molassiotis, A., Boughton, B. J., Burgoyne, T., & van den Akker, O. B. A. (1994). Psychological and physical difficulties in patients post BMT. *EBMT Nurses Group Journal, 1,* 2–6.

Monteiro de Barros, M. C., & Pot-Mees, C. (1994). Enhancing communication: Understanding drawings of bone marrow transplant children. *EBMT Nurses Group Journal, 1,* 56–57.

Morgan, G. (1991). Striking the balance between the need for ongoing research and optimum patient care. *Proceedings of the 7th Meeting of the EBMT Nurses Group* (pp. 49–50). Cortina d'Ampezzo, Italy.

Muir, A. (2000). Sexuality and bone marrow transplantation (BMT)—Considerations for nursing care. *EBMT Nurses Group Journal, 1,* 7–11.

Naylor, N. (1987). Patient's own story. *Proceedings of the 3rd Meeting of the EBMT Nurses Group* (pp. 78–88). Interlaken, Switzerland.

Neyens, M. (1987). Psychological approach of a patient in isolation. *Proceedings of the 3rd Meeting of the EBMT Nurses Group* (pp. 58–59). Interlaken, Switzerland.

Nilsson, U. (1987). Experiences and consequences for families whose child goes through a bone marrow transplantation. *Proceedings of the 3rd Meeting of the EBMT Nurses Group* (pp. 26–33). Interlaken, Switzerland.

Peykerli, G., Bilgen, H., Ozgenc, S., Can, E., Yalman, N., Anak, S., et al. (2002). "Back to School" after pediatric stem cell transplantation. *EBMT Nurses Group Journal, 1,* 14–17.

Planzer, M., & Baumann, D. (1987). Physiotherapy in life-islands. *Proceedings of the 3rd Meeting of the EBMT Nurses Group* (pp. 34–42). Interlaken, Switzerland.

Pot-Mees, C., & Zeitlin, H. (1985). Psychosocial aspects of a bone marrow transplantation for child and family: Some first observations. *Proceedings of the 1st Meeting of the EBMT Nurses Group* (pp. 29–34). Bad Hofgastein (Salzburg), Austria.

Pugh, J., & Toy, A. (1989). Sperm banking: A cause for concern. *Proceedings of the 5th Meeting of the EBMT Nurses Group* (pp. 171–173). Badgastein, Austria.

Rafi, H., Rieux, C., Pautas, C., Beaune, J., Kuentz, M., Bernaudin, F., et al. (1999). To what extent should we inform the patients before stem cell transplant? *EBMT Nurses Group Journal, 2,* 8–9.

Salovaara, H., Riitta, W., Ilves, L., & Kauppila, M. (1999). The coping of a patient after a bone marrow transplantation or a stem cell transplantation. *EBMT Nurses Group Journal, 1,* 20–26.

Saudubray, C., Tellaa, K., Feral, T., Moarau, G., & André, M. (1989). Project for a booklet for patients admitted for a bone marrow transplantation. *Proceedings of the 5th Meeting of the EBMT Nurses Group* (p. 165). Badgastein, Austria.

Simonds, C., Serge Beaussier, P., & Vissuzaine, A. (1994). Clowns in the bone marrow transplant unit: A challenge. *EBMT Nurses Group Journal, 1,* 54–55.

Slater, C., Bass, G. A., Boraks, P. A., Price, J., & Marcus, R. E. (1995). Patients' perceptions of information and support given with regard to fertility pre and post bone marrow transplantation. *EBMT Nurses Group Journal, 1,* 39–41.

Spilker, B. (1990). Introduction. In B. Spilker (Ed.), *Quality of life assessments in clinical trials* (pp. 3–9). New York, NY: Raven Press.

Stotts, M., & Bouchard, M. (1997). Allogeneic bone marrow and blood cell transplantation without protective isolation: A seven year retrospective review. *EBMT Nurses Group Journal, 1,* 13–15.

Svahn, B. M. (1999). Homecare in allogeneic stem cell transplantation. *EBMT Nurses Group Journal, 2,* 17–18.

Toy, A. (1989). Outpatient care following bone marrow transplantation. *Proceedings of the 5th Meeting of the EBMT Nurses Group* (pp. 143–148). Badgastein, Austria.

Valdman, E., & Lundqvist, C. H. (1995). Support groups for relatives to patients with hematological malignancies. *EBMT Nurses Group Newsletter, 1,* 18–19.

Van den Brand, I. (2001). Life after bone marrow transplantation: The paradox between cure and crippling. *EBMT Nurses Group Journal, 2*, 10–12.

van de Loo, F. M. P., & Mentink, C. H. (1987). Life after BMT: Psychological aspects after discharge. *Proceedings of the 3rd Meeting of the EBMT Nurses Group* (pp. 70–77). Interlaken, Switzerland.

Van Nierop, G. (1992). Ethical aspects of patient care in the laminar air flow unit. *EBMT Nurses Group Newsletter, 2*, 34–37.

Vecchi, R., & Coppola, A. (1991). Psychologic observations on the emotional involvement about death in young BMT patients. *Proceedings of the 7th Meeting of the EBMT Nurses Group* (pp. 77–78). Cortina d'Ampezzo, Italy.

Verhoeven, M. J. F. W., & Smiet, T. (1995). Continuity in nursing care: A necessity. *EBMT Nurses Group Journal, 1*, 42–44.

Vickers, P. (1994). Physical and psychological development of children following long-term isolation and matched or haploidentical mismatched bone marrow transplantation for one of the severe immunodeficiency disorders: A preliminary study. *EBMT Nurses Group Journal, 1*, 39–48.

Wendel, K., van Benthem, D., & Fliedner, M. (1991.) Psychological and psychiatric effects of BMT. *Proceedings of the 7th Meeting of the EBMT Nurses Group* (pp. 25–28). Cortina d'Ampezzo, Italy.

Wilke, S., Rudolf, G., Grande, T., Siegert, W., & Sowade, C. (1989). Dealing with interactional conflicts during a bone marrow transplantation in a psychotherapeutic liaison consulting service. *Proceedings of the 5th Meeting of the EBMT Nurses Group* (pp. 115–120). Badgastein, Austria.

Wirén, R., Hämäläinen, T., & Entonen, A. (1993). The BMT patient's mental support in our department. *EBMT Nurses Group Newsletter, 2*, 8–14.

Yang, W. (1990). The quality of life and the power to heal. *Proceedings of the 6th Meeting of the EBMT Nurses Group* (pp. 131–136). The Hague, the Netherlands.

Zhan, L. (1993). Quality of life: Conceptual and measurement issues. *Journal of Advanced Nursing, 17*, 795–800.

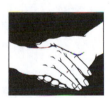

Fatigue and Sleep Disturbances: Symptoms that Cluster and Adversely Affect Quality of Life

MARGARET BARTON-BURKE • MARIA B. CARROLL •
JUDITH A. HEADLEY • JUDITH FRAIN

Some of the factors that contribute to the quality of life are common to all human beings: they are inscribed in the genetic code of the human species and probably have not changed significantly since the Stone Age. Civilized and sophisticated as we may be, we have inherited from our distant ancestors the ability to derive some of our most profound satisfactions from the activities of daily life—when we eat, drink, and love; dream, tell stories or enact imaginings in gesture and pictures; participate in community events where we are both spectators and actors.

—DUBOS (1976)

Introduction

Cancer-related fatigue (CRF) and health-related quality of life (HRQOL) are both considered to be abstract, multidimensional phenomenon with individual meanings and unique attributes; they represent subjective health experiences. The purpose of this chapter is to discuss the symptoms of CRF and sleep disturbances respectively, followed by what is known about these symptoms as a cluster and their impact on HRQOL.

Cancer-Related Fatigue

Bartley (1965) and Bartley and Chute (1947) specified three distinct characteristics of fatigue: (1) fatigue is a self-recognized state; (2) it results from a directly experienced condition; and (3) there is an inferred connection between how tired an individual feels and the amount of exertion experienced by that person. This description of fatigue differs from the definition of cancer-related fatigue, which is "a distressing, persistent, subjective sense of physical, emotional, and/or cognitive tiredness or exhaustion related to cancer or cancer treatment that is not proportional to recent activity and interferes with usual functioning (Berger et al., 2009)." Although tools exist to measure CRF, subjective reporting of the individual's perception continues to be the most common strategy used to ascertain whether a cancer patient is fatigued.

Fatigue is a universal concern of people, healthy and ill (Barton-Burke, 1998). As an illness phenomenon, fatigue affects one's ability to perform everyday activities and increases dependence on others, which ultimately affects the HRQOL for the fatigued individual. This phenomenon of fatigue affects patients in general, but specifically affects individuals with cancer due to the incidence, prevalence, and etiologies of the disease; the treatment sequelae; and the enduring nature of this symptom (Barton-Burke, 2002).

The incidence of CRF ranges from 70% to 100% depending on cancer type and treatment and has been described as the most distressing symptom resulting from cancer and its treatment (Barton-Burke, 2002, 2006a, 2006b; Berger et al., 2009; Blesch et al., 1991; Loge & Kaasa, 1998; Mock et al., 2007; Vogelzang et al., 1997). According to Vogelzang and colleagues (1997), CRF is the longest lasting side effect of cancer and its treatment, continuing for some years after treatment is complete.

Vogelzang and associates' (1997) decade-old national survey of patients, oncologists, and caregivers (i.e., family members and friends who aid in the care of cancer patients) documented that CRF had profound effects on patients, affecting their ability to work, meet family needs, and cope with their disease. This study concluded that patients with cancer experience fatigue during the course of their disease on most days, if not every day. The physicians surveyed believed that CRF was overlooked and under-treated, yet despite the prevalence of CRF and physicians' awareness of it, less than half of all physicians and cancer patients talk about the symptom. Physicians reported their belief that pain is the more debilitating and prevalent side effect, while patients reported that fatigue affected their lives more than pain. The majority of patients claimed fatigue affected their everyday lives and reported that treating their fatigue was as important as treating the cancer itself. Although this study is considered old by scientific standards, current studies continue to corroborate its findings regarding the intensities and adversities of CRF.

Research and Cancer-Related Fatigue

Despite the prevalence of CRF in cancer patients and the growth in published research about this symptom, there is debate about the definitions used, the conceptualizations constructed, and measurement tools used by researchers and clinicians alike. Cancer-related fatigue is a multidimensional, multifactorial symptom that is the most frequent, disturbing complaint for the person with cancer. It is often defined as the subjective feeling of tiredness and lacking physical energy, but CRF is also a symptom with several dimensions of expression and multiple influencing factors. Conceptual and operational definitions of CRF are vital to the study of this phenomenon and to understanding and comparing research results.

However, in most studies the term CRF is used interchangeably to define and describe this symptom, and is used interchangeably as both the definition and a description. Definitions of fatigue vary from terms used to denote a physical sensation or experience (Hart & Frell, 1982; Haylock & Hart, 1979; Rhoten, 1982) to those describing a mental concept such as lack of concentration or deficits in cognitive functioning (Cimprich, 1990, 1993, 1995, 1999). Seldom is the meaning attributed to fatigue by both researchers and study participants made clear to the reader of the study and too often both the conceptual and operational definitions are inconsistent or missing from the published research. Several investigators (Glaus, 1993, 1994; Glaus, Crow, & Hammond, 1996) have attempted to elucidate and define CRF from the patient's perspective.

Definitions of fatigue are inconsistent, numerous, and variable across disciplines and studies (Table 17-1). Broadly, fatigue can be defined as a subjective, multidimensional experience that involves not only pathophysiological causes but also behavioral and psychological aspects (Glaus, 1993). Fatigue is a symptom that interferes with self-care activities (Nail, Jones, Green, Schipper, & Jensen, 1991), the performance of which has gained increased importance with the trend toward outpatient treatment. Increased severity of fatigue has been associated with increased caregiver hours (Jensen & Given, 1993),

---

Table 17-1. A Few Definitions of Fatigue—A Selected List

Fatigue is a decrease in physical performance (Grandjean, 1968).

A state of increased discomfort and decreased efficiency resulting from expenditures of energy reserve (Hart & Frell, 1982).

A subjective sense of weariness or tiredness resulting from exertion or stress or as a condition of impaired efficiency resulting from prolonged mental and/or physical activity or from an attitude of boredom or from disgust with monotonous work (Varricchio, 1985).

Subjective feelings of generalized weariness, weakness, exhaustion, and lack of energy resulting from prolonged stress that is directly or indirectly attributable to the disease process (Aistars, 1987).

A subjective feeling of tiredness influenced by circadian rhythm; it varies in unpleasantness, duration, and intensity. Acute fatigue serves as a protective function. When unusual, excessive, or constant (chronic) fatigue leads to the aversion of activity with the desire to escape (Piper, Lindsay, & Dodd, 1987).

A condition characterized by the subjective feeling of increased discomfort and decreased functional status related to a decrease in energy (Pickard-Holley, 1991).

A state of decreased capacity for physical or mental work, the perception arises from a complex interaction of somatic and psychologic factors (Winningham, 1992).

Fatigue is a subjective phenomenon related to indicators of fatigue such as energy expenditure, sleep disturbances, attentional deficits, decreased endurance, somatic complaints, and weakness. Cancer-related fatigue is a distressing persistent, subjective sense of tiredness or exhaustion related to cancer or cancer treatment that is not proportional to recent activity and interferes with usual functioning (Mock et al., 2007)

Cancer-related fatigue is a distressing persistent, subjective sense of physical, emotional, and/or cognitive tiredness or exhaustion related to cancer or cancer treatment that is not proportional to recent activity and interferes with usual functioning (NCCN Clinical Practice Guidelines in Oncology, 2009).

increased severity of pain (Blesch et al., 1991), diminished cognition (Cimprich, 1992), and depressed mood (Woo, Dibble, Piper, Keating, & Weiss, 1998). Fatigue has been related to inactivity, resulting in loss of muscle mass and reduced cardiac output, leaving the cancer patient in a deconditioned state (Barnes & Bruera, 2002). Winningham and colleagues (1994) found that a cycle of decreasing activity and increasing fatigue led to accelerated deterioration and deconditioning, which resulted in patients fatiguing more quickly when they participated in activity. The relation between fatigue severity and treatment modality has been examined. One study of 322 breast cancer patients found women who had received combination chemotherapy had significantly higher fatigue scores than those who had received radiation therapy only (Woo et al., 1998). The presence of fatigue is associated with dose limitation or discontinuation of therapy in cancer patients. (Winningham et al., 1994; Whedon, Stearns & Mills, 1995; Skalla & Rieger, 1995).

Conceptual Models and Guiding Frameworks of Cancer-Related Fatigue

Fatigue, often conceived of as the subjective feeling of tiredness and lack of physical energy, able to express itself in several different aspects of an individual's life, is influenced by multiple factors. Influencing factors include, but are not limited to, physical and cognitive factors such as activity, hydration, nutrition, motivational factors, and the nature of the fatigue (i.e., acute or chronic) (Berger et al., 2009; Mock et al., 2007; Piper, Lindsay, & Dodd, 1987; Smets, Garssen, Schuster-Uitterhoeve, & de Haes, 1993). There is limited use of conceptual models specifically related to CRF and, when used, these models are underdeveloped. This dearth in the literature regarding conceptual models and guiding frameworks for CRF descriptions, explanations, and predictors about the phenomenon supports the need for further work in theory development, especially because we know that CRF continues after treatment completion (Barton-Burke, 2006a, 2006b).

Fatigue theories can be found in the disciplines of psychology (Grandjean, 1968), physiology (Gibson & Edwards, 1985), ergonomics (Brunier & Graydon, 1993), nursing (Aistars, 1987; Cimprich, 1990; Lee, Lentz, Taylor, Mitchell, & Woods, 1994; Milligan & Pugh, 1994; Pugh & Milligan, 1993; Payne, 2004; Piper et al., 1987; Potempa, Lopez, Reid, & Lawson, 1986; Winningham, 1995), and medicine (Christen, Stage, Galbo, Christensen, & Kehlet, 1989). There are three fatigue theories related to health: the General State of Fatigue Theory (Grandjean, 1968), the science of ergonomics, and Edwards' Theory of Neuromuscular Fatigue (Gibson & Edwards, 1985). All three theories consider fatigue a phenomenon that occurs in healthy individuals.

Grandjean states that "the term fatigue is often used with different meanings and is applied in such a diversity of contexts that it has led to a confusion of ideas" (1968, p. 427). Grandjean, a psychologist, presented general fatigue from a physiological standpoint. In Grandjean's General State of Fatigue Theory, the reticular activating system is the key to an individual's fatigue. He makes a logical case for explaining fatigue from a neuropsychological perspective and, although his model is outdated, his description of symptoms is useful and referred to even today.

Ergonomics seeks to adapt work or working conditions to the worker. It can also be thought of as the study of people adjusting to their environments. Scientists from this discipline examine worker fatigue as it relates to the industrial environment (e.g., fatigue in assembly line workers, fatigue and tiredness associated with computer use). Theoretical descriptions, explanations, or predictions based on the science of ergonomics seem inappropriate to use as a model for persons with cancer.

In Edwards' Theory of Neuromuscular Fatigue, Edwards proposed that both central and peripheral mechanisms of the central nervous system are involved in the fatigue experience (Gibson & Edwards, 1985). This theory offers a logical chain of reasoning to explain fatigue from a physiological perspective. However, it does not explain the relationship of the immune system and other factors such as psychosocial or environmental factors, which may be involved in the fatigue experience.

Other conceptual models or organizing frameworks that discuss the fatigue of individuals who are ill include the following: (1) Aistairs' Organizing Framework for Fatigue (1987), (2) Lee and colleagues' Multidimensional Model of Fatigue (1994), (3) Potempa's General Fatigue Model (1986), (4) Pugh and Mulligan's Childbirth Fatigue Framework (1993), (5) Cimprich's Attentional Fatigue (1990), (6) Piper, Lindsay, and Dodd's Integrated Fatigue Model (1987), (7) Winningham's Psychobiologic Entropy Hypothesis (1992), and (8) Payne's Neuroendocrine-based Regulatory Fatigue Model (2004). Lee and associates (1994) and Potempa and colleagues' (1986) work treats fatigue as an illness phenomenon, while Pugh and Mulligan's (1993) framework focuses on fatigue associated with childbirth.

In oncology nursing the conceptual models and guiding frameworks include the following five models.

Aistars' (1987) Stressor Model examined physiological, psychological, and situational stressors and fatigue. This model helped explain the difference between tiredness and fatigue. It may be useful clinically because Aistairs hypothesized that prolonged stress causes fatigue. This reaction occurs physiologically by activating the reticular activating system and the sympathetic nervous system, resulting in a release of stress hormones. Ultimately, these hormones lead to a depletion of energy stores in the body. This theory tends to describe and explain CRF both in practice or research. However, it does not explain the relationship between the stressors and the response.

Cimprich's Attentional Fatigue is based on attentional theory developed by James, Posner, and Kaplan (Cimprich, 1990). Two kinds of attention (directed attention and involuntary attention) are central to Cimprich's conceptualization. Directed attention reflects a controlled process that supports purposeful activities of daily life and requires mental efforts to sustain. Multiple factors, including informational, affective, and behavioral factors, increase the requirements for directed attention when dealing with a life-threatening illness. If the demands exceed the attentional capacity, the person is at risk for fatigue. The fatigue of directed attention leads to impairment in purposeful activities. This model is prescriptive and contains a conceptual basis for alleviating attentional fatigue, including nursing components to conserve directed attention (Cimprich, 1990). Richardson (1995) suggested that the application of theoretical frameworks addressing components of fatigue, such as Cimprich had done, may enhance understanding of fatigue in persons with cancer.

Piper's Integrated Fatigue Model (Piper et al., 1987) presents a complex framework for explaining the fatigue of cancer. The manifestations, as well as the etiologies of fatigue, are considered in Piper's work. The model has been developed over time specifically for individuals with cancer. Figure 17-1 emphasizes the complex nature of the phenomenon. Piper's theory has many strengths, including offering a comprehensive approach to looking at cancer-related fatigue, blending knowledge about fatigue from several disciplines, grounding in the clinical phenomenon, and applicable for assessing the fatigued individual. However, Figure 17-1 depicts a static theory, lacking specific interactions, theoretical statements, propositions, and outcomes. The lack of theoretical links between categories points to the need for continued development of this theory. A significant theoretical and scientific outgrowth of Piper's Integrated Fatigue Model is the Piper Fatigue Scale, a measurement tool based on the model. This model is clinically relevant and could be developed into a comprehensive assessment tool for fatigue.

Winningham's Psychobiologic Entropy Hypothesis (Winningham, 1992) proposes a model in which any symptom that decreases activity can increase perceptions of fatigue, decrease functional status, promote disability, and result in decreased HRQOL. Winningham, a nurse physiologist, developed this theory to explain fatigue, particularly in the

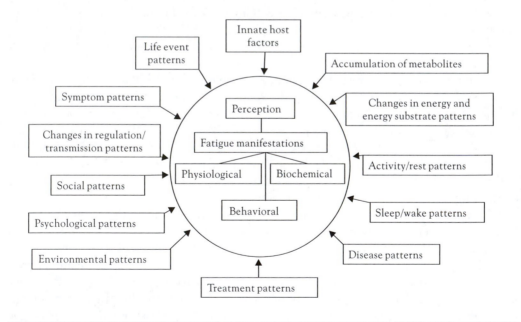

Figure 17-1. **Piper's integrated fatigue model.**

Source: Reprinted from the *Oncology Nursing Forum* with permission from the Oncology Nursing Press, Inc. Piper, B., Lindsey, A., & Dodd, M. 1987. Fatigue mechanisms in cancer patients: Developing nursing theory. *Oncology Nursing Forum* 14(6), 17–23.

cancer patient, by defining fatigue as a symptom that can be influenced by the disease, treatment, and subsequent symptoms (i.e., side effects) of cancer. Figure 17-2 highlights the various factors that contribute to fatigue in the person with cancer; additionally, fatigue is conceptualized as both a primary and secondary phenomenon. Winningham hypothesized if fatigue cannot be alleviated, then another fatigue can occur secondarily to the primary fatigue. This model differs from other nursing theories because it focuses on activity and energetics, thereby offering a different paradigm. In terms of theory, propositional state-ments are offered by Winningham (1992). She contends there is a range of fatigue extending from fatigue-inertia to energy-vigor. If fatigue is allowed to continue, a person will become less energetic and more fatigued. Winningham's Psychobiologic Entropy Hypothesis suggests a systems theory with feedback mechanisms; however, all feedback loops have not been explicated to date. A feedback loop, clearly visible in the model, relates to primary fatigue. If primary fatigue is ablated, there should be no progression to a secondary fatigue. Conversely, if primary fatigue progresses to secondary fatigue, eventually

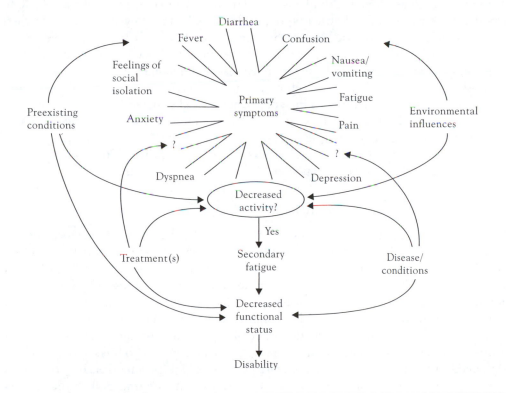

Figure 17-2.   **Winningham's psychobiologic entropy hypothesis.**
  Source: Copyright 1992, 1993 by Maryl L. Winningham. All rights reserved. Used with written con-sent of the author.

the patient will experience a decrease in functional status, and disability will ensue. The model considers environmental factors and preexisting conditions as contributors to CRF, but to what extent these factors influence fatigue is unclear. This theory may be useful clinically for assessment and management of fatigue. Neither Winningham's nor Piper and colleagues' theories have been tested empirically to date.

Payne's Neuroendocrine-based Regulatory Fatigue Model (2004) shifts the paradigm and has brought our thinking about CRF to the biological, cellular level. This model proposes a neuroendocrine-based regulatory fatigue model that can serve as a foundation for interventions to manage fatigue. It suggests biobehavioral systems based on a neuroendocrine regulatory framework.

This new area of exploration and explanation for CRF suggests that proinflammatory cytokines, such as IL-1, IL-6, and TNF have been implicated as possible contributors to the development of common symptoms such as fatigue, depression, and sleep disturbance (Yirmiya et al., 1999). Dysregulated cytokine production has been reported during cancer treatment and is attributed to the effects of chemotherapy, radiation therapy, and surgery (Kristiansson, Saraste, Soop, Sundqvist, & Thörne, 1999; Pusztai et al., 2004). One hypothesis is that, with the destruction of neoplastic cells caused by cancer therapy, there is an accumulation of necrotic tissue, which causes the release of cytokines. This theory may help explain the accumulating evidence of a relationship between chemotherapy, radiation, and surgery, and the development of depression and fatigue in patients with cancer. Depression, and related symptoms such as fatigue, has been associated with inflammatory markers in several chronic illnesses including cancer. Studies have found positive correlations between cytokines (IL-1, IL-6, and TNF) and depression (Musselman et al., 2001), tumor progression (Hussein, Fikky, Bar-Abdel, & Attia, 2004), fatigue (Bower, Ganz, Aziz, & Fahey, 2002; Collado-Hidalgo, Bower, Ganz, Cole, & Irwin, 2006; Costanzo et al., 2005), and sleep disturbance (Illman et al., 2005) in cancer patients.

Measuring Cancer-Related Fatigue

Although there is no standard approach to measure CRF, there is general agreement that objective and subjective items are both necessary to measure the multifactorial and multidimensional nature of CRF (Berger et al., 2009; Meek et al., 2000; Varricchio, 1985, 1995; Wu & McSweeney, 2001). Objective physiologic indicators, such as muscle function, hemoglobin and hematocrit values, and anaerobic metabolism and energy expenditure, have not been routinely used to index CRF. Other clinical indicators such as tumor markers (i.e., CA 125) (Pickard-Holley, 1991), production of cytokines, neuromuscular function, or cellular processes may offer insights into CRF as a physical phenomenon with links to tumor-related byproducts or biochemical processes. Research regarding biological markers may have some type of predictive importance in studying CRF (Ardestani, Inserra, Solkoff, & Watson, 1999; Headley, Ownby, & John, 2004; Payne, 2002, 2004; Payne, Piper, Rabinowitz, & Zimmerman, 2006; St. Pierre, Kasper, & Lindsay, 1992; Wood, Nail, Gilster, Winters, & Elsea, 2006). Other instruments used to measure CRF are either unidimensional, comprised mostly of single items in a general symptom checklist, or multidimensional self-report question-naires (Holley, 2000; McCorkle, 1987; McCorkle & Young, 1978; Piper, Lindsay, et al., 1989; Quick & Fonteyn, 2005; Schwartz, 1998b).

The objective correlates of CRF have not been identified or agreed upon while the subjective nature of fatigue cannot be ignored either. However valid, reliable, psychomet-rically sound scientific instruments are available to measure fatigue in the cancer popula-tion. They include Piper's Fatigue Scale (Piper et al., 1989); the Multifunctional Inventory-20 (MFI-20) by Smets, Garssen, Bonke, and de Haes (1995); Cella's FACIT-F, which has a fatigue subscale (Cella, 1997; Cella & Tulsky, 1990), the Fatigue Symptom Inventory (Hann et al., 1998) and the Schwartz Cancer Fatigue Scale (Schwartz, 1998b). Additionally, Glaus (1993, 1994) reported the development and use of a Visual Analogue Fatigue Scale in her research.

Although research reports regarding fatigue as a side effect of cancer treatments have increased, the diverse ways (e.g., instrument selected, timing of administration) CRF has been measured have made it difficult to determine patterns of CFR within and between treatments for cancer. Questions remain regarding how to best measure CRF and at what times. Meanwhile, CRF is measured in individuals undergoing treatment, in those who have completed treatment and, more recently, in long-term cancer survivors (Andrykowski et al., 1997; Andrykowski, Curran, & Lightner, 1998; Bower et al., 2000; Broeckel, Jacobsen, Horton, Balducci, & Lyman, 1998; Servaes, Verhagen, & Bleijenberg, 2002). What remains unknown is whether all CRF states are the same, and if all forms of CRF have the same causative mechanisms. Also unknown is whether the same interventions work for all individuals experiencing CRF.

Research reports of symptom clusters that include CRF also include sleep disturbances, anemia, pain, and depression as altering conceptualizations of CRF (Anderson et al., 2003; Armstrong, Cohen, Eriksen, & Hickey, 2004; Carpenter et al., 2004; Dodd, Miaskowski, & Paul, 2001). According to Dodd and associates (2001), a symptom cluster is influenced by the timing, occurrence, intensity, and duration of the involved symptoms. The frequency, intensity, and number of symptoms in the cluster can affect outcomes such as HRQOL. Fur-ther study is needed to determine whether these symptoms form a cluster, co-occur, are a clinical syndrome, or are causal to one another. An additional factor needing to be studied for its influence on CRF is anemia. Potentially confounding or intervening variables include the time of day that fatigue is measured, baseline energy levels, changes in fatigue patterns over time, and circadian rhythms. Important issues remain about the direct effects of cancer, the symptom cluster, the effects of cancer treatment, and the strain of dealing with cancer and the relationship to CRF. All these research areas require further study.

In summary, descriptive and interventional studies about CRF exist but there is a lack of well controlled clinical trials regarding strategies to diminish or prevent CRF. In a Cochrane Review of psychosocial interventions in 2009, it was reported there is limited evidence that psychosocial interventions during cancer treatment are effective in reducing fatigue. Several qualitative studies on the effect of these interventions have been completed, but more work regarding CRF in the context of living with cancer is needed.

Published studies include mostly Caucasian adults with a variety of tumors, treatments, sites of treatments, and stages of disease. Few studies include comparison groups. Additionally, these few studies tend to have small samples and emanate from single institutions. Also, there is a lack of understanding of CRF in ethnic and underserved populations (Pud et al., 2008; So et al., 2009). Larger studies targeting ethnically diverse populations from multiple settings are needed. Most CRF research to date is about women with breast cancer; future studies need to include study participants of different ages, different cultural and ethnic backgrounds, with various types of cancer, and at different points in the illness trajectory.

As a final point, although a relationship between a patient's CRF and the fatigue of family caregivers has been documented, the exact mechanism underlying this relationship is not established yet and neither is the mechanism underlying the effect of CRF on family quality of life (Gibson, Garnett, Richardson, Edwards, & Sepion, 2005; Given, Given, & Stommel, 1994; Given, Given, Azzouz, Kozachik, & Stommel, 2001; Given, Given, Azzouz, & Stommel, 2001; Given et al., 2002; Hinds et al., 1999; Hockenberry-Eaton & Hinds, 2000; Hockenberry-Eaton et al., 1998; Jensen & Given, 1991).

Cancer-Related Fatigue as a Clinical Symptom

Fatigue has been identified as one of the most common and disturbing symptoms of cancer and its treatment in patients receiving radiation therapy, chemotherapy, biotherapy, and surgery. Fatigue is most intense in females with ovarian or lung cancer with metastatic disease and poor performance status (Pater et al., 1997). These data corroborate empirical evidence and scientific literature in which younger women with breast cancer or ovarian cancer are reported to be most at risk for fatigue (Irvine et al., 1994; Pickard-Holley, 1991; Vogelzang et al., 1997). Managing symptoms, with methods such as treating with prophylactic antiemetics or proper pain medication, decreases the experience of fatigue (Buchsel, Barton-Burke, & Winningham, 2000; Gaston-Johansson, Fall-Dickson, Bakos, & Kennedy, 1999; Gaston-Johansson, Lachica, Fall-Dickson, & Kennedy, 2004; Graydon, Bubela, Irvine, & Vincent, 1995; Groopman, 1998; Jacobsen et al., 1999; Pater et al., 1997; Winningham, 1995, 1999).

Cancer-related fatigue occurs during and immediately after treatment (Berger & Higginbotham, 2000; Berger, 1998; Boehmke, 2004; Christman, Oakley, & Cronin, 2001; Irvine et al., 1994; Jacobsen et al., 1999; Kolb & Poetscher, 1997; Lovely, Miaskowski, & Dodd, 1999; Miaskowski & Lee, 1999; Piper, Rieger, et al., 1989; Quesada, Talpaz, Rios, Kwizrock, & Gutterman, 1986; Ream & Richardson, 1999; Richardson, Ream, & Wilson-Barnett, 1998) and in long-term survivors (Andrykowski et al., 1998; Bower et al., 2000; Broeckel et al., 1998; Servaes et al., 2002). Some cancer patients have chosen to discontinue treatment because of fatigue. Practitioners may limit doses of various forms of treatment because of patient complaints of fatigue. Also individuals with cancer may attribute impairment of HRQOL to fatigue (Headley et al., 2004). Despite the prevalence of CRF and its clinical effects, its mechanisms are poorly understood, making the effectiveness of

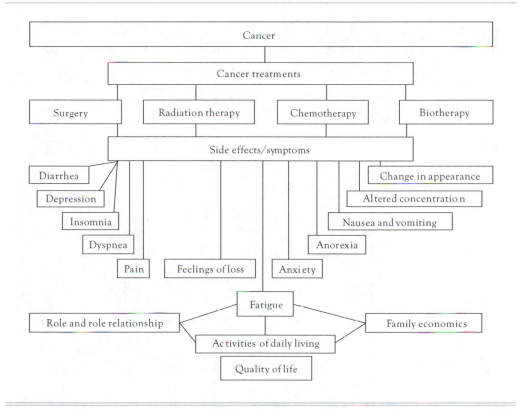

Figure 17-3. **The impact of cancer and its treatments on fatigue and quality of life.**
Source: Copyright 1995 by Margaret Barton-Burke. All rights reserved. Used with written consent of the author.

CRF interventions difficult to explicate fully. Figure 17-3 illustrates various symptoms and side effects resulting from cancer treatment and suggests how CRF impacts HRQOL.

Evidence-based practice is becoming the standard in all clinical care with various organizations developing corresponding clinical practice guidelines (Mock, 2001; Portenoy & Itri, 1999). The National Comprehensive Cancer Network (NCCN) and the Oncology Nursing Society (ONS) are two organizations with evidenced-based guidelines for CRF (Berger et al., 2009; Cella, Davis, Brietbart, & Curt, 2001; Cella, Peterman, Passik, Jacobsen, & Brietbart, 1998; Mitchell, Beck, Hood, Moore, & Tanner, 2007). The guidelines from NCCN, initially developed in 2000, have been updated regularly (For guidelines, go to www.nccn.org or http://www.nccn.org/professionals/physician_gls/f_guidelines.asp).

These guidelines focus on standards of care, a screening algorithm based on mild and moderately severe CRF, and interventions for patients in treatment, in long-term follow-up, and at the end of life. Figures 17-4, 17-5, and 17-6 highlight the evidenced-based interventions for patients with CFR. The NCCN standards for CRF management were

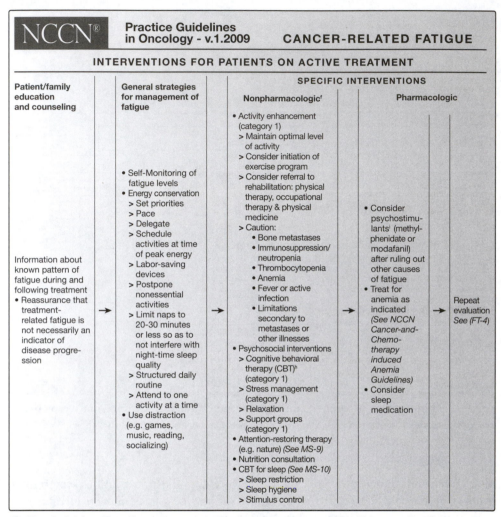

e See Discussion for information on differences between Active treatment, Long term follow-up, and End-of-life treatment. *(See MS-1).*
f Interventions should be culturally specific and tailored to the needs of patients and families because not all patients may be able to integrate these options due to variances in individual circumstances and resources. (Sahler OJZ, Varni JW, Fairclough DL, et ai. Problem-Solving Skills Training for Mothers of Children with Newly Diagnosed Cancer: A Randomized Trial. Journal of Developmental & Behavioral Pediatrics. 23(2):77-86, April 2002).
g Concern is with environment. Limit activity to environments where risk of infection is low.
h A type of psychotherapy that focuses on recognizing and changing maladaptive thoughts and behaviors to reduce negative emotions and facilitate psychological adjustment.
i Pharmacological interventions remain investigational, but have been reported to improve symptoms of fatigue in some patients. There is more evidence for methylphenidate and less for modafinil. These agents should be used cautiously and should not be used until treatment and disease specific morbidities have been characterized or excluded. Optimal dosing and schedule have not been established for use of psychostimulants in cancer patients.
NOTE: All recommendations are category 2A unless otherwise indicated.
Clinical Trials: NCCN believed that the best management of any cancer patient is in a clinical trial. Participation in clinical trials is especially encouraged.

Figure 17-4.   **NCCN interventions for patients on active treatment.**
Source: Reproduced with permission from the NCCN 1.2009 Cancer-Related Fatigue Clinical practice Guidelines in Oncology. Copyright National Comprehensive Cancer Netowkr, 2009. Available
at http://www.nccn.org. Accessed [month, day, year] To view the most recent and complete version
of the guideline, go online to www.nccn.org.

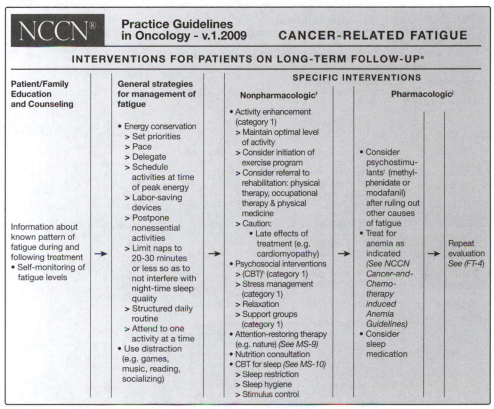

Source: Reproduced with permission from the NCCN 1.2009 Cancer-Related Fatigue Clinical practice Guidelines in Oncology. Copyright National Comprehensive Cancer Netowkr, 2009. Available at http://www.nccn.org. Accessed [month, day, year] To view the most recent and complete version of the guideline, go online to www.nccn.org.

Figure 17-5. NCCN interventions for patients on long-term follow-up.

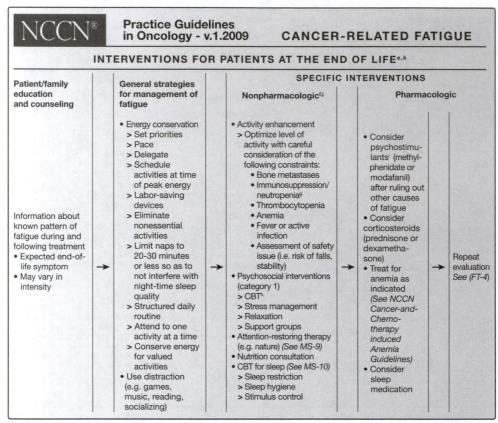

e Discussion for information on differences between Active treatment, Long term follow-up, and End-of-life treatment. *(See MS-1).*

f Interventions should be culturally specific and tailored to the needs of patients and families because not all patients may be able to integrate these options due to variances in individual circumstances and resources. (Sahler OJZ, Varni JW, Fairclough DL, et ai. Problem-Solving Skills Training for Mothers of Children with Newly Diagnosed Cancer: A Randomized Trial. Journal of Developmental & Behavioral Pediatrics. 23(2):77-86, April 2002).

g Concern is with environment. Limit activity to environments where risk of infection is low.

h A type of psychotherapy that focuses on recognizing and changing maladaptive thoughts and behaviors to reduce negative emotions and facilitate psychological adjustment.

i Pharmacological interventions remain investigational, but have been reported to improve symptoms of fatigue in some patients. There is more evidence for methylphenidate and less for modafinil. These agents should be used cautiously and should not be used until treatment and disease specific morbidities have been characterized or excluded. Optimal dosing and schedule have not been established for use of psychostimulants in cancer patients.

k Also See NCCN Palliative Care Guidelines.

NOTE: All recommendations are category 2A unless otherwise indicated.

Clinical Trials: NCCN believed that the best management of any cancer patient is in a clinical trial. Participation in clinical trials is especially encouraged.

Figure 17-6.   **NCCN interventions for patients at the end of life.**

Source: Reproduced with permission from the NCCN 1.2009 Cancer-Related Fatigue Clinical practice Guidelines in Oncology. Copyright National Comprehensive Cancer Netowkr, 2009. Available at http://www.nccn.org. Accessed [month, day, year] To view the most recent and complete version of the guideline, go online to www.nccn.org.

developed to guide care for children, adolescents, and adults. Like the NCCN, ONS worked on practice guidelines for a variety of clinical conditions including CRF. They also have a Web site for their practice guidelines that can be found at http://www.ons.org.

Cancer-related fatigue is not currently assessed systematically with existing assessment tools, but there is movement to make fatigue the sixth vital sign. In that way, healthcare providers would screen every patient for fatigue in the same way that they assess every patient for pain. The NCCN guidelines suggest that clinicians work toward regular assessment of CRF during both inpatient and outpatient encounters and inquire about co-occurring symptoms of pain, anxiety, depression, sleep disturbances, and anemia. Additionally, Piper and colleagues (2008) remind us to assess the gang of seven—anemia, pain, sleep difficulties, nutrition issues, deconditioning or changes in activity patterns, emotional distress (depression or anxiety), and presence of comorbidities.

Implementation of research-based interventions for CRF can be pharmacological or nonpharmacological. Pharmacological interventions include the treatment of fatigue related to anemia resulting from cancer treatment, the use of psycho-stimulants, and the use of antidepressants. Nonpharmacological interventions include exercise or activity enhancement, stress reduction interventions, patient and family education and counseling, attention-restoring activities, and nutrition.

Pharmacological interventions for treating anemia (epoetin alfa, darbepoetin alfa) have increased in use in recent years; their use is guided by national, institutional, and pharmacological guidelines (Rizzo et al., 2008). Psycho-stimulants such as methylphenidate and modafinil may also be considered in the treatment of fatigue (Berger et al., 2009). Antidepressants, like selective serotonin reuptake inhibitors like paroxetine, show no influence on CRF in patients receiving chemotherapy and antidepressants are no longer a recommended option (Mock et al., 2007). The nonpharmacological interventions for CRF include exercise or activity enhancement, stress reduction interventions, patient and family education and counseling, attention restoring activities, and nutrition.

Exercise is well established as a cost-effective intervention for CRF (Headley et al., 2004; Mock et al., 1994, 1997, 2001; Mock, 2003; Schwartz, 1998a, 2000; Schwartz, Thompson, & Masood, 2002; Winningham, 1991, 2001; Young-McCaughan & Sexton, 1991; Young-McCaughan et al., 2003). Studies have demonstrated consistently that physical exercise following cancer diagnosis has a positive effect on QOL, including physical, functional, psychological, and emotional well-being. A meta-analysis of 24 studies published from 1980–1997 (Courneya & Friedenreich, 1999) showed physical activity in patients with cancer resulted in improvements in functional capacity (Dimeo et al., 1996; Dimeo, Fetscher, Lange, Mertelsmann, & Keul, 1997; Dimeo, Tilmann, et al., 1997; MacVicar, Winningham, & Nickel, 1989; Mock et al., 1994, 1997) and improves QOL (Courneya & Friedenreich, 1999; Young-McCaughan & Sexton, 1991). Exercise improves sleep quality and decreases fatigue (Dimeo, Tilmann, et al., 1997; Mock et al., 1997), pain (Dimeo, Fetscher, et al., 1997), and depression (MacVicar & Winningham, 1986; Segar et al., 1999). Furthermore, fatigue is decreased dramatically when the patient has had a good night's sleep. Exercise may also ameliorate both the physical and emotional symptoms associated with cancer (Courneya & Friedenreich, 1999; Pinto, Eakin, & Maruyama, 2000; Pinto & Maruyama, 1999).

Physical and occupational therapists can assist in getting individuals prepared to exercise during and after their treatments. Stress management helps individuals deal with CRF, while patient and family education and counseling helps all members of the family understand what to expect during and after treatment.

Cimprich (1990, 1993, 1995, 1999) developed and tested an attention-restoring intervention she has named *Nature* or *being in a natural environment*. Cimprich's research findings indicate the outcomes of the attention-restoring intervention include improved concentration, problem-solving, and the ability to return to work earlier. Involving a nutritionist or dietitian in the assessment of CRF also can contribute to the overall understanding and treatment of fatigue. Cancer and its treatments can interfere with the physical functioning of patients including nutritional, psychological, and cognitive domains of HRQOL through the development of CRF. Healthcare providers are encouraged to intervene whenever possible using all available evidence to guide their clinical interventions.

Sleep Disturbances and Cancer

Sleep disturbances are another common complaint for the person with cancer (Engstrom, Strohl, Rose, Lewandowski, & Stefanek, 1999; Savard & Morin, 2001). One third to three fourths of people with cancer are thought to experience significant sleep disturbance—a rate twice that experienced by the general population (Berger, 2009; Clark, Cunningham, McMillan, Vena, & Parker, 2004; Koopman et al., 2002). Sleep disturbances are associated with the cancer process itself, as well as its treatment, occurring alongside other physiological and psychological symptoms, including CRF. A sleep disturbance is a disruption in active processes regulated by multiple behavioral, neuroendocrine, and central nervous system factors. Sleep disturbances include, but are not limited to, excessive daytime sleepiness, hypersomnolence, narcolepsy, difficulty falling asleep or awakening during the night, and dyssomnias.

In cancer patients, the most common sleep disturbance is insomnia. The *Diagnostic and Statistical Manual of Mental Disorders*, 4th edition (DSM IV) definition of insomnia is "difficulty initiating or maintaining sleep, or nonrestorative sleep, for at least one month that causes significant distress or impairment in social, occupational, or other important areas of functioning" (American Psychological Association, 1994). The American Academy of Sleep Medicine (2005) adds that the sleep problem occurs despite adequate opportunities and circumstances for sleep. For the majority of cancer patients with insomnia, the complaints are difficulty falling asleep, an inability to maintain sleep with multiple awakenings during the night, and not feeling rested in the morning (Fiorentino & Ancoli-Israel, 2007). Table 17-2 presents a few terms used when discussing sleep disturbances.

There are parallels between CRF and sleep disturbances. Both symptoms are seen in adults and children throughout the cancer disease trajectory and both are known to occur in patients and caregivers alike (Carter, 2003; Carter & Chang, 2000). Research findings

Table 17-2.   Terms Used for Sleep Disturbances

Awakenings during sleep period: The number of awakenings during a sleep period.

Circadian rhythm: Biobehavioral phenomenon associated with fluctuations in light, hormones, eating, and/or socializing that repeats every 24 hours.

Circadian rhythm sleep disorders: Recurrent or chronic patterns of sleep disturbance resulting from alterations of the circadian timing system or misalignment between an individual's rhythm and the 24-hour social and physical environments.

Excessive daytime sleepiness: Episodes of lapses into short-duration sleep, usually when a person is inactive for even brief periods; excessive daytime sleepiness can result from acute or chronic sleep deprivation or loss or other pathophysiologic causes.

Hypersomnias of central origin: Characterized by the primary complaint of daytime sleepiness not related to circadian rhythm sleep disorders, sleep-related breathing disorders, or other causes of disturbed nocturnal sleep.

Insomnias: Disorders that produce repeated difficulty with sleep initiation, duration, consolidation, or quality that occurs despite adequate time and opportunity for sleep and results in some form of daytime impairment.

Isolated symptoms, apparently normal variants, and unresolved issues: Symptoms that either lie at the borderline between normal and abnormal sleep or that exist on a continuum of normal to abnormal events in sleep (e.g., snoring).

Napping during the day: The total number of minutes of sleep during the daytime; may be intentional or unintentional.

Other sleep disorders: Disorders that cannot be classified elsewhere (e.g., other physiologic [organic] sleep disorders).

Parasomnias: Undesirable physical events or experiences that occur during entry into sleep, within sleep, or during arousal from sleep.

Quality of perceived sleep: Multidimensional perceptions of the length and depth of sleep and feelings of being rested on awakening; subjective assessment of sufficiency of sleep for daytime functioning.

Sleep efficiency: The number of minutes of sleep divided by the total number of minutes in bed, multiplied by 100.

Sleep latency: The number of minutes between the time an individual lays down to bed and actually goes to sleep.

Sleep-related breathing disorders: Characterized by disordered respiration during sleep.

Sleep-related movement disorders: Conditions that are characterized primarily by relatively simple, usually stereotyped movements that disturb sleep (e.g., periodic limb movements).

(continues)

Table 17-2. **Terms Used for Sleep Disturbances (continued)**

Sleep-wake disturbances: Perceived or actual alterations in night sleep with resultant daytime impairment. Among the most common sleep disturbances are insomnia, sleep-related breathing disorders, and sleep-related movement disorders (e.g., restless leg syndrome, periodic limb movement disorder). General criteria for insomnia include having difficulty initiating sleep, having difficulty maintaining sleep, and waking too early, as well as sleep that is chronically nonrestorative or poor in quality that occurs despite adequate opportunity and circumstances for sleep.

Total sleep time while in bed: The number of minutes of sleep while in bed.

Wake time after sleep onset: The number of minutes awake or the percentage of time awake after sleep onset during the sleep period.

Source: Adapted from Berger et al., (2005).

and clinical observations link sleep disturbances in cancer patients with CRF. According to Mock and colleagues (2007), CRF affects HRQOL as patients become too tired to participate in meaningful activities. Insomnia is associated with decreased HRQOL for patients, especially those with cancer (Page, Berger, & Johnson, 2006). Sleep disturbance in cancer patients is a unique symptom that has gained attention in recent years (Ancoli-Israel, Moore, & Jones, 2001; Berger, 1998, 2009; Berger et al., 2003; Carpenter et al., 2004; Clark, Cunningham, McMillian, Vena, & Parker, 2004; Davidson, MacLean, Brundage, & Schulze, 2002; Hinds et al., 1999; Roscoe et al., 2002; Vena, Parker, Cunningham, Clark, & McMillian, 2004).

Sleep Disturbances Research and Cancer

The following models and frameworks have guided the study of sleep disturbances related in some way to CRF. Piper's Integrated Fatigue Model has been used consistently by researchers who study sleep disturbances as a result of CRF (Berger & Farr, 1999; Berger & Johnson, 2004; Berger et al., 2002, 2003, 2005). The Wilson and Cleary Conceptual Model of Patient Outcomes (1995) has been used to study fatigue and physical activity in hematopoietic stem transplantation (Hacker et al., 2006). The Theory of Unpleasant Symptoms (Lenz, Suppe, Gift, Pugh, & Milligan, 1995; Lenz, Pugh, Milligan, Gift, & Suppe, 1997) has been used by Carpenter and colleagues (2004), and the Roy Adaptation Model (Roy & Andrews, 1991) was used by Young-McCaughan and associates (2003) and Mock and associates (1997). Losito, Murphy, and Thomas (2006) developed their own multidimensional framework integrating multiple physical and psychological effects of cancer treatment and CRF with group dynamics and exercise. Payne and colleagues (2006) used a biobehavioral conceptual framework that posits both physiological and psychological factors, including neuroendocrine components that are associated with fatigue, sleep disturbance, and depressive symptoms.

The Model of Symptom Management (Dodd, Janson, et al., 2001; Dodd, Miaskowski, 2001) had been gaining wide use and has been used by Lee and colleagues (2001; Lee, Cho, et al., 2004; Lee, Landis, et al., 2004) to study impaired sleep. In that study, they suggest impaired sleep leads to various physiological, cognitive-behavioral, emotional, and social outcomes. A co-occurrence or cluster involving both sleep disturbances and CRF also includes depression or anxiety and pain. It is possible and entirely plausible as our knowledge develops in the area of CRF and sleep disturbances that we will determine the relationships between these two symptoms and all the symptoms that co-occur in cancer patients, especially those of depression or anxiety and pain. Additionally, we should determine the prevalence of sleep disturbance and its association with function and HRQOL.

Two other sleep-specific models are detailed elsewhere (Borbely, 1982; Borbely, Dijk, Acherman, & Tobler, 2001; Spielman & Glovinksy, 2004); they include the Two-Process Model of Sleep Regulation and the Predisposing, Precipitating, and Perpetuating (PPP) Model. A basic understanding of these models, and of sleep architecture, suggests mechanisms affecting sleep in cancer and understanding these models helps make sense of suggested interventions presented later in the chapter.

The Two-Process Model involves process S, the need to sleep, and process C, circadian rhythm. Process S increases as the length of time a person has been awake increases. Sleep onset is delayed if there is stimulation of the sympathetic nervous system or the hypothalamic-pituitary-adrenal axis. In order to maintain sleep without interruption, the thalamus must filter out this type of stimulation continually. Simultaneously, circadian rhythms are generated and synchronized by light and dark cues from the environment. Sleep onset usually begins in conjunction with declining body temperature and one to two hours after an evening rise in melatonin. This process is influenced also by central nervous system neurotransmitter and neuroendocrine factors, including growth hormone and prostaglandins (Berger et al., 2005). The PPP model proposes predisposing, precipitating, and perpetuating factors that increase risk for, trigger, or reinforce insomnia. The Two-Process Model suggests the process involved with sleep, while the PPP Model suggests factors such as biology and situation that contribute to sleep disturbances, specifically insomnia.

A normal, or typical, night of sleep includes four to six cycles of non-rapid eye movement (non-REM) and rapid eye movement (REM) sleep. Sleep begins as non-REM, when mental activity slows, but voluntary muscle control remains intact. Non-REM is a continuum of four stages, with stage one being the lightest level of sleep and four the deepest. After progressing from non-REM stage one to four and back to one, the individual enters REM sleep with increased brain activity and a paralyzed body. Each cycle lasts 90–110 minutes (Vena et al., 2004).

While further research is needed to understand the mechanisms by which cancer affects sleep, as well as the non-REM and REM stages of sleep, studies have demonstrated changes in cortisol production and melatonin secretion in people with certain types of cancers (Berger et al., 2005; Vena et al., 2004). Cytokines produced by cancer cells, and those used to treat it, affect the central nervous system and impact sleep regulation. An increase in cytokines in response to radiation therapy has been thought to promote increased daytime sleepiness and nighttime sleep problems. Hot flashes induced by chemo- or hormonal therapy are associated with awakenings as well (Mormont & Levi, 1997; Vena et al., 2004).

Cancer is a disease of the elderly and changes in sleep architecture are known to accompany old age. People with cancer are likely to be taking one or more medicines known to increase the propensity for sleep problems, such as corticosteroids, benzodiazepines, antiemetics, and opioids. While several classes of drugs increase sleepiness, the associated quality of restorative sleep may be poor as REM sleep and deep sleep actually may be decreased. Psychological distress, pain, and gastrointestinal symptoms are also common and may trigger difficulties with sleep.

Dr. Berger and colleagues (2006) noted biological outcomes of sleep are unsettled and there remain the following challenges: (1) a lack of standard procedures to determine a successful sleep intervention; (2) no agreement on sleep intervention endpoints—is it a good night's sleep, or feeling rested after sleep, or sleeping for a given number of hours, among other less well defined endpoints; (3) discrepancies in how best to measure intended outcomes; and (4) patient self-reports as a proxy for perceived quality of sleep. Our knowledge about quality of sleep as a symptom experience is rudimentary and our exploration of sleep disturbance as a scientific endeavor in persons with cancer is only beginning to emerge. Despite our preliminary stage of understanding about sleep disturbances, cancer, and CRF, several national agencies have identified sleep disturbances as a priority research area (Institute of Medicine, 2005).

Measurement

Scientists recognize the need for randomized, controlled clinical trials that use valid, reliable, and clinically relevant measurement tools. Evidence-based guidelines depend upon the development and use of such instruments in a standardized manner. Measurement tools used in the literature to measure sleep disturbances include biomedical instruments like sleep encephalograms, polysomnography, actigraphy, and a variety of sleep tests and self-reports like the Pittsburgh Sleep Quality Index. Paper and pencil tests like the Piper Fatigue Scale, Symptom Distress Scale of the Profile of Mood States (POMS), the Lee Fatigue Scale, Brief Fatigue Inventory, and Sleep Hygiene Awareness and Practice Scale (Beck, Schwartz, Towsley, Dudley, & Barsevick, 2004; Buysse, Reynolds, Monk, Berman, & Kupfer, 1989; Carpenter & Andrykowski, 1998; Hauri & Wisbey, 1992; Littner et al., 2003; Sadeh, Hauri, Kripke, & Lavie, 1995) are also used.

Polysomnography is considered the gold standard for measuring sleep because it objectively records brain waves, eye movement, muscle tension, and other biological signs such as heart and respiratory rates. Actigraphy is a highly reliable, though indirect, measure of sleep based on a special algorithm and recorded movement with a device about the size of a wrist watch (Fiorentino & Ancoli-Israel, 2007). Actigraphy may be preferable when studying sleep in persons with cancer as it is less cumbersome. Experts propose a collection of nine parameters for measurement in all studies of sleep regarding people with cancer: total sleep time, sleep latency, awakenings, wake time after sleep onset, napping during the day, excessive daytime sleepiness, quality of perceived sleep, stability of circadian rhythms, and sleep efficiency. The Pittsburgh Sleep Quality Index has been validated in patients with cancer and is highly recommended for assessing all nine sleep parameters except sleep efficiency (Berger et al., 2005).

In much of the existing research, sleep disturbances were measured as a correlate of, associated with, or linked in some way to CRF. In a few instances, sleep disturbances are measured as independent variables. More research is needed in this area in order to develop the evidence necessary to treat sleep disturbances effectively. Also, as evidence grows about sleep disturbances, healthcare providers will be able to help cancer patients better understand the effects of sleep disturbances and the impact on CRF, function, and HRQOL.

Clinical Implications

Healthcare providers know cancer patients have disturbed sleep and research supports this clinical observation (Mormont et al., 2000). Providers may not know the extent to which these sleep disturbances affect activities of daily living, function, and HRQOL. Consequences of poor sleep include cognitive impairment, functional decline, fatigue, pain and discomfort, loss of enjoyment, mood disturbance, trouble with relationships, and altered immune and neuroendocrine function. Often a cyclical relationship develops between insomnia and its negative outcomes, in a sense one perpetuating the other. A sleep assessment is fundamental to clinical practice, but is often neglected because of other, possibly more pressing clinical issues. Quite often, if sleep is assessed and found to be a problem, the intervention is pharmacological.

Despite the common experience of sleep disturbance in all phases of cancer care, few cancer patients report this symptom to their care providers. All patients need initial and ongoing screening in both inpatient and ambulatory settings. The Clinical Sleep Assessment for Adults and the Clinical Sleep Assessment for Children are tools that are easily administered for clinical purposes and have excellent face validity. Sleep diaries are also recommended in patients experiencing sleep problems (Berger et al., 2005).

Screening tools that are quick and easy to use should be developed for clinical practice settings. Tools such as the Quick Fatigue Assessment Survey (Quick & Fonteyn, 2005) and others currently are available for use in practice. These screening tools could be integrated into oncology clinical practice, but even easier is asking questions like, "Are you having sleep problems or difficulty staying awake during the day?" (Quick & Fonteyn, 2005). Data gathered from either a formal assessment tool or mere questioning will help providers make referrals for further evaluation, if necessary.

Clinical Interventions

Clinical assessment data gained from either a tool or a question assists healthcare providers in developing appropriate interventions, although to date there is little evidence-based practice from which to design such care. The Oncology Nursing Society (ONS) Putting Evidence into Practice Guidelines (PEP) for sleep and wake disturbances offer a starting point, but there is a need for more research in this area (Page et al., 2006). To date, interventions that increase self-awareness and self-management (e.g., sleep hygiene), or self-monitoring of the negative effects of sleep disturbance (e.g., excessive daytime sleepiness) are the practice standard.

Pharmacological Interventions

Healthcare providers should evaluate the person with cancer for both the need and the effectiveness of pharmacological intervention. Benzodiazepines such as diazepam, triazolam, clonazepam, and nonbenzodiazepines such as zolpidem tartrate, zaleplon, and eszopiclone can contribute to sleep disturbances by causing daytime sleepiness due to half-lives, or possibly as a result of more time spent in non-REM and light sleep stages. Patients should be informed of expected outcomes and risks when prescribed a hypnotic or sedative. Such medications should not be used if the individual has less than eight hours to sleep. Older individuals and those who are at risk for falls must be cautioned in the use of benzodiazepines and hypnotics, as well as their increased risk for subsequent cognitive impairment, functional impairment, falls, and falls with injury. Even shorter acting benzodiazepines and lower dose hypnotics, like 5-mg zolpidem, were once thought to be safer alternatives, yet still carry these risks. (Fick et al., 2003; Wang, Bohn, Glynn, Mogun, & Avorn, 2001).

Diphenhydramine, an anticholinergic antihistamine, is strongly associated with delirium and other adverse events such as urinary catheter placement and increased length of stay when administered to hospitalized older adults (Agostini, Leo-Summers, & Inouye, 2001). A meta-analysis of 20 randomized controlled trials (RCTs) involving more than 2400 older adults concluded that an adverse event is more than twice as likely when this population is administered a sedative or hypnotic (Glass, Lanctot, Herrmann, Sproule, & Busto, 2005). Ramelteon, a melatonin receptor agonist, is a promising alternative as it has no opioid, gabba, benzo, histamine, or dopamine receptor activity. However, it is too early to know its clinical effectiveness.

Additional drugs like tricyclic antidepressants, second-generation antidepressants, antihistamines, chloral derivatives, and neuroleptics are used less commonly, but may be considered to improve sleep. Certain antidepressants may enhance sleep while also treating depression, poor appetite, neuropathic pain, hot flashes, and night sweats. The National Cancer Institute's PDQ Sleep Disorders Web site can be accessed for more information (http://www.cancer.gov/cancertopics/pdq/supportivecare/sleepdisorders/healthprofessional).

In 2004, a panel of experts convened to review the evidence to inform treatment of sleep disturbances in people with cancer. No studies have been designed specifically to measure the efficacy of sedatives or hypnotics in cancer patients. Most studies involve primary insomniacs and healthy volunteers. Five meta-analyses of the effectiveness of hypnotics were published between 1997 and 2004 and indicate that benzodiazepines and non-benzodiazepine hypnotics improve self-reported sleep measures. The clinical significance of these conclusions may be questionable. In a meta-analysis of 45 randomized, controlled trials including 2672 patients, sleep latency was an average of four minutes less and sleep duration one hour longer in those taking a benzodiazepine compared to those taking placebo. Outcome measures across studies were inconsistent and most studies were brief

(Berger et al., 2005). There is widespread use of benzodiazepines with little research to substantiate the efficacy of hypnotic drugs in cancer patients.

Similarly, no published meta-analyses or experimental design studies were found specific to the efficacy of herbal therapy in people with cancer (Holbrook, Crowther, Lotter, Cheng, & King, 2000; Nowell et al., 1997). People with cancer are instructed not to take kava or St. John's wort due to safety concerns, including adverse reactions and herb-drug interactions (Block, Gyllenhaal, & Mead, 2004).

Non-Pharmacological Interventions

One meta-analysis reviewed by the ONS PEP team concluded the duration of effects from behavioral therapy was significantly longer than those from treatment with medication in the general population (Berger et al., 2005; Morin, Culbert, & Schwartz, 1994). Sleep latency decreased by 30% with medication and by 43% with behavioral therapy. Wake time after sleep onset (WTASO) decreased by 46% with medication and by 56% with behavioral therapy.

Given the potential for serious adverse effects of medications in the elderly, efforts must be employed to utilize and study non-pharmacological sleep strategies in older cancer patients experiencing sleep difficulties. In pilot studies, non-pharmacological sleep protocols that combine strategies such as noise reduction, personal hygiene, backrubs, soothing music, and warm non-caffeinated beverages have demonstrated success in reducing the use of hypnotics or sedatives and improving sleep in hospitalized older adults (Inouye, 2000; LaReau, Benson, & Watcharotone, 2008).

Cancer patients should be made aware of the need for sleep as a way to improve their overall function. They should be given information about sleep hygiene (Lacks & Rotert, 1986; Simeit, Deck, & Conta-Marx, 2004) that includes going to bed only when sleepy and at approximately the same time each night, maintaining a regular daily rising time, and avoiding daytime napping. Sleep hygiene techniques (e.g., avoiding caffeine after noon, completing dinner three hours before bedtime, not going to bed hungry, keeping the bedroom cool and the covers light, not keeping a television in the bedroom) are simple tools that can be suggested to patients in an attempt to improve their sleep. A randomized, controlled clinical trial showed favorable sleep outcomes using psychoeducational or informational interventions for both men and women with cancer (Kim, Roscoe, & Morrow, 2002). Although not research-based, complementary care strategies, including expressive therapy, expressive writing, massage, mindfulness-based stress reduction, progressive muscle relaxation, and yoga, offer the person with cancer self-management tools that help them feel in control of what is known in an often out of control situation (Shapiro, Bootzin, Figueredo, Lopez, & Schwartz, 2003).

The Symptom Dyad of CRF and Sleep Disturbances

Clinical experience suggests patients with cancer often present with multiple symptoms. The symptom dyad of CRF and sleep disturbances has been reported along with pain, anxiety, and depression (Ancoli-Israel et al., 2001; Anderson et al., 2003; Armstrong et al., 2004; Berger & Farr, 1999; Berger & Johnson, 2004; Berger et al., 2002, 2003, 2005; Cimprich, 1999; Dodd et al., 2001; Hockenberry-Eaton & Hinds, 2000; Lee, 2001; Lee, Cho, et al., 2004; Lee, Landis, et al., 2004; Sarna, 1993; Visovsky & Schneider, 2003). Other factors affecting CRF and sleep disturbances include night sweats, hot flashes, diarrhea, constipation, and nighttime urination.

Despite a growing body of knowledge, there is limited scientific evidence about the complex interplay between CRF and sleep disturbances. Research findings from several studies suggest sleep disturbance may be part of a syndrome of co-occuring symptoms that includes pain, depression or anxiety, and fatigue (Dodd, Janson, et al., 2001; Dodd, Miaskowski, et al., 2001; Given et al., 2001, 2002; Gift, Stommel, Jablonski, & Given, 2003; Gift, Jablonski, Stommel, & Given, 2004; Redeker, Lev, & Ruggiero, 2000; Sadler et al., 2002). In most of the studies to date, this co-occurring syndrome of pain, depression or anxiety, fatigue, and sleep disturbance was associated with poorer functional status or decreased HRQOL (Given et al., 1994; Given, Given, Azzouz, Kozachik, et al., 2001; Given, Given, Azzouz, & Stommel, 2001; Hockenberry-Eaton & Hinds, 2000; Mock et al., 1997).

The answer to the question of which comes first remains largely unknown. Most research on CRF and sleep disturbances has been conducted during or immediately after treatment, defined as a period of no more than 2 years (Berger & Farr, 1999; Berger & Higginbotham, 2000; Berger et al., 2002, 2003; Boehmke, 2004; Cimprich, 1999; Davidson et al., 2001; Given, Given, Azzouz, Kozachik, et al., 2001; Given, Given, Azzouz, & Stommel, 2001; Hann et al., 1997; Kolb & Poetscher, 1997; Mormont et al., 2000). Information on the symptoms of CRF and sleep disturbances in long-term cancer survivors is limited to a few articles studying women with breast cancer (Andrykowski et al., 1998; Bower et al., 2000; Broeckel et al., 1998; Servaes et al., 2002). Research beyond 5 years is almost nonexistent, leaving substantial gaps in the scientific knowledge about CRF and sleep disturbances (Cella et al., 2001).

Interventions such as exercise, psycho-educational, and structured educational programs are proving to be effective with CRF and sleep disturbances in cancer patients who are in active treatment or the early posttreatment period. Extrapolating these findings, applying them to persons with cancer at varying points in the disease trajectory, and then testing the intervention may prove worthwhile (Allison et al., 2004; Christman et al., 2001; Kim et al., 2002; Mock, 2003; Young-McCaughlin et al., 2003).

Clinical nurses and advanced practice nurses often are the first healthcare team members to hear patient complaints of the co-occurring symptoms of CRF and sleep disturbances. Healthcare providers need to systematically assess cancer patients using consistent tools that are or become familiar to patients. For example, fatigue can be assessed with a 1 to 10 point rating scale similar to those used for pain assessments. An increasing number of patients now are used to answering the fatigue question. Once their fatigue is self-rated, a follow-up question could be asked such as: "How are you sleeping?" Helping patients understand the connection between these two symptoms, and the importance of reporting both CRF and sleep disturbances, may assist healthcare teams (including the patient) to realize that, in many situations, these symptoms remain long after treatment is complete and life resumes.

CONCLUSION

As individuals with cancer and their families focus on managing their disease, their normal lives, including jobs, homes, friends, pursuits of interest, as well as the basic activities of daily living and HRQOL, remain important to them. Fatigue and sleep disturbances often disrupt the patient's ability and desire to accomplish valuable role functioning, thereby diminishing one's perceived HRQOL. The dearth and disparity in the literature regarding theoretical descriptions, explanations, and predictors of CRF and the sleep disturbance phenomenon support the need for ongoing research in the area of HRQOL (Barton-Burke, 1998). Cancer-related fatigue remains a difficult symptom to manage and an illusive concept to study, but it is a real phenomenon to the individual experiencing this symptom and is a constant reminder of cancer. As we learn more about CRF and sleep disturbances, we begin to understand the relationship between CRF and sleep disturbances as co-occurring symptoms. Research supports the fact that CRF is impacted by sleep disturbances, suggesting a more complex phenomenon, such as a symptom cluster. Because there is a significant discrepancy currently existing between a provider's perception of a patient's CRF and a patient's own experience, providers might consider CRF and sleep disturbances as a syndrome that can be treated with a variety of pharmacological and non-pharmacological interventions proposed by evidence-based national guidelines.

An assessment of CRF and sleep disturbances can determine the best therapeutic, prophylactic, and palliative interventions, and research is necessary to test their feasibility. This work should be conducted by multidisciplinary teams of researchers and clinicians. Cancer-related fatigue and sleep disturbances occur in conjunction with other symptoms such as pain, anxiety, and/or depression. A common set of criteria should be developed in order to diagnose the symptom dyad of CRF and sleep disturbances, with or without the concomitant symptoms, as either co-occurring symptoms, a symptom cluster, or as a clinical syndrome.

Current research offers an initial understanding of the complex, multifactorial, and multidimensional problem of CFR. These studies underpin current knowledge about CRF and sleep disturbances and form a basis for understanding the cancer survivorship trajectory. However, data is scarce and what exists is conflicting, making it difficult to understand the phenomenon of CRF and sleep disturbances. Research continues on both CRF and sleep disturbances in order to understand the phenomena, to test interventions, and to add to evidence-based clinical practice, but more work is necessary to understand the interrelationship between CRF and sleep disturbances. Research about the patient's environment is necessary to determine the environment's role as a causal, modifying, or associated variable. Also, outcomes research on irritability, lack of concentration, difficulty making decisions, and the impact on significant aspects of a person's life, including family, family caregivers, and school, work, and social life is important. Ongoing research about the amount of fatigue and/or sleep disturbances, distress or degree of unpleasantness associated with fatigue and/or sleep disturbances, effect of fatigue and/or sleep disturbances on activities of daily living, and associated biological parameters is an important aspect that can be translated into education and practice.

The education of healthcare professionals requires information about CRF and sleep disturbances. Suggestions to incorporate CRF and sleep disturbances into educational curricula are impractical. Instead, healthcare professional students should learn about the side effects and symptoms of cancer therapy, but also realize there are resources such as practice guidelines, standards of practice, and competencies, available for these co-occurring symptoms. Prescribing members of the multidisciplinary team should realize they could and/or should refer patients to accredited sleep disorder centers or a sleep specialist. Staff development offerings, grand rounds, and clinical talks could focus on these symptoms as well. In clinical practice, exercise, psycho-educational, and structured educational programs are proving to be effective interventions during treatment, in the early posttreatment period, and extending into the cancer survivor group as well. Assessing and identifying at-risk populations and developing and testing supportive care measures are important tasks.

Finally, as we become a more multicultural society, we must remember fatigue may not be a word with which the patient population is familiar, and other words, such as Qi (Chi), may be the term necessary for a healthcare provider to use when assessing a person of Chinese descent. Imagine the complexity of the assessment when this individual has CRF and sleep disturbances as co-occurring symptoms.

This chapter offers a snapshot of the research available about the co-occurring symptoms of cancer-related fatigue and sleep disturbances. There is a growing body of research available about both of these symptoms. The knowledge development of each symptom individually and combined will yield evidence and interventions to be used with cancer patients in the future.

References

Agostini, J. V., Leo-Summers, L. S., & Inouye, S. K. (2001). Cognitive and other adverse effects of diphendhydramine use in hospitalized older patients. *Archives of Internal Medicine, 161*, 2091–2097.

Aistars, J. (1987). Fatigue in the cancer patient: A conceptual approach to a clinical problem. *Oncology Nursing Forum, 14*, 25–30.

Allison, P. J., Edgar, L., Nicolau, B., Archer, J., Black, M., & Hier, M. (2004). Results of a feasibility study for a psycho-educational intervention in head and neck cancer. *Psycho-oncology, 13*, 482–485.

American Academy of Sleep Medicine. (2005). *International classification of sleep disorders: Diagnostic and coding manual* (2nd ed.). Westchester, IL: Author.

American Psychological Association. (1994). *Diagnostic and statistical manual of mental disorders* (4th ed.). Washington, DC: Author.

Ancoli-Israel, S., Moore, P. J., & Jones, V. (2001). The relationship between fatigue and sleep in cancer patients: A review. *European Journal of Cancer Care, 10*, 245–255.

Anderson, K. O., Getto, C. J., Mendoza, T., Palmer, S. N., Wang, X. S., Reyes-Gibby, C. C., et al. (2003). Fatigue and sleep disturbances in patients with cancer, patients with clinical depression, and community-dwelling adults. *Journal of Pain and Symptom Management, 25*, 307–318.

Andrykowski, M. A., Carpenter, J. S., Greiner, C. B., Altmaier, E. M., Burish, T. G., Antin, J. H., et al. (1997). Energy level and sleep quality following bone marrow transplantation. *Bone Marrow Transplantation, 20*, 669–679.

Andrykowski, M. A., Curran, S. L., & Lightner, R. (1998). Off-treatment fatigue in breast cancer survivors: A controlled comparison. *Journal of Behavioral Medicine, 21*, 1–18.

Ardestani, S. K., Inserra, P., Solkoff, D., & Watson, R. R. (1999). The role of cytokines and chemokines on tumor progression: A review. *Cancer Detection and Prevention, 23*, 215–225.

Armstrong, T. S., Cohen, M. Z., Eriksen, L. R., & Hickey, J. V. (2004). Symptom management in oncology patients and implications for symptom research in people with primary brain tumors. *Journal of Nursing Scholarship, 36*, 197–206.

Barnes, E. A., & Bruera, E. (2002). Fatigue in patients with advanced cancer. A review. *International Journal of Gynecological Cancer, 12*, 424–431.

Bartley, S. H. (1965). *Fatigue: Mechanism and management.* Springfield, IL: Charles C. Thomas.

Bartley, S. H., & Chute, E. (1947). *Fatigue and impairment in man.* New York, NY: McGraw Hill.

Barton-Burke, M. (1998). Cancer-related fatigue: A holistic view. *Progress in Palliative Care, 6*, 153–159.

Barton-Burke, M. (2002). *Breast cancer experiences: Women's reflections years after diagnosis.* Ann Arbor, MI: UMI Company.

Barton-Burke, M. (2006a). Cancer-related fatigue and sleep disturbances: Further research on the prevalence of these two symptoms in long-term cancer survivors can inform education, policy, and clinical practice. *Cancer Nursing, 29*(2), 72–77.

Barton-Burke, M. (2006b). Fatigue and sleep disturbances in long-term survivors of cancer: State of the science on nursing approaches to manage long-term sequelae of cancer and cancer therapy. *American Journal of Nursing, 106*(3, Suppl.), 71–77.

Beck, S. L., Schwartz, A. L., Towsley, G., Dudley, W., & Barsevick, A. (2004). Psychometric evaluation of the Pittsburgh Sleep Quality Index in cancer patients. *Journal of Pain and Symptom Management, 27*, 140–148.

Berger, A. (1998). Patterns of fatigue and activity and rest during adjuvant breast cancer chemotherapy. *Oncology Nursing Forum, 25*, 51–62.

Berger, A. (2009). Update on the state of the science: Sleep-wake disturbances in adult patients with cancer. *Oncology Nursing Forum, 36*(4), E165–E177.

Berger, A., Abernathy, A. P., Atkinson, A., Barsevick, A. M., Breitbart, W., Cella, D., et al. (2009). Cancer-related fatigue NCCN guidelines, *1.* Retrieved from http://www.canceradvocacy.org/.

Berger, A., & Farr, L. (1999). The influence of daytime inactivity and nighttime restlessness on cancer-related fatigue. *Oncology Nursing Forum, 26*(10), 1663–1671.

Berger, A., & Higginbotham, P. (2000). Correlates of fatigue during and following adjuvant breast cancer chemotherapy: A pilot study. *Oncology Nursing Forum, 27*, 1443–1448.

Berger, A. M., & Johnson, P. J. (2004). Relationship between sleep/wake patterns and fatigue after chemotherapy: A comparison of diary versus actigraphs. Retrieved February 11, 2005, from http://www.nursingsociety.org/education/CS0100/cs0100_index.html.

Blesch, K. S., Paice, J. A., Wickham, R., Harte, N., Schnor, D., Purl, S., et al. (1991). Correlates of fatigue in people with breast or lung cancer. *Oncology Nursing Forum, 18*, 81–90.

Block, K. I., Gyllenhaal, C., & Mead, M. N. (2004). Safety and efficacy of herbal sedatives in cancer care. *Integrative Cancer Therapies, 3*, 128–148.

Boehmke, M. (2004). Measurement of symptom distress in women with early-stage breast cancer. *Cancer Nursing, 27*, 144–152.

Borbely, A. (1982). A two-process model of sleep regulation. *Human Neurobiology, 1*, 195–204.

Borbely, A. A., Dijk, D. J., Acherman, P., & Tobler, I. (2001). Processes underlying the regulation of the sleep-wake cycle. In J. S. Takahashi, F. W. Turek, & R. Y. Moore (Eds.), *Handbook of behavioral neurobiology: Circadian clock* (pp. 458–479). New York, NY: Kluwer Academic/Plenum.

Bower, J. E., Ganz, P. A., Aziz, N., & Fahey, J. L. (2002). Fatigue and proinflammatory cytokine activity in breast cancer survivors. *Psychosomatic Medicine, 64*(4), 604–611.

Bower, J. E., Ganz, P. A., Desmond, K. A., Rowland, J. H., Meyerowitz, B. E., & Belin, T. R. (2000). Fatigue in breast cancer survivors: Occurrence, correlates, and impact on quality of life. *Journal of Clinical Oncology, 18*, 743–753.

Broeckel, J. A., Jacobsen, P. B., Horton, J., Balducci, L., & Lyman, G. H. (1998). Characteristics and correlates of fatigue after adjuvant chemotherapy for breast cancer. *Journal of Clinical Oncology, 16,* 1689–1696.

Brunier, G. M. & Graydon, J. (1993). The influence of physical activity on fatigue in patients with ESRD on hemodialysis. *American Nephrology Nurses Association Journal, 20*(4), 457–461.

Buchsel, P. C., Barton-Burke, M., & Winningham, M. L. (2000). Treatment: An overview. In M. L. Winningham, & M. Barton-Burke (Eds.), *Fatigue in cancer: A multdimensional approach* (pp. 153–169). Sudbury, MA: Jones and Bartlett.

Buysse, D. J., Reynolds, C. F., III, Monk, T. H., Berman, S. R., & Kupfer, D. J. (1989). The Pittsburgh Sleep Quality Index: A new instrument for psychiatric practice and research. *Psychiatry Research, 28,* 193–213.

Carpenter, J. S., & Andrykowski, M. A. (1998). Psychometric evaluation of the Pittsburgh Sleep Quality Index. *Journal of Psychosomatic Research, 45*(1), 5–13.

Carpenter, J. S., Elam, J. L., Ridner, S. H., Carney, P. H., Cherry, G. J., & Cucullu, H. L. (2004). Sleep, fatigue, and depressive symptoms in breast cancer survivors and matched healthy women experiencing hot flashes. *Oncology Nursing Forum, 31,* 591–598.

Carter, P. A. (2003). Family caregivers' sleep loss and depression over time. *Cancer Nursing, 26,* 253–259.

Carter, P. A., & Chang, B. L. (2000). Sleep and depression in cancer caregivers. *Cancer Nursing, 23,* 410–415.

Cella, D. (1997). The Functional Assessment of Cancer Therapy–Anemia (FACT-An) scale: A new tool for the assessment of outcomes in cancer anemia and fatigue. *Seminars in Hematology, 34*(Suppl. 2), 13–19.

Cella, D., Davis, K., Breitbart, W., & Curt, G. For the Fatigue Coalition. (2001). Cancer-related fatigue: Prevalence of proposed diagnostic criteria in a United States sample of cancer survivors. *Journal of Clinical Oncology, 19,* 3385–3391.

Cella, D., Peterman, A., Passik, S., Jacobsen, P. B., & Breitbart, W. (1998). Progress toward guidelines for the management of fatigue. *Oncology, 12,*1–9.

Cella, D. & Tulsky, D. S. (1990). Measuring quality of life today: Methodological aspects. *Oncology, 4*(5), 29–38.

Christen, T., Stage, J. G., Galbo, H., Christensen, N. J., & Kehlet, H. (1989). Fatigue and cardiac and endocrine metabolic response to exercise after abdominal surgery. *Surgery, 105,* 46–50.

Christman, N. J., Oakley, M. G., & Cronin, S. N. (2001). Developing and using preparatory information for women undergoing radiation therapy for cervical or uterine cancer. *Oncology Nursing Forum, 28,* 93–98.

Cimprich, B. (1990). Attentional fatigue in the cancer patient. *Oncology Nursing Forum, 17,* 218.

Cimprich, B. (1992). A theoretical perspective on attention and patient education. *Advances in Nursing Science, 14,* 39–51.

Cimprich, B. (1993). Development of an intervention to restore attention in cancer patients. *Cancer Nursing, 16,* 83–92.

Cimprich, B. (1995). Symptom management: Loss of concentration. *Seminars in Oncology Nursing, 11,* 279–288.

Cimprich, B. (1999). Pretreatment symptom distress in women newly diagnosed with breast cancer. *Cancer Nursing, 22,* 185–194.

Clark, J., Cunningham, M., McMillan, S., Vena, C., & Parker, K. (2004). Sleep-wake disturbances in people with cancer, part II: Evaluating the evidence for clinical decision making. *Oncology Nursing Forum, 31,* 747–771.

Collado-Hidalgo, A., Bower, J. E., Ganz, P. A., Cole, S. W., & Irwin, M. R. (2006). Inflammatory biomarkers for persistent fatigue in breast cancer survivors. *Clinical Cancer Research, 12*(9), 2759–2766.

Costanzo, E. S., Lutgendorf, S. K., Sood, A. K., Anderson, B., Sorosky, J., & Lubaroff, D. M. (2005). Psychosocial factors and interleukin-6 among women with advanced ovarian cancer. *Cancer, 104*(2), 305–313.

Courneya, K. S., & Friedenreich, C. M. (1999). Physical exercise and quality of life following cancer diagnosis: A literature review. *Annals of Behavioral Medicine, 21*(2), 171–179.

Davidson, J. R., MacLean, A. W., Brundage, M. D., & Schulze, K. (2002). Sleep disturbance in cancer patients. *Social Science and Medicine, 54*, 1309–1321.

Davidson, J. R., Waisberg, J. L., Brundage, M. D., & MacLean, A. W. (2001). Nonpharmacologic group treatment of insomnia: A preliminary study with cancer survivors. *Psycho-oncology, 10*, 389–397.

Dimeo, F., Bertz, H., Finke, J., Fetscher, S., Mertelsmann, R., & Keul, J. (1996). An aerobic exercise program for patients with haematological malignancies after bone marrow transplantation. *Bone Marrow Transplantation, 18*, 1157–1160.

Dimeo, F., Fetscher, S., Lange, W., Mertelsmann, R., & Keul, J. (1997). Effects of aerobic exercise on the physical performance and incidence of treatment-related complications after high-dose chemotherapy. *Blood, 90*(9), 3390–3394.

Dimeo, F., Tilmann, M. H. M., Bertz, H., Kanz, L., Mertelsmann, R., & Keul, J. (1997). Aerobic exercise in the rehabilitation of cancer patients after high dose chemotherapy and autologous peripheral stem cell transplantation. *Cancer, 79*(9), 1717–1722.

Dodd, M., Janson, S., Facione, N., Faucett, J., Froelicher, E. S., Humphreys, J., et al. (2001). Advancing the science of symptom management. *Journal of Advanced Nursing, 33*(5), 668–676.

Dodd, M., Miaskowski, C., & Paul, S. M. (2001). Symptom clusters and their effect on the functional status of patients with cancer. *Oncology Nursing Forum, 28*(3), 465–470.

Dubos, R. (1976). The state of health and the quality of life. *The Western Journal of Medicine, 125*, 8–9.

Engstrom, C. A., Strohl, R. A., Rose, L., Lewandowski, L., & Stefanek, M. E. (1999). Sleep alterations in cancer patients. *Cancer Nursing, 22*(2), 143–148.

Fick, D. M., Cooper, J. W., Wade, W. E., Waller, J. L., Maclean, J. R., & Beers, M. H. (2003). Updating the Beers criteria for potentially inappropriate medication use in older adults. *Archives of Internal Medicine, 163*, 2716–2724.

Fiorentino, L., & Ancoli-Israel, S. (2007). Sleep dysfunction in patients with cancer. *Current Treatment Options in Neurology, 9*, 337–346.

Gaston-Johansson, F., Fall-Dickson, J. M., Bakos, A. B., & Kennedy, M. J. (1999). Fatigue, pain, and depression in pre-autotransplant breast cancer patients. *Cancer Practice, 7*(5), 240–247.

Gaston-Johansson, F., Lachica, E. M., Fall-Dickson, J. M., & Kennedy, M. J. (2004). Psychological distress, fatigue, burden of care, and quality of life in primary caregivers of patients with breast cancer undergoing autologous bone marrow transplantation. *Oncology Nursing Forum, 31*(6), 1161–1169.

Gibson, H., & Edwards, R. H. T. (1985). Muscular exercise and fatigue. *Sports Medicine, 2*(2), 120–132.

Gibson, F., Garnett, M., Richardson, A., Edwards, J., & Sepion, B. (2005). Heavy to carry: A survey of parents' and healthcare professionals' perceptions of cancer-related fatigue in children and young people. *Cancer Nursing 28*(1), 27–35.

Gift, A. G., Jablonski, A., Stommel, M., & Given, C. W. (2004). Symptom clusters in elderly patients with lung cancer. *Oncology Nursing Forum, 31*, 202–212.

Gift, A. G., Stommel, M., Jablonski, A., & Given, C. W. (2003). A cluster of symptoms over time in patients with lung cancer. *Nursing Research, 52*, 393–400.

Given, B., Given, C., & Stommel, M. (1994). Family and out-of-pocket costs for women with breast cancer. *Cancer Practice, 2*, 115–120.

Given, C. W., Given, B., Azzouz, F., Kozachik, S., & Stommel, M. (2001). Predictors of pain and fatigue in the year following diagnosis among elderly cancer patients. *Journal of Pain and Symptom Management, 21*, 456–466.

Given, B., Given, C., Azzouz, F., & Stommel, M. (2001). Physical functioning of elderly cancer patients prior to diagnosis and following initial treatment. *Nursing Research, 50,* 222–232.

Given, B., Given, C. W., McCorkle, R., Kozachik, S., Cimprich, B., Rahbar, M. H., et al. (2002). Pain and fatigue management: Results of a nursing randomized clinical trial. *Oncology Nursing Forum, 29,* 949–956.

Glass, J., Lanctot, K. L, Herrmann, N. Sproule, B. A., & Buston, U. E. (2005). Sedative hypnotics in older people with insomnia: Meta-analysis of risks and benefits. *British Medical Journal, 47.*

Glaus, A. (1993). Assessment of fatigue in cancer and non-cancer patients. *Supportive Care in Cancer, 1,* 305–315.

Glaus, A. (1994). Fatigue and cancer—indivisible twins? A comparison between cancer patients, patients with disease other than cancer and healthy people. *Pflege, 7,* 183–197.

Glaus, A., Crow, R., & Hammond, S. (1996). A qualitative study to explore the concept of fatigue/tiredness in cancer patients and in healthy individuals. *European Journal of Cancer Care, 5*(Suppl.), 8–23.

Grandjean, E. (1968). Fatigue: Its physiological and psychological significance. *Ergonomics, 11,* 427–436.

Graydon, J. E., Bubela, N., Irvine, D., & Vincent, L. (1995). Fatigue-reducing strategies used by patients receiving treatment for cancer. *Cancer Nursing, 18,* 23–28.

Groopman, J. E. (1998). Fatigue in cancer and HIV/AIDS. *Oncology, 12,* 335–347.

Hacker, E. D., Ferrans, C. Verlen, E., Ravandi, F., van Besien, K., Gelms, J., et al. (2006). Fatigue and physical activity in patients undergoing hematopoietic stem cell transplant. *Oncology Nursing Forum, 33*(3), 614–624.

Hann, D. M., Jacobsen, P. B., Azzarello, L. M., Martin, S. C., Curran, S. L., Fields, K. K., et al. (1998). Measurement of fatigue in cancer patients: Development and validation of the Fatigue Symptom Inventory. *Quality of Life Research 7,* 301–310.

Hann, D. M., Jacobsen, P. B., Martin, S. C., Kronish, L. E., Azzarello, L. M., & Fields, K. K. (1997). Fatigue in women treated with bone marrow transplantation for breast cancer: A comparison with women with no history of cancer. *Supportive Care in Cancer, 5*(1), 44–52.

Hart, L., & Frell, M. I. (1982). Fatigue. In C. M. Norris (Ed.), *Concept clarification in nursing* (pp. 251–261). Rockville, MD: Aspen.

Hauri, P. J., & Wisbey, J. (1992). Wrist actigraphy in insomnia. *Sleep, 15,* 293–301.

Haylock, P., & Hart, L. (1979). Fatigue in patients receiving localized radiation. *Cancer Nursing, 2,* 461–467.

Headley, J. A., Ownby, K. K., & John, L. D. (2004). The effect of seated exercise on fatigue and qulaity of life in women with advanced breast cancer. *Oncology Nursing Forum, 31*(5), 977–983.

Hinds, P. S., Hockenberry-Eaton, M., Gilger, E., Kline, N., Burleson, C., Bottomley, S., et al. (1999). Comparing patient, parent, and staff descriptions of fatigue in pediatric oncology patients. *Cancer Nursing, 22,* 277–288.

Hockenberry-Eaton, M., & Hinds, P. S. (2000). Fatigue in children and adolescents with cancer: Evolution of a program of study. *Seminars in Oncology Nursing, 16,* 261–272.

Hockenberry-Eaton, M., Hinds, P. S., Alcoser, P., O'Neill, J. B., Euell, K., Howard, V., et al. (1998). Fatigue in children and adolescents with cancer. *Journal of Pediatric Oncology Nursing, 15,* 172–182.

Holbrook, A. M., Crowther, R., Lotter, A., Cheng, C., & King, D. (2000). Meta-analysis of benzodiazepine use in the treatment of insomnia. *Canadian Medical Association Journal, 162,* 225–233.

Holley, S. K. (2000). Evaluating patient distress from cancer-related fatigue: An instrument development study. *Oncology Nursing Forum, 27,* 1425–1431.

Hussein, M. Z., Fikky, A., Abdel Bar, I., & Attia, O. (2004). Serum IL-6 and IL-12 levels in breast cancer patients. *Egypt Journal Immunology, 11*(2), 165–170.

Illman, J., Corringham, R., Robinson, D. Jr., Davis, H. M., Rossi, J. F., Cella, D., et al. (2005). Are inflammatory cytokines the common link between cancer-associated cachexia and depression? *Journal of Supportive Oncology, 3*(1), 37–50.

Inouye, S. K. (2000). Prevention of delirium in hospitalized older patients: Risk factors and targeted intervention strategies. *Annals of Medicine, 32*(4), 257–263.

Institute of Medicine. (2005). *Sleep medicine and research.* Retrieved December 15, 2006, from http://www.iom.edu/project.asp?id=23160.

Irvine, D., Vincent, L., Graydon, J. E., Bubela, N., & Thompson, L. (1994). The prevalence and correlates of fatigue in patients receiving treatment with chemotherapy and radiotherapy. *Cancer Nursing, 17,* 367–378.

Jacobsen, P. B., Hann, D. M., Azzarello, L. M., Horton, J., Balducci, L., & Lyman, G. H. (1999). Fatigue in women receiving adjuvant chemotherapy for breast cancer: Characteristics, course, and correlates. *Journal of Pain and Symptom Management, 18,* 233–242.

Jensen, S., & Given, B. (1991). Fatigue affecting family care givers of cancer patients. *Cancer Nursing, 14,* 181–187.

Jensen, S., & Given, B. (1993). Fatigue affecting family caregivers of cancer patients. *Supportive Cancer Care, 1,* 321–325.

Kim, Y., Roscoe, J. A., & Morrow, G. R. (2002). The effects of information and negative affect on severity of side effects from radiation therapy for prostate cancer. *Supportive Care in Cancer, 10,* 416–421.

Kolb, H. J., & Poetscher, C. (1997). Late effects after allogeneic bone marrow transplantation. *Current Opinions in Hematology, 4,* 401–407.

Koopman, C., Nouriani, B., Erickson, V., Anupindi, R., Butler, L. D., Bachmann, M. H., et al. (2002). Sleep disturbances in women with metastatic breast cancer. *Breast Journal, 8,* 362–370.

Kristiansson, M., Saraste, L., Soop, M., Sundqvist, K. G., & Thörne, A. (1999). Diminished interleukin-6 and C-reactive protein responses to laparoscopic versus open cholecystectomy. *Acta Anaesthesiologica Scandinavica, 43*(2), 146–152.

Lacks, P., & Rotert, M. (1986). Knowledge and practice of sleep hygiene techniques in insomniacs and good sleepers. *Behaviour Research and Therapy, 24,* 365–368.

LaReau, R., Benson, L., & Watcharotone, K. (2008). Examining the feasibility of implementing specific nursing interventions to promote sleep in hospitalized elderly patients. *Geriatric Nursing, 29*(3), 197–206.

Lee, K. A., Lentz, M. J., Taylor, D. L., Mitchell, E. S., & Woods, N. F. (1994). Fatigue as a response to environmental demands in women's lives. *Image: Journal of Nursing Scholarship, 26,* 149–154.

Lee, K. A. (2001) Sleep and fatigue. *Annual Review of Nursing Research, 19,* 249–273.

Lee, K., Cho, M., Miaskowski, C., & Dodd, M. (2004). Impaired sleep and rhythms in persons with cancer. *Sleep Medicine Reviews, 8,* 199–212.

Lee, K. A., Landis, C., Chasens, E. R., Dowling, G., Merritt, S., Parker, K. P., et al. (2004). Sleep and chronobiology: Recommendations for nursing education. *Nursing Outlook, 5,* 126–133.

Lenz, E. R., Pugh, L. C., Milligan, R. A., Gift, A., & Suppe, F. (1997). The middle range theory of unpleasant symptoms: An update. *Advances in Nursing Science, 19,* 14–27.

Lenz, E. R., Suppe, F., Gift, A. G., Pugh, L. C., & Milligan, R. A. (1995). Collaborative development of middle-range theories: Toward a theory of unpleasant symptoms. *Advances in Nursing Science, 17,* 1–13.

Littner, M., Kushida, C. A., Anderson, W. M., Bailey, D., Berry, R. B., Davila, D. G., et al. (2003). Practice parameters for the role of actigraphy in the study of sleep and circadian rhythms: An update for 2002. *Sleep, 26,* 337–341.

Loge, J. H., & Kaasa, S. (1998). Fatigue and cancer prevalence, correlates, and measurement. *Progress in Palliative Care, 6*(2), 43–47.

Losito, J. M., Murphy, S. O., & Thomas, M. L. (2006). The effects of group exercise on fatigue and quality of life during cancer treatment. *Oncology Nursing Forum, 33*(4), 821–825.

Lovely, N., Miaskowski, C., & Dodd, M. (1999). Relationship between fatigue and quality of life in patients with glioblastoma multiforme. *Oncology Nursing Forum, 26*, 921–925.

McCorkle, R. (1987). The measurement of symptom distress. *Seminars in Oncology Nursing, 3*, 248–256.

McCorkle, R., & Young, K. (1978). Development of a symptom distress scale. *Cancer Nursing, 1*, 373–378.

MacVicar, M. G., & Winningham, M. L. (1986). Promoting the functional capacity of cancer patients. *Cancer Bulletin, 38*, 235–239.

MacVicar, M. G., Winningham, M. L., & Nickel, J. L. (1989). Effect of aerobic interval training on cancer patient's functional capacity. *Nursing Research, 38*, 348–351.

Meek, P. M., Nail, L. M., Barsevick, A. M., Schwartz, A. L., Stephen, S., Whitmer, K., et al. (2000). Psychometric testing of fatigue instruments for use with cancer patients. *Nursing Research, 49*(4), 181–190.

Miaskowski, C., & Lee, K. A. (1999). Pain, fatigue, and sleep disturbances in oncology outpatients receiving radiation therapy for bone metastasis: A pilot study. *Journal of Pain and Symptom Management, 17*, 320–332.

Mitchell, S. A., Beck, S. L., Hood, L. E., Moore, K., & Tanner, E. R. (2007). Putting evidence into practice: Evidence-based interventions for fatigue during and following cancer and its treatment. *Clinical Journal of Oncology Nursing, 11*(1), 99–113.

Milligan, R. A., & Pugh, L. C. (1994). Fatigue during the childbearing period. *Annual Review of Nursing Research, 12*, 33–49.

Mock, V. (2001). Fatigue management: Evidence and guidelines for practice. *Cancer, 92*(6, Suppl.), 1699–1707.

Mock, V. (2003). Clinical excellence through evidence-based practice: Fatigue management as a model. *Oncology Nursing Forum, 30*, 787–796.

Mock, V., Abernathy, A. P., Atkinson, A., Barsevick, A. M., Berger, A. M., Cella, D., et al. (2007). *NCCN clinical practice guidelines: Cancer-related fatigue, volume 2.* Retrieved June 1, 2007, from http://www.canceradvocacy.org/.

Mock, V., Barton Burke, M., Sheehan, P., Creaton, E. M., Winningham, M. L., McKenney-Tedder, S., et al. (1994). A nursing rehabilitation program for women with breast cancer receiving adjuvant chemotherapy. *Oncology Nursing Forum, 21*, 899–908.

Mock, V., Dow, K. H., Meares, C. J., Grimm, P. M., Dienemann, J. A., Haisfield-Wolfe, M. E., et al. (1997). Effects of exercise on fatigue, physical functioning, and emotional distress during radiation therapy for breast cancer. *Oncology Nursing Forum, 24*, 991–1000.

Mock, V., Pickett, M., Ropka, M. E., Muscari, E. L., Stewart, K. J., Rhodes, V. A., et al. (2001). Fatigue and quality of life outcomes of exercise during cancer treatment. *Cancer Practice, 9*(3), 119–127.

Morin, C. M., Culbert, J. P., & Schwartz, S. M. (1994). Nonpharmacologic interventions for insomnia: A meta-analysis of treatment efficacy. *American Journal of Psychiatry, 15*, 1172–1180.

Mormont, M. C., & Levi, F. (1997). Circadian-system alterations during cancer processes: A review. *International Journal of Cancer, 70*, 241–245.

Mormont, M. C., Waterhouse, J., Bleuzen, P., Giacchetti, S., Jami, A., Bogdan, A., et al. (2000). Marked 24-h rest/activity rhythms are associated with better quality of life, better response, and longer survival in patients with metastatic colorectal cancer and good performance status. *Clinical Cancer Research, 6*, 3038–3045.

Musselman, D. L., Miller, A. H., Porter, M. R., Manatunga, A., Gao, F., Penna, S., Pearce, B. D., Landry, J., Glover, S., McDaniel, J. S., & Nemeroff, C. B. (2001). Higher than normal plasma interleukin-6 concentrations in cancer patients with depression: preliminary findings. *American Journal of Psychiatry, 158*(8), 1252–1257.

Nail, L., Jones, L. S., Greene, D., Schipper, D. L. & Jensen, R. (1991). Use and perceived efficacy of self-care activities in patients receiving chemotherapy. *Oncology Nursing Forum, 18*(5), 883–887.

National Cancer Institute. (2005). *Sleep disorders.* Retrieved December 15, 2006, from http://www.cancer.gov/cancertopics/pdq/supportivecare/sleepdisorders/healthprofessional.

NCCN Clinical Practice Guidelines in Oncology (2009). *Cancer-Related Fatigue, 1.*

Nowell, P. D., Mazumdar, S., Buysse, D. J., Dew, M. A., Reynolds, C. F., III, & Kupfer, D. J. (1997). Benzodiazepines and zolpidem for chronic insomnia: A meta-analysis of treatment efficacy. *JAMA, 278,* 2170–2177.

Page, M. S., Berger, A. M., & Johnson, L. B. (2006). Putting evidence into practice: Evidence-based intervention for sleep-wake disturbances. *Clinical Journal of Oncology Nursing, 10,* 753–767.

Pater, J. L., Zee, B., Palmer, M., Johnston, D., & Osoba, D. (1997). Fatigue in patients with cancer. Results with National Cancer Institute of Canada Clinical Trial Group studies employing the EROTC HRQOL C-30. *Supportive Care in Cancer, 5,* 410–413.

Payne, J. K. (2002). The trajectory of fatigue in adult patients with breast and ovarian cancer receiving chemotherapy. *Oncology Nursing Forum, 29,* 1334–1340.

Payne, J. K. (2004). A neuroendocrine-based regulatory fatigue model. *Biological Research for Nursing, 6*(2), 141–150.

Payne, J. K., Piper, B. F., Rabinowitz, I., & Zimmerman, M. B. (2006). Biomarkers, fatigue, sleep, and depressive symptoms in women with breast cancer: A pilot study. *Oncology Nursing Forum, 33,* 775–783.

Pickhard-Holley, S. (1991). Fatigue in cancer patients: A descriptive study. *Cancer Nursing, 14,* 13–19.

Pinto, B. M., Eakin, E., & Maruyama, N. C. (2000). Health behavior changes after a cancer diagnosis: What do we know and where do we go from here? *Annals of Behavioral Medicine, 22,* 1–17.

Pinto, B. M., & Maruyama, N. C. (1999). Exercise in the rehabilitation of breast cancer survivors. *Psycho-oncology, 8,* 311–328.

Piper, B. F., Borneman, T., Sun, V. C., Koczywas, M., Uman, G., Ferrell, B., et al. (2008). Cancer-related fatigue: The role of oncology nurses in translating National Comprehensive Cancer Network assesment guidelines into practice. *Clinical Journal of Oncology Nursing, 12*(5, Suppl.), 37–47.

Piper, B. F., Lindsay, A. M., & Dodd, M. J. (1987). Fatigue mechanisms in cancer patients: Developing nursing theory. *Oncology Nursing Forum, 14,* 17–23.

Piper, B., Lindsay, A., Dodd, M., Ferketich, S., Paul, S., & Weller, J. (1989). Development of an instrument to measure the subjective dimension of fatigue. In S. Funk, E. Tournquist, M. Champagne, L. Copp, & R. Wiese (Eds.), *Key aspects of comfort: Management of pain, fatigue and nausea* (pp. 199–208). New York, NY: Springer.

Piper, B. F., Rieger, P. T., Brophy, L., Haeuber, D., Hood, L. E., Lyver, A., et al. (1989). Recent advances in the management of biotherapy-related side effects: Fatigue. *Oncology Nursing Forum, 16,* 27–34.

Portenoy, R. K., & Itri, L. M. (1999). Cancer-related fatigue: Guidelines for evaluation and management. *The Oncologist, 4*(1), 1–10.

Potempa, K., Lopez, M., Reid, C., & Lawson, L. (1986). Chronic fatigue. *Image, 18,* 165–169.

Pud, D., Ben Ami, S., Cooper, B. A., Aouizerat, B. E., Cohen, D., Radiano, R., et al. (2008). The symptom experience of oncology outpatients has a different impact on quality of life outcomes. *Journal of Pain & Symptom Management, 35*(2), 162–170.

Pugh, L. C., & Milligan, R. (1993). A framework for the study of childbearing fatigue. *Advances in Nursing Science, 15,* 60–70.

Pusztai, L., Krishnamurti, S., Perez Cardona, J., Sneige, N., & Esteva, F. J., et al. (2004). Expression of BAG-1 and BcL-2 proteins before and after neoadjuvant chemotherapy of locally advanced breast cancer. *Cancer Investigation, 22*(2), 248–256.

Quesada, J., Talpaz, M., Rios, A., Kwizrock, R., & Gutterman, J. (1986). Clinical toxicity of interferons in cancer patients: A review. *Journal of Clinical Oncology, 4,* 234–243.

Quick, M., & Fonteyn, M. (2005). Development and implementation of a clinical survey for cancer-related fatigue assessment. *Clinical Journal of Oncology Nursing, 9,* 435–439.

Ream, E., & Richardson, A. (1999). From theory to practice: Designing interventions to reduce fatigue in patients with cancer. *Oncology Nursing Forum, 26,* 1295–1303.

Redeker, N. S., Lev, E. L., & Ruggiero, J. (2000). Insomnia, fatigue, anxiety, depression, and quality of life of cancer patients undergoing chemotherapy. *Sch Inquiry in Nurisng Practice, 14,* 275–290.

Rhoten, D. (1982). Fatigue and the post surgical patient. In C. M. Norris (Ed.), *Concept Clarification in Nursing* (pp. 277–300). Rockville, MD: Aspen.

Richardson, A. (1995). Fatigue in cancer patients: A review of the literature. *European Journal of Cancer Care, 4,* 20–32.

Richardson, A., Ream, E., & Wilson-Barnett, J. (1998). Fatigue in patients receiving chemotherapy: Patterns of change. *Cancer Nursing, 21,* 17–30.

Rizzo, J. D., Somerfield, M. R., Hagerty, K. L., Seidenfeld, J., Bohlius, J., Bennett, C. L., et al. (2008). *Journal of Clinical Oncology, 26*(1), 132–149.

Roscoe, J. A., Morrow, G. R., Hickok, J. T., Bushunow, P., Matteson, S., Rakita, D., et al. (2002). Temporal interrelationships among fatigue, circadian rhythm, and depression in breast cancer patients undergoing chemotherapy treatment. *Supportive Care in Cancer, 1,* 329–336.

Roy, S. C., & Andrews, H. A. (1991). *The Roy adaptation model: The definitive statement.* Norwalk, CT: Appleton & Lange.

Sadeh, A., Hauri, P. J., Kripke, D. F., & Lavie, P. (1995). The role of actigraphy in the evaluation of sleep disorders. *Sleep, 18,* 288–302.

Sadler, I. J., Jacobsen, P. B., Booth-Jones, M., Belanger, H., Weitzner, M. A., & Fields, K. K. (2002). Preliminary evaluation of a clinical syndrome approach to assessing cancer-related fatigue. *Journal of Pain and Symptom Management, 23*(5), 406–416.

Sarna, L. (1993). Correlates of symptom distress in women with lung cancer. *Cancer Practice, 1,* 21–28.

Savard, J., & Morin, C. M. (2001). Insomnia in the context of cancer: A review of a neglected problem. *Journal of Clinical Oncology, 19,* 895–908.

Schwartz, A. L. (1998a). Patterns of exercise and fatigue in physically active cancer survivors. *Oncology Nursing Forum, 25,* 485–491.

Schwartz, A. L. (1998b). The Schwartz cancer fatigue scale: Testing reliability and validity. *Oncology Nursing Forum, 25,* 711–717.

Schwartz, A. L. (2000). Daily fatigue patterns and effect of exercise in women with breast cancer. *Cancer Practice, 8,* 16–24.

Schwartz, A. L., Thompson, J. A., & Masood, H. (2002). Interferon-induced fatigue in patients with melanoma: A pilot study of exercise and methylphenidate. *Oncology Nursing Forum, 29,* E85–E90.

Segar, M. L., Katch, V. L., Roth, R. S., Garcia, A. W., Portner, T. I., Glickman, S. G., et al. (1999). The effect of aerobic exercises on self-esteem and depressive and anxiety symptoms among breast cancer survivors. *Oncology Nursing Forum, 25*(1), 107–113.

Servaes, P., Verhagen, C. A., & Bleijenberg, G. (2002). Relations between fatigue, neuropsychological functioning, and physical activity after treatment for breast carcinoma: Daily self-report and objective behavior. *Cancer, 95*(9), 2017–2026.

Shapiro, S. L., Bootzin, R. R., Figueredo, A. J., Lopez, A. M., & Schwartz, G. E. (2003). The efficacy of mindfulness-based stress reduction in the treatment of sleep disturbance in women with breast cancer: An exploratory study. *Journal of Psychosomatic Research, 54,* 85–91.

Simeit, R., Deck, R., & Conta-Marx, B. (2004). Sleep management training for cancer patients with insomnia. *Supportive Care in Cancer, 12,* 176–183.

Skalla, K. A., & Rieger, P. T. (1995). Fatigue. In P. T. Rieger (Ed.), *Biotherapy: A comprehensive review* (pp. 221–242). Sudbury, MA: Jones and Bartlett.

Smets, E. M., Garssen, B., Bonke, B., & de Haes, J. C. (1995). The multidimensional fatigue inventory (MFI): Psychometric qualities of an instrument to assess fatigue. *Journal of Psychosomatic Research, 39*, 315–325.

Smets, E. M. A., Garssen, B., Schuster-Uitterhoeve, A. L., & de Haes, J. C. J. M. (1993). Fatigue in cancer patients. *British Journal of Cancer, 68*, 220–223.

So, W. K. W., Marsh, G., Ling, W. M., Leung, F. Y., Lo, J. C. K., Yeung, M., et al. (2009). The symptom cluster of fatigue, pain, anxiety, and depression and the effect on the quality of life of women receiving treatment for breast cancer: A multicenter study. *Oncology Nursing Forum, 35*(4), 205–214.

Spielman, A. J., & Glovinksy, P. (2004). A conceptual framework of insomnia for primary care practitioners: Predisposing, precipitating, and perpetuating factors. *Sleep Medicine Alerts, 9*, 1–6.

St. Pierre, B., Kasper, C. E., & Lindsay, A. M. (1992). Fatigue mechanisms in patients with cancer: Effects on tumor necrosis factor and exercise skeletal muscle. *Oncology Nursing Forum, 19*, 419–425.

Varricchio, C. G. (1985). Selecting a tool for measuring fatigue. *Oncology Nursing Forum, 12*, 122–127.

Varricchio, C. G. (1995). Measurement issues in fatigue. *Quality of Life—A Nursing Challenge, 4*, 20–23.

Vena, C., Parker, K., Cunningham, M., Clark, J., & McMillan, S. (2004). Sleep-wake disturbances in people with cancer, part I: An overview of sleep, sleep regulation, and effects of disease and treatment. *Oncology Nursing Forum, 31*, 735–746.

Visovsky, C., & Schneider, S. M. (2003). Cancer-related fatigue [Electronic article]. *Online Journal of Issues in Nursing, 8*, 1–23.

Vogelzang, N. J., Breitbart, W., Cella, D., Curt, G. A., Groopman, J. E. & Horning, S. J. (1997). Patient, caregiver, and oncologist perceptions of cancer-related fatigue: Results of a tripart assessment survey. *Seminars in Hematology, 34*(3, Suppl. 2), 4–12.

Wang, P. S., Bohn, R. L., Glynn, R. J., Mogun, H., & Avorn, J. (2001). Zolpidem use and hip fracture in older people. *Journal of the American Geriatrics Society, 49*(12), 1685–1690.

Whedon, M., Stearns, D., & Mills, L. (1995). Quality of life of long-term adult survivors of autologous bone marrow transplantation. *Oncology Nursing Forum, 22*, 1527–1535.

Winningham, M. L. (1991). Walking program for people with cancer: Getting started. *Cancer Nursing, 14*, 270–276.

Winningham, M. L. (1992). *The energetics of activity, fatigue, symptoms management & functional status: A conceptual model.* Paper presented at the 1st International Symposium on Symptom Management, San Francisco, CA.

Winningham, M. L. (1995). Fatigue: The missing link to quality of life. *Quality of Life Research, 4*, 2.

Winningham, M. L. (1999). Fatigue. In C. Yarbro, M. Frogge, & M. Goodman (Eds.), *Cancer symptom management*, 2nd ed. (pp. 58–76). Sudbury, MA: Jones and Bartlett.

Winningham, M. L. (2001). Strategies for managing cancer-related fatigue syndrome: A rehabilitation approach. *Cancer Supplement, 92*, 989–997.

Winningham, M. L., Nail, L. M., Barton-Burke, M., Brophy, L., Cimprich, B., Jones, L. S., et al. (1994). Fatigue and the cancer experience: The state of the knowledge. *Oncology Nursing Forum, 21*(1), 23–36.

Woo, B., Dibble, S. L., Piper, B. F., Keating, S. B., & Weiss, M. C. (1998). Differences in fatigue by treatment methods in women with breast cancer. *Oncology Nursing Forum, 25*, 915–920.

Wood, L. J., Nail, L. M., Glister, A., Winters, K. A., & Elsea, C. R. (2006). Cancer chemotherapy-related symptoms evidence to suggest a role for proinflammatory cytokines. *Oncology Nursing Forum, 33*, 535–542.

Wu, H. S., & McSweeney, M. (2001). Measurment of fatigue in people with cancer. *Oncology Nursing Forum, 28,* 1371–1384.

Yirmiya, R., Weidenfeld, J., Pollak, Y., Morag, M., Morag, A., Avitsur, R., et al. (1999). Cytokines, depression due to a general medical condition, and antidepressant drugs. *Advances in Experimental Medicine and Biology, 461,* 283–316.

Young-McCaughan, S., & Sexton, D. (1991). A retrospective investigation of the relationship between aerobic exercise and quality of life in women with breast cancer. *Oncology Nursing Forum, 18*(4), 751–757.

Young-McCaughan, S., Mays, M. Z., Arzola, S. M., Yoder, L. H., Dramiga, S. A., Leclerc, K. M., et al. (2003). Research and commentary: Change in exercise tolerance, activity and sleep patterns, and quality of life in patients with cancer participating in a structured exercise program. *Oncology Nursing Forum, 30,* 441–454.

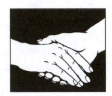

SECTION 5

Patient Perspectives

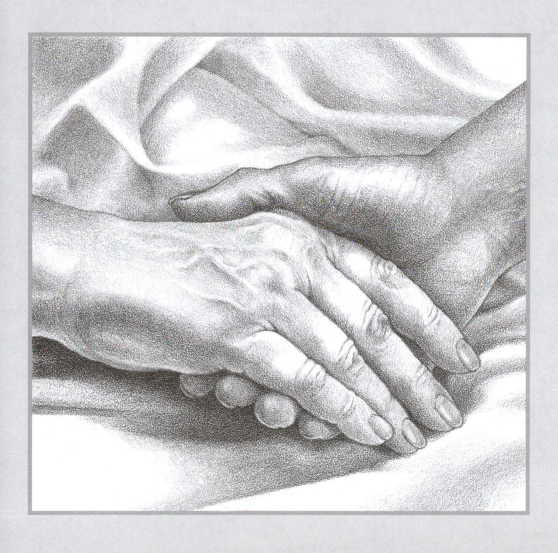

Chapter Eighteen

Cancer Survivorship and Quality for Life

Susan A. Leigh • Ellen L. Stovall

Introduction

Much of the change within our healthcare system is related directly to the miracles and advances of modern medicine. Although the development of sophisticated therapies now offers new hope to people who are diagnosed with cancer, the providers of this potentially miraculous health care are challenged to maintain a focus on the individual concerns of the people under their care. In the midst of complex technology, elaborate delivery systems, complicated protocols, managed care, and fiscal regulations, it is easy to become trapped in the pace, chaos, and frustration of change and to lose sight of the individuality of peoples' needs.

Historical Perspective: From Patienthood to Survivorship

The primary and obvious focus of cancer care over the past few decades has been the eradication of the disease. Objective, quantitative measurements (e.g., blood counts, tumor regression, length of survival) became relevant parameters of success once effective therapies were available. Attending physicians usually made care decisions based solely on information related to the disease, treatment, and potential for response. Physical survival—meaning staying alive—became the utmost goal, while concerns about the quality of that survival remained a luxury. Qualitative concepts of care, though, were hardly novel.

Prior to the explosion of technology and scientific advances in health care, the World Health Organization (1948) defined health as "a state of complete physical, mental, and social well-being and not merely the absence of disease or infirmity" (p. 29). Science and technology may have changed the course of treating and curing a select group of cancers, but nurses, mental health professionals, and patients themselves changed the course of *caring* for people with cancer. Objective measurements and observations remain important but, when used alone, give an incomplete picture of the overall impact of the disease.

As quality of survival is in the eye of the beholder, patient autonomy is of paramount importance. Many researchers and clinicians now recognize the importance of the patient perspective, especially when monitoring fatigue, pain, and psychosocial distress (Clark, 1994). A more recent publication from the National Cancer Institute, *Patient-Centered*

Communication in Cancer Care: Promoting Healing and Reducing Suffering, goes so far as to offer an academic framework for communication between clinicians and their patients (Epstein & Street, 2007). These authors identify three core attributes of this type of individualized care that will help elicit, validate, and create understanding of the patient's perspective of illness; they are careful consideration of patients' needs from their viewpoints, providing patients with real opportunities to participate in their care, and supporting the relationship between the patient and clinicians.

Thus, issues affecting quality of life (QOL) as described by the patient are gaining recognition as major components of cancer care.

Defining Quality of Life

Who Defines Quality of Life?

No matter how many ways QOL is defined, it all boils down to individual perspectives of personal experiences. An individual's answer to the question "What does QOL mean to you?" is highly subjective and personal and can change depending on the specific situation, including time frame, mood, location, family dynamics, and many other variables. The important point is that, no matter how subjective the question may be, it must be asked in order to assess the total patient experience. Frank (1991) writes the following of QOL:

> What happens when my body breaks down happens not just to that body but also to my life, which is lived in that body. When the body breaks down, so does the life. Even when medicine can fix the body, that doesn't always put the life back together again (p. 8).

Incorporating QOL assessments into everyday practice is no longer a luxury, but an important and necessary component of cancer care. As the delivery of care becomes more complicated for the professional caregiver, so does the experience of receiving care for anyone diagnosed with cancer. Complex therapies lead to complicated choices, and the decision making that accompanies these choices warrants a more knowledgeable and assertive healthcare consumer.

Cancer Survivors' Bill of Rights

For many categories of cancer, the potential for extended survival has increased so dramatically patients are compelled to become more informed about their disease and treatment options. An early example of informed consumerism is illustrated in the Cancer Survivors' Bill of Rights (Spingarn, 1988). Published by the American Cancer Society in 1988, this proclamation was written by a cancer survivor for cancer survivors (Spingarn, 1988). The author, Natalie Davis Spingarn, insisted that the consumer voice be heard and not be modified by the medical establishment. Spingarn addressed individual, interpersonal, and social rights to greater care and satisfaction throughout the cancer experience and illustrated a shift from passive patienthood to a more proactive survivorship. Although this statement was written more than two decades ago, it resonates with the needs of survivors today. This also illustrates the many years of hard work and persistence that is needed to bring about social change.

A Shift Toward Survivorship

The concept of survivorship initially was introduced to the field of oncology in 1986 with the founding of the National Coalition for Cancer Survivorship (NCCS) (Leigh & Logan, 1991). Events preceding the initial organizational meeting included a combination of dramatic advances in cancer therapy and an increasing population of cancer survivors, along with changing social trends that saw the development of resource and support networks for patients and their family members.

New therapies to treat cancer elevated the hopes and expectations of surviving this disease. Access to information about scientific breakthroughs became readily available to the general public, and awareness about cancer prevention, early detection, second opinions, and treatment options increased. Many types of cancer shifted from the expected acute disease model to a model of chronic disease, while some patients were actually considered cured. This shift led to a new sense of hope that lives could be extended, and contributed to changes in how decisions were made and who made them.

Historically, the cancer patient's agenda was set less often by patients and more often by healthcare providers, specifically physicians. Eventually, patients decided to exercise more control over all aspects of cancer care that affected their lives, especially those in the frequently neglected psychosocial realm. Thus, a proliferation of support groups, hotlines, resource materials, and patient networks emerged, giving birth to a new social movement that began to inform and empower people with cancer.

This movement remained undefined until NCCS emerged and its leadership began writing about a new concept called survivorship. Life with and after cancer was described as more than black and white, patient versus survivor, cured or not cured. It was seen as a multitude of events and feelings that changed and continued beyond the actual treatment phase. For many people affected by cancer, life after diagnosis was not just about how long one lived, but how well one lived.

Mullan (1990) initially described survivorship as the act of living on, a dynamic concept with no artificial boundaries. Carter (1989) further described this theme as a process of *going through*, suggesting movement through phases. From these models, survivorship came to be viewed as a continual, ongoing process with a focus on quality of life rather than a stage or outcome of survival (Leigh, 1994). Survivorship is not just about remission, cure, or posttreatment survival, which is how the medical profession generally defines it. Rather, when viewed from the perspective of someone diagnosed with this disease, it can be defined as the experience of living with, through, or beyond cancer (Leigh & Logan, 1991). From this reframed point of view, survivorship begins at the moment of diagnosis and continues for the remainder of life (Mullan, 1990).

Defining Survivors

Other semantic discrepancies revolve around who can be considered a cancer survivor. When cancer was considered incurable, the term *survivor* applied to the family members whose loved one died from the disease. This terminology was used for years by the medical profession and insurance companies. When potentially curative therapy became a reality, physicians selected the 5-year parameter to measure survival. Freedom from disease and biomedical longevity became the standard of success when the outcome was measurable and quantifiable.

Quantitative Model: Medical

Even though the 5-year landmark has been modified as a parameter for describing survival, medical professionals still seem inclined to categorize anyone receiving therapy or not completely free of disease as a patient, and everyone who is not under treatment or with no evidence of disease as a survivor. Many survivors, however, feel a conscious and deliberate attempt must be made to resist the urge to pigeonhole the terms cancer survivor and cancer survivorship by using a calculus based on years out of treatment or disease-free survival. Quantitative definitions fail to give recognition to the strenuous efforts of people who are not cured of their disease, require maintenance therapy or periodic changes in treatment modalities, and remain alive for longer than 5 years. Other survivors experience late recurrences, are diagnosed with second malignancies, or develop delayed effects of treatment, requiring further therapy. Additionally, many survivors with poor prognoses struggle day to day attempting to beat the odds and overcome pessimistic expectations about life expectancy.

Yet, there is a renewed desire for the healthcare community to focus more exclusively on the transition from active treatment to posttreatment care. With the release of the Institute of Medicine (IOM) report, *From Cancer Patient to Cancer Survivor: Lost in Transition,* this under-studied area of cancer survival finally is receiving attention that can no longer be denied (Hewitt, Greenfield, & Stovall, 2006). Thus, the focus on survivorship in this IOM report is restricted intentionally to "adult survivors of cancer during the phase of care that follows primary treatment" (Hewitt, Greenfield, & Stovall, 2006, p. 18). Survivorship is narrowly defined for this specific project and report.

Qualitative Model: Consumer

Although the expectation for survival may hold different meanings for all involved, it is the survivors themselves who define survivorship and give meaning to their struggles. Quality of life means significance and purpose to the person living through the experience. A truly patient-centered measure of success would use QOL parameters, with or without measurements of longevity. To help make this transition, healthcare providers should look for ways to eliminate the use of words and descriptions that do the following:

1. *Erect unnecessary boundaries* around the person with cancer (e.g., "He's not a survivor; he's not 5 years posttreatment yet.")
2. *Use terms of clinical measurement* as the only determinant of successful survival (e.g., "She's not cured yet; she's only been in remission for 3 years.")
3. *Impose limitations on hope or take hope away from someone* when few treatment options exist (e.g., "Why do you insist on calling her a survivor? This is her third recurrence, and you need to face the reality that she's going to die.")

The act of defining the word survivor is one of empowerment, as noted by Gray (1992) in *Persons with Cancer Speak Out.* Over the past few decades, the language of cancer has evolved to the point where the term *cancer victim* is the oddity and *cancer survivor* is more the norm. Although it is arguable that the term *patient* somehow belongs in the science and practice of medical and psychosocial oncology, few will disagree that the term *survivor* evokes a more powerful image.

As the concept of the empowered survivor has encouraged a shift from paternalism to partnership, cancer support and advocacy organizations around the country have enlarged the language of survivorship to include other qualitative descriptors of this population. Many survivors favor powerful labels (e.g., veteran, victor, advocate, activist, warrior) (Leigh, 2001). Others dislike the use of warlike metaphors and prefer a more gentle or spiritual label (e.g., thriver, graduate, blessed, triumpher). Some who may be living with recurrent or metastatic disease have an extreme dislike for the term survivor and express anger about oversimplifying survivorship while emphasizing only the positive aspects of recovery (Mayer, 1998). Though this may sound confusing, or even insignificant to some, an important point is that survivors themselves should be allowed to define themselves within the context of their own illness experience rather than rely solely on the agendas and descriptives of the healthcare community (Leigh, 1994).

Cancer survivors are hardly the only ones adding to this labeling confusion. Due to the current rise in managed care, survivors are also called *clients, consumers,* or *customers.* These labels reflect the influence of business in our current healthcare marketplace. This new influence is not without its problems; a most unfortunate addition to this cadre of labels has been a long-term survivor's use of the term *beggar* when describing her- or himself within the health maintenance system.

None of these descriptives is right or wrong necessarily. As the potential for surviving cancer expands, so must the language describing this expansion. Whether using quantitative or qualitative descriptives, survivors and practitioners simply need to define these terms within the context they are used. Thus, the term *survivor* in this chapter reflects the NCCS definition, "from the time of its discovery and for the balance of life, an individual diagnosed with cancer is a survivor" (Mullan, 1990, p. 1).

Stages of Survival and Quality of Life

Obviously, cancer survivors have different issues and concerns depending on their circumstances along the survival continuum. In the classic article "Seasons of Survival: Reflections of a Physician with Cancer," Mullan (1985) was the first to propose a model of survival that includes acute, extended, and permanent stages. Quality-of-life issues are of paramount importance in all of these stages. It must also be noted, though, that cancer survivors can die in any of the three stages. Some advocates, including this author, now describe end of life as the "final stage of survival." Although QOL issues are of paramount importance at end of life, this chapter will not address death and dying as a separate entity.

Acute Stage

The acute (or immediate) stage of survival begins at the time of the diagnostic workup and continues through the initial courses of medical treatment. The survivor commonly is called a patient during this stage, and initially the primary focus is on physical survival: "How long will I live?" "Will I be cured?" "Will I lose my hair?" Usually, without any prior training, those who are ill are required to make sophisticated medical decisions about therapy at a time of intense vulnerability, fear, and pressure. Inexperienced in navigating the complicated culture of medicine or advocating for themselves, many people continue to delegate treatment-related decisions to their physicians. Others, however, are not so quick to surrender the decisions about their lives to any one person. They ask for information, explanations, second opinions, and more effective communication in an attempt to understand the choices and decisions before them.

Many supportive care resources and services are more available for patients in the acute stage. Access to the healthcare team, counselors, patient support networks, resource libraries, hotlines, and family support systems help survivors navigate this stage. *Navigation* has become a specialized service in many settings, as navigators act as personal guides to the newly diagnosed in our increasingly complicated healthcare systems and situations. In order to improve their chances for quality survival, many survivors are taught that advocating for oneself can be as important as receiving the right therapy. *The Cancer Survival Toolbox* (NCCS, 2009) is an example of just one resource that offers self-navigation tools to survivors and their loved ones. However, the picture changes, sometimes dramatically, once treatment ends.

Extended Stage

If the disease responds during the initial course of therapy, the survivor will transition into the extended (or intermediate) stage of survival. This stage often is described as watchful waiting, limbo, or remission, as survivors monitor their bodies for symptoms of disease recurrence. Uncertainty about the future prevails as medically based support systems are no longer readily available, and survivors must learn to deal with the unknowns by themselves. Common questions include, "How many times a day should I examine myself?" "Is this symptom a sign of recurrence, or is it normal?" "Why do I still feel tired/fearful/depressed?" Recovery entails dealing with the physical and emotional effects of treatment, while reestablishing social roles can be challenged by ignorance and discrimination. The quality of one's life after cancer becomes a major concern.

While no longer a patient, the person may not feel entirely healthy and may have difficulty feeling like a survivor. Ambiguity defines this stage as survivors find themselves afloat in a mixture of joy and fear—happy to be alive and finished with treatments, yet afraid of what the future may hold.

The need for continued supportive care during this transitional stage was highlighted as early as the 1980s (Leigh, 1994; Mullan, 1990; Welch-McCaffrey, Loesher, Leigh, Hoffman, & Meyskens, 1989). Community and peer networks often replace institutional support, and recovery entails regaining both physical and psychological stamina. Time frames for curing the body and healing the spirit are individualized, and may or may not occur in harmony. Survivors must continue to advocate for themselves, often within the context of a group or recovery program, but may also begin advocating for others through support networks.

An example of support and resources during this phase of survival is the Lance Armstrong Foundation Web site, Livestrong.org. This site offers social networking along with practical information about exercise, nutrition, and general recovery. It also assists survivors with the development of personalized survivorship care plans. These care plans, which include treatment summaries (historical) and follow-up (future) plans, offer guidelines to help with the transition to life after cancer.

Permanent Stage

As a certain level of trust and comfort gradually returns, survivors enter the permanent (or long-term) stage of survival. This is equivalent roughly to what the medical establishment calls cure or sustained remission. Although most survivors experience a gradual evolution from a state of "surviving to thriving," as described by Dow (1990), others must deal with the chronic, debilitating, or delayed effects of therapy. Quality of life becomes a major focus of long-term survival: "I guess I shouldn't complain about my infertility. After all, I'm alive." "How will I get health insurance if I lose this job?" "Will I get cancer again?" Although many long-term survivors have no physical evidence of disease and appear to have recovered fully, all remain at risk for recurrence of the original disease or for the development of other malignancies. With an ever expanding population of long-term survivors, the fallout from cancer therapies is becoming more evident; still there is no systematic follow-up after cancer treatment ends. Once again, the use of survivorship care planning will help identify long-term risks and the need for continued follow-up, especially with primary care providers.

Meanwhile, the life-threatening experience of cancer is never forgotten. In many ways, survival enhances appreciation for life, while at the same time reminding survivors of their vulnerability. The metaphor of the Damocles syndrome illustrates this dichotomy. Dressed in royal fineries and surrounded by good food and fine wine, Damocles could not eat or drink, as he imagined that the thin thread holding the sword above his head might break at any moment (Koocher & O'Malley, 1981). A more current view of this syndrome might be interpreted as post-traumatic stress disorder, or PTSD. How individual survivors interpret this metaphor of life or psychological diagnosis will influence the quality of their survival.

For many long-term survivors, a lack of guidelines—both evidence-based and consensus-based—to ensure or enhance disease-free survival has been a major concern. Pediatric oncology is far beyond adult oncology in the systematic follow-up of long-term survivors, so that potential pitfalls can be identified early and interventions can be instituted when needed. Adults, on the other hand, often feel burdened by what Siegal and Christ (1990) called the glorification of recovery, whereby survivors are praised for overcoming diversity and sometimes scolded for complaining. The identification of real problems can be hampered when survivors appear healthy. No one wants to believe that something may be wrong, whether physically, emotionally, or socially (Siegal & Christ, 1990; Smith, 1981). Symptoms of distress, both biomedical and psychosocial, must be taken seriously. In this age of cost containment, managed care, and potential healthcare reform, long-term survivors need continued access to appropriate specialists more than ever, yet they are often denied referrals when the seriousness of their complaints are misunderstood, minimized, or considered too expensive.

As the population of long-term cancer survivors increases, attention to survival issues must be encouraged. Even if the disease is eradicated, the psychosocial sequelae of surviving a life-threatening experience must be recognized as a barrier to full recovery. Advocacy at national levels must continue to direct attention to these issues by involving survivors in the legislative process and in guiding public policy.

Survivor-Related Advocacy

While many healthcare providers see themselves as advocates for their patients, the idea of advocacy often intimidates survivors because they do not understand it. At a basic level though, advocacy has little to do with public policy or politics; it means "active support on behalf of . . ." (Stovall & Clark, 1996, p. 276). Thus, physicians, nurses, and social workers act on behalf of their patients. Lawyers act on behalf of their clients. Members of the clergy act on behalf of their congregations. But more important, survivors and their families need to learn how to act on their own behalf in order to ensure quality survival from their perspectives. The NCCS model of advocacy is three-tiered: advocacy for self, advocacy for others, and advocacy for community.

For Self

When survivors act on behalf of themselves, it becomes self-advocacy. Alternatively, family members can advocate for their loved ones, especially in cultures where bringing attention to one's self may be inappropriate. Although a person may feel paralyzed, inarticulate, and extremely vulnerable when first diagnosed with cancer, this state usually does not last forever. It is imperative that survivors and their supporters overcome their initial state of inertia, develop plans of action, and make decisions that affect both the quality and quantity of their lives. Effective communication with healthcare personnel and family members is the first step toward effectual self-advocacy.

Other examples of self-advocacy include asking appropriate questions, seeking second opinions, accessing understandable information about treatments, and requesting culturally relevant support. These examples potentially can help survivors feel more empowered.

Other reasons for encouraging self-advocacy include the following:

- Gaining a sense of stability and control during unpredictable times
- Building confidence in the face of seemingly insurmountable challenges
- Seeking out others in the same situation for peer support
- Improving chances for better and longer survival
- Diminishing feelings of hopelessness and helplessness

By transforming apprehensions and anxieties into productive energy, survivors not only obtain up-to-date and accurate information, but also become more adept at advocating for themselves and others.

For Others

Many survivors who have recovered from their disease or are coexisting with cancer as a chronic illness have a need to "give something back" and assist their fellow survivors. Having learned first-hand how powerful it was to arm themselves with the nonmedical tools of survival, such as information gathering, effective communication, and peer support, there is a willingness to share the road maps of survival that may have been unavailable to them. This is the veteran–rookie connection—the experienced traveler paving the way for the newly diagnosed. This model of mutual aid is the foundation of the survivorship movement and is poignantly illustrated below by a survivor who had just been diagnosed with Hodgkin's disease:

> I would need to find the *right* doctor and the *right* medical facility to meet my new, critical needs. And yet I was paralyzed. I needed to find someone immediately who knew my terror; someone I could talk with on a personal—rather than clinical—level; someone who had "been there." I needed to find a survivor (Morrison, 1983, p. B5).

Most survivors are more than willing to talk to other survivors about cancer, usually enhancing the QOL for both parties. The veteran survivor feels good about being helpful and the rookie survivor gains much needed support, along with the glimpse of a possible future. Two cancer veterans may support each other when no one else seems to understand the occasional or continuing trauma of surviving a once fatal disease. Some survivors use their personal experiences in other ways, including the following:

- Starting or joining support groups
- Manning local cancer hotlines
- Speaking publicly to raise awareness about cancer to religious and civic groups and to the media

- Encouraging community libraries and bookstores to update their cancer resources
- Teaching medical students, healthcare professionals, and the business community about the many facets of surviving cancer
- Raising funds for cancer research or support
- Sitting on program, funding, or research committees as a patient advocate
- Helping to create community resource, retreat, and healing centers

The point must be made, however, that not all survivors feel altruistic. While some survivors feel a need to remain attached to the cancer community, many others do not. They exhibit no visible scars or problems. For them, cancer is past history and private. Still other survivors may fear discrimination at work or in social settings if their medical history becomes known. Anticipated rejection can keep the most vocal survivor silent and can diminish greatly the quality of that person's life. Obviously survivors who do not fear recrimination are still needed to advocate on behalf of those who do.

For Community

With the rapid growth of cancer-related advocacy over the past decade, especially on a national level, many successes can be reported. Community advocacy often focuses on national agendas and public policy. For example, advocates representing pediatric oncology have raised community awareness about the increasing population of adult survivors of childhood cancers, many whom now have chronic health problems, are unable to find affordable insurance, or suffer discrimination in school or in the workplace. These young survivors are not only outspoken but also extremely effective when recommending changes in health policy.

Another potent example of a national initiative is illustrated by the work of breast cancer advocates. In less than 3 years during the early 1990s, a well organized, informed, articulate, and sometimes angry group of women challenged the United States government to earmark millions of dollars from the Department of Defense for breast cancer research. It worked! Although highly controversial, this was unprecedented in the history of research funding and exemplified the power of the masses. Today, these funds are targeted for other types of cancer, including ovarian and prostate cancers.

When problems surrounding cancer care are identified, anyone can tell his or her story to the media. Anyone can write to politicians. And many survivors can and are testifying before legislative bodies in an effort to change public opinion and public policy around cancer.

Quality Cancer Care

As the United States moves away from a healthcare system of predominantly fee-for-service insurance plans to those under managed care, and the unknowns of healthcare reform are addressed, national cancer advocacy organizations must be on the alert to issues affecting cancer care. Early on in this quest for healthcare reform in relation to cancer,

NCCS surveyed healthcare providers, scientists, government officials, and professional and advocacy organizations about the critical issue of quality cancer care. Besides addressing the strengths and weaknesses of the old and new systems, NCCS (1995) called for several fundamental issues to be reflected in standards and guidelines for reliable measurements of care.

In our current climate of managed care, disease repair, and bottom-line systems of cost containment, care is time and time is money. Convincing the powers that hold the purse strings to finance programs and projects that focus on QOL has become one of our major challenges. The concept of QOL is called an endangered species by Ferrell (1993), and "may be lost during healthcare reform and amidst what [he or she has] termed the 'dehumanization' of cancer" (p. 1471).

CONCLUSION

The impact of the cancer experience permeates all aspects of a person's life and must be measured in terms of both quantity *and* quality. Although the lives of many cancer survivors have been saved or extended, they have also been permanently altered. Survivors themselves must identify their needs, voice their concerns, and advocate for needed social changes and continued support throughout the continuum of cancer care. Only after acknowledging the full spectrum of survivorship can survivors truly celebrate and appreciate quality of life *for* life.

REFERENCES

Carter, B. (1989). Going through: A critical theme in surviving breast cancer. *Innovations in Oncology Nursing, 5*, 2–4.

Clark, E. J. (1994). Parameters for conducting quality of life research. In B. Rabinowitz, E. J. Clark, & J. Hayes (Eds.), *Demystifying oncology research: A handbook for psychosocial and nursing practitioners* (pp. 21–24). Trenton, NJ: State of New Jersey Commission on Cancer Research.

Dow, K. H. (1990). The enduring seasons in survival. *Oncology Nursing Forum, 17*, 511–516.

Epstein, R. M., & Street, R. L. (2007). *Patient-centered communication in cancer care* (Monograph, NIH Publication No. 07-6225). Bethesda, MD: National Cancer Institute.

Ferrell, B. R. (1993). To know suffering. *Oncology Nursing Forum, 20*, 1471–1477.

Frank, A. W. (1991). *At the will of the body.* Boston, MA: Houghton Mifflin.

Gray, R. E. (1992). Persons with cancer speak out: Reflections on an important trend in Canadian health care. *Journal of Palliative Care, 8*, 30–37.

Hewitt, M., Greenfield, S., & Stoval, E. (2006). *From cancer patient to cancer survivor: Lost in transition.* Washington, DC: The National Academies Press.

Koocher, G., & O'Malley, J. (Eds.). (1981). *The Damocles syndrome: Psychosocial consequences of surviving childhood cancer.* New York, NY: McGraw Hill.

Leigh, S. (1994). Cancer survivorship: A consumer movement. *Seminars in Oncology, 21*, 783–786.

Leigh, S. (2001). Preface: The culture of survivorship. In C. H. Yarbro (Ed.), *Seminars in Oncology Nursing, 17*(4), 234–235.

Leigh, S., & Logan, C. (1991). The cancer survivorship movement. *Cancer Investigation, 9*, 571–579.

Mayer, M. (1998). Advanced breast cancer: A guide to living with metastatic disease (2nd ed.). Sebastopol, CA: O'Reilley & Assoc.

Morrison, J. (1983, March 9). Perspective: The survivor as advocate. *The Washington Post*, p. B5.

Mullan, F. (1985). Seasons of survival: Reflections of a physician with cancer. *New England Journal of Medicine, 313*, 270–273.

Mullan, F. (1990). Survivorship: An idea for everyone. In F. Mullan & B. Hoffman (Eds.), *Charting the journey: An almanac of practical resources for cancer survivors* (pp. 1–4). Mount Vernon, NY: Consumers Union.

National Coalition for Cancer Survivorship (NCCS). (1995). *Briefing paper: Quality cancer care*. Silver Spring, MD: Author.

National Coalition for Cancer Survivorship (NCCS). (2009). *Cancer Survival Toolbox*. Retrieved January 6, 2010 from www.canceradvocacy.org/toolbox

Siegal, K., & Christ, G. H. (1990). Hodgkin's disease survivorship: Psychosocial consequences. In M. J. Lacher & J. R. Redman, Jr. (Eds.), *Hodgkins' disease: Consequences of survival* (pp. 383–399). Philadelphia, PA: Lea & Febiger.

Smith, D. W. (1981). *Survival of illness*. New York, NY: Springer.

Spingarn, N. D. (1988). *The cancer survivors' bill of rights*. Atlanta, GA: The American Cancer Society.

Stovall, E., & Clark, E. J. (1996). Survivors as advocates. In B. Hoffman (Ed.), *A cancer survivor's almanac: Charting your journey* (pp. 273–280). Minneapolis, MN: Chronimed Publishing.

Welch-McCaffrey, D., Loescher, L. J., Leigh, S. A., Hoffman, B., & Meyskens, F. (1989). Surviving adult cancer, Part 2: Psychosocial implications. *Annals of Internal Medicine, 3*, 517–524.

World Health Organization (1948). World Health Organization constitution. In *Basic Documents* (p. 29). Geneva, Switzerland: WHO.

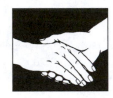

Chapter Nineteen

Quality-of-Life Stories Told by Patients and Families

Quality of Life from a Survivor of Childhood Cancer

Margaret Gunther Lee

Cancer is an amazing thing. It can cause you to realize how precious life is while at the same time, tearing you apart inside. Whether you are the patient or the caregiver, one cannot walk away the same after dealing with such a life-threatening illness. As a patient, I know that my experience with cancer has had a profound effect on my life physically, emotionally, socially, and spiritually.

I was diagnosed with Philadelphia chromosome positive acute lymphocytic leukemia at the age of 12. Upon my diagnosis in June 1992, I faced two and a half years of weekly chemotherapy as well as many procedures and medications, and 2 weeks of cranial radiation. These years brought new challenges, suffering, and victory that I had never experienced before. As a Christian, I found the strength to face the hardships and challenges that my cancer brought in my relationship with the Lord.

During these years, I was constantly reminded of the battle that was going on within my body. I often asked myself, "Is this really happening?" and wondered "Why me?" I felt so different from other kids my age. While they were worried about clothes, social events, and the opposite sex, I was concerned with staying in remission, keeping up in school, and how sick I would get from my next chemo. During this time, the hospital was my comfort zone. Here, there were many other kids who, like me, had no hair and were sick from chemo. However, these individuals had a spark inside them to press on, to endure the fire, and to make it through another day.

After getting used to the cancer routine, it became a way of life for my family and me. I enjoyed seeing my doctors and nurses, and my port-o-cath was my best friend. During these years, I spent so much time at the hospital that I referred to it as my "second home." However, this new way of life was not easy. I was often physically tired and sick, especially after receiving chemo, and I missed anywhere from a day to a week of school after treatment each week. While the doctors, nurses, and other staff at the hospital worked diligently to restore my physical quality of life, my social quality of life declined. So many people were there to support me and pray for me, but as the months went by and it was obvious that I was not going to "Get Well Soon," some of my friends dropped by the wayside. I learned from experience that any serious illness will show you who your true friends are. While I did lose some very special friends during these years, I made many new friends at the hospital. Talking with others at the hospital who had cancer was so helpful to me. Often, these individuals were the only people who could understand how difficult it was to undergo countless treatments and procedures.

After completing treatment in November 1994, I was drained of energy and was finishing out the first semester of my ninth grade year at home. At the age of 14, I was excited about the days to come and the energy that I would be getting back. However, 6 weeks after I finished treatment, I learned that my cancer had returned. Still exhausted, I was not sure that I was up for any more treatment. The next blow came when my doctor told me that my chance of survival with the only treatment option available, a bone marrow transplant, was only 20%.

Here is where the importance of quality of life comes into play. From an outsider's perspective, you probably would not understand why a 14-year-old cancer patient would refuse treatment. However, do not ever assume that you know what is best until you have been faced with the decision yourself. Chemotherapy and all the other treatment regimens that a cancer patient faces are often more difficult and more thoroughly draining than anything one will face here on earth. This was my mindset as I faced this relapse. However, I chose to have the bone marrow transplant and soon began chemo and a rigorous schedule of treatment to hopefully achieve remission once again.

There was no quality of life in those months before my transplant. Preparation for the bone marrow transplant was so much harder than my leukemia treatment. However, I survived the rigorous treatment and received my sister's bone marrow 4 months after the news of my initial relapse. I was in the hospital for a total of 7½ weeks, during which I incurred many devastating side effects, some of which required ICU care on the ventilator. Wheeling out of the hospital for the first time in 7½ weeks was truly amazing. Surrounded by my parents, my brother, and my sister, I marveled at the beauty of the sky, the trees, and the birds that I had only viewed through a distant hospital window for so many weeks. God was so good to me. I know that it is solely by His grace that I was even able to leave the hospital.

Even though I was able to return home in June, I still had a very long road ahead of me. Because my immune system was still weak, I spent the next year primarily at home and wore a hepa-filter mask when I went out in public. The side effects from my 2½ years of treatment and from my bone marrow transplant were really affecting me. I began to experience severe headaches for 80 to 90% of each day. In addition, my energy level began to decrease. In December 1995, a year after I had relapsed, I developed shingles directly above and behind my right eye. This launched a round of extreme pain due to post-herpetic neuralgia and a lifetime of eye problems from the damage from the shingles and the radiation treatments I had received. Years of cancer treatment and a bone marrow transplant, which were meant to restore my health, had left me with very little physical and social quality of life. With continual pain, extreme loneliness, and other daily struggles, I often wondered why the Lord had even brought me through the transplant. However, the Lord reminded me that He had a very special purpose and plan for my life here on earth.

Throughout the years, the support of my family has had a profound impact on my quality of life. They have always been right behind me 110% throughout my treatment.

Both of my parents sought to be involved in my treatment, whether it was taking me to the hospital each week, standing beside me during my procedures, or staying with me when I was an inpatient. They were right there supporting me as I finished chemo as well as when I relapsed and had to decide whether or not I would receive any more treatment. We cried, laughed, and grew together during these difficult years.

During 1996, my parents and I began searching for the reason why my energy level continued to decrease. After months of seeing doctors, having many tests, and changing medication dosages, my parents and I still did not have an answer as to why I was so exhausted. I spent much of my day around the house in bed or doing very low energy tasks. In addition, I continued my studies through a homebound program, doing my best to stay caught up in school.

In November 1996, I saw an endocrinologist who suggested that my fatigue might be due to low growth hormone levels. A few weeks later I underwent a series of inpatient tests. My growth hormone levels were indeed lower than the normal level, but I chose not to begin growth hormone shots due to the possible chance of relapse. However, by June I had no quality of life; I was bedridden with exhaustion and only "existed." My doctor suggested that I go in for growth hormone testing again. The test results showed that my growth hormone levels had decreased significantly. At this point, my quality of life was so poor that I was willing to risk the small possibility of relapse from growth hormone replacement if I could have several good months or years of life. So on June 13, 1997, I began the daily injections. Around August of that same year I began to have a little more energy. As time went on and we increased the dosage I gained even more energy. I cannot express how much these shots affected my quality of life. I continually thank the Lord for the brilliant individuals who determined how to produce growth hormones. Many people do not understand how I can give myself a shot everyday, but they have never experienced the extreme unending and debilitating exhaustion that I lived with for so long.

As my energy improved, I was able to take one or two classes a semester at my high school and complete the rest of my classes through the homebound program. I spent much of my time studying, as I was driven to do well in school. When I relapsed I had taken a semester off from school, and so I was now in class with the grade below me. The combination of only attending one or two classes at school as well as not knowing many people in my new class was difficult. My social quality of life continued to decline, and I experienced severe loneliness. Because I was at home so much, I was extremely thankful to have siblings with whom I could interact. My sister, Catherine, and I had become very close, especially after she donated the bone marrow for my transplant. I considered Catherine to be my best friend and my link to the outside world.

Looking back, I can see that my doctors and nurses did everything in their power for so many years to bring me through my treatment. However, after being in my hospital bubble for so many years, I was not prepared to go back into the real world. I was left hanging, trying to figure out how to be a teenager. I felt so different; I had dealt with struggles and issues no child or teenager should ever have to face and I had watched countless friends die. This had really changed my priorities and my outlook on life and had caused me to become an adult at age 12.

Outwardly, I struggled to fit in with a group of people from whom I had been disconnected during my years of treatment. Entering my treatment as a petite girl, the extensive chemotherapy, steroids, and radiation had stunted my growth, leaving me at four feet eleven inches tall. I was often mistaken for a 12-year-old child, offered a kid's menu, or teased about my height. However, I have learned to laugh at the many comments that people feel compelled to make about my height. In addition, I know that one day I will appreciate looking much younger than I actually am.

After graduating from high school in May 1999, I chose to attend Union University that fall. Still struggling with headaches, much eye pain, and a less than normal energy level, I only took 11 hours my first semester. Attending college was a tremendous milestone in my life. The Lord brought me through so much and improved my quality of life through the years, but my family and I did not know if I would be able to handle the demands of college. However, driven to succeed, I finished my freshman year with 28 credit hours.

Going to college allowed me to step out of a world where everyone knew that I had had cancer. It also allowed me to meet many new people and make new friends. I remember standing in the hall one day before class thinking, "I actually feel comfortable standing around with a large group of people my age." During my junior high and high school years, I spent so much time with adults that I felt more comfortable with these more mature individuals. So, another milestone was reached; I had a greater social quality of life and was comfortable interacting with my peers.

At 22 years old I became a senior at Union University, and I completed a double major in psychology and family studies. I had a wonderful quality of life with plenty of energy, minimal pain, great friends, and a God who continued to amaze me. I now hope to use my skills, both from school and from my life experiences, to work in missions. Looking back, I can thank the Lord for allowing me to have cancer. I feel that I have grown so much as an individual in all qualities of life. I know that my experience with cancer has made me who I am today. While I do not know what my quality of life will be like a year from today or even a week from today, for me, this does not really matter. I do not know what the future holds, but I know the One who holds the future.

A Journey Through Cancer

Michael C. Sullivan

"No way would I let them nuke me or dump toxic waste into my bloodstream if I ever got cancer!" Such was my macho litany when discussions arose of people fighting cancer. The summer of 1987 provided me with a reality check and an ongoing discovery of my own values and strengths—which continues to this day. Along the way, I discovered the true meaning of love, enhanced my spirituality, and came to know what friendship *really* is.

In June of 1987, I injured my back moving a large booth container while closing our exhibit area at a trade show in Washington, DC. I flew home in agony. I called a friend who was a neurosurgeon, and he scheduled a CAT scan and appointment. At that appointment, we determined the back problem was going to resolve itself without surgery. Having become very aware of my body during this painful episode, I had noticed a lump in my left inguinal area and asked him about it. My doctor was unsure of what it was and suggested that I should see a surgeon. The next morning I received a call in my office from the surgeon. He wanted to schedule an appointment. Cool, a doctor calling *me* for an appointment, rather than the other way around. We agreed to meet the following Monday. At that time, after poking and prodding, he said that we couldn't be sure of anything without minor surgery to either fix the hernia (which I was convinced was the problem) or "biopsy" the lump. The procedure was scheduled for Friday, the first day of the longest three days of my life. Biopsies should be illegal on Fridays! You can't get the results before Monday or Tuesday.

Interestingly, when we came home from the outpatient center on Friday, and I went to bed, we saw something new in the actions of Max, our golden retriever. Before, when we wanted Max to get on the bed, it required extensive coaxing (if not an engraved invitation) to convince him it was okay. This day, however, Max immediately joined me on the bed and rested his large head and front paws on my leg, just below the dressing over the incision site. My wife Lynne came in to check the dressing and site, but when she reached for the area, Max firmly pushed her hand away with his nose. *He* was going to take care of the old man! (Later, he relented and allowed her to do her ministrations.)

Tuesday we got the dreaded news: lymphoma! (non-Hodgkin's). The fact that my wife worked at an NCI-designated Comprehensive Cancer Center was the first of many blessings I experienced during my journey. At first, it didn't seem to be a blessing, however. With her background in critical care nursing, she could only relate my cancer to her experiences with the terminally ill patients who she had cared for. We were devastated.

One of the benefits of being married to a nurse is that the compulsiveness, assertiveness, and perfectionism of the profession spills over into the personal life as well. Starting Tuesday afternoon, and continuing throughout my journey, Lynne was "on top" of arranging, scheduling, monitoring, and following up on every specialist I was to see and every procedure I was to undergo. Actually, my role in this journey was easy—I just sat (or lay) back and appreciated whatever was my fate for that day, and that I had gotten through *one* more day.

Initially, we decided that because my lymphoma was a low-grade "indolent" type, we could not pursue a "cure." Shortly thereafter, however, the cancer center added a new radiation oncologist to the staff. He was an expert in a new inverted-Y type of radiation therapy. Because my disease was rated as a Stage II, we decided to "shoot the works" with a course of radiation.

The doctor may have been a technical expert, but his understanding of patient concerns and fears left a lot to be desired. He refused to prescribe an antiemetic because he didn't want to "create a self-fulfilling prophesy!" Naturally, after the first 140 rads to my abdomen, I came home and threw up. It took Lynne almost three hours to get a prescription filled for compazine—while I retched and reconsidered my decision to undergo therapy.

Eventually, I became somewhat used to the Monday through Friday nausea and vomiting. The nausea and vomiting became a part of my life. I learned that the compazine tablets and suppositories, if taken around the clock, slightly ameliorated these symptoms, as did eating immediately after arriving home. After that first treatment, I asked the radiation oncologist to decrease the dose. At a lower dose (120 rads per treatment), I tended to better tolerate the therapy. Because my symptoms were less intense with the lower dose, the radiation oncologist wanted to raise the dose back to 140 rads. I adamantly refused his efforts to persuade me that a higher dose was better for me. Later, I found out that he wrote on my chart that I was a noncompliant patient.

Throughout the 8 weeks of radiation, Max provided me with unconditional love and attention. If the truth be known, Max was often in the way. He was so concerned with my vomiting that he stayed *very* close with his nose near my face. He stayed with me for the first 20 minutes or so after I arrived home, always placing his body between me and Lynne, preventing her from caring for me. We quickly realized that Max had his own routine and concerns for my care. Whenever I could, I walked Max twice a day, discussing my thoughts and feelings with him. I really think he understood.

I was disturbed by the constant fatigue I experienced during radiation. The fatigue affected my ability to carry out routine activities—the walks with Max were slower and shorter, weekends were spent taking *long* naps, and driving to work was a major effort. All my efforts were aimed at getting through each day. I didn't have the energy for any extra activities.

Throughout the radiation, I had the false impression that when radiation was completed, my life would return to normal. But that wasn't the case. I was discouraged and depressed. I wanted to feel better. I wanted to be normal. It took several months to regain some energy. In fact, my energy and stamina are less now than before the radiation.

In 1989, my lymphoma recurred. I had several enlarged axillary nodes and one under the jaw. It was disquieting, to say the least, but easily managed with an oral agent (Chlorambusol). Taking an oral agent that had no side effects allowed Lynne and I to maintain a normal life style—notwithstanding the continued nagging fear of recurrence.

In July 1992, my cancer came back with a vengeance. That same week, we discovered that Max had an inoperable liver tumor, with metastatic pleural effusions that caused labored breathing. His symptoms came on so suddenly! The quality of his life was diminished—he wasn't able to take walks, eat, or rest comfortably. We had Max put to sleep a few days after he was diagnosed. I still miss him. (It was not a good summer.) Luckily, a two-year-old golden retriever, Trigger, was in need of a good home, and we adopted him. He stepped right into Max's footsteps in boosting my spirits, exercising me, and showering me with unconditional love.

After a discussion with my oncologist, I decided to have a bone marrow transplant. Although my marrow had been harvested shortly after diagnosis, he decided that I should have a peripheral stem cell transplant instead. Preparatory to the procedure, I had to undergo a course of CHOP (chemotherapy involving cyclophosphamide, hydroxydaunorubicin [doxorubicin], Oncovin [vincristine], and prednisone/prednisolone). During this chemotherapy, I would schedule my business trips for the weeks between treatments. On Monday I would go to the hospital to have a blood test, then go on to the airport for my flight. I had a small insulated bag in which I carried my Neupogen, syringes, needles—and later, when I had my central line in, the catheter care items. The flight attendants would give me ice to keep the Neupogen cool, and I would get ice at the hotel to continue the cooling task. Each morning I would give myself a shot and tend to my catheter care. We discovered that old 35-mm film containers were perfect receptacles for the needles. As cumbersome as it all may seem, my little "freedom kit" allowed me a return to normalcy by permitting me to return to my peripatetic travel schedule.

The transplant is still a hazy memory to me. With the agreement of my physicians, I stayed "zonked" on Ativan and left the daily decisions on care to Lynne. I had a difficult time with the ablative chemotherapy. That, coupled with a stubborn fever, makes me grateful now for my decision to take an amnesiac. During the first 2 weeks, Lynne was at my bedside. Her every-20-minutes mouth care resulted in my being the first patient in the unit to have no mouth sores at all. Engraftment was a long, slow process because the radiation to my pelvis had diminished marrow production in the radiated area. I waited for over 40 days before my AGC climbed above 500. I was astounded by the fatigue I experienced! Reading the morning paper was an all day effort—and seldom completed. TV was of little interest, except for *Jeopardy* and *Wheel of Fortune*. Surprisingly, though, I did not feel bored. Between trying to read the paper, listening to tapes, and going over my many cards and letters, I seemed to have a pretty full day. Every day Lynne would arrive at 6:30 a.m. to help with my shower and breakfast. She would stay until rounds and then go to work—after reviewing my plan of care for the day with my nurse. At 6:30 p.m. she would arrive again and stay until I nodded off around 10 p.m.

Finally, I got to go home, and that certainly raised my spirits. But, again, I was astounded at my lack of stamina and overwhelming fatigue. The week after my arrival home, Lynne had to go to a conference in Florida. I was sure I could handle everything on my own. That idea, naturally, was disposed of and replaced with a plan to have her father stay with me. The concept was further refined by her mother, who was convinced that the "boys" would fail miserably at attempted bachelorhood. She joined Lynne's dad, and the three of us had a great time! Although we all kept forgetting that I should wear a mask at the grocery store. The time was special because I was able to interact with them on subjects other than my disease and care. There were some good laughs—beginning the first night when Lynne's dad flew out of bed after being awakened by Trigger's wet muzzle in his ear!

Although I have had another recurrence posttransplant, my spirits and hopes are up! I have faced the dreaded "C-word" and survived—and will continue to do so. However, I was shaken by a very good friend's diagnosis of non-Hodgkin's lymphoma. His doctor was never able to get Ken into remission. In the brief span of 18 months, Ken's health declined. He died the day I flew to Florida to be with him.

Why Ken? Why not me? These are questions that keep running through my head. Every experience on this journey has given me a much stronger appreciation for the fragility and preciousness of life. Not only will I never again hunt for sport, but also I won't even step on bugs when Trigger and I are out on our walks!

I have adjusted to a life without the stamina I had before my treatments. It was difficult to accept the fact that my mountaineering days are over. It took me several years before I finally was willing to give away my backpacking and rock-climbing gear.

Lynne is a nurse researcher who focuses on quality-of-life issues. As I prepared this article, I thought a lot about that subject. What *is* quality of life? When I was sick, quality of life was being as symptom-free as possible. It was being able to live as normal a life as possible. It was enduring the various procedures and forms of treatment with the least amount of difficulty and loss of dignity. It was the knowledge that I had an excellent healthcare team. It was the complete support and prayers of family, friends—and even strangers—to help pull me through the experience. I am so very fortunate, because the good Lord provided me with these excellent resources.

Now that I'm through the process, I realize that quality of life has an all new meaning. As a cancer survivor, I feel that I must repay that gift of survival with a life of quality. I owe a great deal to a lot of people—many to whom I'll probably never be able to express sufficient gratitude for their contribution to my survival. I feel an obligation to contribute something in return for this extra time that has been given to me. How do I do this? I believe that I have an obligation to ensure that other cancer survivors are provided with support, encouragement, and prayer. All cancer survivors and their families and friends receive a terrifying education. *Now,* I have the opportunity to be the educator. I can also help healthcare personnel understand that I—and all cancer survivors—have had a life before cancer and will have a life after cancer. I believe that we must remind our doctors and nurses to listen to our stories, and to learn what is important to us.

Shortly after my peripheral stem cell transplant, a friend—who, by the way, had kept me inundated with cards, calls, and good wishes—was diagnosed with breast cancer. Lynne and I were able to help guide Rosemari through her battle with cancer by sharing our own experiences and tips for care. Just being there to take her to chemotherapy, or spending time with her so she was not alone, was an opportunity to repay those who had done the same for me.

We must also ensure that newly diagnosed patients understand the importance of gaining and maintaining some control over their treatment—and, thus, over their disease—and their lives. I was lucky—I had my favorite nurse at my bedside throughout the process. But it doesn't require a nurse or medically trained family member to realize that we *do* need that modicum of control over a situation that has the potential for spinning us out of control so easily.

All of us who have been treated for cancer are fortunate in having a caring and understanding staff to meet our needs. But what many people forget (both laypeople and health professionals) is the fact that cancer doesn't just strike the patient—it strikes the entire family. Spouses and loved ones should not be forgotten in the support process.

In 1981, shortly after Lynne and I began dating, her family had a picnic at a local park. As an only child who had little contact with aunts or uncles, I was unprepared to walk into a gathering of nearly a hundred assorted relatives of her clan! However, that clan was a tremendous support to me as I've wended my way through this 9-year journey. Also, my parents, family, friends, neighbors, and fellow church members were of immeasurable value and contributed significantly to the positive outcomes of my treatments. No words, however, can fully express the awe, respect, and, of course, the love I feel for my bride. She was—and is—the reason I am here now. I live because of her. I live *for* her. Lynne is the *quality* of my life!

(*Author note:* Michael has died since writing this piece.)

Life's Presents

Lynne M. Rivera

On that fateful day in July 1987, I did not realize that my life would change so dramatically. For several months following Mike's diagnosis of cancer, I felt that my life was falling apart. I felt out of control. Eventually, I have come to realize that Mike's cancer has changed my life in many positive ways.

Life is fragile and temporary, but grand! How many times in a day do I think about how fortunate I am to have had Mike alive and healthy to share another day with me? We were very fortunate to have the resources that provided us with the physicians, the nurses, and the medical technology that continued to give us another chance at remission.

Nine years and three recurrences later, I realized that every day was a gift from God. This was not to say that my life was perfect and without the usual deadlines and little frustrations. Believe me, there were still days when I would like to twitch my nose and make a troublesome colleague, friend, family member, or husband disappear from sight; or maybe they would have liked me to disappear. However, every day *was* special and enhanced by the love of family and friends, and the love and companionship of my wonderful husband (who finally succumbed to cancer).

A Personal Perspective on Quality of Life

Anonymous Patient

Having cancer at 35 years old is an especially traumatic experience because it occurred very suddenly, and it is a rare type of oral cancer usually found in males over 45 who have a history of smoking or drinking. I was in good health at the time of diagnosis, and I did not smoke or drink. My career was starting to take off, as I was getting good reviews of my work as a consultant. A new relationship was going okay as well. Then it happened. When diagnosed, I thought that it was sure death. My experience with cancer from family history was that if you have cancer, you die. Mother, grandmother, grandfather, great uncle, all had cancer and died a short while after diagnosis. I cried and was in a state of shock for days. A few days later, I had the surgery and then went home. A few weeks later, I returned to work. At first, I was disoriented at work, but within 6 months, my work was better than before. I was stronger, more confident, and took more risks. Later, I left my job due to political reasons, boredom, lack of opportunity (I kind of topped out), and my relationship ended (she had feelings for another man). I moved to a nearby city in search of another job/career and a relationship.

There are some themes that emerged for me 6 months to a year after the surgery and continue to be driving yet divergent forces guiding my life. The most upfront theme is the continuous awareness of vulnerability, both physically and emotionally—a vulnerability that I had not felt before. The cancer could reoccur at any time; my life could be shortened at any time. Stronger values emerged or became more prominent for me. First, the defense mechanism of denial does not work very well for me anymore. I do not hide things well from myself or others. I am pretty much aware of things as they are, for better or worse. Being honest with oneself becomes the norm. This can be good and bad. Good, in that I do not waste time and energy on things that will get me nowhere. Bad, in the sense that I am constantly hit with reality head on, with no time for escape or assimilation. I see things in life quite clearly for the most part. I see through the deception and the facades. I think I have always been this way, but now it is more pronounced.

Another thing that happened for me is the emerging conflicting feelings, that things that were important in the past are not as important now. But, in a sense, things important in the past are even more important now. Let me explain. Let's take my career. I do not really care anymore what I do for a living. I do not have dreams of being a success in business, climbing the corporate ladder, etc. (this development has been in motion for a while, but has intensified since the cancer). My self-worth is not based as much on work as it was in the past. On the other hand, things that I value in work, that I feel I need in order to feel good about myself in work are now more pressing than ever to find. Being paid for my value, being respected as a person, being respected as a professional, doing something I believe in, that is ethical and makes a difference—these are the things that are most important to me now. A tough combination of things to find in the workplace in America in the 1990s. When I work, I need these things more than ever. Also, in terms of a relationship, the need for someone that thinks and lives like me is more needed than ever. A "soulmate" is very critical at this time in my life. Along with the need for a soulmate is the high level of vulnerability that I feel; vulnerability due to financial instability, the various losses I have experienced, and the physical vulnerability.

I have always been an introspective person to some extent. But, the cancer experience has forced me to examine myself internally more intensely and extensively than ever before. When you have cancer, there is nowhere to hide, no place to escape to, to postpone self-examination. Life hits you between the eyes each and every day. The awareness of possible reoccurrence, this time not being so lucky to be alive and healthy, comes to your mind and guides your thoughts and actions each and every day. Risking everything and anything for some sense of peace, inner power, contentment, and the feeling of doing the right thing is the mode of living that guides me each and every day. I have always felt this way, but now I feel compelled to act this way, even though the fears, doubts, and anxieties are still there to confront me in regard to relationships and career, aging, family, finances, etc. Feel the fear and do it anyway, I guess, is the motto.

I have also felt that I live outside the mainstream of society. But now, I feel an even stronger alienation from society's values and norms and ways of doing things. I have been fighting this internally; I would like to be one of the many. But gradually, internally, I am accepting that this will never happen because of who I am and, in large part, for what the cancer experience has forced me to face.

The cancer experience makes you feel and think and act in a way that says there is nothing to lose. When your life has been threatened and continues to be threatened every day—you live, what more is there to lose? That is the ultimate loss, isn't it? But, if you are still here on earth, it seems important to keep finding yourself and being honest with yourself. I feel constantly driven to take paths that will help me to become a stronger me, a more content me. These paths are scary, and I want to turn back or avoid or deny them. But then, the force comes again, putting a sign in front of you saying that you cannot settle for less. I may not be here much longer. I cannot put it off. I do not want any regrets at the end of my life. The pain of dealing with cancer and the fact that life is terminal is traumatic enough. To have regret and not be able to do anything about it, when your energy is drained and you're sick and in pain, would be more horror than I could imagine. I want to feel when I am on my deathbed that I have done it all, I have tried it all, I have explored the world and myself and myself with others, and I have learned a lot and shared a lot and accomplished a lot, and now I am ready to go to wherever it is we go.

Since I last told my story in this book, I have experienced a recurrence of tongue cancer. Time passed quickly as life moves on. Now I am considered cured. Has my life changed much?

I did start my own business doing what I really enjoy doing. I put forth much energy to get it up and running. I did fairly well with it, although the economy has been on the decline, and it has turned into a struggle to get business. I have developed a great relationship with my wife and best friend. I am continuing my business in a new location and things have gone okay. I have aged and I feel that I am on a good path with my life, although it is still scary pursuing a career in organizational development, which is helping employees to communicate better with each other and managers to lead better. I like the fact that I help surface unresolved conflicts that employees may have with each other or with their manager. My goal is to get the truth, which is elusive and hidden. Maybe I am an idealist, but I believe that people can work well with each other and have some joy in the workplace. After all, we spend so many of our waking hours at work. We need to have some feeling of fulfillment from what we do for so much of our waking hours. Cancer is not staring me in the face right now, but I am a changed person forever. Having cancer makes you used to experiencing continuous feelings of anxiety, which is what we have in the workplace today. But hopefully, I can help others live with the uncertain times and know that it is okay to feel uncertain, to feel anxious, and to feel that you are not sure where you are going.

Oncology and Spirituality: A Spouse's Story

Anonymous Spouse

This is the first anniversary of the discovery of her malignant tumor. I offer a silent prayer of thanks to God with quiet relief that she is doing well and that we as a couple are able to celebrate this date, even though the beast still stalks her. With ambivalence I stare at the refrigerator magnet: "National Cancer Survivors Day, A Celebration of Life." The brightly colored words and dancing image mock me, for my gratitude is contingent and my hope is qualified.

The events of 12 months ago are terribly vivid. Memory replays them in slow motion in distinct contradiction to the racing emotions that accompany the mental narrative. Her surgeon's intervention was direct, quick, and effective, like his New York City street speech and manners. His style reassured her—no easy task—and that was sufficient for me. He performed the excision, and no other treatment was required. Behind large doors deep in the bowels of the hospital, the shadow on the radiologist's image was erased in the last surgery of the night. We had allowed for the worst possibilities, but she would be spared the wretched therapies of chemo and radiation. For us, it was a Passover event, as real as the Biblical story of the deliverance of the people of Israel from the bondage of the pharaoh's slavery. The dark angel did not visit our house. The dread of our adolescent children's fears would remain only anticipatory. We all went home and began living in our collective recovery.

We began a series of cycles. For 2 months and 3 weeks, the credo of "no bad news is good news" put her cancer in perspective and sustained us. We were appreciative for a competent clinician/researcher and for nurses whose competencies included caring. We were humbly mindful of our access to good health care, and acutely aware of the poor distribution of resources in this country. The support of friends and faith was precious. We enjoyed the sweet, dull routines of our former lives. And then, at the end of 3 months, her follow-up appointment with the surgeon climaxed the cycle. In the outpatient waiting area, we were never alone. As intrusive and discomforting as a drunk staggering onto a crowded bus, the figure of anxiety sat prominently between us. Wondrously, the surgeon's prognosis of encouragement dispelled the uninvited specter, and we began the cycle anew. The prayers of thanks were offered again, but this continuing encouragement now weighs upon her and, domino-like, on me.

She feels guilty that she is doing as well as she is. She does not suffer the physical afflictions of others who carry the diagnosis of cancer. Others are more stigmatized in their flesh and blood and bones, literally bearing the stigmata of disease or treatment. Does a survivor who thrives deserve the sympathy or attention offered to those who have been more authentically victimized? She takes the measure of her fears and contrasts them to the fears of those whose prognoses are truly frightening, and then lays hers aside. The effect on me is inhibiting; my dance for joy is performed solo and in private. And yet I know there is more at work in her.

Abused sexually as a child, she never expected to fall in love and marry, or give birth to two dear children, or work as a professional and contribute to her community. The first days of the diagnosis threatened her with losing all. She discovered then that she could be profoundly content with her life, that at long last there was a legacy of which she could be proud. Regardless of the future, she had found God's blessing for her. I was touched, surprised, and cried.

We go on now, like Sarah and Abraham, in faith and into a land unknown, uncertain of the future and sure that we are sustained, nevertheless. Fear comingles with hope, and with guilt, with gratitude. She is fiercely resilient and tenacious in her vulnerability. The cancer is not living her; God is, and we are both blessed.

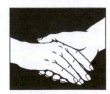

Conclusion

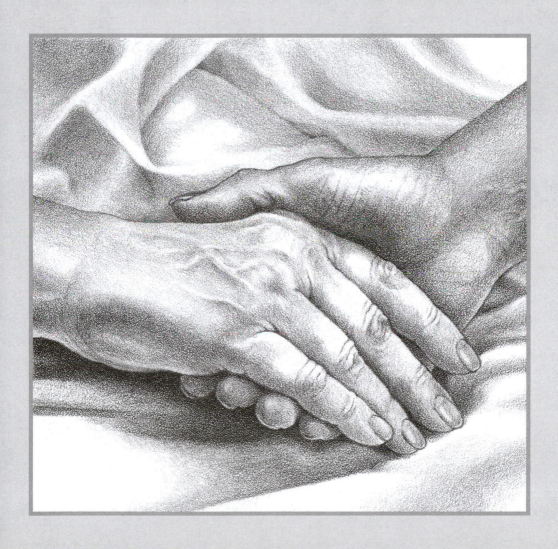

Chapter Twenty

Nursing and Patient Perspectives on Quality of Life

Pamela S. Hinds • Cynthia R. King

Introduction

In this closing chapter, impressions and recommendations regarding nursing and patient perspectives on quality of life (QOL) during illness-related experiences will be summarized. These impressions and recommendations have application for theory, research, and practice. For future research, and clinical, educational, and administrative efforts, to sufficiently reflect the nursing and patient perspectives on QOL, most, if not all, of the recommendations need to be incorporated. The purposeful combining of the two perspectives in this text and in this chapter is not to deny the unique aspects of each, but to emphasize their conceptual commonalities and the link between patient and nurse perspectives that directly influences care given to patients. The link represents the merger of nurses' knowledge of disease, health, human development, and respect for patients with the perceptions, values, and preferences of patients. This merger influences care, the patients' response to their care, and, ultimately, the outcomes of the care. A second reason for combining both perspectives in the same text is to further promote the commitment of nurses to solicit from patients their views on QOL and to do so in a way that convinces patients that their perspectives are heard, respected, and integrated into their care.

More than two dozen definitions and descriptions of QOL are contained in this text. This implies that nursing as a discipline has found multiple though differing conceptualizations to be useful. Most of these are not derived directly from patients, but rather from available literature and clinical observations. The latter two sources are valid and valuable, but the direct participation of patients in defining their QOL adds to the validity and value of the existing definitions. Given the varying and diverse conceptualizations being used, it is important to state clearly the definition of QOL being used in any future work and to include a brief rationale for the selection of that conceptualization (see Table 20-1). Efforts to develop consensus definitions that best convey QOL for defined groups need to continue, but until such agreements on definitions are achieved, the conceptual basis for QOL needs to be explicitly stated. The incomplete conceptual analysis of QOL is most notable in pediatric populations (see Chapter 7), in situations in which the family rather than the individual is the unit of analysis (see Chapter 10), and in survivor populations (see Chapter 18). Rather than include a definition of QOL in their work, some authors imply a definition by the scale or scales used to measure QOL. It is inaccurate to assume that the term QOL evokes a shared understanding among nurses or other healthcare professionals.

Table 20-1. **QOL-Related Recommendations for Future Research or Projects to Ensure that Nursing and Patient Perspectives Are Sufficiently Reflected**

1. Solicit from patients their views on their QOL.
2. Include an explicit definition of QOL.
3. Provide a rationale for the definition of QOL included.
4. Use a definition of QOL that corresponds with the scope of the research or project.
5. Match the breadth of the conceptualization (global or focused) of QOL with a measurement approach.
6. Specify the domains of QOL and their definitions.
7. Provide a rationale for the domains of QOL included.
8. Distinguish the essential characteristics of QOL from variables that influence or are associated with QOL.
9. Make explicit the QOL model being used, including its domains, associated variables, and underlying assumptions.
10. Reflect the dynamism of QOL in the model used.
11. Avoid measuring QOL at a single point.
12. Avoid relying solely on a single, global item to measure QOL.
13. Solicit patient QOL ratings at true change points and not just at stable points during and after care.
14. Use established measures (those with known psychometric properties) of QOL.
15. Avoid using a standardized weighting system for the domains of QOL so that true change will not be obscured.
16. Quality of life at end of life needs to include the perspectives of patients and their significant others.

It seems equally inaccurate to assume that patients share a common conceptualization of the term QOL until this has been documented or refuted through systematically solicited input from patients. The contributors to this text who are patients have offered the following key characteristics of QOL in the cancer experience:

1. A profound sense of personal vulnerability
2. An inability to deny that which is frightening
3. Changing perceptions of what is important in life
4. A desire to make a difference in the lives of others
5. A need to be respected by others
6. A loving connection with a special person
7. Learning to tolerate feeling alienated from a societal norm or value
8. A greater appreciation of daily activities
9. A need to be taken seriously
10. A profound sense of spirituality

More specifically for healthcare providers, these contributors have indicated a desire to be honestly involved in decisions about their care without risk of being labeled "difficult" or "noncompliant." The contributors have also conveyed that key characteristics of QOL can change in importance during and after treatment for cancer. The essential characteristics of QOL offered by patients are somewhat different from those described by nurses and other professionals, although the difference may be strictly semantic. Nevertheless, the need remains for a direct comparison of these differences and more direct solicitations of QOL definitions from patients at the point of diagnosis of a life-threatening illness to cure or from diagnosis to death (see Table 20-1).

Although achieving consensus definitions of QOL is a priority, such definitions may legitimately differ by breadth and specificity according to the scope of the research or project. A broad, global definition will provide valuable flexibility when cultures or other large groups are being compared (see Chapter 4). The broad conceptual approach will need to be matched by an equally broad measurement approach (or use of global measures of QOL). Such a matched conceptual and measurement approach will likely yield findings that will invite us as nurses to view groups of patients and other individuals in new ways, or to further refine our previous impressions and understandings. This is the benefit of comparing groups on a similar basis—using a consensus definition of QOL. In contrast, a consensus definition and conceptualization that is narrowly focused can be matched with an equally focused measurement approach, for example, QOL in 7- to 12-year-old pediatric oncology patients experiencing pain. The benefit of the narrowly focused approach is that findings may translate more readily into direct care practices tailored for the studied group. The recommendations here are to use a consensus definition that corresponds to the scope of the research or project, and to match the breadth of the conceptualization with a corresponding measurement approach (see Table 20-1).

Whether the conceptual and measurement approach is broad and global or narrow and focused, the essential domains (along with the conceptual definitions of QOL and the attributes of QOL) need to be specified. The rationale for considering the essential domains also needs to be included (see Table 20-1). At present, four domains are most commonly included in the nursing literature: physical functioning, emotion or psychological functioning, social functioning, and disease- or treatment-related symptoms. However, the definitions of these domains vary across studies and projects. Current work in nursing with the domains of QOL indicates that the one or more domains that represent what is of greatest meaning to a patient or group at the time of measurement are those that most accurately convey QOL (see Chapter 8). Which domains convey meaning may vary by patient or by time and events. Padilla, Kagawa-Singer, and Ashing-Giwa (Chapter 6) and Taylor and Davenport (Chapter 5) suggest that the domain of spirituality used by some researchers may be the domain that most sensitively measures meaning. Although not yet confirmed by research data, this is an example of a rationale for considering spirituality an essential domain of QOL.

The careful effort put into clarifying the conceptual nature of QOL, including its essential characteristics and domains, will also benefit efforts to distinguish these from external sources of influence on QOL, such as antecedent and mediating variables (see Chapter 4).

Distinguishing the features or characteristics that comprise QOL from the variables that affect QOL will further nurses' understanding of what QOL is for patients and what can be done to positively influence their QOL during care for cancer (Table 20-1). This effort will also result in a specification of relationships between QOL and other variables, or model-building, thus contributing to our theoretical understanding of this construct.

Models that seek to convey the context and the characteristics of QOL in the lives of patients receiving care related to cancer will need to reflect the dynamism of QOL over time and events, and the influence of both internal and external factors on QOL. Such dynamism could be conveyed by a feedback loop in the model or some other feature that would prevent the misrepresentation of QOL as occurring in linear, sequential fashion. The recommendation is that a model of QOL be specified or depicted in future work, that the underlying assumptions be made explicit, and that the dynamism of QOL be conveyed (Table 20-1).

Both patient and nursing perspectives indicate that QOL changes in degree or intensity and is time- and event-dependent. Not yet established is whether the intensity is also disease- and treatment-dependent. This change can be in an overall, general sense or in a particular domain or characteristic of QOL. Such change (or lack thereof) needs to be documented. Considering the dynamism of QOL, multiple measurement points with the same respondents, or a cross-sectional approach with very carefully delineated and justified measurement points, will be required. Measuring QOL at a single point will not suffice for full understanding of the nature of QOL, nor will it contribute information that could be used to guide clinical care (see Table 20-1).

Similarly, it is anticipated that as advances continue in the treatment of cancer, as the number of cancer survivors increases, and as supportive care improves, QOL may change form, or the standards of comparison previously used may change. This idea of changing form is consistent with the idea that the concept of QOL is in part social and influenced and shaped by the context within which it exists (Toulmin, 1972). The likelihood of change means that QOL will need to be examined over time both conceptually and empirically.

Sufficiency in empirical measurement of QOL from nursing and patient perspectives is unlikely to be met by a single, global item (see Chapter 8). Although a patient's response to the item may give an indication of a general perception at that moment, the response would not identify the source or domain that accounts for the change. This, then, would not provide a basis for a care intervention from nurses or other healthcare professionals, or a basis for not initiating an intervention. The single item would make minimal demands on the patient, but that benefit is offset by the lack of clinically useful information. Therefore, the recommendation is to avoid relying solely on a single, global item to measure QOL when the intent is to gather information that will be helpful in providing clinical care (Table 20-1).

The potential burden on patients of measuring their QOL is increased by the need to have repeated measures and by the timing of those measures. Key measurement points are those at which a change in QOL is anticipated, such as during confirmed progression of disease or nadirs. The balance between burden and the opportunity for a patient to express perceptions and values in a way that could benefit him or her or others is important to achieve. Seeking patients' QOL only at stable points may prevent healthcare professionals from learning essential information about QOL that may only be evident at change points, and prevent patients from sharing their views at critical times (Table 20-1).

Several psychometrically sound QOL instruments are available for use with adults. These are available in global forms and disease-specific modular forms. It is important to use these instruments consistently (rather than develop new measures) to document their ability to accurately measure QOL in different groups at varying time points (see Chapter 8). Similarly, general and disease-specific QOL instruments are now available for pediatric patients and their parents. As a result, researchers tend to use a battery of measures in an attempt to document all domains of quality of life.

Accuracy of interpreting QOL scores and capturing change in the domains of QOL also have implications for scoring QOL measures. Composite scores could obscure change in individual domains. Assigning weights to domains may also obscure the true change in intensity being obscured. Individual scores for each domain may be the more appropriate scoring method with QOL (Table 20-1).

CONCLUSION

Nursing's commitment is to support and influence in a positive manner the QOL of patients during and following care for cancer. This commitment reflects our belief that QOL is a process that changes over time and situations and that it can be altered by both internal factors (e.g., cellular response to treatment) and external factors (e.g., nursing care interventions). That commitment, combined with knowledge of patients' perspectives on their QOL, will most assuredly result in care that assists patients in achieving the most positive outcomes possible in the physical, psychological, symptom-related, social, and spiritual domains.

REFERENCE

Toulmin, S. (1972). *Human understanding*. Princeton, NJ: Princeton University Press.

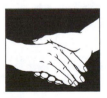

Quality of Life Measurements

Selected instruments used to measure quality of life (QOL) are contained in this appendix. The instruments represent diverse approaches to quantifying QOL. These approaches include the global single-item, generic , and cancer-specific measures.

Quality of Life
Visual Analogue Scale (VAS)

KATE LORIG

Contact person: Kate Lorig, RN, DrPH, Director, Stanford Patient Education Research Center, 1000 Welch Road, Suite 204, Palo Alto, CA 94304.

Quality of Life Visual Analogue Scale (VAS)

Take a moment and think of the best possible life and the worst possible life. Now, on the line below, place an "X" to indicate where your life is now:

Best
possible
life

Worst
possible
life

Scoring. Measure in centimeters with ruler, "10" being "Worst possible life" and "0" being "Best possible life." Enter the number where the middle of the "X" is located. Enter whole numbers, not decimals. If the "X" is between centimeters, round down if below 0.5, round up if 0.5 and above, and if exactly at 0.5, round to the nearest even number.

Note: The line must be *exactly* 10 cm long. When reproducing, make sure your printer or copy machine reproduces at exactly 100 percent. You cannot have a reliable measurement if the line is not exactly the same length each time. A small, clear, plastic ruler will make it easier to see the scoring point. Make sure all scoring is done with identical rulers.

The McCorkle and Young Symptom Distress Scale

RUTH MCCORKLE • KATHY YOUNG GRAHAM

Contact person: Ruth McCorkle, PhD, FAAN, Professor, The Florence S. Wald Professor of Nursing, Director, Center for Excellence in Chronic Illness Care, Chair, Doctoral Program, Yale University School of Nursing, 100 Church Street, South, PO Box 9740, New Haven, CT, 06536. Used with permission from Ruth McCorkle, PhD, FAAN.

ID# _____ DATE _____

(SDS) Each of the following sections lists 5 different statements. Think about what each statement says, then place a circle around the one statement that most closely indicates how you have been feeling during the past 7 days. Please circle one statement for each section.

1. Appetite

1. I have my normal appetite.
2. My appetite is usually, but not always, pretty good.
3. I don't really enjoy my food like I used to.
4. I have to force myself to eat my food.
5. I cannot stand the thought of food.

2. Insomnia

1. I sleep as well as I always have.
2. I have occasional spells of sleeplessness.
3. I frequently have trouble getting to sleep and staying asleep.
4. I have difficulty sleeping almost every night.
5. It is almost impossible for me to get a decent night's sleep.

3. Pain (a)

1. I almost never have pain.
2. I have pain once in a while.
3. I frequently have pain—several times a week.
4. I am usually in some degree of pain.
5. I am in some degree of pain almost constantly.

4. Pain (b)

1. When I do have pain, it is very mild.
2. When I do have pain, it is mildly distressing.
3. The pain I do have is usually fairly intense.
4. The pain I have is usually very intense.
5. The pain I have is almost unbearable.

5. Fatigue

1. I am usually not tired at all.
2. I am occasionally rather tired.
3. There are frequently periods when I am quite tired.
4. I am usually very tired.
5. Most of the time, I feel exhausted.

6. Bowel

1. I have my normal bowel pattern.
2. My bowel pattern occasionally causes me some discomfort.
3. I frequently have discomfort from my present bowel pattern.
4. I am usually in discomfort because of my present bowel pattern.
5. My present bowel pattern has changed drastically from what was normal for me.

7. *Concentration*

1 — I have my normal ability to concentrate.

2 — I occasionally have trouble concentrating.

3 — I often have trouble concentrating.

4 — I usually have at least some difficulty concentrating.

5 — I just can't seem to concentrate at all.

8. *Appearance*

1 — My appearance has basically not changed.

2 — My appearance has gotten a little worse.

3 — My appearance is definitely worse than it used to be, but I am not greatly concerned about it.

4 — My appearance is definitely worse than it used to be, and I am concerned about it.

5 — My appearance has changed drastically from what it was.

9. *Breathing*

1 — I usually breathe normally.

2 — I occasionally have trouble breathing.

3 — I often have trouble breathing.

4 — I can hardly ever breathe as easily as I want.

5 — I almost always have severe trouble with my breathing.

10. *Outlook*

1 — I am not fearful or worried.

2 — I am a little worried about things.

3 — I am quite worried, but unafraid.

4 — I am worried and a little frightened about things.

5 — I am worried and scared about things.

11. *Cough*

1 — I seldom cough.

2 — I have an occasional cough.

3 — I often cough.

4 — I often cough and occasionally have severe coughing spells.

5 — I often have persistent and severe coughing spells.

12. *Nausea (a)*

1 — I seldom feel any nausea at all.

2 — I am nauseous once in a while.

3 — I am often nauseous.

4 — I am usually nauseous.

5 — I suffer from nausea almost continually.

13. *Nausea (b)*

1 — When I do have nausea, it is very mild.

2 — When I do have nausea, it is mildly distressing.

3 — When I have nausea, I feel pretty sick.

4 — When I have nausea, I feel very sick.

5 — When I have nausea, I am as sick as I could possibly be.

Demands of Illness Inventory

MEL R. HABERMAN

Contact person: Mel Haberman, PhD, RN, FAAN, Associate Dean for Research, Washington State University College of Nursing, 2917 W. Fort George Wright Drive, Spokane, WA 99224-5291. Used with permission from Dr. Mel Haberman.

Demands of Illness Inventory: Patient Version

Below is a list of events and thoughts that describe experiences some individuals have when they experience a health problem. Read each item carefully and determine the extent to which you have had the experience as the result of your health problem *during the last two weeks including today.*

Note: Please mark NA only if the item is not applicable to your particular situation, otherwise mark 0 to 4. Please do not skip any items. Thank you!

NA	= Not Applicable
0	= Not at All
1	= A Little Bit
2	= Moderately
3	= Quite a Bit
4	= Extremely

As the result of my illness I have experienced:

		NA	0	1	2	3	4
1.	Headaches.	NA	0	1	2	3	4
2.	Faintness or dizziness.	NA	0	1	2	3	4
3.	Pains in heart or chest.	NA	0	1	2	3	4
4.	Pains in lower back.	NA	0	1	2	3	4
5.	Nausea or upset stomach.	NA	0	1	2	3	4
6.	Soreness of muscles.	NA	0	1	2	3	4
7.	Hot or cold spells.	NA	0	1	2	3	4
8.	Numbness or tingling in parts of my body.	NA	0	1	2	3	4
9.	Feeling weak in parts of my body.	NA	0	1	2	3	4
10.	Heavy feelings in my arms or legs.	NA	0	1	2	3	4
11.	Feeling rundown.	NA	0	1	2	3	4
12.	Inability to stay at my usual weight.	NA	0	1	2	3	4

As the result of my illness I think about:

		NA	0	1	2	3	4
13.	The value my life has for me.	NA	0	1	2	3	4
14.	How long I might live.	NA	0	1	2	3	4
15.	Not being able to achieve my goals in life.	NA	0	1	2	3	4
16.	How I might reorder the priorities in my life.	NA	0	1	2	3	4
17.	My own mortality.	NA	0	1	2	3	4
18.	How unprepared I've been for this experience.	NA	0	1	2	3	4

Note: Patient version, Woods, Haberman, & Packard, copyright © 1984, 1987, 1993.

19. The uncertainties I face.	NA	0	1	2	3	4
20. Whether my life will ever return to normal.	NA	0	1	2	3	4
21. What will happen to my family in the future.	NA	0	1	2	3	4
22. Whether my children will face the same illness.	NA	0	1	2	3	4
23. Not having any past experience to relate this one to.	NA	0	1	2	3	4
24. How my experience compares with others having the same or a similar experience.	NA	0	1	2	3	4
25. Why is this happening to me?	NA	0	1	2	3	4
26. How unfair this experience has been.	NA	0	1	2	3	4
27. My odds of getting this illness.	NA	0	1	2	3	4
28. What has caused the illness.	NA	0	1	2	3	4

As the result of my illness our family:

29. Income has gone down.	NA	0	1	2	3	4
30. Doesn't have enough time or energy for recreational activities outside our home.	NA	0	1	2	3	4
31. Doesn't have enough money to support our usual lifestyle.	NA	0	1	2	3	4
32. Doesn't have enough time or energy to entertain friends at home.	NA	0	1	2	3	4
33. Doesn't have enough money for our healthcare bills.	NA	0	1	2	3	4
34. Doesn't have enough time or energy to go out with friends.	NA	0	1	2	3	4
35. Has had to change our old meal patterns.	NA	0	1	2	3	4
36. Has had to change our child care arrangements.	NA	0	1	2	3	4

As the result of my illness:

37. The children have had to take responsibility for household tasks.	NA	0	1	2	3	4
38. My partner has had to take responsibility for household tasks.	NA	0	1	2	3	4
39. The quality of my sexual activities has changed.	NA	0	1	2	3	4

40. The frequency of my sexual activities has changed.	NA	0	1	2	3	4
41. There isn't time or energy for sexual activities.	NA	0	1	2	3	4
42. I worry about how my children are reacting to my illness.	NA	0	1	2	3	4
43. The children need more emotional support.	NA	0	1	2	3	4
44. The children need more information.	NA	0	1	2	3	4
45. I need more emotional support from my family.	NA	0	1	2	3	4
46. There is a strain on my relationship with my partner.	NA	0	1	2	3	4
47. My partner has had difficulty understanding my feelings.	NA	0	1	2	3	4
48. I worry about how my partner is responding to my illness.	NA	0	1	2	3	4
49. I wish my partner were handling the illness situation better.	NA	0	1	2	3	4
50. I need to be more sensitive to my partner's moods.	NA	0	1	2	3	4
51. I need to provide more emotional support to my partner.	NA	0	1	2	3	4
52. I need to protect my partner from stress.	NA	0	1	2	3	4
53. I need my partner to be more sensitive to my moods.	NA	0	1	2	3	4
54. I need my partner to help me with my treatment.	NA	0	1	2	3	4
55. My partner has had to change his work patterns.	NA	0	1	2	3	4
56. I'm not able to work at my job.	NA	0	1	2	3	4
57. I've had to miss more time at work than usual.	NA	0	1	2	3	4
58. I'm not able to do my usual amount of work.	NA	0	1	2	3	4
59. I've had trouble finding a job.	NA	0	1	2	3	4

As the result of my illness our family has had to:

60. Make new decisions about running the house.	NA	0	1	2	3	4
61. Revise the rules for the children.	NA	0	1	2	3	4

62. Discuss things concerning the children more.	NA	0	1	2	3	4
63. Decide what is really important to us.	NA	0	1	2	3	4

As the result of my illness:

64. I go out with friends less often.	NA	0	1	2	3	4
65. My social life has decreased.	NA	0	1	2	3	4
66. I often have to help others understand my illness.	NA	0	1	2	3	4
67. It's hard to keep up with my usual pace or routine.	NA	0	1	2	3	4
68. People have been overprotective.	NA	0	1	2	3	4
69. People seem less supportive as time goes on.	NA	0	1	2	3	4
70. I find that I need to help others accept my illness.	NA	0	1	2	3	4
71. Others do not really know or understand what I am going through.	NA	0	1	2	3	4
72. Others act differently toward me.	NA	0	1	2	3	4
73. It's hard to plan social activities because I don't know how I'll feel.	NA	0	1	2	3	4

As the result of my illness I:

74. Feel self-conscious about my body.	NA	0	1	2	3	4
75. Feel less attractive.	NA	0	1	2	3	4
76. Feel dissatisfied with the way I look.	NA	0	1	2	3	4
77. Feel I cannot always rely on my body.	NA	0	1	2	3	4
78. Think more about my own sexual appeal.	NA	0	1	2	3	4
79. Think about the disfigurement caused by surgery/treatment.	NA	0	1	2	3	4
80. Think about possibly needing to undergo surgery that would result in disfigurement.	NA	0	1	2	3	4
81. Think about the possibility of undergoing surgery to improve my appearance.	NA	0	1	2	3	4
82. Think about not being able to be pregnant and have a child.	NA	0	1	2	3	4
83. Feel more susceptible to other illnesses.	NA	0	1	2	3	4
84. Concentrate on new bodily sensations that may indicate illness.	NA	0	1	2	3	4
85. Worry my illness may reoccur with its initial severity.	NA	0	1	2	3	4

86. Tend to be preoccupied with the symptoms of my illness. NA 0 1 2 3 4
87. Think about how I'm handling my illness situation. NA 0 1 2 3 4
88. Wonder if the illness can be controlled in the future. NA 0 1 2 3 4
89. Wonder if the illness is spreading undetected. NA 0 1 2 3 4
90. Wonder why I still receive treatments even though my symptoms have subsided. NA 0 1 2 3 4
91. Think about the illness being unending. NA 0 1 2 3 4
92. Worry my health will get progressively worse. NA 0 1 2 3 4
93. Worry the illness will involve other parts of my body in the future. NA 0 1 2 3 4

As the result of my medical treatment:

94. I find it difficult to continue with follow-up appointments. NA 0 1 2 3 4
95. I find it difficult to continue the treatments. NA 0 1 2 3 4
96. I sometimes think the adverse effects of treatment outweigh the possible benefits. NA 0 1 2 3 4
97. I worry about the expense of treatment. NA 0 1 2 3 4
98. I've changed my diet. NA 0 1 2 3 4
99. I'm more regimented in the time I eat. NA 0 1 2 3 4
100. My whole life is more regimented. NA 0 1 2 3 4
101. I'm adjusting the way I exercise. NA 0 1 2 3 4
102. It's difficult to find suitable clothing. NA 0 1 2 3 4
103. I'm considering the need to undergo more treatment. NA 0 1 2 3 4
104. I'm considering if I should try a different treatment. NA 0 1 2 3 4
105. It's difficult waiting for the results of my medical tests. NA 0 1 2 3 4
106. It's difficult waiting to undergo treatment or surgery. NA 0 1 2 3 4

At times, my healthcare providers:

107. Are not sensitive to my preferences for treatment. NA 0 1 2 3 4

108. Act as if my opinions are unimportant.　　NA　0　1　2　3　4
109. Make decisions without my best interests in mind.　　NA　0　1　2　3　4
110. Do not tell me the truth about my health status.　　NA　0　1　2　3　4
111. Do not show concern for me as a person.　　NA　0　1　2　3　4

As I've experienced my illness situation:

112. I do not want my health providers to tell me the truth if my health takes a turn for the worse.　　NA　0　1　2　3　4
113. I want more facts about the treatments.　　NA　0　1　2　3　4
114. I have questions that I want to ask but just can't.　　NA　0　1　2　3　4
115. I feel rushed to make a hasty treatment decision.　　NA　0　1　2　3　4
116. I want to be more assertive about expressing the direction my treatment should take.　　NA　0　1　2　3　4
117. I want to be told the reason why, when asked to do something for treatment.　　NA　0　1　2　3　4
118. I sometimes don't understand the treatment I'm receiving.　　NA　0　1　2　3　4
119. I'm not satisfied with the progress of my treatment.　　NA　0　1　2　3　4
120. I'm not satisfied with my hospital care.　　NA　0　1　2　3　4
121. I feel my illness is being incorrectly managed.　　NA　0　1　2　3　4
122. I'm not confident my health problems will be correctly managed in the future.　　NA　0　1　2　3　4

As the result of my medical treatments:

123. I worry about the physical side effects of treatment.　　NA　0　1　2　3　4
124. I worry I'll develop new physical symptoms in the future.　　NA　0　1　2　3　4
125. I often feel worse rather than better after treatment.　　NA　0　1　2　3　4

Demands of Illness Inventory: Scoring Procedures

Scoring: Both the frequency of demands (number or incidence of demands) and intensity of experienced demands can be computed for each item and subscale or for the total instrument.

The *frequency of occurrence score* can be calculated at several levels. At the most basic level, each item can be converted to a "Yes/No" categorical variable. As such, "item frequencies" represent the number of subjects that rated an item 1 or greater. We usually report these as percentages of the total sample. For example, if 75 out of 100 subjects rated an item 1 or greater, then 75 percent of the sample experienced that demand.

At the next level, a similar item analysis can be conducted for each subscale by summing the items rated 1 or greater within a subscale. Subscale frequencies can be reported for each subject or for the sample as a whole. The theoretical range for this score is from zero to the number of items in each subscale (or from zero to 125 for the total instrument). These scores can be expressed as whole numbers or as percentages. For example, if 2 out of a possible 4 items in a subscale are rated 1 or greater by the subject, the frequency of experienced demands for that subscale may be expressed as a 2 or as 50 percent. Similarly, if 50 out of a total of 125 items are rated 1 or greater by the subject, the frequency score for the total instrument may be expressed as a 50 or as 40 percent (50/125).

Lastly, means can be calculated from the aforementioned distributions of subscale or total instrument frequency scores. These means represent the average number of demands experienced by the sample as a whole for each subscale or for the total instrument (see Table 4, Haberman, Woods, & Packard, 1990). These means can also be rank ordered (see Table 5, Haberman, Woods, & Packard, 1990).

A variation of reporting the frequency of demands is the calculation of *incidence rates*. Incidence rates describe the percent of items in a scale marked as a demand of illness, i.e., as problematic. They represent the number of items scored a 1 or greater, divided by the number of items in the subscale (or in the total instrument) × 100. The incidence rate is insensitive to gradations in the intensity of individual items, treating ratings of "a little bit," "moderately," "quite a bit," and "extremely" identically.

For the *intensity of demands scores,* we generally use item and subscale mean scores. However, a mean intensity score also can be calculated for the total instrument. The intensity score has a theoretical range of 0 to 4 per item or per subscale. To calculate the mean intensity score for each item, sum the intensity ratings by item for the entire sample and divide by the total sample size. To calculate the mean intensity score for each subscale, sum the intensity ratings for all the items in the subscale and divide by the number of items in the subscale. Subscale intensity means for the sample as a whole can be calculated from these distributions of the individual subject's subscale intensity scores. Sample means represent the average intensity of demands experienced by the sample as a whole for each subscale dimension. The means can be reported directly or rank ordered (same format as Tables 4 and 5, Haberman, Woods, & Packard, 1990).

Note: Scoring procedures, Woods, Haberman, & Packard, copyright © 1987, 1993.

Demands of Illness Inventory: Patient's Version

Standardized Item Alphas

Subscale	Frequency	Intensity
Physical symptoms	.8484	.8646
Personal meaning	.8457	.9179
Family functioning	.9120	.9228
Social relationship	.8227	.8747
Self-image	.8027	.8709
Monitoring symptoms	.7835	.9104
Treatment issues	.8892	.9164
Total instrument	.9621	.9717

Sample: 96 women with breast cancer
29 women with diabetes
Total = 125

Demands of Illness Inventory: Revision of the 1987 Version

Item change: The 1993 version has 1 item change from the 1987 version.

- 1987 Version, Item #112. *"Not thoroughly explained my health status to me."*
- 1993 Version, Item #112. *"I do not want my health providers to tell me the truth if my health takes a turn for the worse."*

Because of this item change, the Treatment Relationships Subscale lost an item and the Treatment Information Exchange Subscale gained an item (#112).

All of the remaining changes are editorial and not substantive. Minor wording changes were made to several items to improve the grammar and clarity of the items.

1. The introduction was changed, deleting an Example item and changing the Note to read: *Please mark NA only if the item is not applicable to your particular situation, otherwise mark 0 to 4. Please do not skip any items. Thank you!*
2. Not Applicable was added as a response choice. The 0 to 4 rating scale remains unchanged.
3. References to "cancer and diabetes" were removed from the tool.
4. Items #94 to 125 were changed from the past to the present tense. The present tense is more relevant especially when using the tool in a repeated measures design. The change is more consistent with the instructions, which tell respondents to answer the questions *based on the last two weeks including today.*
5. Items were changed that were formally reverse scored. All the items are now scored in the same direction. The higher the item score, the greater the intensity of demand.

Demands of Illness Inventory: Patient and Partner Versions

Subscale	Total items	Item numbers
I. Physical Symptoms	12	1–12
II. Personal Meaning	16	13–28
III. Family Functioning		
A. Adaptation	8	29–36
B. Integration	13	37–49
C. Partner Caretaking	5	50–54
D. Work Situation	5	55–59
E. Decision Making	4	60–63
IV. Social Relationships	10	64–73
V. Self-Image	9	74–82
VI. Monitoring Symptoms, Self, & Others	11	83–93
VII. Treatment Issues		
A. Accommodation	13	94–106
B. Relationships	5	107–111
C. Information Exchange	7	112–118
D. Evaluation	4	119–122
E. Direct Effects	3	123–125
		Total = 125

REFERENCES

Haberman, M. R., Woods, N. F., & Packard, N. J. (1990). Demands of chronic illness: Reliability and validity assessment of a demands of illness inventory. *Holistic Nursing Practice*, 5(1), 25–35.

Lewis, F. M., & Hammond, M. A. (1992). Psychosocial adjustment of the family to breast cancer: A longitudinal analysis. *Journal of the American Medical Women's Association*. 47(5), 194–200.

Lewis, F. M., Hammond, M. A., & Woods, N. F. (1993). The family's functioning with newly diagnosed breast cancer in the mother: The development of an explanatory model. *Journal of Behavioral Medicine*, 16(4), 351–370.

Packard, N. J., Haberman, M. R., Woods, N. F., & Yates, B. C. (1991). Demands of illness among chronically ill women. *Western Journal of Nursing Research*, 13(4), 434–457.

Woods, N. F., Haberman, M. R., & Packard, N. J. (1990). Demands of illness inventory: Relationship to individual, dyadic and family adaptation to chronic illness. *Western Journal of Nursing Research*, 15(1), 10–30.

Quality of Life Index

GERALDINE V. PADILLA • MARCIA M. GRANT

Contact person: Geraldine Padilla, PhD, Associate Dean for Research, University of California, San Francisco, School of Nursing, Box 0604, N 339, San Francisco, CA, 94122. Used with permission from Geraldine Padilla, PhD, and Marcia Grant, RN, DNSc.

Pt. No. _____

Time given: _____

Agency: _____

1. How easy is it to adjust to your radiation treatment to date?
   not at all   very easy

2. How much fun do you have (hobbies, recreation, social activity)?
   none   a great deal

3. Do you worry about the cost of your medical care?
   not at all   extremely

4. If you have pain, how distressing is it?
   not at all   extremely

5. How useful do you feel?
   not at all   extremely

6. How much happiness do you feel?
   none at all   a great deal

7. How satisfying is your life?
   not at all   extremely

8. Is your sexual activity sufficient to meet your needs?
   not at all   extremely

9. Is your radiation treatment interfering with your sexual activity?
   not at all   a great deal

10. Are you worried (fearful or anxious) about your radiation treatment?
    not at all   constantly

11. How much can you work at your usual tasks?
    not at all   a great deal

12. How is your present ability to concentrate?
    extremely poor   excellent

13. How much strength do you have?
    none at all   a great deal

14. Do you tire easily?
    not at all   a great deal

15. Is the amount of time you sleep sufficient to meet your needs?
    not at all   completely

16. How is your quality of life?
    extremely poor   excellent

17. How is your appetite?
    extremely poor   excellent

18. Is the amount you eat sufficient to meet your needs?
    not at all   completely

19. Are you worried about your weight?
    not at all   a great deal

20. If you have nausea, how distressing is it?
    not at all   extremely

21. If you vomit, how distressing is it?
    not at all   extremely

Information on Quality-of-Life Index (QLI-RT)

The following information is for a Quality-of-Life Index that includes 21 linear analogue scale items.

Pelvic Radiation Sample

In the Padilla and Grant studies (Padilla, 1990, 1992; Padilla et al., 1992), studies that focus on cancer patients receiving radiation treatment to the pelvic area, the QLI is measured three times: N = 186 during Radiation Treatment week one (RT Week 1); N = 174 during Radiation Treatment week three (RT Week 3); N = 146 during the first follow-up (FU) after the completion of radiation treatment (RT 1st FU).

Internal consistency thetas for the total scale are as follows: during the first week of radiation treatment = 0.86; during the third week of treatment = 0.90; during the first follow-up visit = 0.92.

Internal consistency alphas for subscales during the radiation treatment follow-up period are as follows: psychological well-being = 0.87, physical well-being = 0.87, symptoms = 0.86, sexual activity = 0.97, and worry over weight and cost of treatment = 0.42.

Source: Padilla, 1992; Padilla, 1990; Padilla, Grant, Lipsett et al., 1992.

Validity: Factor analysis is based on an N of 85 from the first week of radiation treatment. The regression analysis is based on an N of 101.

Factor analytic construct validity: Five factors (psychological, physical, symptoms, sexual activity, and worry over weight and cost of radiation treatment).

Concurrent validity: Significant *r*s of 0.58 between tension-anxiety and psychological well-being subscale; and 0.60 between fatigue and physical well-being subscale.

Head and Neck Radiation Sample

In the Padilla and Grant studies (Padilla, 1992; Padilla et al., 1992) that focus on cancer patients receiving radiation treatment to the head and neck area, the QLI is measured 6 times: N = 181 RT week 1; N = 176 RT week 3; N = 156 end of RT; N = 129 RT 1st FU; N = 109 3 month FU; N = 82 18 month FU.

Internal consistency theta 0.88 for the total scale (based on an N of 110 at RT week 1).

Validity: Factor analysis is based on an N of 110 at RT week 1.

Factor analytic construct validity: Six factors (psychological, physical, nutrition and pain distress, other symptom distress, sleep and worry over cost, treatment anxiety-adjustment).

REFERENCES

Padilla, G. V. (1992). Validity of health-related quality of life subscales. *Progress Cardiovascular Nursing*, 7(1), 13–20.

Padilla, G. V., Grant, M. M., Lipsett, J., Anderson, P. R., Rhiner, M., & Bogen, C. (1992). Health quality of life and colorectal cancer. *Cancer, 70*(5 Suppl.), 1450–1456.

Padilla, G. V. (1990). Gastrointestinal side effects and quality of life in patients receiving radiation therapy. *Nutrition, 6*(5), 367–370.

Padilla, G. V. , Grant, M. M., Ferrell, B. R., & Presant, C. (1996). Quality of life—cancer. In Spilker, B. (Ed.), *Quality of life and pharmacoeconomics in clinical trials* (2nd ed.), (pp. 301–308). New York, NY: Raven Press.

Caregiver Quality of Life
Self-Assessment Scale©

The caregiver role for a person with cancer is important. When responding to the following questions think about your caregiving experience over the last week. Respond to each question based on a "best estimate" of the impact of the occurrence or event.

Check the response category that best describes how caregiving has influenced you.

Social Relationships

	Almost Never	A Little	Half the Time	Most of the Time	Almost Always
1. I feel I cannot leave my relative alone.	[ ]	[ ]	[ ]	[ ]	[ ]
2. I get what I need from my family and friends.	[ ]	[ ]	[ ]	[ ]	[ ]
3. I feel cut off from other people.	[ ]	[ ]	[ ]	[ ]	[ ]
4. I feel a loss of privacy.	[ ]	[ ]	[ ]	[ ]	[ ]
5. Caregiving for ____ puts a strain on my relationship with him/ her.	[ ]	[ ]	[ ]	[ ]	[ ]

Economic Situation

	Almost Never	A Little	Half the Time	Most of the Time	Almost Always
1. Caregiving has put a financial strain on us.	[ ]	[ ]	[ ]	[ ]	[ ]
2. I worry about medical expenses.	[ ]	[ ]	[ ]	[ ]	[ ]
3. There is enough money to meet our needs.	[ ]	[ ]	[ ]	[ ]	[ ]

Emotional/Psychological Reactions

	Almost Never	A Little	Half the Time	Most of the Time	Almost Always
1. I resent having to take care of _____.	[ ]	[ ]	[ ]	[ ]	[ ]
2. Caring for _____ makes me feel good.	[ ]	[ ]	[ ]	[ ]	[ ]
3. I feel overwhelmed.	[ ]	[ ]	[ ]	[ ]	[ ]
4. I feel calm and peaceful.	[ ]	[ ]	[ ]	[ ]	[ ]
5. It upsets me to see what is happening to _____.	[ ]	[ ]	[ ]	[ ]	[ ]
6. I feel sad.	[ ]	[ ]	[ ]	[ ]	[ ]
7. I have trouble keeping my mind on what I am doing.	[ ]	[ ]	[ ]	[ ]	[ ]
8. I feel confined by caregiving.	[ ]	[ ]	[ ]	[ ]	[ ]
9. I worry about the future.	[ ]	[ ]	[ ]	[ ]	[ ]

Physical Reactions

	Almost Never	A Little	Half the Time	Most of the Time	Almost Always
1. I am taking care of my own health.	[ ]	[ ]	[ ]	[ ]	[ ]
2. I get enough sleep.	[ ]	[ ]	[ ]	[ ]	[ ]
3. I am tired.	[ ]	[ ]	[ ]	[ ]	[ ]
4. I have enough physical strength to take care of _____.	[ ]	[ ]	[ ]	[ ]	[ ]
5. I am eating regular meals (e.g. sitting down, balanced diet, no fast food).	[ ]	[ ]	[ ]	[ ]	[ ]
6. I take care of my own needs last.	[ ]	[ ]	[ ]	[ ]	[ ]

Spiritual Issues

	Almost Never	A Little	Half the Time	Most of the Time	Almost Always
1. My personal beliefs give me the strength to face difficulties.	[ ]	[ ]	[ ]	[ ]	[ ]

Overall Personal Health and Quality of Life

	Better	About the Same	Worse
1. Since I began providing care for ____, my quality of life is:	[ ]	[ ]	[ ]
2. My current personal health is ____ than this time last year.	[ ]	[ ]	[ ]

	Poor	Fair	Satisfactory	Very Good	Excellent
3. I would rate my overall quality of life as:	[ ]	[ ]	[ ]	[ ]	[ ]

Thank you for completing this assessment.

Quality of Life Scale
Bone Marrow Transplant

BETTY R. FERRELL • MARCIA M. GRANT

Contact person: Betty R. Ferrell, PhD, RN, FAAN, Associate Research Scientist, City of Hope National Medical Center, 1500 East Duarte Road, Duarte, CA 91010-0269. Version 1. Used with permission from Betty R. Ferrell, PhD, RN, FAAN, and Marcia Grant, DNSc, RN, FAAN.

Quality of Life in Bone Marrow Transplant Survivors

Thank you for taking the time to complete this questionnaire.

We want to ensure that your responses are anonymous and confidential. Once your completed questionnaires are received, a number will be assigned and your name will not appear on any questionnaires.

All results will go directly to the Department of Nursing Research. *Your individual responses will not be reported to your nurse, physician, or social worker.* Therefore, if you have any specific concerns, please contact your nurse, physician, or social worker directly. See the enclosed colored sheet for their telephone numbers.

Name _____ Date _____

Current address, if changes have occurred within the last year.

_____

_____

Current telephone number including area code _____

Please complete the following information.

1. Marital status prior to your bone marrow transplant (BMT).
   Single ___   Married ___   Divorced ___   Widowed ___   Separated ___
   Marital status now.
   Single ___   Married ___   Divorced ___   Widowed ___   Separated ___

2. Age_____

3. Height_____

4. Current weight_____

5. Are you satisfied with your current weight?
   No ___   Yes ___

6. Has a substantial weight change occurred since your BMT?
   No ___   Yes ___
   If yes, has it been an:
   Increase_____   Please identify the number of pounds ____
   Decrease _____   Please identify the number of pounds ____

7. How many colds and episodes of flu do you have per year? _____
   Is this more than ___, less than ____, or the same as ____ before your BMT?

8. List all medications you are currently taking.

Medication Name and Dose	Physician's Instructions for Taking the Medication	How Are You Taking the Medication?
Example: Advil 200 mg	1 tablet 4 times a day	1 tablet 3 times a day

9. Do you have chronic graft-versus-host disease?
   No ___   Yes ___

10. Have you been able to return to work since your BMT?
    No ___   Yes (part-time) ___   Not applicable ___
    Yes (full-time) ___

11. If you have not been able to return to work, why not? _____
    _____
    _____

12. If you have returned to work, are you employed in the same occupation as before your BMT?
    No ___   Yes ___
    If no, why did you change your occupation? _____
    _____
    _____

13. Have you been able to return to school since your BMT?

    No ___   Yes (part-time) ___   Not applicable ___

    Yes (full-time) ___

14. If you have not been able to return to school, why not? _____

    _____

    _____

15. Are you using any home treatments or remedies?

    No ___   Yes ___

    If yes, please identify what you are using. _____

    _____

    _____

16. Please identify any activities that you participate in such as exercise, sports, or other recreational activities. _____

    _____

    _____

17. Do you currently have health insurance?

    No ___   Yes ___

18. Have you experienced any difficulty with acquiring or maintaining health insurance?

    No ___   Yes ___

    If yes, please explain. _____

    _____

    _____

19. Have you experienced any problems with your employer related to your disease or treatment?

    No ___   Yes ___

    If yes, please explain. _____

    _____

    _____

20. Do you belong to a support group?

    No ___   Yes ___

    If yes, to which group do you belong? _____

    _____

    _____

Directions: We are interested in knowing how your experience of having cancer and having a BMT affects your Quality of Life. Please answer all of the following questions based on *your life at this time*.

Please *circle* the number from 0–10 that best describes your experiences.
NA = not applicable to me/doesn't apply to me

Physical Well-Being

To what extent are the following a problem for you:

21. Skin changes
no problem   0   1   2   3   4   5   6   7   8   9   10   a severe problem   NA

22. Bleeding problems
no problem   0   1   2   3   4   5   6   7   8   9   10   a severe problem   NA

23. Mouth dryness
no problem   0   1   2   3   4   5   6   7   8   9   10   a severe problem   NA

24. Changes in vision
no problem   0   1   2   3   4   5   6   7   8   9   10   a severe problem   NA

25. Hearing loss
no problem   0   1   2   3   4   5   6   7   8   9   10   a severe problem   NA

26. Fatigue
no problem   0   1   2   3   4   5   6   7   8   9   10   a severe problem   NA

27. Ringing in your ears
no problem   0   1   2   3   4   5   6   7   8   9   10   a severe problem   NA

28. Appetite changes
no problem   0   1   2   3   4   5   6   7   8   9   10   a severe problem   NA

29. Physical strength
no problem   0   1   2   3   4   5   6   7   8   9   10   a severe problem   NA

30. Sleep changes
no problem   0   1   2   3   4   5   6   7   8   9   10   a severe problem   NA

31. Sexual activity
no problem   0   1   2   3   4   5   6   7   8   9   10   a severe problem   NA

32. Pain or aches
no problem   0   1   2   3   4   5   6   7   8   9   10   a severe problem   NA

33. Loss of feeling, tingling, or pain in your hands or feet
no problem   0   1   2   3   4   5   6   7   8   9   10   a severe problem   NA

34. Shortness of breath or difficulty breathing

no problem 0 1 2 3 4 5 6 7 8 9 10 a severe problem NA

35. Constipation

no problem 0 1 2 3 4 5 6 7 8 9 10 a severe problem NA

36. Nausea

no problem 0 1 2 3 4 5 6 7 8 9 10 a severe problem NA

37. Fertility changes

no problem 0 1 2 3 4 5 6 7 8 9 10 a severe problem NA

38. Rate your overall physical health

extremely poor 0 1 2 3 4 5 6 7 8 9 10 excellent NA

Psychological Well-Being

39. Do you have any distress from visual changes?

not at all 0 1 2 3 4 5 6 7 8 9 10 a great deal NA

40. Has it been difficult for you to adjust to your illness?

very difficult 0 1 2 3 4 5 6 7 8 9 10 not at all NA

41. How good is your overall quality of life?

extremely poor 0 1 2 3 4 5 6 7 8 9 10 excellent NA

42. How much enjoyment are you getting out of life?

none at all 0 1 2 3 4 5 6 7 8 9 10 a great deal NA

43. How is your present ability to concentrate or to remember things?

extremely poor 0 1 2 3 4 5 6 7 8 9 10 excellent NA

44. How useful do you feel?

not at all 0 1 2 3 4 5 6 7 8 9 10 extremely NA

45. How much happiness do you feel?

none at all 0 1 2 3 4 5 6 7 8 9 10 complete NA

46. Do you feel like you are in control of things in your life?

none at all 0 1 2 3 4 5 6 7 8 9 10 completely NA

47. Do you enjoy the things in life now that you used to take for granted?

not at all 0 1 2 3 4 5 6 7 8 9 10 a great deal NA

48. How satisfying is your life?

not at all 0 1 2 3 4 5 6 7 8 9 10 extremely NA

49. How much have you been able to focus on being well again?

not at all 0 1 2 3 4 5 6 7 8 9 10 a great deal NA

50. Has your illness or treatment caused unwanted changes in your appearance?

not at all   0 1 2 3 4 5 6 7 8 9 10   a great deal   NA

51. Are you fearful of recurrence of your cancer?

not at all   0 1 2 3 4 5 6 7 8 9 10   extremely   NA

52. How difficult is it for you to cope as a result of your disease and treatment?

not at all   0 1 2 3 4 5 6 7 8 9 10   extremely   NA

53. Has your illness or treatment decreased your self-concept (the way you see yourself)?

not at all   0 1 2 3 4 5 6 7 8 9 10   extremely   NA

54. How distressing was the initial diagnosis of your cancer?

not at all   0 1 2 3 4 5 6 7 8 9 10   extremely   NA

55. How distressing were your cancer treatments (i.e., chemotherapy, radiation, BMT, or surgery)?

not at all   0 1 2 3 4 5 6 7 8 9 10   extremely   NA

56. How distressing has the time been since your treatment ended?

not at all   0 1 2 3 4 5 6 7 8 9 10   extremely   NA

57. How much anxiety do you have?

none at all   0 1 2 3 4 5 6 7 8 9 10   severe   NA

58. How much depression do you have?

none at all   0 1 2 3 4 5 6 7 8 9 10   severe   NA

59. Are you fearful of a second cancer?

not at all   0 1 2 3 4 5 6 7 8 9 10   extremely   NA

60. Are you fearful of the spreading (metastasis) of your cancer?

not at all   0 1 2 3 4 5 6 7 8 9 10   extremely   NA

61. Rate your overall psychological well-being.

extremely poor   0 1 2 3 4 5 6 7 8 9 10   excellent   NA

Social Concerns

62. How much financial burden resulted from your illness or treatment?

none   0 1 2 3 4 5 6 7 8 9 10   extreme   NA

63. How distressing has your illness been for your family?

not at all   0 1 2 3 4 5 6 7 8 9 10   extremely   NA

64. Has your illness or treatment interfered with your personal relationships?

not at all   0 1 2 3 4 5 6 7 8 9 10   completely   NA

65. Is the amount of affection you receive sufficient to meet your needs?

not at all   0   1   2   3   4   5   6   7   8   9   10   completely   NA

66. Is the amount of affection you give sufficient to meet your needs?

not at all   0   1   2   3   4   5   6   7   8   9   10   completely   NA

67. Has your illness or treatment interfered with your sexuality?

not at all   0   1   2   3   4   5   6   7   8   9   10   completely   NA

68. Has your illness or treatment interfered with your plans to have children?

not at all   0   1   2   3   4   5   6   7   8   9   10   a great deal   NA

69. Has your illness or treatment interfered with your employment?

not at all   0   1   2   3   4   5   6   7   8   9   10   completely   NA

70. Has your illness or treatment interfered with your family goals?

not at all   0   1   2   3   4   5   6   7   8   9   10   completely   NA

71. Is the amount of support you receive from others sufficient to meet your needs?

not at all   0   1   2   3   4   5   6   7   8   9   10   completely   NA

72. Has your illness or treatment interfered with your activities at home?

not at all   0   1   2   3   4   5   6   7   8   9   10   completely   NA

73. How much isolation is caused by your illness or treatment?

none   0   1   2   3   4   5   6   7   8   9   10   complete   NA

74. Rate your overall social well-being.

extremely poor   0   1   2   3   4   5   6   7   8   9   10   excellent   NA

Spiritual Well-Being

75. How much uncertainty do you feel about your future?

none at all   0   1   2   3   4   5   6   7   8   9   10   extreme   NA

76. Do you sense a purpose/mission for your life or a reason for being alive?

not at all   0   1   2   3   4   5   6   7   8   9   10   a great deal   NA

77. Do you have a sense of inner peace?

not at all   0   1   2   3   4   5   6   7   8   9   10   completely   NA

78. How hopeful do you feel?

not at all   0   1   2   3   4   5   6   7   8   9   10   extremely   NA

79. Is the amount of support you receive from personal spiritual activities such as prayer or meditation sufficient to meet your needs?

not at all   0   1   2   3   4   5   6   7   8   9   10   completely   NA

80. Is the amount of support you receive from religious activities such as going to church or synagogue sufficient to meet your needs?

not at all   0   1   2   3   4   5   6   7   8   9   10   completely   NA

81. Has your illness made positive changes in your life?

none at all   0   1   2   3   4   5   6   7   8   9   10   extreme   NA

82. Rate your overall spiritual well-being.

extremely poor   0   1   2   3   4   5   6   7   8   9   10   excellent   NA

83. Would you recommend a bone marrow transplant to a family member or close friend with the same illness?

not at all   0   1   2   3   4   5   6   7   8   9   10   definitely yes   NA

84. Has filling out this tool been useful to you?

not at all   0   1   2   3   4   5   6   7   8   9   10   extremely   NA

REFERENCES

Grant, M., Ferrell, B., Schmidt, G. M., Fonbuena, P., Niland, J. C., & Forman, S. J. (1992). Measurement of quality of life in bone marrow transplantation survivors. *Quality of Life Research*, 1(6), 375–384.

Ferrell, B., Grant, M., Schmidt, G. M., Rhiner, M., Whitehead, C., Fonbuena, P., et al. (1992a). The meaning of quality of life for bone marrow transplant survivors. Part 1: The impact of bone marrow transplant on quality of life. *Cancer Nursing*, 15(3), 153–160.

Ferrell, B., Grant, M., Schmidt, G. M., Rhiner, M., Whitehead, C., Fonbuena, P., et al. (1992b). The meaning of quality of life for bone marrow transplant survivors. Part 2: Improving quality of life for bone marrow transplant survivors. *Cancer Nursing*, 15(4), 247–253.

Schmidt, G. M., Niland, J. C., Forman, S. J., Fonbuena, P., Dagis, A. C., Ferrell, B. R., et al. Extended follow up in 201 long-term allogeneic bone marrow transplant survivors: Addressing issues of quality of life. *Transplantation*, 55(3), 551–557.

Grant, M., Ferrell, B., Schmidt, G., Fonbuena, P., Niland, J., & Forman, S. (1992). Researching quality of life indicators: Their impact on the daily life of bone marrow transplant patients. In C. D. Bailey (Ed.), *Proceedings of the Seventh International Conference on Cancer Nursing* (Cancer Nursing Changing Frontiers, Vienna) (pp. 80–84). Oxford, UK: Rapid Communications.

Quality of Life Components for Pediatric Oncology Group (POG) Protocols

ANDREW BRADLYN

Contact person: Andrew Bradlyn, PhD, Department of Behavioral Medicine and Psychiatry, Robert C. Byrd Health Sciences Center, West Virginia University, 930 Chestnut Ridge Road, Morgantown, WV 26505. Used with permission from Andrew Bradlyn, PhD.

Rand Health Status Measure (Modified) for Children Ages 0–4 Years (Day 7, Post Surgery: 1-Week Report)

Instructions

1. Read each question carefully.
2. *Circle the number* of the *one answer* that most closely fits this child.

Example:

    1. Has this child ever had a cold?

       Yes   1

       No   2

Follow any instructions next to the number you circled, which tell you to go to another question or another page.

Example:

    2. Does this child wear glasses?

       Yes   1 - Answer 2-a

       No   2 - Go to 3

  2-a. How long has this child been wearing glasses?

       Less than 1 year   1

       About 1 year   2

       About 2 years   3

       More than 2 years 4

If there are no instructions after your answer, go to the very next question.

What time is it now?_____   What is the date today? _____

During the past week (not including today):

    1. Was this child in bed for all or most of the day because of health?

       Yes   1 - Answer 1-a

       No   2 - Go to 2

  1-a. How long has this child been in bed for all or most of the day because of health?

       1 to 2 days   1

       3 to 4 days   2

       5 to 7 days   3

    2. Has this child been in a hospital or other medical facility because of health?

       Yes   1 - Answer 2-a

       No   2 - Go to 3

2-a. How long has this child been in a hospital or other medical facility because of health?

1 to 2 days	1
3 to 4 days	2
5 to 7 days	3

FL/MOB _____

3. Was this child unable to walk unless assisted by an adult or by crutches, artificial limb, or braces?

Yes, unable to walk unless assisted	1 - Answer 3-a
No, no trouble walking	2 - Go to 4
Not walking yet because of age	3 - Go to 4

3-a. How long has this child been unable to walk without assistance?

1 to 2 days	1
3 to 4 days	2
5 to 7 days	3

FL/PA _____

During the past week *(not including today)*:

4. Does this child's health limit the *kind* or *amount* of ordinary play he or she can do?

Yes	1 - Answer 4-a
No	2 - Go to 5

4-a. How long has the child's health limited the kind or amount of play he or she could do?

1 to 2 day	1
3 to 4 days	2
5 to 7 days	3

5. Does this child's health keep him from taking part in ordinary play?

Yes	1 - Answer 5-a
No	2 - Go to 6

5-a. How long has this child's health kept him or her from taking part in ordinary play?

1 to 2 days	1
3 to 4 days	2
5 to 7 days	3

FL/RA _____

6. Because of health, did this child need more help than normal for children of the same age in eating, dressing, bathing, or using the toilet?

Yes	1 - Answer 6-a
No	2 - Go to 7

6-a. How long has this child needed extra help with eating, dressing, bathing, or using the toilet?

1 to 2 days	1
3 to 4 days	2
5 to 7 days	3

FL/SC _____

During the past week *(not including today):*

7. Considering this child's progress in sitting up, walking, and talking, how do you feel about the way he or she is growing up or developing?

Very satisfied	1
Somewhat satisfied	2
Neither satisfied nor worried	3
Somewhat worried	4
Very worried	5

8. How do you feel about this child's eating habits?

Very satisfied	1
Somewhat satisfied	2
Neither satisfied nor worried	3
Somewhat worried	4
Very worried	5

9. How do you feel about this child's sleeping habits?

Very satisfied	1
Somewhat satisfied	2
Neither satisfied nor worried	3
Somewhat worried	4
Very worried	5

10. How do you feel about this child's bowel habits?

Very satisfied	1
Somewhat satisfied	2
Neither satisfied nor worried	3
Somewhat worried	4
Very worried	5

SAT DEV _____

11. Please read each of the following statements, and then *circle one of the numbers on each line* to indicate whether the statement is true or false for this child. There are no right or wrong answers. Some of the statements may look or seem like others, but each statement is different and should be rated by itself.

> If a statement is *definitely true* for this child, circle 1.
> If a statement is *mostly true* for this child, circle 2.
> If you *don't know* whether it is true or false, circle 3.
> If it is *mostly false* for this child, circle 4.
> If it is *definitely false* for this child, circle 5.

	Definitely true	Mostly true	Don't know	Mostly false	Definitely false
A. This child's health is excellent.	1	2	3	4	5
B. This child was so sick once, I thought he or she might die.	1	2	3	4	5
C. This child seems to resist illness very well.	1	2	3	4	5
D. This child seems to be less healthy than other children I know.	1	2	3	4	5
E. This child has never been seriously ill.	1	2	3	4	5
F. When there is something going around, this child usually catches it.	1	2	3	4	5

What time is it now?_____

TOTAL HP _____   TOTAL RAND _____

Parent Satisfaction with Questionnaire

1. How much of a burden was this questionnaire for you?

1	2	3	4	5

Required
minimal effort
            Required
            extreme effort

2. How difficult were the questions to understand?

1	2	3	4	5

Extremely
easy
            Extremely
            difficult

3. How well did this questionnaire describe how your child has been doing over the past week?

1	2	3	4	5

Not well
at all
            Somewhat
            well
                        Extremely
                        well

Thank you for your assistance!

Parent Form

Overall health rating

1	2	3	4	5	6
Very poor	Poor	Somewhat poor	Somewhat good	Good	Very good

Using this scale (1–6), how would you rate your child's overall health during the past two weeks?

Quality-of-Life Rating

1	2	3	4	5	6
Very poor	Poor	Somewhat poor	Somewhat good	Good	Very good

Using this scale (1–6), how would you rate your child's quality of life during the past two weeks? By "quality of life," we mean how your child is doing overall (their physical, psychological, and social well-being).

Play-Performance Scale for Children (Parent Form)

Child's name: _____

Your name: _____

    Relationship: Mother ❑ Father ❑ Other ❑

Today's date: _____

Directions: On this form are a series of descriptions. Each description has a number beside it. Think about your child's play and activity over the past *two weeks*. Think about both good and bad days. Average out this period. Now read the descriptions and pick the one that best describes your child's play during the past *two weeks*. *Circle the number beside that one description.*

100	Fully active, normal.
90	Minor restrictions in physically strenuous activity.
80	Active, but tires more quickly.
70	Both greater restriction of, and less time spent in, active play.
60	Up and around, but minimal active play; keeps busy with quieter activities.
50	Gets dressed, but lies around much of the day; no active play; able to participate in all quiet play and activities.
40	Mostly in bed; participates in quiet activities.
30	In bed; needs assistance even for quiet play.
20	Often sleeping; play entirely limited to very passive activities.
10	No play; does not get out of bed.
0	Unresponsive.

The Bush Bone Marrow Transplant Symptom Inventory

NIGEL BUSH

Contact person: Nigel Bush, PhD, Research Scientist, Fred Hutchinson Cancer Research Center, Mail Stop M-224, 1124 Columbia Street, Seattle, WA 98104-2092. Copyright © 1994. Used with permission from Nigel Bush, PhD.

Late Complications of BMT Module

Origin: The BMT module is an original instrument compiled following exhaustive reviews of BMT literature and from inservice discussions with staff at the Fred Hutchinson Cancer Research Center in Seattle, WA (USA). However, the BMT module is not strictly a stand-alone QOL instrument. Rather we developed it as a BMT-specific addendum or module to the European Organization for Research and Treatment of Cancer (EORTC) QLQ-C30 quality-of-life questionnaire (4), and as part of a battery of seven instruments encompassing four domains of QOL in BMT (physical, psychological, and social functioning, and disease/treatment symptoms).

Purpose: To complement the QLQ-C30 as a disease-specific addendum module for assessing primarily, but not exclusively, the symptomatology of long-term recovery from BMT over time in large samples of adult bone marrow and stem cell transplantation patients.

Population: Adult patients undergoing and recovering from bone marrow or stem cell transplantation. All types of transplant and treatment regimens are represented. The diseases represented in the sample may include all types of acute and chronic leukemia, preleukemia, multiple myeloma, nonHodgkins lymphoma, Hodgkins disease, aplastic anemia, and solid tumor patients receiving BMTs or stem cell transplantations.

Administration:
Rater: Has been administered and collected by mail or in person by general administrative staff or healthcare professionals. Questionnaire is self-assessed by patient. Scoring and assessment require relatively competent data entry and analysis person.
Time Required: Approximately 5–10 minutes. Time for self-assessed completion of entire battery of which it is a part has averaged 90 minutes.
Training: Is an integral part of a larger battery with detailed instructions. Questions are self-explanatory. Little or no guidance on the part of the patient is required.
Scoring: Follows the scoring convention of the QLQ-C30. Most of the fifty items, scaled identically to the EORTC QLQ-C30 with four-point Likert scales linearly transformed to 0–100 scales, are rated for occurrence/severity of symptoms.

Description: The module includes items that primarily index the disease/treatment symptoms domain of health-related quality of life (QOL), although the remaining three domains commonly defined (physical, psychological, and social functioning) are also represented. Multiple items are categorized by: skin, eyes, mouth/throat, joints/muscles involvement, pulmonary problems, sex/warmth/intimacy, cognitive dysfunction, infections, and fear of relapse/dying. When calculating composite scores, items from two categories, pulmonary problems and cognitive dysfunction, are combined with items from the EORTC QLQ-C30 to form more complete BMT-specific subscales. Items already included in the EORTC QLQ-C30 are omitted from the module. Single items index physical appearance, hair and nail loss, teeth problems, abnormal sense of taste, heartburn and abdominal pain, sinusitis and runny nose, chronic GVHD, and minor symptoms/ailments.

Coverage: We have employed this instrument as a component of a much larger research assessment battery. However, we intend that a future, more refined battery will be employed by clinicians as a more comprehensive clinical outcome assessment tool.

Reliability: We recently tested the module as part of a large QOL assessment packet on 125 subjects surviving 6–18 years after BMT, and calculated alpha coefficients for the various categories. The overall Cronbach's alpha for the BMT module was 0.87 with category alphas ranging from 0.71–0.89 with four exceptions (skin = 0.55, mouth/throat = 0.69, infections = 0.32, fear of relapse/dying = 0.66). Current, ongoing use in a four-year longitudinal study of patients from pretreatment to five-year post-BMT appears, from very cursory examination, to be yielding similar figures.

Validity: Generally face valid. Content validity for the fifty items has been derived from inservice discussions with staff at the Fred Hutchinson Cancer Research Center in Seattle, WA, and from the BMT literature.

Responsiveness: Too early to tell. Longitudinal assessment ongoing.

Strengths: Extremely comprehensive in assessing the symptomatology of long-term recovery from BMT. Easy to administer and simple enough for self-assessment. We believe the instrument complements well the QLQ-C30 as a disease/treatment specific module.

Weaknesses/Caution: The BMT module is still under development. In its present form, the BMT module does not contain rigorously psychometric scales. It includes aforementioned categories of items (e.g., eyes, skin, etc.) grouped by site or topic for convenience. We have calculated simple descriptive data such as incidences and frequencies from this instrument. At its present stage of development, we regard the module as a comprehensive *descriptive* inventory of late complications of BMT. We are currently testing it in longitudinal studies of BMT patients with yearly repeated measures at one to five years and will be using data from our QOL battery to develop new statistical methods for QOL outcome assessment. These include novel techniques (mixed effects models) for dealing with unconditional estimates of QOL trends that are not subject to attritional biases over time (missing data). We hope to develop new endpoints for BMT that will superficially resemble Q-TWIST. On completion of that study we hope to be able to shorten and refine the questionnaire.

EORTC Core Quality of Life Questionnaire (QLQ-C30) by Mail

We are interested in some things about you and your health. *Please answer all the questions yourself by circling the number that best applies to you.* There are no right or wrong answers. The information that you provide will remain strictly confidential.

Today's date (day, month, year) _____ /_____ /_____

	No	Yes
1. Do you have any trouble doing strenuous activities, like carrying a heavy shopping bag or a suitcase?	1	2
2. Do you have any trouble taking a *long* walk?	1	2
3. Do you have any trouble taking a *short* walk outside of the house?	1	2
4. Do you have to stay in a bed or a chair for most of the day?	1	2
5. Do you need help with eating, dressing, washing yourself, or using the toilet?	1	2
6. Are you limited in any way in doing either your work or doing household jobs?	1	2
7. Are you completely unable to work at a job or do household jobs?	1	2

During the past *two weeks*:

	Not at all	A little bit	Quite a bit	Very much
8. Were you short of breath?	1	2	3	4
9. Have you had pain?	1	2	3	4
10. Did you need to rest?	1	2	3	4
11. Have you had trouble sleeping?	1	2	3	4
12. Have you felt weak?	1	2	3	4
13. Have you lacked appetite?	1	2	3	4
14. Have you felt nauseated?	1	2	3	4
15. Have you vomited?	1	2	3	4
16. Have you been constipated?	1	2	3	4
17. Have you had diarrhea?	1	2	3	4
18. Were you tired?	1	2	3	4
19. Did pain interfere with your daily activities?	1	2	3	4

	Not at all	A little bit	Quite a bit	Very much
20. Have you had difficulty in concentrating on things, like reading a newspaper or watching television?	1	2	3	4
21. Did you feel tense?	1	2	3	4
22. Did you worry?	1	2	3	4
23. Did you feel irritable?	1	2	3	4
24. Did you feel depressed?	1	2	3	4
25. Have you had difficulty remembering things?	1	2	3	4
26. Has your physical condition or medical treatment interfered with your *family* life?	1	2	3	4
27. Has your physical condition or medical treatment interfered with your *social* life?	1	2	3	4
28. Has your physical condition or medical treatment caused you financial difficulties?	1	2	3	4

For the following questions please circle the number between 1 and 7 that best applies to you.

29. How would you rate your overall physical condition during the past *two weeks?*

1	2	3	4	5	6	7

Very poor   Excellent

30. How would you rate your overall quality of life during the past *two weeks?*

1	2	3	4	5	6	7

Very poor   Excellent

Former bone marrow or stem cell transplant patients sometimes report that they have the following symptoms. Please indicate the extent to which you have experienced these symptoms during the past *two weeks.*

	Not at all	A little bit	Quite a bit	Very much
31. Skin problems (overall)?	1	2	3	4
a. Rashes	1	2	3	4
b. Dryness	1	2	3	4
c. Sweating	1	2	3	4
d. Painful skin	1	2	3	4
e. Skin ulcers	1	2	3	4
32. Hair loss	1	2	3	4

	Not at all	A little bit	Quite a bit	Very much
33. Nail loss	1	2	3	4
34. Eye problems (overall)?	1	2	3	4
a. Dryness	1	2	3	4
b. Grittiness	1	2	3	4
c. Burning	1	2	3	4
d. Blurring	1	2	3	4
e. Sensitivity to light	1	2	3	4
f. Cataracts	1	2	3	4
35. Mouth/throat problems (overall)?	1	2	3	4
a. Dryness	1	2	3	4
b. Soreness	1	2	3	4
c. Burning	1	2	3	4
36. Teeth problems (dental caries, etc.)	1	2	3	4
37. Abnormal sense of taste for food or drink	1	2	3	4

During the past *two weeks*, to what extent have you experienced:

	Not at all	A little bit	Quite a bit	Very much
38. Heartburn	1	2	3	4
39. Abdominal pain	1	2	3	4
40. Weight loss	1	2	3	4
41. Sinusitis	1	2	3	4
42. Runny nose	1	2	3	4
43. Breathing problems (overall)?	1	2	3	4
a. Coughing	1	2	3	4
b. Wheezing	1	2	3	4
c. Bronchitis	1	2	3	4
d. Asthma	1	2	3	4
44. Painful joints (overall)?	1	2	3	4
a. Hip joints	1	2	3	4
b. Other joints	1	2	3	4
45. Painful muscles	1	2	3	4
46. Infections (overall)?	1	2	3	4
a. Varicella zoster (VZV)	1	2	3	4
b. Herpes simplex	1	2	3	4
c. Cytomegalovirus (CMV)	1	2	3	4
d. Pneumonia	1	2	3	4
e. Measles	1	2	3	4

	Not at all	A little bit	Quite a bit	Very much
f. Chickenpox	1	2	3	4
g. Shingles	1	2	3	4
47. Chronic graft-versus-host disease (GVHD)	1	2	3	4
48. Minor symptoms or ailments? (common cold, flu, migraine, etc.) Please describe	1	2	3	4

_____

_____

	Not at all	A little bit	Quite a bit	Very much
49. Compared with your appearance before your transplant, how satisfied are you now with your appearance?	1	2	3	4
50. Have you been satisfied with your own sexual appeal?	1	2	3	4
51. Have you been satisfied with your ability to share warmth and intimacy?	1	2	3	4
52. Have you been interested in sexual thoughts or feelings?	1	2	3	4

53. Do you have any physical problems that reduce your satisfaction with sex and intimacy?   Yes   No

Please describe (remember that your answers will be treated with the strictest confidence).

_____

_____

	Not at all	A little bit	Quite a bit	Very much
54. Have you been worried by fear of infection?	1	2	3	4
55. Have you been worried by thoughts about relapse or dying?	1	2	3	4
56. Have you had difficulty in maintaining your attention and train of thought?	1	2	3	4
57. Have you had difficulty in reasoning and thinking clearly?	1	2	3	4

58. Are there any other things that have affected the quality of your life over the past *two weeks*?

_____

_____

_____

59. Has the quality of your life over the past two weeks been typical of the past five or six months, or has it been unusual? If the past two weeks have been unusual, please describe how, in more detail.

_____

_____

_____

Please check to make sure that you have answered all of the questions.

Please use the space below for any additional comments you might have:

_____

_____

_____

REFERENCES

Aaronson, N. K., Ahmedzai, S., Bergman, B., Bullinger, M., Cull, A., Duez, N. J., et al. (1993). The European organization for research and treatment of cancer QLQ-C30: A quality of life instrument for use in international clinical trials in oncology. *Journal of National Cancer Institute, 85*, 356–376.

Bush, N. E., Haberman, M., Donaldson, G., & Sullivan, K. M. (1995). Quality of life of 125 adults surviving 6–18 years after bone marrow transplantation. *Social Science and Medicine, 40*, 479–490.

Haberman, M., Bush, N. E., Young, K., & Sullivan, K. M. (1993). Quality of life of adult long-term survivors of bone marrow transplantation: A qualitative analysis of narrative data. *Oncology Nursing Forum, 20*, 1545–1553.

PedsQL™
Pediatric Quality of Life
Inventory for Young Children
(ages 5–7)

Contact person: James W. Varni, PhD, Professor and Senior Scientist, Center for Child Health Outcomes, Children's Hospital and Health Center, 3020 Children's Way, MC 5053, San Diego, CA, 92123, telephone: 858-966-4907. jvarni@chsd.org

PedsQL™
Pediatric Quality of Life Inventory

Version 4.0

PARENT REPORT for YOUNG CHILDREN (ages 5–7)

DIRECTIONS

On the following page is a list of things that might be a problem for **your child**. Please tell us **how much of a problem** each one has been for **your child** during the **past ONE month** by circling:

0 if it is **never** a problem

1 if it is **almost never** a problem

2 if it is **sometimes** a problem

3 if it is **often** a problem

4 if it is **almost always** a problem

There are no right or wrong answers.

If you do not understand a question, please ask for help.

In the past **ONE month**, how much of a **problem** has your child had with . . .

PHYSICAL FUNCTIONING (problems with . . .)	Never	Almost Never	Some-times	Often	Almost Always
1. Walking more than one block	0	1	2	3	4
2. Running	0	1	2	3	4
3. Participating in sports activity or exercise	0	1	2	3	4
4. Lifting something heavy	0	1	2	3	4
5. Taking a bath or shower by him or herself	0	1	2	3	4
6. Doing chores, like picking up his or her toys	0	1	2	3	4
7. Having hurts or aches	0	1	2	3	4
8. Low energy level	0	1	2	3	4

EMOTIONAL FUNCTIONING (problems with . . .)	Never	Almost Never	Some-times	Often	Almost Always
1. Feeling afraid or scared	0	1	2	3	4
2. Feeling sad or blue	0	1	2	3	4
3. Feeling angry	0	1	2	3	4
4. Trouble sleeping	0	1	2	3	4
5. Worrying about what will happen to him or her	0	1	2	3	4

SOCIAL FUNCTIONING (problems with . . .)	Never	Almost Never	Some-times	Often	Almost Always
1. Getting along with other children	0	1	2	3	4
2. Other kids not wanting to be his or her friend	0	1	2	3	4
3. Getting teased by other children	0	1	2	3	4
4. Not able to do things that other children his or her age can do	0	1	2	3	4
5. Keeping up when playing with other children	0	1	2	3	4

SCHOOL FUNCTIONING (problems with . . .)	Never	Almost Never	Some-times	Often	Almost Always
1. Paying attention in class	0	1	2	3	4
2. Forgetting things	0	1	2	3	4
3. Keeping up with school activities	0	1	2	3	4
4. Missing school because of not feeling well	0	1	2	3	4
5. Missing school to go to the doctor or hospital	0	1	2	3	4

PedsQL™
Pediatric Quality of Life Inventory

Version 4.0

YOUNG CHILD REPORT (ages 5–7)

Instructions for interviewer:

I am going to ask you some questions about things that might be a problem for some children. I want to know how much of a problem any of these things might be for you.

Show the child the template and point to the responses as you read.

If it is <u>not at all</u> a problem for you, point to the smiling face

If it is <u>sometimes</u> a problem for you, point to the middle face

If it is a problem for you <u>a lot</u>, point to the frowning face

I will read each question. Point to the pictures to show me how much of a problem it is for you. Let's try a practice one first.

	Not at all	Sometimes	A lot
Is it hard for you to snap your fingers?	☺	😐	☹

Ask the child to demonstrate snapping his or her fingers to determine whether or not the question was answered correctly. Repeat the question if the child demonstrates a response that is different from his or her action.

Think about how you have been doing for the last few weeks. Please listen carefully to each sentence and tell me how much of a problem this is for you.

After reading the item, gesture to the template. If the child hesitates or does not seem to understand how to answer, read the response options while pointing at the faces.

PHYSICAL FUNCTIONING (problems with . . .)	Not at all	Sometimes	A lot
1. Is it hard for you to walk?	0	2	4
2. Is it hard for you to run?	0	2	4
3. Is it hard for you to play sports or exercise?	0	2	4
4. Is it hard for you to pick up big things?	0	2	4
5. Is it hard for you to take a bath or shower?	0	2	4
6. Is it hard for you to do chores (like pick up your toys)?	0	2	4
7. Do you have hurts or aches? (*Where?* _____)	0	2	4
8. Do you ever feel too tired to play?	0	2	4

Remember, tell me how much of a problem this has been for you for the last few weeks.

EMOTIONAL FUNCTIONING (problems with . . .)	Not at all	Sometimes	A lot
1. Do you feel scared?	0	2	4
2. Do you feel sad?	0	2	4
3. Do you feel mad?	0	2	4
4. Do you have trouble sleeping?	0	2	4
5. Do you worry about what will happen to you?	0	2	4

SOCIAL FUNCTIONING (problems with . . .)	Not at all	Sometimes	A lot
1. Is it hard for you to get along with other kids?	0	2	4
2. Do other kids say they do not want to play with you?	0	2	4
3. Do other kids tease you?	0	2	4
4. Can other kids do things that you cannot do?	0	2	4
5. Is it hard for you to keep up when you play with other kids?	0	2	4

SCHOOL FUNCTIONING (problems with . . .)	Not at all	Sometimes	A lot
1. Is it hard for you to pay attention in school?	0	2	4
2. Do you forget things?	0	2	4
3. Is it hard to keep up with schoolwork?	0	2	4
4. Do you miss school because of not feeling good?	0	2	4
5. Do you miss school because you have to go to the doctor's or hospital?	0	2	4

How much of a problem is this for you?

Not at all

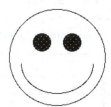

Sometimes

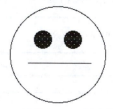

A lot

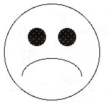

PedsQL™
Cancer Module

Version 3.0

PARENT REPORT for YOUNG CHILDREN (ages 5–7)

DIRECTIONS

Children with cancer sometimes have special problems. On the following page is a list of things that might be a problem for **your child**. Please tell us how **much of a problem** each one has been for **your child** during the **past ONE month** by circling:

0 if it is **never** a problem

1 if it is **almost never** a problem

2 if it is **sometimes** a problem

3 if it is **often** a problem

4 if it is **almost always** a problem

There are no right or wrong answers.

If you do not understand a question, please ask for help.

In the past **ONE month**, how much of a **problem** has your child had with . . .

PAIN AND HURT (problems with . . .)	Never	Almost Never	Some-times	Often	Almost Always
1. Aches in joints and/or muscles	0	1	2	3	4
2. Having a lot of pain	0	1	2	3	4

NAUSEA (problems with . . .)	Never	Almost Never	Some-times	Often	Almost Always
1. Becoming nauseated during medical treatments	0	1	2	3	4
2. Food not tasting very good to him or her	0	1	2	3	4
3. Becoming nauseated while thinking about medical treatments	0	1	2	3	4
4. Not feeling hungry	0	1	2	3	4
5. Some foods and smells making him or her nauseous	0	1	2	3	4

PROCEDURAL ANXIETY (problems with . . .)	Never	Almost Never	Some-times	Often	Almost Always
1. Needle sticks (i.e., injections, blood tests, IVs) causing him or her pain	0	1	2	3	4
2. Getting anxious about having blood drawn	0	1	2	3	4
3. Getting anxious about having needle sticks (i.e., injections, blood tests, IVs)	0	1	2	3	4

TREATMENT ANXIETY (problems with . . .)	Never	Almost Never	Some-times	Often	Almost Always
1. Getting anxious when waiting to see the doctor	0	1	2	3	4
2. Getting anxious about going to the doctor	0	1	2	3	4
3. Getting anxious about going to the hospital	0	1	2	3	4

WORRY (problems with . . .)	Never	Almost Never	Some-times	Often	Almost Always
1. Worrying about side effects from medical treatments	0	1	2	3	4
2. Worrying about whether or not his or her medical treatments are working	0	1	2	3	4
3. Worrying that the cancer will reoccur or relapse	0	1	2	3	4

In the past **ONE month**, how much of a **problem** has your child had with . . .

COGNITIVE PROBLEMS (problems with . . .)	Never	Almost Never	Some-times	Often	Almost Always
1. Figuring out what to do when something bothers him or her	0	1	2	3	4
2. Solving math problems	0	1	2	3	4
3. Writing school papers	0	1	2	3	4
4. Difficulty paying attention to things	0	1	2	3	4
5. Remembering what is read to him or her	0	1	2	3	4

PERCEIVED PHYSICAL APPEARANCE (problems with . . .)	Never	Almost Never	Some-times	Often	Almost Always
1. Feeling that he/she is not good looking	0	1	2	3	4
2. Not liking other people to see his or her scars	0	1	2	3	4
3. Being embarrassed about others seeing his or her body	0	1	2	3	4

COMMUNICATION (problems with . . .)	Never	Almost Never	Some-times	Often	Almost Always
1. Telling the doctors and nurses how he or she feels	0	1	2	3	4
2. Asking the doctors or nurses questions	0	1	2	3	4
3. Explaining his or her illness to other people	0	1	2	3	4

PedsQL™
Cancer Module

Version 3.0

YOUNG CHILD REPORT (ages 5–7)

Instructions for interviewer:

I am going to ask you some questions about things that might be a problem for some children. I want to know how much of a problem any of these things might be for you.

Show the child the template and point to the responses as you read.

If it is <u>not at all</u> a problem for you, point to the smiling face

If it is <u>sometimes</u> a problem for you, point to the middle face

If it is a problem for you <u>a lot</u>, point to the frowning face

I will read each question. Point to the pictures to show me how much of a problem it is for you. Let's try a practice one first.

	Not at all	Sometimes	A lot
Is it hard for you to snap your fingers?	☺	😐	☹

Ask the child to demonstrate snapping his or her fingers to determine whether or not the question was answered correctly. Repeat the question if the child demonstrates a response that is different from his or her action.

Think about how you have been doing for the last few weeks. Please listen carefully to each sentence and tell me how much of a problem this is for you.

After reading the item, gesture to the template. If the child hesitates or does not seem to understand how to answer, read the response options while pointing at the faces.

PAIN AND HURT (problems with . . .)	Not at all	Sometimes	A lot
1. Do you ache or hurt in your joints and/or muscles?	0	2	4
2. Do you hurt a lot?	0	2	4

NAUSEA (problems with . . .)	Not at all	Sometimes	A lot
1. Do you get sick to your stomach when you have medical treatments?	0	2	4
2. Does food taste bad to you?	0	2	4
3. Do you get sick to your stomach when you think about medical treatments?	0	2	4
4. Do you not feel hungry?	0	2	4
5. Do some foods and smells make your stomach upset?	0	2	4

PROCEDURAL ANXIETY (problems with . . .)	Not at all	Sometimes	A lot
1. Do needle sticks (i.e., injections, blood tests, IVs) hurt you?	0	2	4
2. Do you get scared when you have to have blood tests?	0	2	4
3. Do you get scared about having needle sticks (i.e., injections, blood tests, IVs)?	0	2	4

TREATMENT ANXIETY (problems with . . .)	Not at all	Sometimes	A lot
1. Do you get scared when you are waiting to see the doctor?	0	2	4
2. Do you get scared when you have to go to the doctor?	0	2	4
3. Do you get scared when you have to go to the hospital?	0	2	4

WORRY (problems with . . .)	Not at all	Sometimes	A lot
1. Do you worry about side effects from medical treatments?	0	2	4
2. Do you worry about whether or not your medical treatments are working?	0	2	4
3. Do you worry that your cancer will come back?	0	2	4

Think about how you have been doing for the last few weeks. Please listen carefully to each sentence and tell me how much of a problem this is for you.

COGNITIVE PROBLEMS (problems with . . .)	Not at all	Sometimes	A lot
1. Is it hard for you to figure out what to do when something bothers you?	0	2	4
2. Do you have trouble solving math problems?	0	2	4
3. Do you have trouble writing school papers?	0	2	4
4. Is it hard for you to pay attention to things?	0	2	4
5. Is it hard for you to remember what is read to you?	0	2	4

PERCEIVED PHYSICAL APPEARANCE (problems with . . .)	Not at all	Sometimes	A lot
1. Do you feel you are not good looking?	0	2	4
2. Do you not like other people to see your scars?	0	2	4
3. Are you embarrassed when others see your body?	0	2	4

COMMUNICATION (problems with . . .)	Not at all	Sometimes	A lot
1. Is is hard for you to tell the doctors and nurses how you feel?	0	2	4
2. Is it hard for you to ask the doctors and nurses questions?	0	2	4
3. Is it hard for you to explain your illness to other people?	0	2	4

How much of a problem is this for you?

Not at all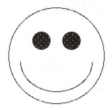

Sometimes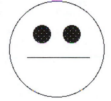

A lot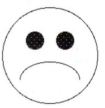

PedsQL™
Pediatric Quality of Life
Inventory for Children
(ages 8–12)

PedsQL™
Pediatric Quality of Life Inventory

Version 4.0

PARENT REPORT for CHILDREN (ages 8–12)

DIRECTIONS

On the following page is a list of things that might be a problem for **your child**. Please tell us **how much of a problem** each one has been for **your child** during the **past ONE month** by circling:

> 0 if it is **never** a problem
>
> 1 if it is **almost never** a problem
>
> 2 if it is **sometimes** a problem
>
> 3 if it is **often** a problem
>
> 4 if it is **almost always** a problem

There are no right or wrong answers.

If you do not understand a question, please ask for help.

In the past **ONE month**, how much of a **problem** has your child had with . . .

PHYSICAL FUNCTIONING (problems with . . .)	Never	Almost Never	Some-times	Often	Almost Always
1. Walking more than one block	0	1	2	3	4
2. Running	0	1	2	3	4
3. Participating in sports activity or exercise	0	1	2	3	4
4. Lifting something heavy	0	1	2	3	4
5. Taking a bath or shower by him or herself	0	1	2	3	4
6. Doing chores around the house	0	1	2	3	4
7. Having hurts or aches	0	1	2	3	4
8. Low energy level	0	1	2	3	4

EMOTIONAL FUNCTIONING (problems with . . .)	Never	Almost Never	Some-times	Often	Almost Always
1. Feeling afraid or scared	0	1	2	3	4
2. Feeling sad or blue	0	1	2	3	4
3. Feeling angry	0	1	2	3	4
4. Trouble sleeping	0	1	2	3	4
5. Worrying about what will happen to him or her	0	1	2	3	4

SOCIAL FUNCTIONING (problems with . . .)	Never	Almost Never	Some-times	Often	Almost Always
1. Getting along with other children	0	1	2	3	4
2. Other kids not wanting to be his or her friend	0	1	2	3	4
3. Getting teased by other children	0	1	2	3	4
4. Not able to do things that other children his or her age can do	0	1	2	3	4
5. Keeping up when playing with other children	0	1	2	3	4

SCHOOL FUNCTIONING (problems with . . .)	Never	Almost Never	Some-times	Often	Almost Always
1. Paying attention in class	0	1	2	3	4
2. Forgetting things	0	1	2	3	4
3. Keeping up with schoolwork	0	1	2	3	4
4. Missing school because of not feeling well	0	1	2	3	4
5. Missing school to go to the doctor or hospital	0	1	2	3	4

PedsQL™
Pediatric Quality of Life Inventory

Version 4.0

CHILD REPORT (ages 8–12)

DIRECTIONS

On the following page is a list of things that might be a problem for you. Please tell us **how much of a problem** each one has been for you during the **past ONE month** by circling:

> 0 if it is **never** a problem
>
> 1 if it is **almost never** a problem
>
> 2 if it is **sometimes** a problem
>
> 3 if it is **often** a problem
>
> 4 if it is **almost always** a problem

There are no right or wrong answers.

If you do not understand a question, please ask for help.

In the past **ONE month**, how much of a **problem** has this been for you . . .

ABOUT MY HEALTH AND ACTIVITIES (problems with . . .)	Never	Almost Never	Some-times	Often	Almost Always
1. It is hard for me to walk more than one block	0	1	2	3	4
2. It is hard for me to run	0	1	2	3	4
3. It is hard for me to do sports activity or exercise	0	1	2	3	4
4. It is hard for me to lift something heavy	0	1	2	3	4
5. It is hard for me to take a bath or shower by myself	0	1	2	3	4
6. It is hard for me to do chores around the house	0	1	2	3	4
7. I hurt or ache	0	1	2	3	4
8. I have low energy	0	1	2	3	4

ABOUT MY FEELINGS (problems with . . .)	Never	Almost Never	Some-times	Often	Almost Always
1. I feel afraid or scared	0	1	2	3	4
2. I feel sad or blue	0	1	2	3	4
3. I feel angry	0	1	2	3	4
4. I have trouble sleeping	0	1	2	3	4
5. I worry about what will happen to me	0	1	2	3	4

HOW I GET ALONG WITH OTHERS (problems with . . .)	Never	Almost Never	Some-times	Often	Almost Always
1. I have trouble getting along with other kids	0	1	2	3	4
2. Other kids do not want to be my friend	0	1	2	3	4
3. Other kids tease me	0	1	2	3	4
4. I cannot do things that other kids my age can do	0	1	2	3	4
5. It is hard to keep up when I play with other kids	0	1	2	3	4

ABOUT SCHOOL (problems with . . .)	Never	Almost Never	Some-times	Often	Almost Always
1. It is hard to pay attention in class	0	1	2	3	4
2. I forget things	0	1	2	3	4
3. I have trouble keeping up with my schoolwork	0	1	2	3	4
4. I miss school because of not feeling well	0	1	2	3	4
5. I miss school to go to the doctor or hospital	0	1	2	3	4

PedsQL™
Cancer Module

Version 3.0

PARENT REPORT for CHILDREN (ages 8–12)

DIRECTIONS

Children with cancer sometimes have special problems. On the following page is a list of things that might be a problem for **your child**. Please tell us **how much of a problem** each one has been for **your child** during the **past ONE month** by circling:

0 if it is **never** a problem

1 if it is **almost never** a problem

2 if it is **sometimes** a problem

3 if it is **often** a problem

4 if it is **almost always** a problem

There are no right or wrong answers.

If you do not understand a question, please ask for help.

In the past **ONE month**, how much of a **problem** has your child had with . . .

PAIN AND HURT (problems with . . .)	Never	Almost Never	Some-times	Often	Almost Always
1. Aches in joints and/or muscles	0	1	2	3	4
2. Having a lot of pain	0	1	2	3	4

NAUSEA (problems with . . .)	Never	Almost Never	Some-times	Often	Almost Always
1. Becoming nauseated during medical treatments	0	1	2	3	4
2. Food not tasting very good to him or her	0	1	2	3	4
3. Becoming nauseated while thinking about medical treatments	0	1	2	3	4
4. Not feeling hungry	0	1	2	3	4
5. Some foods and smells making him or her nauseous	0	1	2	3	4

PROCEDURAL ANXIETY (problems with . . .)	Never	Almost Never	Some-times	Often	Almost Always
1. Needle sticks (i.e., injections, blood tests, IVs) causing him or her pain	0	1	2	3	4
2. Getting anxious about having blood drawn	0	1	2	3	4
3. Getting anxious about having needle sticks (i.e., injections, blood tests, IVs)	0	1	2	3	4

TREATMENT ANXIETY (problems with . . .)	Never	Almost Never	Some-times	Often	Almost Always
1. Getting anxious when waiting to see the doctor	0	1	2	3	4
2. Getting anxious about going to the doctor	0	1	2	3	4
3. Getting anxious about going to the hospital	0	1	2	3	4

WORRY (problems with . . .)	Never	Almost Never	Some-times	Often	Almost Always
1. Worrying about side effects from medical treatments	0	1	2	3	4
2. Worrying about whether or not his or her medical treatments are working	0	1	2	3	4
3. Worrying that the cancer will reoccur or relapse	0	1	2	3	4

In the past **ONE month**, how much of a **problem** has your child had with . . .

COGNITIVE PROBLEMS (problems with . . .)	Never	Almost Never	Some-times	Often	Almost Always
1. Figuring out what to do when something is bothering him or her	0	1	2	3	4
2. Solving math problems	0	1	2	3	4
3. Writing school papers or reports	0	1	2	3	4
4. Difficulty paying attention to things	0	1	2	3	4
5. Remembering what he or she reads	0	1	2	3	4

PERCEIVED PHYSICAL APPEARANCE (problems with . . .)	Never	Almost Never	Some-times	Often	Almost Always
1. Feeling that he or she is not good looking	0	1	2	3	4
2. Not liking other people to see his or her scars	0	1	2	3	4
3. Being embarrassed about others seeing his or her body	0	1	2	3	4

COMMUNICATION (problems with . . .)	Never	Almost Never	Some-times	Often	Almost Always
1. Telling the doctors and nurses how he or she feels	0	1	2	3	4
2. Asking the doctors or nurses questions	0	1	2	3	4
3. Explaining his or her illness to other people	0	1	2	3	4

PedsQL™
Cancer Module

Version 3.0

CHILD REPORT (ages 8–12)

DIRECTIONS

Children with cancer sometimes have special problems. Please tell us **how much of a problem** each one has been for you during the **past ONE month** by circling:

> 0 if it is **never** a problem
>
> 1 if it is **almost never** a problem
>
> 2 if it is **sometimes** a problem
>
> 3 if it is **often** a problem
>
> 4 if it is **almost always** a problem

There are no right or wrong answers.

If you do not understand a question, please ask for help.

In the past **ONE month**, how much of a **problem** has this been for you . . .

PAIN AND HURT (problems with . . .)	Not at all	Sometimes	A lot
1. I ache or hurt in my joints and/or muscles	0	2	4
2. I hurt a lot	0	2	4

NAUSEA (problems with . . .)	Not at all	Sometimes	A lot
1. I become sick to my stomach when I have medical treatments	0	2	4
2. Food does not taste very good to me	0	2	4
3. I become sick to my stomach when I think about medical treatments	0	2	4
4. I don't feel hungry	0	2	4
5. Some foods and smells make my stomach upset	0	2	4

PROCEDURAL ANXIETY (problems with . . .)	Not at all	Sometimes	A lot
1. Needle sticks (i.e., injections, blood tests, IVs) hurt	0	2	4
2. I get scared when I have to have blood tests	0	2	4
3. I get scared about having needle sticks (i.e., injections, blood tests, IVs)	0	2	4

TREATMENT ANXIETY (problems with . . .)	Not at all	Sometimes	A lot
1. I get scared when I am waiting to see the doctor	0	2	4
2. I get scared when I have to go to the doctor	0	2	4
3. I get scared when I have to go to the hospital	0	2	4

WORRY (problems with . . .)	Not at all	Sometimes	A lot
1. I worry about side effects from medical treatments	0	2	4
2. I worry about whether or not my medical treatments are working	0	2	4
3. I worry that my cancer will come back	0	2	4

In the past **ONE month**, how much of a **problem** has this been for you . . .

COGNITIVE PROBLEMS (problems with . . .)	Never	Almost Never	Some-times	Often	Almost Always
1. It is hard for me to figure out what to do when something bothers me	0	1	2	3	4
2. I have trouble solving math problems	0	1	2	3	4
3. I have trouble writing school papers or reports	0	1	2	3	4
4. It is hard for me to pay attention to things	0	1	2	3	4
5. It is hard for me to remember what I read	0	1	2	3	4

PERCEIVED PHYSICAL APPEARANCE (problems with . . .)	Never	Almost Never	Some-times	Often	Almost Always
1. I feel I am not good looking	0	1	2	3	4
2. I don't like other people to see my scars	0	1	2	3	4
3. I am embarrassed when others see my body	0	1	2	3	4

COMMUNICATION (problems with . . .)	Never	Almost Never	Some-times	Often	Almost Always
1. It is hard for me to tell the doctors and nurses how I feel	0	1	2	3	4
2. It is hard for me to ask the doctors and nurses questions	0	1	2	3	4
3. It is hard for me to explain my illness to other people	0	1	2	3	4

PedsQL™
Pediatric Quality of Life
Inventory for Teens
(ages 13–18)

PedsQL™
Pediatric Quality of Life Inventory

Version 4.0

PARENT REPORT for TEENS (ages 13–18)

DIRECTIONS

On the following page is a list of things that might be a problem for **your teen**. Please tell us how much of a problem each one has been for **your teen** during the past ONE month by circling:

> 0 if it is **never** a problem
>
> 1 if it is **almost never** a problem
>
> 2 if it is **sometimes** a problem
>
> 3 if it is **often** a problem
>
> 4 if it is **almost always** a problem

There are no right or wrong answers.

If you do not understand a question, please ask for help.

In the past **ONE month**, how much of a **problem** has your teen had with . . .

PHYSICAL FUNCTIONING (problems with . . .)	Never	Almost Never	Some-times	Often	Almost Always
1. Walking more than one block	0	1	2	3	4
2. Running	0	1	2	3	4
3. Participating in sports activity or exercise	0	1	2	3	4
4. Lifting something heavy	0	1	2	3	4
5. Taking a bath or shower by him or herself	0	1	2	3	4
6. Doing chores around the house	0	1	2	3	4
7. Having hurts or aches	0	1	2	3	4
8. Low energy level	0	1	2	3	4

EMOTIONAL FUNCTIONING (problems with . . .)	Never	Almost Never	Some-times	Often	Almost Always
1. Feeling afraid or scared	0	1	2	3	4
2. Feeling sad or blue	0	1	2	3	4
3. Feeling angry	0	1	2	3	4
4. Trouble sleeping	0	1	2	3	4
5. Worrying about what will happen to him or her	0	1	2	3	4

SOCIAL FUNCTIONING (problems with . . .)	Never	Almost Never	Some-times	Often	Almost Always
1. Getting along with other teens	0	1	2	3	4
2. Other teens not wanting to be his or her friend	0	1	2	3	4
3. Getting teased by other teens	0	1	2	3	4
4. Not able to do things that other teens his or her age can do	0	1	2	3	4
5. Keeping up when playing with other teens	0	1	2	3	4

SCHOOL FUNCTIONING (problems with . . .)	Never	Almost Never	Some-times	Often	Almost Always
1. Paying attention in class	0	1	2	3	4
2. Forgetting things	0	1	2	3	4
3. Keeping up with schoolwork	0	1	2	3	4
4. Missing school because of not feeling well	0	1	2	3	4
5. Missing school to go to the doctor or hospital	0	1	2	3	4

PedsQL™
Pediatric Quality of Life Inventory

Version 4.0

TEEN REPORT (ages 13–18)

DIRECTIONS

On the following page is a list of things that might be a problem for you. Please tell us **how much of a problem** each one has been for you during the **past ONE month** by circling:

0 if it is **never** a problem

1 if it is **almost never** a problem

2 if it is **sometimes** a problem

3 if it is **often** a problem

4 if it is **almost always** a problem

There are no right or wrong answers.

If you do not understand a question, please ask for help.

In the past **ONE month**, how much of a **problem** has this been for you . . .

ABOUT MY HEALTH AND ACTIVITIES (problems with . . .)	Never	Almost Never	Some-times	Often	Almost Always
1. It is hard for me to walk more than one block	0	1	2	3	4
2. It is hard for me to run	0	1	2	3	4
3. It is hard for me to do sports activity or exercise	0	1	2	3	4
4. It is hard for me to lift something heavy	0	1	2	3	4
5. It is hard for me to take a bath or shower by myself	0	1	2	3	4
6. It is hard for me to do chores around the house	0	1	2	3	4
7. I hurt or ache	0	1	2	3	4
8. I have low energy	0	1	2	3	4

ABOUT MY FEELINGS (problems with . . .)	Never	Almost Never	Some-times	Often	Almost Always
1. I feel afraid or scared	0	1	2	3	4
2. I feel sad or blue	0	1	2	3	4
3. I feel angry	0	1	2	3	4
4. I have trouble sleeping	0	1	2	3	4
5. I worry about what will happen to me	0	1	2	3	4

HOW I GET ALONG WITH OTHERS (problems with . . .)	Never	Almost Never	Some-times	Often	Almost Always
1. I have trouble getting along with other teens	0	1	2	3	4
2. Other teens do not want to be my friend	0	1	2	3	4
3. Other teens tease me	0	1	2	3	4
4. I cannot do things that other teens my age can do	0	1	2	3	4
5. It is hard to keep up with my peers	0	1	2	3	4

ABOUT SCHOOL (problems with . . .)	Never	Almost Never	Some-times	Often	Almost Always
1. It is hard to pay attention in class	0	1	2	3	4
2. I forget things	0	1	2	3	4
3. I have trouble keeping up with my schoolwork	0	1	2	3	4
4. I miss school because of not feeling well	0	1	2	3	4
5. I miss school to go to the doctor or hospital	0	1	2	3	4

PedsQL™

Cancer Module

Version 3.0

PARENT REPORT for TEENS (ages 13–18)

DIRECTIONS

Teens with cancer sometimes have special problems. On the following page is a list of things that might be a problem for **your teen**. Please tell us how much of a problem each one has been for **your teen** during the **past ONE month** by circling:

> 0 if it is **never** a problem
>
> 1 if it is **almost never** a problem
>
> 2 if it is **sometimes** a problem
>
> 3 if it is **often** a problem
>
> 4 if it is **almost always** a problem

There are no right or wrong answers.

If you do not understand a question, please ask for help.

In the past **ONE month**, how much of a **problem** has your teen had with . . .

PAIN AND HURT (problems with . . .)	Never	Almost Never	Some-times	Often	Almost Always
1. Aches in joints and/or muscles	0	1	2	3	4
2. Having a lot of pain	0	1	2	3	4

NAUSEA (problems with . . .)	Never	Almost Never	Some-times	Often	Almost Always
1. Becoming nauseated during medical treatments	0	1	2	3	4
2. Food not tasting very good to him or her	0	1	2	3	4
3. Becoming nauseated while thinking about medical treatments	0	1	2	3	4
4. Not feeling hungry	0	1	2	3	4
5. Some foods and smells making him or her nauseous	0	1	2	3	4

PROCEDURAL ANXIETY (problems with . . .)	Never	Almost Never	Some-times	Often	Almost Always
1. Needle sticks (i.e., injections, blood tests, IVs) causing him or her pain	0	1	2	3	4
2. Getting anxious about having blood drawn	0	1	2	3	4
3. Getting anxious about having needle sticks (i.e., injections, blood tests, IVs)	0	1	2	3	4

TREATMENT ANXIETY (problems with . . .)	Never	Almost Never	Some-times	Often	Almost Always
1. Getting anxious when waiting to see the doctor	0	1	2	3	4
2. Getting anxious about going to the doctor	0	1	2	3	4
3. Getting anxious about going to the hospital	0	1	2	3	4

WORRY (problems with . . .)	Never	Almost Never	Some-times	Often	Almost Always
1. Worrying about side effects from medical treatments	0	1	2	3	4
2. Worrying about whether or not his or her medical treatments are working	0	1	2	3	4
3. Worrying that the cancer will reoccur or relapse	0	1	2	3	4

In the past **ONE month**, how much of a **problem** has your teen had with . . .

COGNITIVE PROBLEMS (problems with . . .)	Never	Almost Never	Some-times	Often	Almost Always
1. Figuring out what to do when something is bothering him or her	0	1	2	3	4
2. Solving math problems	0	1	2	3	4
3. Writing school papers or reports	0	1	2	3	4
4. Difficulty paying attention to things	0	1	2	3	4
5. Remembering what he or she reads	0	1	2	3	4

PERCEIVED PHYSICAL APPEARANCE (problems with . . .)	Never	Almost Never	Some-times	Often	Almost Always
1. Feeling that he or she is not good looking	0	1	2	3	4
2. Not liking other people to see his or her scars	0	1	2	3	4
3. Being embarrassed about others seeing his or her body	0	1	2	3	4

COMMUNICATION (problems with . . .)	Never	Almost Never	Some-times	Often	Almost Always
1. Telling the doctors and nurses how he or she feels	0	1	2	3	4
2. Asking the doctors or nurses questions	0	1	2	3	4
3. Explaining his or her illness to other people	0	1	2	3	4

PedsQL™
Cancer Module

Version 3.0

TEEN REPORT (ages 13–18)

DIRECTIONS

Teens with cancer sometimes have special problems. Please tell us **how much of a problem** each one has been for you during the **past ONE month** by circling:

0 if it is **never** a problem

1 if it is **almost never** a problem

2 if it is **sometimes** a problem

3 if it is **often** a problem

4 if it is **almost always** a problem

There are no right or wrong answers.

If you do not understand a question, please ask for help.

In the past **ONE month**, how much of a **problem** has this been for you . . .

PAIN AND HURT (problems with . . .)	Not at all	Sometimes	A lot
1. I ache or hurt in my joints and/or muscles	0	2	4
2. I hurt a lot	0	2	4

NAUSEA (problems with . . .)	Not at all	Sometimes	A lot
1. I become sick to my stomach when I have medical treatments	0	2	4
2. Food does not taste very good to me	0	2	4
3. I become sick to my stomach when I think about medical treatments	0	2	4
4. I don't feel hungry	0	2	4
5. Some foods and smells make my stomach upset	0	2	4

PROCEDURAL ANXIETY (problems with . . .)	Not at all	Sometimes	A lot
1. Needle sticks (i.e., injections, blood tests, IVs) hurt	0	2	4
2. I get scared when I have to have blood tests	0	2	4
3. I get scared about having needle sticks (i.e., injections, blood tests, IVs)	0	2	4

TREATMENT ANXIETY (problems with . . .)	Not at all	Sometimes	A lot
1. I get scared when I am waiting to see the doctor	0	2	4
2. I get scared when I have to go to the doctor	0	2	4
3. I get scared when I have to go to the hospital	0	2	4

WORRY (problems with . . .)	Not at all	Sometimes	A lot
1. I worry about side effects from medical treatments	0	2	4
2. I worry about whether or not my medical treatments are working	0	2	4
3. I worry that my cancer will come back or relapse	0	2	4

In the past **ONE month**, how much of a **problem** has this been for you . . .

COGNITIVE PROBLEMS (problems with . . .)	Never	Almost Never	Some-times	Often	Almost Always
1. It is hard for me to figure out what to do when something bothers me	0	1	2	3	4
2. I have trouble solving math problems	0	1	2	3	4
3. I have trouble writing school papers or reports	0	1	2	3	4
4. It is hard for me to pay attention to things	0	1	2	3	4
5. It is hard for me to remember what I read	0	1	2	3	4

PERCEIVED PHYSICAL APPEARANCE (problems with . . .)	Never	Almost Never	Some-times	Often	Almost Always
1. I feel I am not good looking	0	1	2	3	4
2. I don't like other people to see my scars	0	1	2	3	4
3. I am embarrassed when others see my body	0	1	2	3	4

COMMUNICATION (problems with . . .)	Never	Almost Never	Some-times	Often	Almost Always
1. It is hard for me to tell the doctors and nurses how I feel	0	1	2	3	4
2. It is hard for me to ask the doctors and nurses questions	0	1	2	3	4
3. It is hard for me to explain my illness to other people	0	1	2	3	4

Index